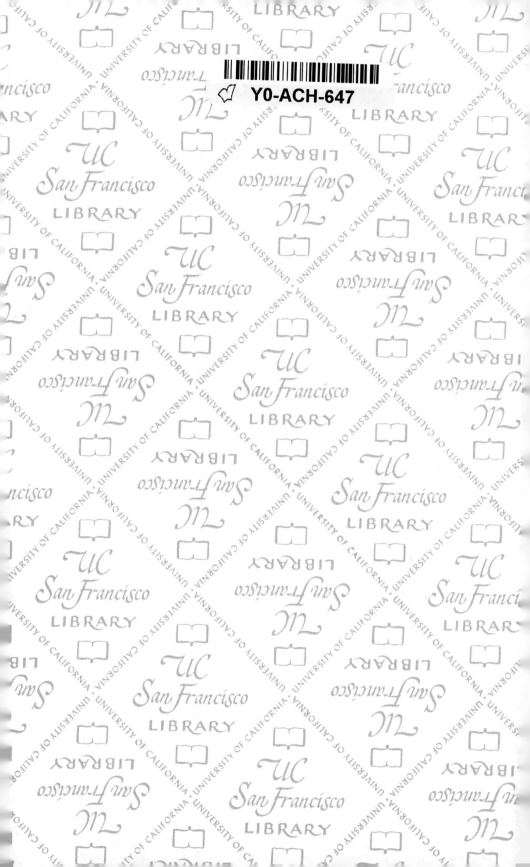

Series in Laboratory Medicine
Leo P. Cawley, M.D., *Series Editor*

Electrophoresis and Immunoelectrophoresis
Leo P. Cawley, M.D.

Practical Blood Transfusion
Douglas W. Huestis, M.D.
Joseph R. Bove, M.D.
Shirley Busch, M.P.H., BB SPEC. (ASCP)

Clinical Laboratory Statistics
Roy N. Barnett, M.D.

Laboratory Management
Jack E. Newell, M.D.

Fluorometric Techniques in Clinical Chemistry
Franklin R. Elevitch, M.D.

Sickle Cell Hemoglobin: Molecule to Man
Makio Murayama, Ph.D.
Robert M. Nalbandian, M.D.

Legal Aspects of Laboratory Medicine
John R. Feegel, M.D., J.D.

Organ Preservation for Transplantation
Armand M. Karow, Jr., Ph.D.
George J. M. Abouna, M.B., F.R.C.S.
Arthur L. Humphries, Jr., M.D.

Laboratory Procedures in Clinical Microbiology
John A. Washington II, M.D.

Laboratory Diagnostic Procedures in the
Rheumatic Diseases, Second Edition
Alan S. Cohen, M.D.

The Diagnosis of Bleeding Disorders,
Second Edition
Charles A. Owen, Jr., M.D., Ph.D.
E. J. Walter Bowie, M.A., B.M., F.A.C.P.
John H. Thompson, Jr., Ph.D.

Immunopathology: Clinical Laboratory
Concepts and Methods
Robert M. Nakamura, M.D.

Immunopathology
Clinical Laboratory
Concepts and Methods

Immunopathology
Clinical Laboratory
Concepts and Methods

Robert M. Nakamura, M.D.

Department of Molecular Immunology, Scripps Clinic and Research Foundation;
Head, Department of Pathology, Hospital of Scripps Clinic, La Jolla,
California; Adjunct Professor of Pathology, University of
California, Irvine, California College of Medicine,
Irvine, California

With 9 Contributing Authors

Little, Brown and Company
Boston

Contributing Authors

Carol A. Bell, M.D.
Associate Clinical Professor of Pathology, University of California, Irvine, California College of Medicine, Irvine, California; Director of Clinical Laboratories, Daniel M. Brotman Memorial Hospital, Culver City, California

Gerald A. Beathard, M.D., Ph.D.
Assistant Professor of Medicine, Division of Nephrology, and Associate Professor of Pathology, Division of Experimental Pathology and Immunology, The University of Texas Medical Branch at Galveston, Galveston, Texas

Jerry C. Daniels, M.D., Ph.D.
Research Fellow in Medicine, Harvard Medical School and Robert B. Brigham Hospital, Boston, Massachusetts

Marianne L. Egan, Ph.D.
Associate Research Scientist, Department of Immunology, City of Hope National Medical Center, Duarte, California

Stephan E. Ritzmann, M.D.
Professor of Medicine and Pathology, Director of Division of Experimental Pathology and Immunology, and Co-Director, Transplantation Immunology Laboratory, The University of Texas Medical Branch at Galveston, Galveston, Texas

Hideto Sakai, M.D.
Instructor in Medicine and Pathology, and Chief, Nucleoprotein Laboratory, Division of Experimental Pathology and Immunology, The University of Texas Medical Branch at Galveston, Galveston, Texas

Courtney M. Townsend, Jr., M.D.
Resident Physician, Section of Transplantation Surgery, The University of Texas Medical Branch at Galveston, Galveston, Texas

Ernest S. Tucker, III, M.D.
Associate Clinical Professor of Pathology and Pediatrics, University of California, San Diego, La Jolla, California; Director of Laboratories, Immuno-Diagnostics, Inc., San Diego, California

Theona M. Vyvial, A.A.
Research Technologist and Supervisor, Transplantation Immunology Laboratory, Section of Experimental Pathology and Immunology, The University of Texas Medical Branch at Galveston, Galveston, Texas

Preface

Within the past few years several books on the basic elements and general concepts of immunology and immunopathology have been published. The pathologists and hospital clinical laboratory personnel, however, have needed a text with primary emphasis on (1) practical available laboratory methods and (2) information on proper standardization and on monitoring and interpreting test results together with underlying concepts of the immune disorders.

This book is written to fill that need. Emphasis is on clinical laboratory methods and concepts that are necessary for the interpretation of tests. The text is designed to supplement the basic texts and serve as a reference for solving problems.

The chapters were written with a disease-oriented approach. Part I deals with diagnostic patterns of immunologic disorders, while Part II assesses specific autoimmune disorders. Transplantation and tumor immunology are covered in Part III. Part IV provides supplemental information and methods. Every effort has been made to have all the necessary information concerning a specific problem within the pertinent chapter.

The contributing authors and I acknowledge the help of Drs. W. O. Weigle, E. M. Tan, H. Inami, S. J. Hayashi, R. Walwick, and Leo P. Cawley who gave advice and encouragement and reviewed portions of the manuscript. The secretarial help of Mrs. Barbara Davis and Mrs. Barbara Wilson is greatly appreciated. Many of the medical illustrations were prepared by Mr. Jack Regnier and Mrs. Sandy Kessler. Mr. J. Alexander and Mr. L. C. Shockey made an inspiring contribution with their photographic work. Any errors that may have slipped by their careful scrutiny must remain the responsibility of the author.

R. M. N.

Contents

III   Transplantation and Tumor Immunology

IV   Supplemental Information and Methods

I

Diagnostic Patterns of Immunologic Disorders

1

Approach of the Pathologist to the Clinical Immunology Problem

How should the general pathologist approach the rapidly expanding field of immunology and program the various new tests to meet the needs and demands of clinicians? In the field of immunology, advances have been in (a) immunologic concepts and (b) immunologic methods. Pathologists are asked to be familiar with and to coordinate the concepts and methods of immunology. Many conceptual advances have been in the clarification of immunopathologic mechanisms in a wide variety of diseases. Areas of immunology, which frequently overlap, may be briefly defined as follows [11]:

A. *Immunobiology* deals with the origin, inducement, and mechanisms of the immune response.

B. *Immunochemistry* is concerned with the physicochemical structure and molecular actions of antigen and antibody either in vivo or in vitro.

C. *Immunopathology* can be broadly defined as the study of diseases induced or resulting from immune mechanisms. It is primarily concerned with untoward consequences in immunologic responses.

D. *Serology* classically has dealt with antibodies and their reactions with antigens outside the host.

E. *Immunohematology* encompasses immunology and immunochemistry of certain constituents of the blood.

F. *Clinical immunology* in general covers the various autoimmune disorders, immune deficiency diseases, allergic disorders, transplantation, and problems of neoplastic diseases.

Clinical laboratory sections may be organized as follows:

A. *Immunochemistry* is organized to conduct the numerous tests for the serum protein abnormalities and includes the competitive binding and radioimmunoassay procedures.

B. *Immunohematology* performs tests for blood group and leukocyte antigens and antibodies, and tests for hemolytic blood disorders.

C. *Microbiology* comprises the many immunologic tests related to infectious diseases.

D. *Clinical immunology* encompasses the laboratory tests oriented toward the diagnosis and follow-up of autoimmune disorders, immune deficiency diseases, allergic disorders, transplantation problems, and neoplastic diseases.

It is not important whether clinical immunology is organized in one area of the laboratory or distributed in more than one area. Tests for a certain disorder group such as autoimmune diseases should be placed in one section on a disease-oriented basis. Concepts and methods of immunology should be coordinated and the test results interpreted by the clinical pathologist. A particular immunologic test should be interpreted in light of the various other tests performed on the same patient. Correlation of results of different tests with an interpretation of the results has recently been utilized in the laboratory diagnosis of hyperlipoproteinemias. Electrophoretic analysis of lipoproteins is performed along with the quantitative determination of triglycerides and cholesterol; the report entails an interpretation.

One can consider the various immunologic methods as assay techniques with many advantages and disadvantages. The pathologist is required to be familiar with the many pitfalls, particularly the deficiencies in the specificity and sensitivity of the various tests. He is asked to correlate the tests with newer immunologic concepts to provide the clinician with a meaningful answer.

A wide spectrum of different methods is now available to the clinical pathologist. Specific antibodies differ in their specificity and sensitivity but have made possible the development of tests sensitive in the nanogram to picogram per milliliter range. We are now in the age of quantitation, and the relative or quantitative values require interpretation in light of particular disease processes. Furthermore, variation in standardization and specificity of immunologic methods is common knowledge. For example, antibodies which have a high affinity and are potent may give unwanted cross reactions, and weak antiserum may be specific but lack sensitivity (Fig. 1-1). Because of the difficulty with standardization of immunologic tests, each laboratory should attempt to standardize carefully each particular antiserum and antigen used. Test results should be considered on a relative value basis unless compared with acceptable international standards.

Varying sensitivity is well illustrated by the numerous immunologic tests available for the detection of hepatitis-associated antigen (HAA). Antibody reactions of primary, secondary, and tertiary types vary in their relative sensitivities. The agar gel diffusion test may be considered to be a precipitin test with a sensitivity value of 1. The cross electrophoretic or electroimmunodiffusion (EID) method increases that sensitivity 10 times, whereas the radioimmunoassay procedure (RIA) for HAA [21] will increase the sensitivity 10,000 times. One may wonder about the significance of a positive radioimmunoassay test for HAA in donors. What is the incidence of hepatitis in recipients who receive donor blood with a positive RIA test and a negative EID test? These questions of significance for hepatitis incidence remain to be elucidated.

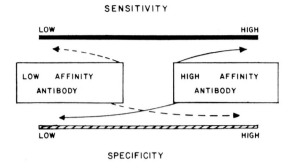

Figure 1-1
Variable properties of antibodies. Antisera made in the same animal or different animal to a specific antigen vary in their specificity and sensitivity. An antiserum containing high affinity antibodies will show greater sensitivity, and specificity will be decreased because of the tendency to cross react with other related antigens. On the other hand, antiserum with low affinity antibodies will be more specific and less sensitive than an antiserum containing high affinity antibodies.

Detection of alpha$_1$ fetoprotein by agar gel diffusion is diagnostic for hepatocellular carcinoma or an embryonal cell carcinoma. The sensitivity of the agar gel test is in the range of 3,000 ng per milliliter whereas a current radioimmunoassay procedure results in sensitivity at one nanogram per milliliter level [15]. With the more sensitive tests for alpha$_1$ fetoprotein one can obtain values in a normal person, and for liver diseases such as hepatitis [20]. Thus, with the increasing complexity of various tests of different specificities and sensitivities, each laboratory must characterize the antiserum and antigen involved in the particular test and provide information as to the sensitivity and significance of results.

Pathologists are faced with a difficult problem of obtaining well-characterized and standardized immunological reagents [6]. Investigators have noted that many commercially available antisera to human IgM and IgG showed inappropriate specificities when assayed with a panel of antigens under conditions of high sensitivity [16].

Eleven laboratories, well known internationally, were involved in a cooperative study in which they measured immunoglobulin levels and standards. There was an extremely large ratio between the highest and lowest reported values: 2.2 for IgG, 3.2 for IgA, and 5.0 for IgM [17]. In contrast, when an international reference preparation was used as a standard, the ratios between the highest and lowest reported values were 1.36 for IgG, 1.17 for IgA, and 1.31 for IgM. Because of the serious discrepancies, international experts recommended substituting units for milligram values related to international standards for the various immunoglobulins [1, 5].

Recently, there has been much effort for international standardization of antisera and reagents. Several detailed recommendations on the characterization and clinical use of immunologic reagents have been made by various groups of investigators and the World Health Organization [1, 4]. Also, workers have been active in establishing standards for fluorescein-conjugated antisera [2, 3, 9]. However, one must remember that there are no definite standards in fluorescence microscopy procedures. Characterization of antisera and instrumentation, including filters, would be extremely difficult.

Today, standardization of the immunologic test is a serious challenge to the pathologist. Current problems in the standardization of immunologic tests make it difficult to use a computer printout approach in reporting of results [6].

Laboratory tests are usually performed to aid in the determination of one of the following: (a) diagnosis, (b) therapeutic results, and (c) prognosis. To illustrate the complexity of the clinical immunology problem, we may consider the various laboratory tests which are available for the diagnosis and therapeutic monitoring of systemic lupus erythematosus and related collagen diseases. Currently available are the following tests for antinuclear antibodies [14]:

A. LE cell preparation
B. Antiglobulin consumption
C. Precipitin
D. Agglutination
E. Complement fixation
F. Indirect immunofluorescent tests
G. Enzyme-labeled antibody
H. Radio-labeled DNA antigen-binding capacity

What is the value and relative sensitivity of each of these tests? The tests are designed to detect the following nuclear antigens:

A. Native DNA which is double-stranded
B. Single-stranded DNA
C. Nucleoprotein
D. Saline soluble antigens—Sm antigen (carbohydrate containing protein), ribonucleoprotein, extractable nuclear antigen (ENA)
E. RNA
F. Nucleolar RNA

What significance have these various antigens? When present, antibodies to native DNA, specific nucleohistone determinant, or Sm antigen are highly indicative of systemic lupus erythematosus. Patients with a high antibody titer to ribonucleoprotein or ENA respond to corticosteroid therapy and have a much better prognosis with a benign course of the kidney disease [18], and may have a mixed connective tissue disorder [19]. Recommended screening tests in the routine clinical laboratory for the diagnosis of lupus and related diseases are the immunofluorescent and immunoenzyme tests. Well-controlled procedures show that a negative test rules out the diagnosis of systemic lupus erythematosus if the patient is not treated with corticosteroids or immunosuppressive agents. A positive fluorescent test should be titered and followed up with a sensitive test for DNA antibodies as well as antibodies to other nuclear antigens. The fluorescent pattern is helpful in evaluation of the type of antinuclear antibodies present.

Immune complexes play a key role in the pathogenesis of lupus erythematosus, and anti-DNA is the pathogenic antibody [10, 13]. Cryoglobulins tend to have biological action similar to immune complexes, and they also play a role in the pathogenesis of lupus nephritis [10]. Acute symptoms in systemic lupus are related to immune complex formation resulting from the binding of antibody to DNA released into the circulation. Thus, in the monitoring of therapy, useful tests are the detection and quantitation of DNA antibody, cryoglobulins, immune complexes, and serum complement levels. As stated above, patients with a high titer of antibody to ENA in general have a better prognosis and respond to corticosteroid therapy [18].

Clinical immunology not only involves clinical pathology, but extends into the areas of surgical and anatomic pathology. Laboratory tests should be correlated with results from these disciplines; the general pathologist is in the best position to combine findings of the surgical and anatomic areas with clinical laboratory results. This is illustrated by the various immunologic renal diseases [12] which have been characterized as follows:

A. Antiglomerular basement membrane nephritis of Goodpasture's type
B. Immune complex glomerulonephritis in which immunofluorescent studies of the kidney biopsy can be correlated with serum complement level, serum immune complex determination, and serum protein electrophoresis and immunoelectrophoresis
C. Chronic membranoproliferative glomerulonephritis with hypocomplementemia
D. Nephropathy with IgG and IgA deposits
E. Immune complex tubular disorders
F. Nephrosis with IgE immunoglobulin deposits [8].

In the work-up of immune deficiency diseases one must perform tests to evaluate humoral and cellular immunity and correlate their results with lymphatic tissue biopsy examinations [7].

In summary, the important points for a pathologist are:

A. He must become familiar with the new concepts and methods of immunology. One can learn this by reading, by attending workshops, and by initiating the various laboratory tests and solving the problems.
B. He should be aware of the difficulties with standardization of tests involving immunologic methods. Because of the variable properties of antibodies and antisera, the results may be relative rather than absolute quantitative values.

C. The clinical laboratory tests in clinical immunology should be clustered and organized with disease orientation. Each department of the laboratory should be monitoring the various tests performed, and when there is a significant result on a particular test, it should be correlated with other tests to provide a meaningful answer to help the clinician and the patient.

D. Requests for clinical immunologic procedures should be regarded as similar to surgical pathology requests with all of the implications for pursuit of meaningful answers. In surgical pathology, one performs further studies such as special stains or seeks help from a consultant. If there is a diagnostic problem in clinical immunology it would seem appropriate for the pathologist to perform other ancillary tests which may provide definitive answers. A puzzling problem would best be handled by referral to an established expert.

References

1. Anderson, S. E., Bangham, D. R., Batty, I., Becker, W., Cinader, B., Van der Giessen, M., Hymes, F., Long, D., Peetoom, F., Pondman, K., Raynaud, M., Reimer, C. B., Rowe, D. S., Schwick, H. G., and Vrancheva, S.   Measurement of the concentration of human serum immunoglobulins. *J. Immunol.* 107:1798, 1971.
2. Barnett, E. V.   Staining activity of conjugates in relation to their antibody content. In E. J. Holborow (ed.), *Standardization of Immunofluorescence*. Oxford, England: Blackwell, 1970.
3. Beutner, E. H., Sepulveda, M. R., and Barnett, E. V.   Quantitative studies of immunofluorescent staining: II. Relationships of characteristics of unabsorbed anti-human IgG conjugates to their specific and nonspecific staining properties in an indirect test for antinuclear factors. *Bull. WHO* 39:587, 1968.
4. Characterization of antisera as reagents, recommendations made by the MRC Working Party on the clinical use of immunological regents. *Immunology* 20:3, 1971.
5. Editorial Comment: Standards for immunoglobulins. *Lancet* 2:82, 1971.
6. Fudenberg, H. H.   Problems in standardization of immunological laboratory results. In E. R. Gabrieli (ed.), *Clinically Oriented Documentation of Laboratory Data*. New York: Academic, 1972, p. 359.
7. Gatti, R. A., and Good, R. A.   The immunological deficiency diseases. *Med. Clin. North Am.* 54:281, 1970.
8. Gerber, M. A., and Paronetto, F.   IgE in glomeruli of patients with nephrotic syndrome. *Lancet* 1:1097, 1971.
9. Holborow, E. J., et al.   Report by a subcommittee on the discussion of requirements for specification of anti-immunoglobulin conjugates that took place during the conference. In E. J. Holborow (ed.), *Standardization of Immunofluorescence*. Oxford, England: Blackwell, 1970, p. 275.
10. Koffler, D., Agnello, V., Thoburn, R., and Kunkel, H. G.   Systemic lupus erythematosus: Prototype of immune complex nephritis in man. *J. Exp. Med.* 134:169s, 1971.
11. Kwapinski, J. B. G.   A concept of modern immunology. In J. B. G.

Kwapiński (ed.), *Research in Immunochemistry and Immunobiology.* Baltimore: University Park Press, 1972, vol. 2, p. *vii.*
12. McCluskey, R. T.   The value of immunofluorescence in the study of human renal disease. *J. Exp. Med.* 134:242s, 1971.
13. Nakamura, R. M., and Allen, H. J.   Immunopathologic mechanisms and recent concepts in the pathogenesis of systemic lupus erythematosus. *Cutis* 11:607, 1973.
14. Nakamura, R. M., and Allen, H. J.   Laboratory tests for diagnosis of systemic lupus erythematosus and related disorders. *Cutis* 11:655, 1973.
15. Purves, L. R., and Geddes, E. W.   A more sensitive test for alpha feto-protein. *Lancet* 1:47, 1972.
16. Reimer, C. B., Phillips, D. J., Maddison, S. E., and Shore, S. L.   Comparative evaluation of commercial precipitating antisera against human IgM and IgG. *J. Lab. Clin. Med.* 76:949, 1970.
17. Rowe, D. S., Anderson, S. E., and Grab, B.   A research standard for human serum immunoglobulins—IgG, IgA, and IgM. *Bull. WHO* 43:535, 1970.
18. Sharp, G. C., Irvin, W. S., La Roque, R. L., Velez, C., Daly, V., Kaiser, A. D., and Holman, H. R.   Association of autoantibodies to different nuclear antigens in clinical patterns of rheumatic disease and responsiveness to therapy. *J. Clin. Invest.* 50:350, 1971.
19. Sharp, G. C., Irvin, W. S., Tan, E. M., Gould, R. G., and Holman, H. R.   Mixed connective tissue disease—an apparently distinct rheumatic disease syndrome associated with a specific antibody to an extractable nuclear antigen (ENA). *Am. J. Med.* 52:148, 1972.
20. Smith, J. B.   Occurrence of alpha fetoprotein in acute viral hepatitis. *Int. J. Cancer* 8:421, 1971.
21. Walsh, J. H., Yalow, R. S., and Berson, S. A.   Radioimmunoassay of Australia antigen. *Vox Sang.* 19:217, 1970.

2

Major Constituents of the Immune System and Immune Deficiency Diseases

General Aspects of the Immune System

In humans and higher animals, the lymphoid system consists of a central component (thymus and bursa equivalent) and a peripheral component (spleen and lymph nodes) [37, 38, 62]. The thymus, which is essential for the development and maintenance of a normal immune system, is primarily responsible for cellular defenses (delayed hypersensitivity) and transplantation immunity. In birds, antibody production is dependent upon the lymphoid cells of the bursa. The mammalian counterpart of the bursa of birds may be represented by the tonsils, appendix, and Peyer's patches of the small intestine [37, 38]. In mammals the bone marrow has been found to contain a significant amount of antibody-producing cells (B-lymphocytes).

In humans, the stem cells originating in bone marrow differentiate into two distinct cell lines, one dependent on the presence of the thymus (T-lymphocytes) and the other (B-lymphocytes) independent of the thymus. The T-lymphocytes, which make up the largest part of the recirculatory pool of small lymphocytes, localize in the paracortical areas of the lymph nodes and spleen. The T-cells are lymphocytes which have differentiated under the influence of the thymus and which are responsible for mediating cellular immune reaction. The B-lymphocytes appear in the follicles of the outer cortex and medulla of lymph nodes. Both populations of T and B cells contain antigen sensitive cells.

The immune responses to many antigens involve the participation of (a) T-lymphocytes, (b) B-lymphocytes, and (c) macrophages. The role of the macrophage appears to be nonspecific, for the macrophage handles various antigens without immunologic discrimination [136]. The macrophage may serve to present the antigen to the reactive T- and B-lymphocytes in a physical state such that the committed lymphocyte may interact and select the antigen molecules.

There are many types of T-cells [60]. T-cells which are antigen reactive and capable of being stimulated by antigen to proliferate and

10

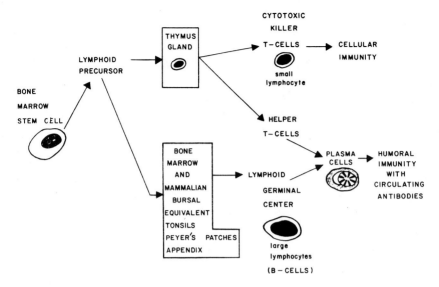

Figure 2-1
Differentiation of lymphoid cells.

differentiate can be called "educated T-cells" [78]. T-cells which are activated by various means and produce biochemical mediators of cellular immunity should be called "activated T-cells" [78]. T-cells may be activated by certain nonspecific agents as well as by specific antigens.

The T-lymphocytes interact and stimulate B-lymphocytes to antibody production in response to certain antigens. The cooperation of T-lymphocytes and B-lymphocytes, in the IgM hemolysin response to sheep cells in mice, was observed by Claman and co-workers [31]. The T-cells may act by (a) binding antigen in its surface to provide a higher localized antigen concentration for stimulation of B-cells [99]; or (b) production by the specific antigen reactive T-cells of a mitogenic factor which causes proliferation of the antigen reactive B-cells [50]. High doses of antigen obviate the need for T-cells in the antibody production by B-cells. Certain antigens with repeated determinants as polysaccharides do not require the T-cell interaction for antibody production [100].

The B-lymphocyte system is characterized as follows:
A. The B-lymphocytes can differentiate, proliferate, and mature into plasma cells with antibody production.
B. Any defect of the B-cell system will lead to a deficiency in immunoglobulins.
C. B-lymphocytes may be intact with a defective T-lymphocyte system, and the individual may demonstrate a poor antibody response in conditions where T-lymphocytes play a role in antigen recognition.

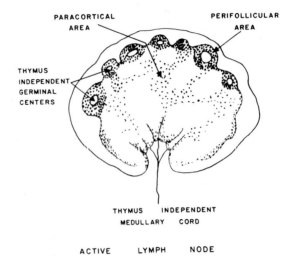

Figure 2-2
Schematic diagram showing localization of thymus dependent and thymus
independent lymphoid cells in lymph node. The thymus dependent (T-cells)
are found in the paracortical areas and with thymus dependent cell stimulation, follicles may appear. The antibody producing (B-cells) lymphoid cells
are seen in follicles with germinal centers along the outer cortical areas and
also B-cells are seen in the medullary areas. The perifollicular area of the
follicle is the area surrounding the germinal center.

D. B-lymphocytes have been demonstrated to show significant amounts
   of surface immunoglobulins.
E. B-cells and not T-cells have the capacity to bind antigen-antibody
   complexes [20, 102]. This property has been utilized to separate
   T-cells from B-cells [14].
   The T-lymphocytes show the following features:
A. They may be stimulated in culture with blast transformation by
   phytohemagglutinin (PHA).
B. They can proliferate to form a population of antigen sensitive cells
   which have a long life span and play a role in immunologic memory
   (educated T-cells).
C. The T-lymphocytes can be cytoxic for graft target cells.
D. They release a number of soluble factors which are chemotactic for
   mononuclear cells, inhibit migration of macrophages, are mitogenic
   for other lymphocytes, and increase vascular permeability.
E. The T-lymphocytes interact and stimulate B-lymphocytes to antibody production in response to certain antigens.
F. Human T-cells tend to form rosettes with sheep red blood cells in
   vitro [10, 24, 35, 77, 85, 150]. The rosette formation with sheep red

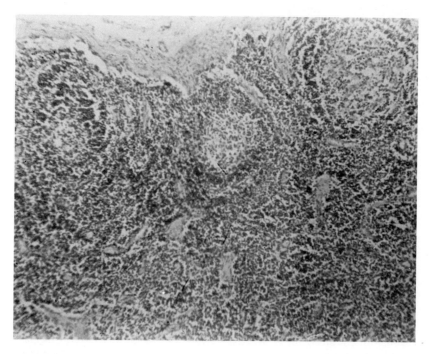

Figure 2-3
Microscopic section of lymph node. There are several follicles with active germinal centers. (H&E section, 100×, before 5% reduction.)

cells has been used as a marker for human thymus-derived cells [77, 150].

Cellular Immunity

Immunity may be defined as the specific protection against a noxious agent or organism due to previous exposure to the same agent or organism. The thymic immune system is concerned with cellular immunity. This is mediated by the thymic lymphocyte or T-cell. Numerous systems have been proposed to classify lymphocytes on the basis of size and other morphologic properties. Ultrastructurally, the lymphocyte is represented by a very large nucleus occupying the major portion of the cell's volume. In the cytoplasm can be found a few organelles such as mitochondria, a Golgi apparatus, a few vacuolar structures, and a few ribosomal structures. In contrast to the plasma cell, the lymphocyte has no organized system of endoplasmic reticulum. Lymphocytes represent a highly mobile population of cells widely distributed in the body, being found in blood, lymph, lymphoid organs, and body fluids.

Lymphocytes participate in cellular defense reactions which include [16, 138] (a) delayed hypersensitivity reactions, (b) transplantation immunity, (c) defense against the development of neoplasia, (d) resistance to certain intracellular pathogens such as tuberculosis, fungal, and certain viral infections, and (e) autoimmune diseases.

The cell-mediated immune reactions involve various steps as (a) the recognition of antigens encountered by circulating lymphoid cells, (b) cell proliferation, and (c) liberation of biochemical and pharmacologic mediators which can result in cellular damage to the target, foreign or native host tissue.

Delayed Hypersensitivity, Antimicrobial, and Antitissue Cellular Immunity

Delayed-type hypersensitivity has been characterized as a cell-mediated or cellular immune skin reaction in which (a) a delayed skin reaction with erythema and induration is observed 24 to 48 hours after a second exposure of a specific antigen, as tuberculin; (b) the skin reaction is characterized by the accumulation of mononuclear cells consisting of macrophages and lymphocytes; (c) the lesions are observed in the absence of detectable circulating antibodies; and (d) the reaction can be transferred by intact cells.

Mackaness has noted that effector cells in cell-mediated reactions against infectious agents are exclusively of the monocyte-macrophage type because phagocytosis is an essential step in the process of bacterial inactivation [91, 92]. On the other hand, the antitissue type of cellular immune reactions involves both lymphocytes and monocyte-macrophage type of cells. Mackaness has cited considerable evidence that a cell-associated, noncirculating IgM immunoglobulin may play a role in the mediation of the cellular immune reactions [91, 92]. Passive sensitization of a specific IgM will provide mononuclear phagocytes with the ability to accumulate at a particular infective site or target tissue. The IgG immunoglobulins which can circulate may interfere with cellular immune mechanisms (a) by interreaction with the antigen and subsequent sequestration; and (b) by suppressing the production of specific IgM with peculiar biological properties.

Soluble Mediators of Cellular Immunity

The T-cell reactions are known to release a variety of biochemical mediators. The factors include [81, 107, 138] (a) migration inhibitory factor, (b) lymphotoxin, (c) transfer factor, (d) lymphocyte-transforming factor, (e) mononuclear cell chemotactic factor, (f) skin reactive factor, (g) interferon, and (h) factor involved in eosinophil chemotaxis.

A. Migration inhibitory factor (MIF) [42]. This factor is nondialyzable and heat stable (56°C), and will inhibit the migration of a population of macrophages. The MIF will cause the macrophages to round up and become more sticky and vacuolated [111].

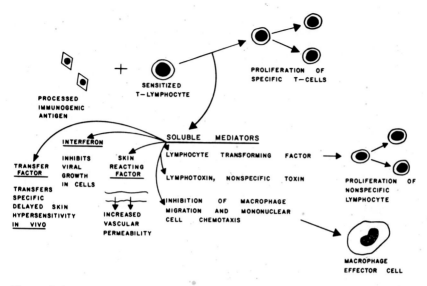

Figure 2-4
Soluble mediators in cellular immune reactions.

B. Lymphotoxin. This appears to be a protein or proteins of varying molecular weight (80,000–90,000) which are heat sensitive and are toxic to various nonspecific target cells [64, 65, 107, 118].

C. Transfer factor. This factor has a small molecular weight, is a compound of less than 10,000, is dialyzable, and is most likely a polynucleotide [82, 83]. The factor may be isolated from circulating leukocytes and/or lymphocytes from one individual and may be passively administered to another. In humans, it is possible to transfer cellular sensitivity of prolonged duration with the administration of a specific transfer factor. The transfer factor is resistant to the exogenous addition of DNase, RNase, and trypsin. The passive transfer of the transfer factor will induce a specific delayed sensitivity reaction with evidence of concomitant circulating or cell-bound antibody.

D. Lymphocyte transforming factor. This factor is produced by the interaction of sensitized T-cells with specific antigen. The factor will then cause the transformation of normal, nonsensitive lymphocyte blast cells [137].

E. Mononuclear cell chemotactic factor. The supernatants containing the above factors also contain a substance chemotactic for monocytes and macrophages [146]. This factor may play a role in attracting macrophages to the site of interaction of the antigen.

F. Skin reactive factor. After the reaction of sensitized lymphocytes and antigen, another chemical mediator which has been detected is the factor which induces a skin lesion at 8–12 hours when injected intradermally into the skin of guinea pigs [17, 106]. The lesion is characterized by infiltration with mononuclears and neutrophils.

G. Interferon. This substance is produced by cells infected with certain viruses. The interferon produced will render other tumor cells so they become resistant to infection by a variety of unrelated viruses. Recently, interferon production has been seen when lymphocytes are stimulated by a specific antigen or by phytohemagglutinin (PHA) [66].

H. Factor involved in eosinophil chemotaxis. Stimulated lymphocytes release biologically active substances which interact with immune complexes to generate eosinophil chemotactic factors [34].

In Vitro Correlates of Cellular Immunity

There are several in vitro reactions which are believed to parallel cellular immune reactions in vivo. Some of the techniques are as follows:

TRANSFORMATION AND PROLIFERATION OF LYMPHOCYTES [23, 111]. Lymphocytes from an antigen sensitive donor will transform into blast cells and proliferate when cultured in vitro with the specific antigen. Lymphocytes from patients with athymic or lymphopenic immune deficiency diseases do not respond to antigens in culture and have a severely impaired response to the nonspecific stimulation with phytohemagglutinin (PHA).

CYTOTOXICITY OF LYMPHOID CELLS IN VITRO [64, 65, 118]. Sensitized lymphocytes, as in cases of cancerous patients, may be cytotoxic for the specific tumor cells. Also lymphocytes may become cytotoxic and produce lymphotoxin when stimulated by a nonspecific mitogen as PHA. The nonantigen reactive lymphocytes may also be stimulated by proliferating antigen reactive lymphocytes and become cytotoxic. Thus, an immunologically specific interaction of antigen with specific lymphocytes will stimulate other nonspecific lymphocytes to participate in the destruction of bystander target cells.

INHIBITION OF MACROPHAGE MIGRATION. The migration of macrophages out of a capillary tube is inhibited by a macrophage inhibitory factor which is produced by the interaction of sensitized lymphocytes with specific antigen [23, 42, 111].

In the study of humans, two methods have been employed. First, the migration of human buffy coat cells has been applied to study many cellular sensitivity reactions [122]. However, a two-step approach is a more sensitive and reproducible system. In the first step, the human blood lymphocytes are cultured with the specific antigen and the amount of MIF produced is tested. The cell-free culture medium is tested for its ability to inhibit the migration of guinea pig macrophages in a test system first described by David [114].

Children with congenital thymic aplasia were unable to produce MIF, and children with agammaglobulinemia had a normal response [114].

Humoral Immunity

Plasma cells constitute one of the major sources of antibodies which are the effector mechanisms for the humoral system. There is evidence that T-cells are involved in antigen recognition and sensitization of B-cells. The B-cells proliferate and differentiate into plasma cells with the production of antibodies.

Based upon the reactivity of immunoglobulins with specific antisera, as well as other properties, 5 classes of human immunoglobulins have been described [18, 33, 51, 95, 112, 135]. There are three major immunoglobulins, IgG, IgA, IgM, and two minor immunoglobulins, IgD and IgE. These globulins constitute 20 to 25% of the total serum proteins. The various classes of immunoglobulins show a marked degree of heterogeneity, with respect to their function, structure, and genetic properties. The recommended nomenclature of human immunoglobulins by the Subcommittee for Human Immunoglobulins of the IUIS Nomenclature Committee is to eliminate the existing dual terminology of Ig and γ [133]. The symbols L and K are recommended to be discontinued since L and K are confused with light chains and lambda type. The terms kappa type (κ) and lambda type (λ) should be used to indicate the type of whole molecules or isolated chains [133]. The light chains were formerly described as K type and L type. Therefore the notations as IgG (λ) or IgM (κ), etc., should be used.

The concentrations of different serum immunoglobulins vary from birth to adulthood [3, 26, 28, 76, 126, 130]. The level of IgG decreases rapidly after birth, from the adult level to a low level at 3–4 months of age. The initial high level represents to a large extent the passively transferred antibody from the infant's mother. Then it gradually increases and reaches an average adult level before the age of 16. Normally IgA is not detectable in umbilical cord serum. The IgA level increases slowly during infancy and reaches about 25% of the adult value at the end of the first year. It continues to increase gradually and reaches an average adult level at approximately 16 years of age. The IgM level is detected in small quantities in umbilical cord serum and is apparently produced by the fetus. The IgM level increases rapidly after birth and reaches an average adult level before those of IgG or IgA. It has attained 50% of the normal adult level by the age of 4 months.

IgG immunoglobulins have a molecular weight of 160,000 with a 7S sedimentation coefficient in the ultracentrifuge [51]. The IgG serum concentration in a normal adult is about 1200 mg per 100 ml. The IgG

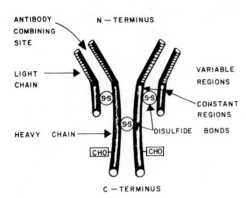

Figure 2-5
Schematic model of IgG immunoglobulin.

fraction contains the majority of antibacterial, antiviral, and antitoxic antibodies [33].

Serum IgA immunoglobulins have a molecular weight of 170,000 [135]. The serum IgA concentration in normal persons is approximately 200 mg per 100 ml. The IgA immunoglobulins contain a wide variety of different functional antibodies which include antitoxins, antibacterial agglutinins, isoagglutinins, and skin-sensitizing antibodies. IgA immunoglobulins are synthesized by plasma cells found within the lamina propria of the mucous membranes of the respiratory and gastrointestinal tracts. The mucous secretions contain the immunoglobulin in the form represented by two IgA molecules linked by a protein called the secretory or transport piece. This complex molecule, called *secretory IgA*, plays a significant role of local immune reactions in the mucous membrane surfaces, especially against viruses [68]. IgA deficiency may be associated with gastrointestinal malabsorption, respiratory tract infections, and a high incidence of autoimmune disease [5, 6].

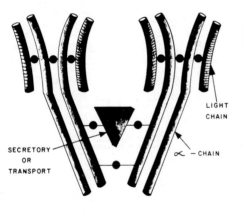

Figure 2-6
Schematic model of secretory IgA immunoglobulin.

The third class of immunoglobulins is IgM. These are large complex molecules, with a molecular weight of approximately 900,000 and a sedimentation coefficient in ultracentrifuge of 19S [95]. They exist in the serum in a concentration of approximately 140 mg per 100 ml. The IgM class of immunoglobulins contains many natural antibodies, that is, the ABO blood group, isoantibodies, rheumatoid factors, anti-thyroglobulin antibodies, and heterophile antibodies. Many of the antibacterial antibodies directed against gram-negative microorganisms are also IgM immunoglobulins.

The fourth class of immunoglobulins is IgD. The molecular weight of this globulin is approximately 150,000. IgD has a sedimentation coefficient in the ultracentrifuge of 7S, and is found in the serum in a concentration of approximately 3 mg per 100 ml. Most of the evidence for the antibody activity of IgD has been obtained by indirect antibody or antigen binding tests [123]. Direct proof of specific antibody activity in a purified preparation of IgD still remains to be elucidated. A surprisingly large fraction of human peripheral blood lymphocytes bear surface IgD immunoglobulins. With immunofluorescence studies, 2.7% of the peripheral blood lymphocytes showed membrane-associated IgD [139]. This is apparently 18% of all lymphocytes bearing surface immunoglobulins [139].

A fifth class of immunoglobulins has been described and is referred to as IgE [18]. The IgE immunoglobulin possesses skin-sensitizing properties responsible for the Prausnitz-Kuestner (P-K) reaction observed in humans. IgE has a specific affinity to bind to surface receptors on the mast cells and basophiles [18, 76]. The IgE immunoglobulins appear to play a role in immediate allergic reactions in humans; however, the

Figure 2-7
Schematic model of IgM immunoglobulin.

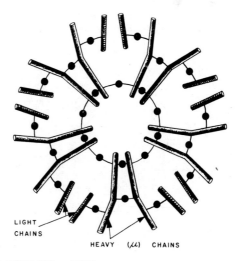

LIGHT CHAINS

HEAVY (μ) CHAINS

● = DISULFIDE   BONDS

Table 2-1. Immunoglobulins.

	IgG	IgA	IgM	IgD	IgE
Molecular weight	160,000	170,000 (serum) 390,000 (secretory)	900,000	160,000	200,000
Sediment coefficient (S units)	7	7, 11	19	7	8
Electrophoretic mobility	γ	slow β	between γ and β	between γ and β	slow β
Heavy chain nomenclature	γ	α	μ	σ	ε
Number of heavy chains	2	2	10	2	2
Number of light chains (K or λ)	2	2	10	2	2
Subclasses	$\gamma1, \gamma2, \gamma3, \gamma4$	$\alpha1, \alpha2$	μ (several)	two	—
Bind complement	+, +, +, −	−	+	−	—
Normal serum concentration (mg/100 ml) range	700–1700	70–350	70–210	3	0.03
mean value	1,200	210	140		

clinical significance of the IgE immunoglobulin still remains to be evaluated [76].

Classification of Primary or Congenital Immune Deficiency Diseases

The immune deficiency diseases may be regarded as either genetically determined (primary disorders) or acquired in association with certain disease processes (secondary disorders). In general, primary immune deficiencies are seen mainly in children, whereas secondary disorders are usually seen in adults.

Classification of Congenital or Primary Immune Deficiency Diseases
A. Nonspecific cellular deficiency—defect in phagocytosis and inflammation
B. Nonspecific humoral deficiency—defects in complement and chemotactic functions
C. Specific cellular deficiency—thymic dysplasia syndromes
D. Specific humoral deficiency—antibody deficiency syndrome, i.e., Bruton's syndrome
E. Combined specific cellular and humoral deficiency—i.e., alymphopenic agammaglobulinemia

Nonspecific Cellular Deficiency—Defects in Phagocytosis and Inflammation

The phagocytic system includes both fixed macrophages of the reticuloendothelial system and the circulating monocytes and polymorphonuclear leukocytes. The clinical entities may fall within two classes which are due to either quantitative or qualitative defects in the cells.

Quantitative Defect [15, 115]
A. Congenital neutropenia: (a) maternal antibodies; (b) infantile agranulocytosis—recessive—usually fatal; (c) benign chronic granulocytopenia of children—dominant; (d) children with severe depression of granulocytes often get necrotic tonsils and recurrent staphylococcal infections
B. Acquired neutropenia—from drugs, etc.
C. Quantitative deficiency of the macrophage (RES) system from splenectomy or invasion by tumor

Qualitative Defects of the Phagocytic System [48, 49, 87, 110, 149]
A clinical picture of recurrent infections is seen in a heterogeneous group of conditions in which the number of polymorphonuclear leukocytes is

Table 2-2. Congenital or Primary Immune Deficiency Diseases.

Cellular, Nonspecific (neutrophil)	Humoral, Nonspecific (complement)	Cellular, Specific (lymphocyte)	Humoral, Specific (antibody)	Combined Cellular and Humoral Defects
A	B	C	D	E
Chediak-Higashi	Essential hypocomplementemia	Thymic alymphoplasia, DiGeorge syndrome	Primary hypogammaglobulinemia	Swiss type agammaglobulinemia
Fatal granulomatous disease of childhood	Familial angioedema		Transient hypogammaglobulinemia	Wiskott-Aldrich syndrome
Neutropenias	C'3 deficiency		Dysgammaglobulinemias	Ataxia telangiectasia
	C'5 deficiency		Selective IgG subgroup deficiency	
			Salivary IgA deficiency	

Table 2-3. Classification of Primary Immune Deficiency Diseases.
(World Health Organization Committee Recommendations) [53, 54]

Type	Suggested Cellular Defect		
	B-Cells	T-Cells	Stem Cells
Infantile X-linked agammaglobulinemia	+		
Selective immunoglobulin deficiency (IgA)	+*		
Transient hypogammaglobulinemia of infancy	+		
X-linked immunodeficiency with hyper-IgM	+*		
Thymic hypoplasia (pharyngeal pouch syndrome, DiGeorge)		+	
Episodic lymphopenia with lymphocytotoxin		+	
Immunodeficiency with normal or hyperimmunoglobulinemia	+	+†	
Immunodeficiency with ataxia telangiectasia	+	+	
Immunodeficiency with thrombocytopenia and eczema (Wiskott-Aldrich)	+	+	
Immunodeficiency with thymoma	+	+	
Immunodeficiency with short-limbed dwarfism	+	+	
Immunodeficiency with generalized hematopoietic hypoplasia	+	+	+
Severe combined immunodeficiency			
(a) autosomal recessive	+	+	+
(b) X-linked	+	+	+
(c) sporadic	+	+	+
Variable immunodeficiency	+	+†	

* Involve some but not all B-cells
† Encountered in some but not all patients

normal but the cells demonstrate a qualitative defect. The cellular defect may manifest changes and affect (a) complement dependent chemotaxis of inflammatory cells [147]; (b) opsonization-removal of foreign particles; and (c) digestion and killing of bacteria after the ingestion by phagocytes.

One complicated case of a 3½-year-old child with a history of recurrent infections had evidence of a cellular defect of neutrophils with agammaglobulinemia [125]. The neutrophils had an impaired chemotaxis and were unable to phagocytize *Staphylococcus aureus* bacteria.

A case of a 23-year-old female adult who had a history of recurrent infections had monocytes which were unresponsive to autologous migration inhibitory factor (MIF) and to heterologous MIF from 2 of 3 healthy adults [90]. Humoral immunity, complement, and bacteriocidal functions were intact in the patient [90].

Neutrophilic Dysfunction Syndrome (chronic granulomatous disease of childhood)
These patients suffer from recurrent bacterial infections by organisms which usually are not pathogenic to normal people. The neutrophils can ingest bacteria but cannot kill phagocytized bacteria. The patients have eczema and enlarged spleen, liver, and lymph nodes, and form granulomas in many organs including lung, liver, kidney, hair, and skin. The condition generally leads to death, often before the age of 10 years. The disease was originally described in males as a sex-linked recessive trait and transmitted by heterozygote females. Recently, chronic granulomatous disease has also been described as a probable recessive trait in females with the same disease. This condition can be diagnosed by means of the quantitative tetrazolium test [12]. The sex-linked recessive cases in males were demonstrated to be deficient in nicotinamide adenine denucleotide (NADH) oxidase and nicotinamide adenine denucleotide phosphate (NADPH) oxidase [11].

The defect in chronic granulomatous disease primarily involves the hexose monophosphate shunt. Without this shunt, white cells have diminished O_2 consumption and decreased hydrogen peroxide production, which causes them to have a decreased capacity to kill intracellular catalase-positive organisms. Patients with chronic granulomatous disease are susceptible to infections with organisms such as *Staph. aureus, Serratia,* and *Aerobacter* organisms which are usually not pathogenic in normal persons. These bacteria produce catalase. The polymorphs of these patients are able to phagocytize the bacteria and have been shown to have decreased hydrogen peroxide production [110, 149]. This property may be related to the inability to kill catalase-producing bacteria such as streptococci and pneumococci.

MYELOPEROXIDASE DEFICIENCY [86, 119]. A deficiency in myeloperoxidase of neutrophils and monocytes. White blood cells killed the bacteria at slower than normal rate. The white blood cells of such patients were unable to kill *Candida albicans* at the rate observed in normal controls.

JOB'S SYNDROME [43]. A disorder characterized by recurrent cold staphylococcal abscesses and eczema. The process etiology is unknown, and the disease has been described only in females and believed to be transmitted as an autosomal recessive.

CHEDIAK-HIGASHI SYNDROME [148].   In this condition there are chronic infections and albinism of skin, hair, and eyes. There appears to be an abnormality of lysosomal and melanin granules. These patients have a high incidence of lymphomas or leukemias. Granulocytes and monocytes contain giant cytoplasmic peroxidase granules which are believed to be giant lysosomes. The phagocytosis of paraffin oil by leukocytes from two patients with Chediak-Higashi syndrome was doubled in relation to normal cells [131], whereas in chronic granulomatous disease the phagocytic ratio is not abnormal. It is possible that in Chediak-Higashi syndrome there is a degranulation defect which results in giant cytoplasmic inclusion granules [131].

Nonspecific Humoral Deficiency

The complement system, consisting of at least 11 different serum protein substances [101, 117], plays an important role in immunologic disease. Components of complement or split products are involved as follows.

Immune Adherence

This is an agglutination phenomenon which is based on the ability of antigen-antibody-complement complexes to adhere to the surface of nonsensitized particles such as red cells, leukocytes, and platelets. This results in the attachment of sensitized bacteria or viruses to cellular elements and makes them vulnerable to phagocytic cells. Opsonification is also based upon immune adherence, since a particle which adheres to the surface of a phagocyte is engulfed more easily. Both immune adherence and opsonification are dependent upon cell C3 (third component of complement). Binding sites for complement components have been detected on the surfaces of neutrophils and macrophages [73, 84]. The mononuclear phagocytes have receptor sites with specificity for C3 [74].

Leukocyte Chemotactic Factors

Chemotactic factors for neutrophils are heterogeneous in origin and structure [142, 145, 147]. C3a, produced by C3 convertase and other enzymes, and C5a, produced by sequential interaction of the complement system, are chemotactic for neutrophils. The activated trimolecular complex of C5, C6, and C7 is a potent chemotactic factor for polymorphonuclear leukocytes, which are attracted to an area of antigen antibody reaction with subsequent inflammation. In addition, factors chemotactic for mononuclear cells have been observed [146].

A patient with a serum inhibitor which results in impaired chemotaxis of neutrophils had a history of recurrent infections [144]. Similarly, defective chemotaxis associated with a serum inhibitor was observed in patients with liver cirrhosis [44]. This defect in chemotaxis of neutrophils may help explain the increased susceptibility to infections in cirrhosis [44].

Anaphylatoxin
Anaphylatoxin may be derived from C3 and C5 [101, 117]. It is a substance of low molecular weight which can cause increased vascular permeability, smooth muscle contraction, and release histamine from mast cells or tumor basophils.

Complement Defect in C3 Metabolism
An adult male with Klinefelter's syndrome and recurrent bacterial infections has been described [4]. The defect was not believed to be simply a result of C3 deficit but resulted from a defect in a serum substance which stabilized C3.

Familial Dysfunction of C5
Two cases of C5 deficiency were identified in patients with recurrent bacterial infections [98]. With deficiencies of any of the components C1 to C5, in vitro assays of complement activity usually show impaired activity. In humans, C1q deficiencies have been associated with some immunoglobulin deficiencies and suggest a relationship between serum C1q and IgG synthesis [117].

Primary Cellular-Specific Immune Deficiency Diseases

Thymic Dysplasia Syndromes
There are a number of syndromes that have been described involving the thymus, resulting in thymic dysplasia or agenesis. The classic example of thymic dysplasia is DiGeorge's syndrome [47, 80]. This condition is characterized by a failure of the derivatives of the third and fourth pharyngeal pouches to develop, and it results in an absence or partial absence of the thymus and parathyroid glands. The peripheral lymphoid tissue shows an absence of lymphocytes in the paracortical thymic dependent areas. The numbers of plasma cells present in lymphoid tissue is normal, and germinal centers are intact. On the other hand, the lymphocytes present in the circulating blood may be normal in number. There is no deficiency of immunoglobulins. However, the primary immune response is often deficient since this response does apparently involve T-lymphocytes in some way. Cellular immunity is markedly defective. These infants usually die in infancy. Generalized tetany is often present in the newborn, and cardiovascular malformations resulting from hypocalcemia are common. The infants have frequent viral, fungal, and parasitic infections such as pneumocystis, and there is also a defect in primary humoral immune responses in some cases due to the role that T-lymphocytes play in underdeveloped thymus, the absence of delayed hypersensitivity, and the inability to reject skin allografts.

The patient will demonstrate a negative skin test to a variety of bacterial, viral, and fungal proteins and to chemicals such as dinitrochlorobenzene (DNCB). The lymphocytes will fail to transform in vitro in the presence of phytohemagglutinin (PHA). The serum immunoglobulin levels are normal. These patients are prone to infection with low-grade pyogenic bacteria and other intracellular pathogens such as tubercle bacilli, listeriae, and salmonellae. They are prone to viral and fungal infections, as vaccinia, rubeola, cytomegalic inclusion disease, and *C. albicans*.

Gatti et al. [56] have reported a case of DiGeorge syndrome with combined immunodeficiency. The patient had an absent in vitro lymphocyte response to phytohemagglutinin and a normal mixed lymphocyte culture response after 3 weeks of age.

Lischner and DiGeorge [89] have suggested that the humoral immune function may sometimes be more severely impaired than formerly believed. They feel that complete absence of the thymus is associated with severe impairment of antibody formation, and certain patients with DiGeorge's syndrome, in whom humoral immunity is largely intact, may have incomplete defects and have small thymic remnants which support some humoral immune functions. Thymus grafting has restored cellular immune functions in thymic dysplasia [7, 8, 32]. The restoration was established quickly and was long lasting. Human fetal thymic tissue 13 to 16 weeks old has been found to be beneficial, although tissue from fetuses older than 16 weeks may cause a graft virus host reaction [97]. Thymic reconstitution has been tried by implanting in one infant thymic cells from another fetus which had been placed in a millipore diffusion chamber [124]. Thymic cell function was induced as measured by thymidine incorporation after stimulation of the lymphocytes with PHA [124]. The infant died of aspiration pneumonia. Whether thymic cell function can be induced in man with humoral fetal-thymic factors still may be debatable [97]. Since the patients lack the ability to initiate homograft reaction, blood transfusions with viable leukocytes may initiate a graft versus host reaction [72]. Thus, precautions must be taken to avoid transfusion of these patients with viable leukocytes.

Primary Humoral, Specific Immune Deficiency Diseases

Bruton's Type of Agammaglobulinemia
This was the first type of classifiable immune deficiency disorder reported by Bruton in 1952, following his study of a patient with this disease, a young boy who had a marked deficiency of the humoral defense mechanism [25]. There is a deficiency of circulating immunoglobulins with an inability to form antibodies to an antigenic challenge. Plasma cells and germinal centers are absent in lymphoid tissues. Im-

munologic phenomena associated with the cellular immune system are usually normal, so that the individual is able to effect allograft rejection and other lymphocytic functions. The thymic structure is normal. This disease is transmitted as a sex-linked recessive trait.

These patients are particularly susceptible to repeated infections with high-grade encapsulated pyogenic pathogens. Patients are prone to *Haemophilus influenzae,* streptococcal, meningococcal, and *Pseudomonas aeruginosa* infections [15]. In contrast, these patients have little trouble with recurrent viral or fungal infections and usually have a normal reaction to vaccinia virus [79].

Bruton's type of agammaglobulinemia has a high incidence of chronic polyarthritis similar to rheumatoid arthritis [13]. Subcutaneous nodules resembling those of rheumatoid arthritis are seen.

Isohemagglutinin titers are usually zero, and the Schick test with diphtheria toxoid is positive. The Schick test may be negative if the patient is receiving exogenous γ immunoglobulin therapy.

Patients with this form of congenital agammaglobulinemia usually reject skin grafts, develop delayed skin reactions to antigens such as *Candida,* streptokinase-streptodornase, and 2,4,dinitrochlorobenzene.

The patients with Bruton's type of agammaglobulinemia respond well to monthly injections of γ-globulin except with progressive sinopulmonary disease. The exogenous administration of γ-globulins is often supplemented with short courses of antibiotics to eliminate certain pathogenic bacteria.

Dysgammaglobulinemia

A number of instances in which an individual plasma cell line is deficient has been reported. Normal or increased amounts of other plasma cell lines may lead to an imbalance of the immunoglobulin concentrations, giving rise to the term dysgammaglobulinemia. The immunoglobulin deficiency can occur in various ways—as a complete deficiency in immunoglobulins, or as specific IgG, IgM, or IgA deficiencies [53, 67]. There are also different combined deficiencies as well as IgG subgroup deficiencies which have resulted in the patient being susceptible to repeated pyogenic infections [120].

SELECTIVE IGA DEFICIENCY.   The isolated deficiency of IgA is very common and may occur as part of another disease process, such as hereditary telangectasia [5, 6]. This occurs with a frequency of about 1:600 [132] or 1:1000 [58]. The number of circulating lymphocytes found in the individual's blood is normal, and immunoglobulin antibody responses of the individual are normal except for the production of IgA antibodies. Cellular immunity is normal. Since IgA is the primary antibody secreted onto the mucosal surfaces, these individuals may have episodes of bronchitis and sinusitis. In addition, they may have gastrointestinal dysfunctions associated with malabsorption and steatorrhea.

Although several of the individuals are apparently normal, there is an extremely high incidence of autoimmune diseases [5, 6] and particularly rheumatoid arthritis and systemic lupus erythematosus among the patients with selective IgA deficiencies [30].

IGE DEFICIENCY.   Individuals with IgE concentrations in serum of less than 15 ng/ml are considered to be IgE deficient [108]. The geometric mean IgE level of a normal population was reported to be 105 ng/ml with a range of 5 to 2045 ng/ml. Specific IgE deficiency was noted in 7 of 73 patients and was not associated with respiratory tract disease.

Serum IgE levels in patients with adult-acquired hypogammaglobulinemia were reduced and 7 of 50 first-degree relatives had low IgE levels [129]. The IgE levels varied with patients with selective IgA deficiency and a combined deficiency did not necessarily predispose the patient to recurrent infections [108, 129].

Primary Combined Cellular and Humoral Deficiency Diseases

Swiss Type of Agammaglobulinemia

This disorder was first described by Swiss investigators and appears to be transmitted as a single autosomal recessive trait [19]. Generally death occurs before the age of 2 years. Smallpox vaccination leads to progressive vaccinia in these infants. Most investigators feel that the stem cells are defective in this disorder. The immunologic defect in these patients consists of a combined deficiency in both humoral and cellular defenses. The humoral aspect of this disease is reflected by a deficiency of all classes of immunoglobulins and the absence of plasma cells from lymphoid tissue. Cellular deficiency is confirmed by the abnormally low number of peripheral blood lymphocytes. This disorder is probably due to a failure of the specific differentiation of lymphoid stem cells into thymic-dependent lymphocytes.

A significant number of these patients will have an adverse reaction to vaccination with smallpox of BCG and to administration of fresh whole blood with viable lymphocytes [67, 72]. Some of these patients have been successfully treated, with complete restoration of immunologic functions, by grafts of histocompatible marrow cells [96, 128]. It appears that when appropriate stem cells are provided the patients are capable of developing functional T-cells.

Buckley et al. [27] employed lymphocytotoxic antibodies to an infant's lymphocytes, obtained from the mother, to circumvent fatal acute graft-versus-host disease, when incompatible bone marrow transplants were given in a case of severe combined immunodeficiency. The infant was treated with maternal plasma containing the lymphocytotoxic antibodies before and after infusion of maternal bone marrow cells. The therapeutic approach may be useful since the infant survived for 14 months, which is a much longer period than any other reported severe combined deficiency disease case treated with incompatible bone marrow transplants.

Wiskott-Aldrich Syndrome

This is a sex-linked recessive disease characterized by thrombocytopenia, eczema, and recurrent infections [21, 36]. The numbers of circulating lymphocytes are usually quite low; however, the numbers of plasma cells present in lymphoid tissue are within normal limits. An immunoglobulin deficit is usually present, but the class of immunoglobulin involved and the degree of deficiency is variable. A low IgM level and a high IgA level are frequent findings. A high IgE level is seen and may reflect chronic stimulation by antigens which these patients cannot process normally [141]. Cellular immunity is also deficient. The thymus architecture is normal and germinal centers are present in lymphoid tissue, although they may be decreased in numbers. The number of lymphocytes in thymic-dependent areas of lymphoid tissue is deficient.

These patients have a deficiency in their capacity to process pneumococcal polysaccharide and may have an abnormal A-cell or phagocytic cell function [22, 36]. They are susceptible to (a) infections with herpes simplex, varicella, pneumocystis carinii, and many different bacterial infections; (b) massive bleeding secondary to thrombocytopenia; and (c) lymphoreticular malignancies.

A case of Wiskott-Aldrich syndrome has been treated with HL–A-compatible bone marrow transplant with some improvement [9]. The bone marrow transplant was not as successful as certain transplants in cases of lymphopenic immunologic deficiency. Levin et al. [88] have treated Wiskott-Aldrich syndrome with dialyzable transfer factor (dialysate of donor peripheral leukocytes). They reported excellent clinical improvement with successful transfer of delayed cutaneous reactivity to certain antigens. After treatment of the patient with transfer factor, the patient's lymphocytes produced migration inhibitory factor without concomitant DNA synthesis. The experiment supports the evidence that factors responsible for skin test sensitivity and activity of migration inhibitory factor may be different from in vitro lymphocyte transformation.

Ataxia-Telangiectasia

These patients have deficient immunologic responses in both humoral and cell-mediated reactions [105, 116]. The cardinal features of the disease are (a) progressive ataxia with onset at infancy, (b) subcutaneous telangiectasia, and (c) apraxia of eye movements. Approximately 60% of the patients show a deficiency of IgA in their serum, saliva, and both nasopharyngeal and gastrointestinal secretions. In addition, a significant percentage of patients have IgE deficiency [108].

The most consistent immunologic deficiency in ataxia-telangiectasia is the deficiency of cell-mediated reactions [57]. The underlying defect in this disease has not been clearly delineated. The possibilities are (a) defective T-cells in the cellular immunity as well as in support of IgA and IgE immunoglobulin production and (b) defective interaction of primitive endodermal mesodermal elements.

Implantation of the thymus and spleen of fetal donors has been attempted without significant results [63]. It appears that thymic dysplasia may not be the crucial defect in this disease.

Acquired Immune Deficiency Diseases

The acquired disorders are predominantly seen in adults. Although they very often occur secondary to another primary disease state, in general they play a very prominent role in the disease process.

Primary Acquired Hypogammaglobulinemia
This condition is usually seen in adults and the level of circulating IgG is less than 500 mg per 100 ml [103]. It is probably not inherited and affects both sexes. The hypogammaglobulinemia is often found to be associated with other immunologic disorders, such as systemic lupus erythematosus, hemolytic anemia, and thrombocytopenia. This is probably the most common immune deficiency disorder. The incidence of malignancy is extremely high in this disorder.

Secondary Acquired Hypogammaglobulinemia
This condition can occur in a number of other disease states, as exfoliative dermatitis, and renal and gastrointestinal disorders which are accompanied by an excessive loss of serum proteins. The causes of secondary hypogammaglobulinemia may be due to a wide variety of diseases which affect the synthesis of immunoglobulins, such as (a) increased catabolism and loss of immunoglobulins (nephrotic syndrome, protein-losing enteropathy, intestinal lymphangiectasia); (b) bone marrow disorders and reticuloendothelial tumors; and (c) toxic conditions [127].

Hodgkin's Disease [1, 2]
There are several kinds of lymphoma, and one of the most common types is Hodgkin's disease. Patients with Hodgkin's disease show normal or elevated levels of immunoglobulins and are capable of a normal antibody response. However, cell-mediated immunity is defective and lymphopenia may occur late in the disease. The lymphocytes that are present in circulation in patients with Hodgkin's disease are abnormal by in vitro tests. This is confirmed since the delayed hypersensitivity to various antigens is impaired. Patients reject skin allografts poorly, and there is increased susceptibility to tuberculous, fungal, and viral infections. The immunologic defect is explained by defective T-lymphocytes. In a functional sense, it may represent the acquired analogue of the congenital absence of the thymus.

Sarcoidosis [121]

Sarcoidosis is a systemic granulomatous inflammatory reaction of un-known etiology. The characteristic histologic lesion is a granuloma with-out caseous necrosis. Patients with this disorder characteristically have a deficiency of cellular immunity with defective delayed skin hypersensi-tivity reactions, decreased ability to reject transplants, and an abnormal in vitro testing of lymphocytes. The humoral immune system is normal, and normal or increased amounts of immunoglobulins may be present.

Uremia [41]

Uremia is a syndrome characterized by azotemia or the retention of nitrogenous waste material, acidosis, and generally anemia. Patients with chronic uremia often have altered cellular immunity. Allograft rejection and cutaneous hypersensitivity have been found to be impaired. Lympho-cytes from individuals with chronic uremia may have shortened life spans. Lymphocytopenia of the peripheral blood and atrophy of the thymus have been described. Defective lymphocytes have been demon-strated by in vitro testing.

Chronic Lymphocytic Leukemia [69, 70]

Patients with chronic lymphocytic leukemia demonstrate a combined cellular and humoral immune defect. The serum immunoglobulin levels are often decreased, particularly during the terminal phase of the dis-ease. The combined cellular and humoral immune defect may be due to a faulty differentiation of either the bone marrow or lymphoid stem cell. It appears that the lymphocytes circulating in the patient's blood stream in very large numbers are actually immunologically incompetent cells. In chronic lymphocytic leukemia, the circulating lymphocytes are unable to become sensitized and may have a longer life span than im-munocompetent lymphocytes, which can become sensitized, committed, and destroyed in various immunologic pathways.

Monoclonal Gammopathies [40, 109, 113]

In patients with monoclonal gammopathies, it is postulated that one clone of plasma cells proliferates and results in the production of a homogeneous single type of immunoglobulin. The remainder of the plasma cell lines and their normal immunoglobulin products are either normal or decreased. The ability of patients with this disorder to pro-duce normal antibodies is often markedly decreased. The classic ex-ample is multiple myeloma; and with defective production of specific protective antibodies, the patients are susceptible to bacterial infections.

Immune Deficiency Disease and Malignancy

Patients with immune deficiencies have a very high incidence of malig-nancy [59, 69, 140]. Also certain forms of malignancies are regularly seen with immunologic defects [59, 140].

Primary immune deficiencies have a high incidence of malignancy as well as a great susceptibility to infections [52, 58, 59, 61, 141]. An increased incidence of leukemia has been seen with sex-linked infantile agammaglobulinemia [59]. A wide variety of tumors has been observed to accompany diseases as ataxia-telangiectasia and Wiskott-Aldrich syndrome.

Secondary immune deficiencies as seen in prolonged immunosuppressive therapy are also accompanied by an increase in the incidence of cancer [58, 61, 94]. The malignancies have been of the epithelial and lymphoreticular types [94]. It is apparent that all immunosuppressive agents may enhance the development of cancer. A case with reticulum cell sarcoma developing at the site of local injection of antilymphocyte globulin has been reported [45].

There apparently is a loss of homeostatic defense mechanisms against neoplasia with a failure of immune surveillance mechanisms [24]. Genetic factors likely play a role in the susceptibility to neoplasms by immune deficient patients. The inability to mount an immune response to specific oncogenic, virus, or tumor antigens on the surface of the cells is probably linked to genetic control mechanisms.

Association of Immune Deficiency Diseases and Autoimmune Disorders

The presence of autoimmune reactivity in cases of immune deficiency diseases has been well documented in isolated IgA deficiency [5, 6, 30] and agammaglobulinemia [52]. Patients with agammaglobulinemia have an unusually high incidence of an arthritis which resembles rheumatoid arthritis [13]. Subcutaneous nodules are seen, and upon biopsy examination the nodule shows features of a rheumatoid nodule with a paucity of mononuclear cells and an absence of plasma cells.

The development of autoantibodies in patients with immune deficiency diseases is probably the result of the action of environmental pathogens, such as bacteria and viruses in an immunologically deficient host [104]. Mice thymectomized at birth and raised in the normal environment will develop "wasting disease" [93] with the development of autoimmune manifestations similar to those found in systemic lupus erythematosus [46]. On the other hand, if the mice were thymectomized at birth and placed in a germ-free environment, they do not develop the autoimmune manifestations until after they are placed in the normal conventional environment.

There is evidence that genetic factors, which are involved in immune deficiency diseases, also may play a role in the pathogenesis of autoimmune complications. Relatives of patients with immune deficiency diseases have a very high frequency of autoimmune disease [53].

The possible role of viruses in autoimmunity is currently under much investigation. Definite proof of viral etiology in many of these diseases awaits further investigation. In humans, viral infections have been associated with autoimmune hemolytic anemia [39]. Evidence has been accumulating for the interplay of viral and genetic factors in the pathogenesis of systemic lupus erythematosus [134].

References

1. Aisenberg, A. C.   Studies of lymphocyte transfer reactions in Hodgkin's disease. *J. Clin. Invest.* 44:555, 1965.
2. Aisenberg, A. C.   Immunological status of Hodgkin's disease. *Cancer* 19:385, 1966.
3. Allansmith, M., McClellan, B. H., Butterworth, M., and Maloney, J. R. The development of immunoglobulin levels in man. *J. Pediatr.* 72:726, 1968.
4. Alper, C. A., Abramson, M., Johnston, R. B., Jandl, J. H., and Rosen, F. S.   Increased susceptibility to infection associated with abnormalities of complement mediated functions and of the third component of complement (C3). *N. Engl. J. Med.* 282:349, 1970.
5. Ammann, A. J., and Hong, R.   Selective IgA deficiency and autoimmunity. *Clin. Exp. Immunol.* 7:833, 1970.
6. Ammann, A. J., and Hong, R.   Selective IgA deficiency: Presentation of 30 cases of review of the literature. *Medicine* 50:223, 1971.
7. August, C. S., Rosen, F. S., Filler, R. M., Janeway, C. A., Markowski, B., and Kay, H. E. M.   Implantation of a foetal thymus, restoring immunological competence in a patient with thymic aplasia (DiGeorge syndrome). *Lancet* 2:210, 1968.
8. August, C. S., Berkel, A. I., Levey, R. H., Rosen, F. S., and Kay, H. E. M.   Establishment of an immunological competence in a child with congenital thymic aplasia by a graft of fetal thymus. *Lancet* 1:1080, 1970.
9. Bach, F. H., Albertini, R. J., Joo, P., Anderson, J. L. Y., and Bortin, M. M.   Bone marrow transplantation in a patient with Wiskott-Aldrich syndrome. *Lancet* 2:1364, 1968.
10. Bach, J. F., Dormont, J., Dardenne, M., and Balner, H.   In vitro rosette formation inhibition by antihuman antilymphocyte serum. Correlation with skin graft prolongation in subhuman primates. *Transplantation* 8:265, 1969.
11. Baehner, R. L., and Nathan, D. G.   Quantitative nitroblue tetrazolium test in chronic granulomatous disease. *N. Engl. J. Med.* 27:971, 1968.
12. Baehner, R. L., and Karnovsky, M. C.   Deficiency of reduced nicotinamideadenine dinucleotide oxidase in chronic granulomatous disease. *Science* 162:1277, 1968.
13. Barnett, E. V., Winkelstein, A., and Weinberger, H.   Agammaglobulinemia with polyarthritis and subcutaneous nodules. *Am. J. Med.* 48:40, 1970.
14. Basten, A., Sprent, J., and Miller, J. F. A. P.   Receptor for antibody-antigen complexes used to separate T-cells from B-cells. *Nature* [*New Biol.*] 235:178, 1972.
15. Bellanti, J. A., and Schlegel, R. J.   The diagnosis of immune deficiency diseases. *Pediatr. Clin. North Am.* 18:49, 1971.
16. Benacerraf, B., Biozzi, G., Bloom, B. R., Brunner, T., David, J. R., Gell,

P. G. H., Johanovsky, J., and Perlmann, P.   Cell mediated immune responses—Report of a WHO Scientific Group. World Health Organization Tech. Report. No. 423. Geneva: WHO, 1969.

17. Bennett, B., and Bloom, B. R.   Reactions in vivo and in vitro produced by a soluble substance associated with delayed type hypersensitivity. *Proc. Natl. Acad. Sci. U.S.A.* 59:756, 1968.

18. Bennich, H., and Johansson, S. G. O.   Structure and function of human immunoglobulin E. *Adv. Immunol.* 13:1, 1971.

19. Bergsma, D., and Good, R. A.   *Immunologic Deficiency Diseases in Man.* New York: The National Foundation, 1968.

20. Bianco, C., Patrick, R., and Nussenzweig, V.   A population of lymphocytes bearing a membrane receptor for antigen-antibody complement complexes: I. Separation and characterization. *J. Exp. Med.* 132:702, 1970.

21. Blaese, R. M., Brown, R. S., Strober, W., and Waldman, T. A.   The Wiskott-Aldrich syndrome: A disorder and possible defect in antigen processing or recognition. *Lancet* 1:1056, 1968.

22. Blaese, R. M., Oppenheim, J. J., Seeger, R. J., et al.   Lymphocyte macrophage interaction in antigen induced in vitro lymphocyte transformation in patients with the Wiskott-Aldrich syndrome and other diseases with anergy. *Cell. Immunol.* 4:228, 1972.

23. Bloom, B. R.   In vitro approaches to the mechanisms of cell mediated immune reactions. *Adv. Immunol.* 13:101, 1971.

24. Brain, P., Gordon, J., and Willets, W. A.   Rosette formation by peripheral lymphocytes. *Clin Exp. Immunol.* 6:681, 1970.

25. Bruton, O. C.   Agammaglobulinemia. *Pediatrics* 9:722, 1952.

26. Buckley, C. E., III, and Dorsey, F. C.   Serum immunoglobulin levels throughout the life span of the healthy man. *Ann. Int. Med.* 75:653, 1971.

27. Buckley, R. H., Dees, S. C., and O'Fallon, W. M.   Serum immunoglobulins: I. Levels in normal children and in uncomplicated childhood allergy. *Pediatrics* 41:600, 1968.

28. Buckley, R. H., Amos, B., Kremer, W. B., and Stickel, D. L.   Incompatible bone marrow transplantation in lymphopenic immunologic deficiency—circumvention of fatal graft vs. host disease by immunologic enhancement. *N. Engl. J. Med.* 285:1035, 1971.

29. Burnet, F. M.   *Immunological Surveillance.* Oxford: Pergamon, 1970.

30. Cassidy, J. T., Burt, A., Petty, R., and Sullivan, D.   Selective IgA deficiency in connective tissue diseases. *N. Engl. J. Med.* 280:275, 1968.

31. Claman, H. N., and Chaperon, E. A.   Immunologic complementation between thymus and bone marrow cells: A model for the two cell theory of immunocompetence. *Transplant. Rev.* 1:92, 1969.

32. Cleveland, W. W., Fogel, B. J., Brown, W. T., and Kay, H. E. M.   Foetal thymic transplant in a case of DiGeorge syndrome. *Lancet* 2:1211, 1968.

33. Cohen, S., and Porter, R. R.   Structure and biological activity of immunoglobulins. *Adv. Immunol.* 4:237, 1964.

34. Cohen, S., and Ward, P. A.   In vitro and in vivo activity of a lymphocyte and immune complex dependent chemotactic factor for eosinophils. *J. Exp. Med.* 131:1288, 1971.

35. Coombs, R. R. A., Gurner, B. W., Wilson, A. B., Holm, G., and Lind-

gren, B.   Rosette formation between human lymphocytes and sheep red cells not involving immunoglobulin receptors. *Int. Arch. Allergy Appl. Immunol.* 39:658, 1970.

36. Cooper, M. D., Chase, H. P., Lowman, J., Krivit, W., and Good, R. A. Wiskott-Aldrich syndrome—an immunologic deficiency disease involving the afferent limb of immunity. *Am. J. Med.* 44:499, 1968.

37. Cooper, M. D., Kincade, P. W., and Lawton, A. R.   Thymus and bursal function in immunologic development. B. M. Kagen and E. R. Stiehm (eds.), *Immunologic Incompetence.* Chicago: Year Book, 1971, p. 81.

38. Cooper, M. D., and Lawton, A. R.   The mammalian "Bursa Equivalent": Does lymphoid differentiation along plasma cell lines begin in the gut-associated lymphoepithelial tissues (GALT) of mammals? In M. E. Hanna, Jr. (ed.), *Contemporary Topics in Immunobiology.* New York: Plenum Press, 1972, vol. 1, chap. 3.

39. Dacie, J. V.   III. Haemolytic anaemia following or associated with known virus infections. In *The Haemolytic Anaemias.* Part II: *The Autoimmune Anaemias.* London: Churchill, 2nd ed., 1962.

40. Dammacco, F., and Clausen, J.   Antibody deficiency in paraproteinemia. *Acta Med. Scand.* 179:755, 1966.

41. Daniels, J. C., Sakai, H., Remmers, A. R., Sarles, H. E., Fish, J. C., Cobb, E. K., Levin, W. C., and Ritzmann, S. E.   In vitro reactivity of human lymphocytes in chronic uraemia: Analysis and interpretation. *Clin. Exp. Immunol.* 8:213, 1971.

42. David, J. R., Lawrence, H. S., and Thomas, L.   Delayed hypersensitivity in vitro: II. Effect of sensitive cells on normal cells in the presence of antigen. *J. Immunol.* 93:247, 1964.

43. Davis, S. D., Schaller, J., and Wedgewood, R. J.   Job's syndrome: Recurrent "cold" staphyloccal abscesses. *Lancet* 1:1013, 1966.

44. De Meo, A. N., and Andersen, B. R.   Defective chemotaxis associated with a serum inhibitor in cirrhotic patients. *N. Engl. J. Med.* 286:735, 1972.

45. Deodhar, S. D., Kuklinca, A. G., Vidt, D. G., Robertson, A. L., and Hazard, J. B.   Development of reticulum cell sarcoma at the site of antilymphocyte globulin injection in a patient with renal transplant. *N. Engl. J. Med.* 280:1104, 1969.

46. DeVries, M. J., van Putten, L. M., Balner, H., and van Bekkum, D. W. Lesions suggérant une réactivité autoimmune chez des souris atteintes de la "runt" disease: Après thymectomie neonatale. *Rev. F. Etud. Clin. Biol.* 9:381, 1964.

47. DiGeorge, A. M.   Congenital absence of the thymus and its immunologic consequences: Concurrence with congenital hypoparathyroidism. In R. A. Good and D. Bergsma (eds.), *Immunologic Deficiency Disease in Man.* New York: National Foundation Press, 1968, vol. 4, p. 116.

48. Douglas, S. D., and Fudenberg, H. H.:   Host defense failure: The role of phagocytic dysfunction. *Hosp. Practice* 4:29, 1969.

49. Douglas, S. D.   Analytic review: Disorders of phagocytic function. *Blood* 35:851, 1970.

50. Dutton, R. W., Falkoff, R., Hirst, J. A., Hoffmann, M., Koppler, J. W., Kettman, J. R., Lesley, J. F., and Vann, D.   Is there evidence for a non-antigen specific diffusable chemical mediator from a thymus derived cell in the initiation of the immune response? In B. Amos (ed.), *Progress*

in Immunology. 1st International Congress of Immunology. New York and London: Academic, 1971, p. 355.
51. Fahey, J. L.   Heterogeneity of γ-globulins. *Adv. Immunol.* 2:42, 1962.
52. Fraser, K. J., and Rankin, J. G.   Selective deficiency of IgA immunoglobulins associated with carcinoma of the stomach. *Aust. Ann. Med.* 19:165, 1970.
53. Fudenberg, H. H., et al.   Classification of the primary immune deficiencies. World Health Organization Recommendations. *N. Engl. J. Med.* 283:656, 1970.
54. Fudenberg, H. H., et al.   Primary immunodeficiencies: Report of World Health Organization Committee. *Pediatrics* 47:935, 1971.
55. Fudenberg, H. H.   Genetically determined immune deficiency as the predisposing cause of "autoimmunity" and lymphoid neophasia. *Am. J. Med.* 51:295, 1971.
56. Gatti, R. A., and Good, R. A.   The immunological deficiency diseases. *Med. Clin. North Am.* 54:281, 1970.
57. Gatti, R. A., and Good, R. A.   Occurrence of malignancy in immunodeficiency disease: A literature review. *Cancer* 28:89, 1971.
58. Gatti, R. A., Gershanik, J. J., Levkoff, A. H., Wertelecki, W., and Good, R. A.   DiGeorge syndrome associated with combined immunodeficiency-dissociation of phytohemagglutinin and mixed leucocyte response. *J. Pediatr.* 81:920, 1972.
59. Good, R. A., and Gabrielson, A. E. (eds.)   *The Thymus in Immunobiology*. New York: Hoeber Med. Div., Harper & Row, 1964.
60. Good, R. A., and Finstad, J.   An essential relationship between the lymphoid system, immunity and cancer. *J. Natl. Cancer Inst.* 31:41, 1969.
61. Good, R. A., Biggar, W. D., and Park, B. H.   Immunodeficiency diseases in man. In B. Amos (ed.), *Progress in Immunology*. 1st International Congress of Immunology. New York: Academic, 1971, p. 700.
62. Good, R. A.   Relations between immunity and malignancy. *Proc. Natl. Acad. Sci. U.S.A.* 69:1026, 1972.
63. Goya, H., Fujimoto, T., and Sumiyoshi, A.   Congenital immunologic deficiency diseases. *Acta Haematol. Jap.* 30:11, 1967.
64. Granger, G. A.   Mechanisms of lymphocyte induced cell and tissue destruction in vitro. *Am. J. Pathol.* 60:469, 1970.
65. Granger, G. A., and Williams, T. W.   Lymphocyte effector molecules: Mechanism of human lymphotoxin induced in vitro target cell destruction and role in PHA induced lymphocyte target cell cytolysis. In B. Amos (ed.), *Progress in Immunology*. 1st International Congress of Immunology. New York and London: Academic, 1971, p. 437.
66. Green, J. A., Cooperband, S. R., and Kibrick, S.   Immune specific induction of interferon production in cultures of human blood lymphocytes. *Science* 164:1415, 1969.
67. Gustafson, S. R., and Coursin, D. B.   Immunologic deficiency states. In S. R. Gustafson and D. B. Coursin (eds.), *The Pediatric Patient*. Philadelphia: Lippincott, 1969, pp. 13–66, 262–271.
68. Hanson, L. A., Borssen, R., Holmgren, J., Jodal, V., Johansson, B. G., and Kaijser, B.   Secretory IgA. In B. M. Kagen and E. R. Stiehm (eds.), *Immunologic Incompetence*. Chicago: Year Book, 1972.

38   I: Diagnostic Patterns of Immunologic Disorders

69. Harris, J. E., and Sinkovics, J. E. *The Immunology of Malignant Diseases.* St. Louis: Mosby, 1970.
70. Harris, J., and Bagai, R. C. Immune deficiency states associated with malignant disease in man. *Med. Clin. North Am.* 56:501, 1972.
71. Holmes, B., Park, B. H., Malawista, S. E., Quie, P. G., Nelson, D. C., and Good, R. A. Chronic granulomatous disease in females: A deficiency of leucocyte glutathione peroxidase. *N. Engl. J. Med.* 283:217, 1970.
72. Hong, R., Gatti, R. A., and Good, R. A. Hazards and potential benefits of blood transfusion in immunologic deficiency. *Lancet* 2:388, 1968.
73. Huber, H., Polley, M. J., Linscott, W. D., Fudenberg, H. H., and Müller-Eberhard, H. J. Human monocytes: Distinct receptor sites for the third component of complement and for immunoglobulin G. *Science* 162:128, 1968.
74. Huber, H., and Fudenberg, H. H. The interaction of monocyte and macrophages with immunoglobulins and complement. *Ser. Haematol.* 1970, vol. III, p. 160.
75. Johansson, S. G. O., and Berg, T. Immunoglobulin levels in healthy children. *Acta Paediatr. Scand.* 56:572, 1967.
76. Johansson, S. G. O., Bennich, H. H., and Berg, T. The clinical significance of IgE. In R. S. Schwartz (ed.), *Progress in Clinical Immunology.* New York: Grune & Stratton, 1972, vol. 1, p. 157.
77. Jondal, M., Holm, G., and Wigzell, H. Surface markers on human T and B lymphocytes: I. A large population of lymphocytes forming nonimmune rosettes with sheep red blood cells. *J. Exp. Med.* 136:207, 1972.
78. Katz, D., and Benacerraf, B. The regulatory influence of activated T-cells on B-cells response to antigen. *Adv. Immunol.* 15:1, 1972.
79. Kempe, C. H. Studies on smallpox and complications of smallpox vaccination. *Pediatrics* 26:176, 1960.
80. Kretschmer, R., Say, B., Brown, D., and Rosen, F. S. Congenital aplasia of the thymus gland (DiGeorge syndrome). *N. Engl. J. Med.* 279:1295, 1968.
81. Lawrence, H. S., and Landy, M. *Mediators of Cellular Immunity.* New York: Academic, 1969.
82. Lawrence, H. S. Transfer factor. *Adv. Immunol.* 11:195, 1969.
83. Lawrence, H. S. Transfer factor and cellular immune disease. *N. Engl. J. Med.* 283:411, 1970.
84. Lay, W. H., and Nussenzweig, V. Receptors for complement on leucocytes. *J. Exp. Med.* 128:991, 1968.
85. Lay, W. H., Mendes, N. F., Bianco, C., and Nussenzweig, V. Binding of sheep red blood cells to a large population of human lymphocytes. *Nature* 230:531, 1971.
86. Lehrer, R. I., and Cline, M. J. Leucocyte myeloperoxidase deficiency and disseminated candidiasis: The role of myeloperoxidase in resistance to *Candida* infections. *J. Clin. Invest.* 48:1478, 1969.
87. Lehrer, R. I. The role of phagocytic function in resistance to infection. *Calif. Med.* 114:17, 1971.
88. Levin, A. S., Spitler, L. E., Stites, D. P., and Fudenberg, H. H. A genetically determined cellular immune deficiency: Clinical and laboratory response to therapy with "transfer factor." *Proc. Natl. Acad. Sci. U.S.A.* 67:821, 1970.

89. Lischner, H. W., and DiGeorge, A. M.   Role of thymus in humoral immunity. *Lancet* 2:1044, 1969.
90. Louie, J. S., and Goldberg, L. S.   Lymphocyte-monocyte defect associated with anergy and recurrent infection. *Clin. Exp. Immunol.* 11:469, 1972.
91. Mackaness, G. B., and Blanden, R. V.   Cellular immunity. *Prog. Allergy* 11:89, 1967.
92. Mackaness, G. B.   The monocyte in cellular immunity. *Semin. Hematol.* 7:172, 1970.
93. McIntire, K. R., Sell, S., and Miller, J. F. A. P.   Pathogenesis of postnatal thymectomy wasting syndrome. *Nature* 204:151, 1964.
94. McKhann, C. F.   Primary malignancy in patients undergoing immunosuppression for renal transplantation. *Transplantation* 8:209, 1969.
95. Metzger, H.   Structure and function of γ M macroglobulins. *Adv. Immunol.* 12:57, 1970.
96. Meuwissen, H. J., Gatti, R. A., Terasaki, P. I., Hong, R., and Good, R. A.   Treatment of lymphopenic hypogammaglobulinemia and bone marrow aplasia by transplantation of allogenic marrow. *N. Engl. J. Med.* 281:691, 1969.
97. Miller, J. F. A. P.   Thymic tissue as a therapeutic measure. *N. Engl. J. Med.* 287:218, 1972.
98. Miller, M. E., and Nilsson, U. R.   A familial deficiency of the phagocytosis enhancing activity of serum related to a dysfunction of the fifth component of complement (C5). *N. Engl. J. Med.* 282:354, 1970.
99. Mitchison, N. A.   Immunocompetent cell populations. In M. Landy and W. Braun (eds.), *Immunological Tolerance.* New York: Academic, 1969.
100. Möller, G.   Immunocyte triggering. *Cell Immunol.* 1:573, 1970.
101. Müller-Eberhard, H. J.   Chemistry and reaction mechanism of complement. *Adv. Immunol.* 8:1, 1968.
102. Nussenzweig, V., Bianco, C., Dukor, P., and Eden, A.   Receptors for C3 on B lymphocytes: Possible role in the immune response. In B. Amos (ed.), *Progress in Immunology.* 1st International Congress of Immunology. New York and London: Academic, 1971, p. 73.
103. O'Loughlin, J. M.   Immunologic deficiency states. *Med. Clin. North Am.* 56:747, 1972.
104. Osoba, O.   Thymic function, immunologic deficiency, and autoimmunity. *Med. Clin. North Am.* 56:319, 1972.
105. Peterson, R. D. A., Cooper, M. D., and Good, R. A.   Lymphoid tissue abnormalities associated with ataxia telangiectasia. *Am. J. Med.* 41:342, 1966.
106. Pick, E., Krejci, J., and Turk, J. L.   Release of skin reactive factor from guinea pig lymphocytes by mitogens. *Nature* 225:236, 1970.
107. Pick, E., and Turk, J. L.   The biological activities of lymphocyte products: A review. *Clin. Exp. Immunol.* 10:1, 1972.
108. Polmar, S. H., Waldmann, T. A., Balestra, S. T., Jost, M. C., and Terry, W. D.   Immunoglobulin E in immunologic deficiency diseases: I. Relation of IgG and IgA to respiratory tract disease in isolated IgE deficiency, IgA deficiency and ataxia telangiectasia. *J. Clin. Invest.* 51:326, 1972.
109. Pruzanski, W., and Orgryzlo, M. A.   The changing pattern of disease associated with M components. *Med. Clin. North Am.* 56:371, 1972.

110. Quie, P. E.   Chronic granulomatous disease of childhood. *Adv. Pediatr.* 16:287, 1969.
111. Revillard, J. P.   *Cell Mediated Immunity—In Vitro Correlates.* Basel: Karger, 1971.
112. Ritzmann, S. E., and Levin, W. C.   II. Polyclonal and monoclonal gammopathies. In H. R. Dettelbach and S. E. Ritzmann (eds.), *Lab Synopsis.* Somerville, N.J.: Behring, 1969, vol. 2.
113. Ritzmann, S. E., Daniels, J. C., Lawrence, M. C., Beathard, G. A., and Levin, W. C.   Monoclonal gammopathies: Present status. *Tex. Med.* 68:91, 1972.
114. Rocklin, R. E., Rosen, F. S., and David, J. R.   In vitro lymphocyte response of patients with immunologic deficiency disease. *N. Engl. J. Med.* 282:1340, 1970.
115. Rosen, F. S., and Janeway, C. A.   The gammaglobulins: III. The antibody deficiency syndromes. *N. Engl. J. Med.* 275:709, 1966.
116. Rosenthal, I. M., Markowitz, A. S., and Madenis, R.   Immunologic incompetence in ataxia telangiectasia. *Am. J. Dis. Child.* 110:69, 1965.
117. Ruddy, S., Gigli, I., and Austen, K. F.   The complement system of man. *N. Engl. J. Med.* 287:489, 545, 591, and 641, 1972.
118. Russell, S. W., Rosenau, W., Goldberg, M., and Kunitomi, G.   Purification of human lymphotoxin. *J. Immunol.* 109:784, 1972.
119. Salmon, S. E., Cline, M. J., Schultz, J., and Lehrer, R. I.   Myeloperoxidase deficiency: Immunologic study of a genetic defect. *N. Engl. J. Med.* 282:250, 1970.
120. Schur, P. H., Borel, H., Gelfand, E. W., Alper, C. A., and Rosen, F.   Selective gamma G globulin deficiency in patients with recurrent pyogenic infection. *N. Engl. J. Med.* 283:631, 1970.
121. Siltzbach, L. E.   Sarcoidosis. In M. Samter (ed.), *Immunological Diseases.* Boston: Little, Brown, 1971, 2nd ed., vol. 1, p. 581.
122. Soborg, M.   The leucocyte migration technique for in vitro detection of cellular sensitivity in man. In B. R. Bloom and P. R. Glade (eds.), *In Vitro Methods of Cell Mediated Immunity.* New York: Academic, 1971.
123. Spiegelberg, H. L.   γ D Immunoglobulins. In F. P. Inman (ed.), *Contemporary Topics in Immunochemistry.* New York: Plenum Press, 1972, vol. 1, p. 165.
124. Steele, R. W., Limas, C., Thurman, G. B., Schuelein, M., Bauer, H., and Bellanti, J. A.   Familial thymic aplasia: Attempted reconstitution with fetal thymus in a millipore diffusion chamber. *N. Engl. J. Med.* 287:787, 1972.
125. Steerman, R. L., Snyderman, R., Leikin, S. L., and Colten, H. R.   Intrinsic defect of the polymorphonuclear leucocyte resulting in impaired chemotaxis and phagocytosis. *Clin. Exp. Immunol.* 9:939, 1971.
126. Stiehm, E. R., and Fudenberg, H. H.   Serum levels of immune globulins in health and disease: A survey. *Pediatrics* 37:715, 1966.
127. Stiehm, E. R.   The gamma globulins. In *Brennemann's Practice of Pediatrics.* Hagerstown, Md.: Harper & Row, 1970, vol. 2, p. 1.
128. Stiehm, E. R., Lawlor, G. J., Kaplan, M. S., Greenwald, H. L., Neerhout, R. C., Sengar, P. S. D., and Terasaki, P. I.   Immunologic reconstitution in severe combined immunodeficiency without bone marrow chromosomal chimerism. *N. Engl. J. Med.* 286:797, 1972.

129. Stites, D. P., Ishizaki, K., and Fudenberg, H. H.   Serum IgE concentrations in hypogammaglobulinaemia and selective IgA deficiency— studies on patients and family members. *Clin. Exp. Immunol.* 10:391, 1972.
130. Stoop, J. W., Zegers, B. J. M., Sander, P. C., and Ballieux, R. E. Serum immunoglobulin levels in healthy children and adults. *Clin. Exp. Immunol.* 4:101, 1969.
131. Stossel, T. P., Root, R. K., and Vaughan, M.   Phagocytosis in chronic granulomatous disease and the Chediak-Higashi syndrome. *N. Engl. J. Med.* 286:118, 1972.
132. Strober, W., Blaese, R. M., and Waldmann, T. A.   Immunologic deficiency diseases. *Bull. Rheum. Dis.* 22:686, 1971–1972.
133. Subcommittee for Human Immunoglobulins of the IUIS Nomenclature Committee.   Recommendations for the nomenclature of human immunoglobulins. *J. Immunol.* 108:1733, 1972.
134. Talal, N.   Immunologic and viral factors in the pathogenesis of systemic lupus erythematosus. *Arthritis Rheum.* 13:887, 1970.
135. Tomasi, T. B., Jr., and Bienenstock, J.   Secretory immunoglobulins. *Adv. Immunol.* 9:1, 1968.
136. Unanue, E. R.   The regulatory role of macrophages in antigenic stimulation. *Adv. Immunol.* 15:95, 1972.
137. Valentine, F. T., and Lawrence, H. S.   Lymphocyte stimulation: Transfer of cellular hypersensitivity to antigen in vitro. *Science* 165:1014, 1969.
138. Valentine, F. T., and Lawrence, H. S.   Cell mediated immunity. *Adv. Intern. Med.* 17:51, 1971.
139. Van Borel, J. A., Paul, W. E., Terry, W. D., and Green, I.   IgD bearing human lymphocytes. *J. Immunol.* 109:648, 1972.
140. Waldmann, T. A., Strober, W., and Blaese, R. M.   Immunodeficiency disease and malignancy: Various immunologic deficiencies of man and the role of immune processes in the control of malignant disease. *Ann. Intern. Med.* 77:605, 1972.
141. Waldmann, T. A., Polmar, S. H., Balestra, S. T., Jost, M. C., Bruce, R. M., and Terry, W. D.   Immunoglobulin E in immunologic deficiency diseases: II. Serum IgE concentrations of patients with acquired hypogammaglobulinemia, thymoma, and hypogammaglobulinemia, myotonic dystrophy, intestinal lymphangiectasia and Wiskott-Aldrich syndrome. *J. Immunol.* 109:304, 1972.
142. Ward, P. A., Cochrane, C. G., and Müller-Eberhard, H. J.   The role of serum complement in chemotaxis of leucocyte in vitro. *J. Exp. Med.* 122:322, 1965.
143. Ward, P. A., Cochrane, C. G., and Müller-Eberhard, H. J.   Further studies on the chemotactic factor of complement and its formation in vivo. *Immunology* 11:141, 1966.
144. Ward, P. A., and Schlegel, R. J.   Impaired leukotactic responsiveness in a child with recurrent infections. *Lancet* 1:344, 1969.
145. Ward, P. A., and Newman, L. J.   A neutrophilic chemotactic factor from human C'5. *J. Immunol.* 102:93, 1969.
146. Ward, P. A., Remold, H. G., and David, J. R.   The production by antigen stimulated lymphocytes of a leukotactic factor distinct from migration inhibitory factor. *Cell. Immunol.* 1:162, 1970.

147. Ward, P. A.   Neutrophilic chemotactic factors and related clinical disorders. *Arthritis Rheum.* 13:181, 1970.
148. Windhorst, D. B., Zelickson, A. S., and Good, R. A.   Chediak-Higashi syndrome: Hereditary giantism of cytoplasmic organelles. *Science* 151:81, 1966.
149. Windhorst, D. B.   Functional defects of neutrophils. *Adv. Intern. Med.* 16:329, 1970.
150. Wybran, J., Carr, M. C., and Fudenberg, H. H.   The human rosette-forming cell as a marker of a population of thymus derived cells. *J. Clin. Invest.* 51:2537, 1972.

3

Approach to the Diagnosis of Immune Deficiency Diseases

History

R ecurrent infections usually bring the patient to the attention of the physician. The following types of infections may suggest an immunologic defect [6]: (a) recurrent infections caused by bacteria of *high grade* virulence (e.g., *Diplococcus pneumoniae, Hemophilus influenzae*); (b) those caused by *low grade* virulence or unusual organisms such as *Serratia marcescens* and paracolon bacilli; (c) those caused by fungi (i.e., *Candida albicans*); and (d) unusual reactions to vaccines, as progressive vaccinia. A history of repeated respiratory viral infections is common, and usually there is no underlying immune defect. A history of several episodes of pneumonia confirmed by x-ray or repeated occurrences of otitis media would make one suspicious of an underlying immune defect in the patient. Other nonimmunologic disease states which predispose to current infection should be excluded by history and physical examination. Examples are cystic fibrosis and diabetes.

Other points which should be investigated are [6, 39]:

A. History of allergy and tests that have been done.

B. Prior surgery, particularly tonsillectomy, adenoidectomy, and appendectomy. The results of histologic examination on excised tissue may help in the assessment of the immune system. Absence of lymphocytes in the paracortical thymus dependent areas in lymph nodes indicates a cellular immune defect, while absence of germinal centers and plasma cells indicates a humoral immune defect.

C. X-ray evaluation of (a) lateral chest for visualization of thymic shadow. A small thymic shadow in children must be cautiously interpreted, since children with severe infections may have a small thymic shadow [32]; (b) lateral nasopharynx for pharyngeal lymphoid tissue. Absence of lymphoid tissue is typical of congenital hypogammaglobulinemia.

D. Radiation therapy to thymus or nasopharynx.

E. Sites of infections and organisms recovered; age of onset of infections.

F. Previous immunizations and reactions to them.

G. Prior γ-globulin treatment with details as to dosage, frequency, and date last given and the source of γ-globulin, as placental or serum.
H. Family history of collagen diseases, endocrine disorders, tumor, or early death.
I. History of congenital rubella [65].

Physical Examination

A. General appearance—children with cellular or combined cellular and humoral deficiencies look malnourished and debilitated.
B. Skin—search for monilial rash, eczema, telangiectasis, petechial hemorrhages.
C. Lymphoid tissue—note lymph nodes, tonsillar tissue, liver and spleen.
D. Joints—arthritis may be present.
E. Evaluate patient for active infection.
F. Search for possible malignancy since a high incidence is seen in immune deficiency diseases [108].

It cannot be overemphasized that in most cases of immune deficiency diseases, a good history and physical examination will often be sufficient to make the diagnosis. Many of the various tests enumerated below are of confirmatory value.

Tests for Inflammatory Response and Phagocytic Function

TESTS FOR INFLAMMATORY RESPONSE

WBC count, Differential, and Hemoglobin
A white blood count and morphologic examination of peripheral blood can provide a great deal of information. An absolute neutrophil count below 1,800 cells/mm³ or absolute lymphocyte counts below 1,500 cells/mm³ may indicate significant cellular deficiency [24, 32, 43]. Normally infants should show a total of greater than 1,500 *small* lymphocytes/mm³ [43]. Some children with cellular deficiency have normal numbers of lymphocytes, but these are of the medium and large types which resemble monocytes.

Often existing neutropenia is associated with thrombocytopenia or thrombocytosis [43]. Cyclic neutropenia may be seen at intervals of about 21 days in cases such as recurring stomatitis [32]. Neutrophilic cells which contain giant cytoplasmic granules may be from a patient with Chediak-Higashi syndrome. Eosinophilia and monocytes may be seen in certain immune diseases [32, 43]. The hemoglobin, red cell morphology, and presence of Howell-Jolly bodies may suggest the presence of autoimmune hemolytic anemia and help evaluate splenic function.

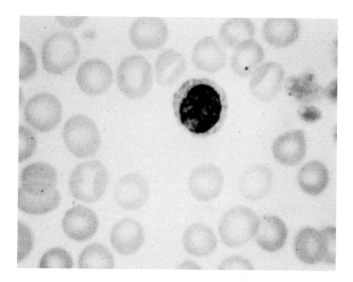

a

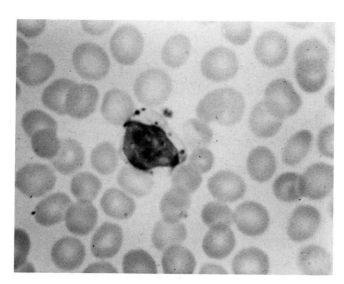

b

Figure 3-1
Circulating lymphocytes. (a) Small lymphocytes; (b) large lymphocytes.
(Wright's stained blood smear; 1,000× before 25% reduction.)

Sedimentation Rate and C-Reactive Protein
These tests are indicators for the presence of an existing inflammation.

Serum Complement Activity, Total and/or C3, C4, C5
These tests are performed to evaluate complement function if a non-specific humoral defect is suspected and is helpful in the case of existing severe autoimmune diseases coexisting with the immune deficiency syndrome.

Rebuck Skin Window Technique [94]
This test measures cell morphology and function in an inflammatory response. The skin window tests will uncover overall defects in the inflammatory response, including defects in chemotaxis secondary to complement deficiency.

In Vitro Test for Defective Leukocyte Chemotaxis [25]
This test is performed in suspected cases of nonspecific intrinsic cellular defect or nonspecific humoral defect (including the presence of serum inhibitors) in patients which may result in defective inflammatory response.

TESTS FOR PHAGOCYTIC FUNCTION
A. Histochemical Nitroblue Tetrazolium Test (NBT) [66].
B. NBT test stimulated with endotoxin [67].
C. Quantitative NBT test [4].
D. Bacteriocidal test for the diagnosis of chronic granulomatous disease [75].

Histochemical Nitroblue Tetrazolium Test (NBT)
When leukocytic function is normal, the cells are able to reduce NBT dye at a normal rate during in vitro phagocytosis of particles as latex [4]. During the course of a natural bacterial infection, the organism may be engulfed in vivo and metabolic changes are induced in the neutrophils which can cause a spontaneous in vitro reduction of NBT dye [59, 66]. The test was initially proposed as a means to differentiate bacterial infections from other nonbacterial diseases.

Thus, the NBT test is an in vitro test which gives an indication of the amount of in vivo phagocytic activity of the neutrophils occurring in the patient at the time the specimen was drawn. The NBT-positive neutrophils increased strikingly in bacterial infections as *Streptococcal pneumoniae, H. influenzae, Neisseria meningitides,* Group A streptococci, and *Escherichia coli* infections, as well as *C. albicans* septicemia [67]. The test has appeared to be positive in malaria, miliary tuberculosis, and certain parasitic diseases [62]. Increased NBT reduction was found in newborn infants [30] and in patients with osteogenesis imperfecta [30].

In normal controls, the absolute number of NBT-positive neutrophils was found by Park et al. [67] to be between 145 and 720/mm^3 with a mean percentage of 8.5. No deviation from the normal was seen in patients [67] with (a) rheumatoid arthritis; (b) systemic lupus erythematosus—patients may show a normal or low value [30]; (c) a variety of viral diseases, including measles, chickenpox, mumps, or mumps meningoencephalitis confirmed by spinal fluid examination; or (d) patients with primary tuberculosis.

Low NBT indices are seen in (a) patients with chronic granulomatous diseases [4, 30, 62, 67]; (b) congenital agammaglobulinemia [68]; (c) systemic lupus erythematosus; or (d) patients treated with corticosteroids [61], phenylbutazone [98], or aspirin [30]. Patients under treatment with indomethacin show NBT indices which are normal or elevated [30].

NBT Test Stimulated with Endotoxin [67]

Patients with chronic granulomatous disease secondary to a defective neutrophilic function will show a negative NBT test. In addition, a negative result can be expected in patients with a defect in the humoral and cellular component of the phagocytic system. It was noticed that with the regular NBT test, very low values were noted in normal controls and patients with infections after treatment with systemic antibiotics [69]. In order to differentiate the negative results of dysfunction of the phagocytic system and negative results due to the absence of bacteria, an endotoxin-stimulated NBT test was devised [67].

With endotoxin stimulation approximately one-half of the neutrophils are NBT-positive in normal controls, whereas dye reduction is totally absent in chronic granulomatous disease. A negative endotoxin-stimulated NBT test in patients with proved bacterial infection in the blood should indicate that there is a defect in either the humoral or the cellular component of the phagocytic system.

The stimulation of NBT reduction by neutrophils is lower when EDTA was used as an anticoagulant instead of heparin [67]. Thus, it appears that complement is required for endotoxin stimulation of NBT dye reduction, and that the interaction of bacterial endotoxin products with neutrophils during natural infection may contribute to increased reduction of NBT dye.

Quantitative NBT Test

A quantitative NBT test permits precise identification of patients, carrier, and unaffected persons [4]. In this test, a standard number of the patients' neutrophils are exposed to a known amount of latex particles. The phagocytic reaction is allowed to proceed, and normally the neutrophils will activate enzymes which will reduce NBT. The reaction is

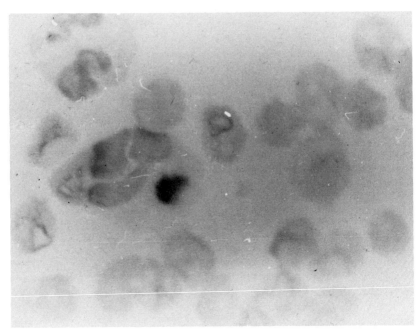

a

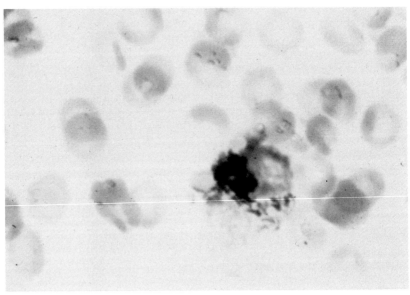

b

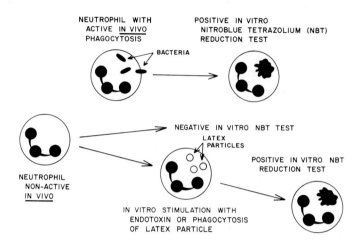

c

Figure 3-2
Neutrophils showing positive nitroblue tetrazolium test. Reduced NBT formazan granules in neutrophils may be discrete as in (a) or irregular as in (b).
Positive NBT formazan granules are differentiated from toxic granulations by
their size and doubly refractile borders. (1,000×.) (c) Significance of nitroblue tetrazolium (NBT) reduction test.

allowed to proceed for 15 min at 37° C and stopped by the addition of dilute HCl [4]. After centrifugation, the supernatant is aspirated and the visible purple granular button is extracted with pyridine. The color is measured in a spectrophotometer. The same procedure is carried out on the patient's leukocytes after 15 min exposure at 37° C to heat-killed *Staphlococcus aureus*.

Bacteriocidal Test for the Diagnosis of
Chronic Granulomatous Disease

Patients with CGD can ingest bacteria normally, but there is a defect in the intracellular killing of certain bacteria, especially the types which contain the enzyme catalase and which have a low concentration of hydrogen peroxide, such as *Staph. aureus, S. marcescens,* paracolon bacilli, and *Aerobacter aerogenes* [55, 109]. Patients with CGD are able to phagocytize streptococcal organisms without difficulty. Streptococci produce hydrogen peroxide. It seems possible that the metabolic abnormality in the polymorphs of patients with CGD is a decreased hydrogen peroxide production [55, 76, 109], which is related (a) to the ability of the polymorphs to kill hydrogen peroxide-producing bacteria such as streptococci, and (b) to defective killing of catalase-producing bacteria, as *Staph. aureus* and *S. marcescens.*

The bacteriocidal test, such as described by Quie et al. [75], consists of incubating leukocytes and *Staph. aureus* in fresh frozen, pooled human serum and Hank's solution. The mixture is incubated at 37° C with shaking, and aliquots are removed at 0, 30, 60, and 120 min. Distilled water is added to the aliquots with lysis of the leukocytes and then cultured in agar plates. After incubation, bacterial colony counts are performed.

The leukocytes of patients with chronic granulomatous disease can phagocytize nonhydrogen peroxide-producing bacteria as *Staph. aureus* but are unable to kill the bacteria. The defective monocytes and neutrophils of these patients fail to show enhanced aerobic metabolism during phagocytosis and do not produce hydrogen peroxide or reduce NBT dye. The nonproduction of hydrogen peroxide will allow survival of bacteria within the phagocytic cells in chronic granulomatous disease [29, 42]. It is best to perform the bacteriocidal test with the same bacteria from the patient with suspected CGD.

Tests Used Primarily for the Evaluation of Humoral Immunity

A. Tests for the presence of immunoglobulin and existing antibodies to common antigens.
B. Tests for assessment of antibody formation following active immunization [34].

TESTS FOR THE PRESENCE OF IMMUNOGLOBULINS AND EXISTING ANTIBODIES TO COMMON ANTIGENS

Schick Test

If an individual has been previously immunized with diphtheria toxoid and his humoral immune system is normal, the Schick test will be negative. A positive Schick test in such cases is presumptive evidence of IgG deficiency.

Presence of Natural A and B Isohemagglutinins

The isohemagglutinin titer during the first 2 years of life is low [35]. Isohemagglutinins are occasionally found at birth and in 100% of normal infants by 10 months of age; they reach adult titers by 2 years of age [100]. In infants over 2 years of age, the anti-A and anti-B titers are 1:32 and 1:16 or higher, respectively [24].

Children with recurrent infections, whose isohemagglutinins are lower than reported normals, usually suffer a defect of humoral immunity. The complete absence of isohemagglutinins is presumptive evidence of IgM deficiency. Absent or diminished isohemagglutinin titers are found also in cellular or combined cellular and humoral defects [100]. Isohemagglutinin titers have been reported as low as zero in the Wiskott-Aldrich syndrome [51].

Serum Protein Electrophoresis and Immunoelectrophoresis

Serum protein electrophoresis is performed for the detection of dysproteinemias, such as monoclonal gammopathies. Immunoelectrophoresis will determine only qualitative levels of immunoglobulins IgG, IgM, IgA, and help in the diagnosis of dysproteinemias. In the newborn the immunoelectrophoretic pattern shows a normal absence of IgM and IgA.

It should be emphasized here that a serum protein electrophoresis is *not* a quantitative method for the determination of immunoglobulins. When the concentration of IgG is low, as it is in normal infancy, the serum electrophoresis is often inaccurate [24]. The concentration of immunoglobulin correlates with IgG concentration only when the concentration of IgG is normal. The routine electrophoresis will not distinguish the various major immunoglobulins.

Quantitative Radial Immunodiffusion of Immunoglobulins, as IgG, IgM, IgA, IgD

Immunoelectrophoresis and serum protein electrophoresis cannot replace the quantitative determination of immunoglobulins. The most common deficiency is the isolated IgA deficiency [36]. A low serum value of a specific immunoglobulin is critically examined. However, an abnormally *high* value noted in one or more immunoglobulins should make one suspect that the patient may have some underlying primary

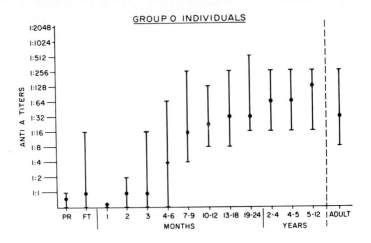

a

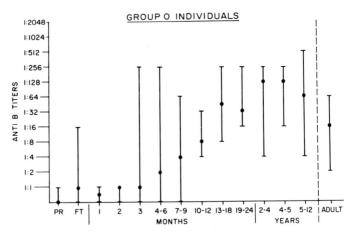

b

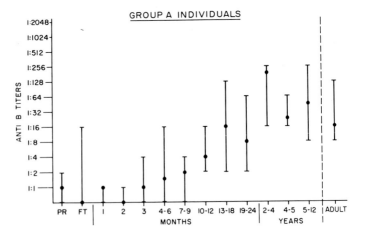

c

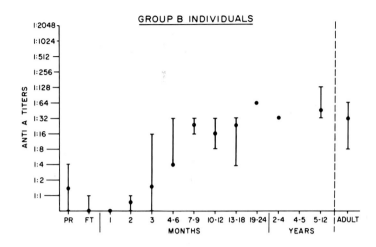

d

Figure 3-3

Median and range of anti-A (a) and anti-B (b) isohemagglutinins found in group O prematures (PR), term infants (FT), children, and adults. Median and range of anti-B isohemagglutinins found in group A (c) and of anti-A isohemagglutinins found in group B (d) prematures (PR), term infants (FT), children, and adults. (From Taylor et al. [100], *Annals of Allergy* 29:378, 1971, with permission.)

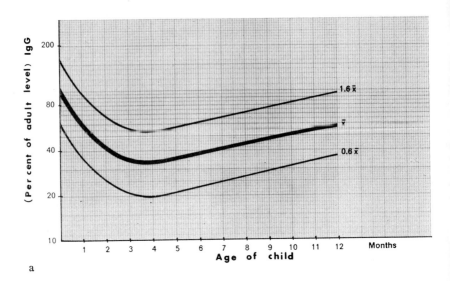

a

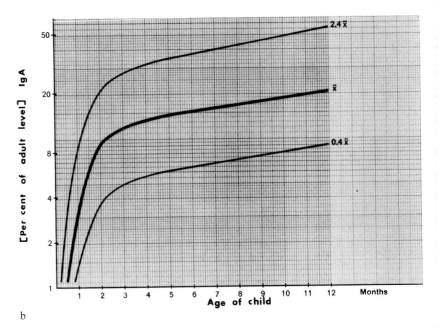

b

Figure 3-4
Serum immunoglobulin levels in healthy infants from birth to 1 year of age.
Mean values $\bar{x}$; statistical variation as given on each graph. (a) IgG; (b) IgA;
(c) IgM. Serum immunoglobulin levels in healthy children from 1 to 15
years of age. Mean values $\bar{x}$; statistical variation as given on each graph.
(d) IgG; (e) IgA; (f) IgM. At birth, the levels of IgA, IgM, IgD, and IgE

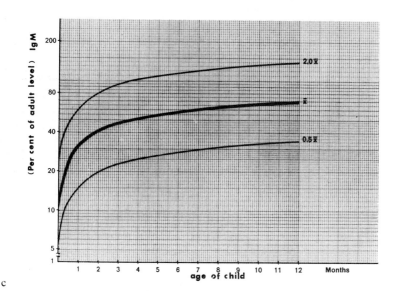

c

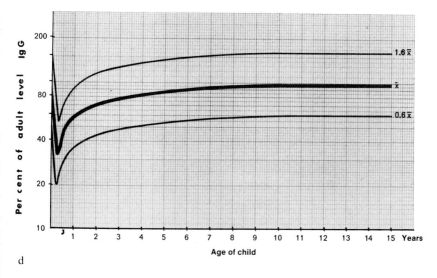

d

immunoglobulins are very low. The IgG level is comparable to the maternal level due to passive placental transfer. The infant immunoglobulin levels in the chart are expressed as percentage of the normal adult. The mean adult levels ± 2 S.D. in mg per 100 ml are as follows: IgG, 1,200 (700–1,700); IgA, 210 (70–350); and IgM, 140 (70–120). Adult IgD and IgE levels are 3 mg per 100 ml and 0.03 mg per 100 ml, respectively. (Slightly modified and reproduced with permission from Behring Diagnostics, Somerville, N.J. Tables compiled by W. Becker of Behringwerke, Marburg/Lahn, West Germany.)

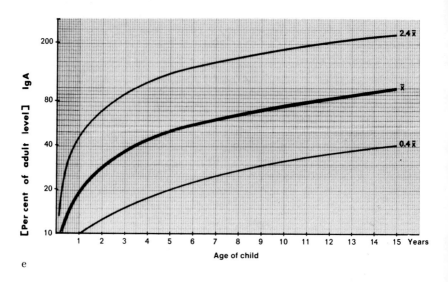

e

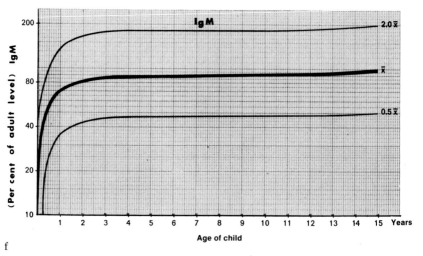

f

Figure 3-4 (*continued*)

or secondary immune defect also. An IgG concentration of 200 mg/100 ml is considered the practical threshold value [34]. An IgA deficiency shows less than 5 mg/100 ml of serum [2]. Normal values of children at different ages have been published [1, 17, 18, 44, 95, 97, 103].

Detection of IgA Antibodies in Parotid Gland Salivary Secretions [11, 13]

This procedure may be helpful in the evaluation of immune mechanisms of mucosal resistance [11]. It is of interest to note that two patients have been reported to show deficiency of serum IgA with normal levels of secretory IgA [2].

The secretory IgA is an 11S sedimenting protein which consists of a dimer 7S IgA plus a transport piece (T component). The IgA molecules are found in saliva, urine, and mucosal linings when examined, and contain the IgA determinant and the T component [101, 102].

Quantitation of IgG Subclasses

Patients with a history of recurrent pyogenic infections may be associated with selective IgG subclass deficiencies [87, 88]. The serum from these patients showed a normal total immunoglobulin level when examined by routine protein electrophoresis. Immunoelectrophoresis revealed a marked deficiency of IgG immunoglobulins. Three patients were reported [87]. One patient had normal levels of IgA and IgM immunoglobulins; IgG3 subclass was increased; and IgG1, IgG2, and IgG4 were decreased. The second patient had a normal IgA level, an increased IgM level, a normal IgG4 level, and deficient levels of IgG1, IgG2, and IgG3. The third patient had normal IgA, IgM, IgG3, and IgG4 levels while the IgG1 and IgG2 levels were markedly decreased.

Rectal Biopsy Examination for Antibody-Producing Cells

A biopsy may be taken for routine histology and immunofluorescent localization of IgG, IgM, and IgA immunoglobulins [85]. Rectal tissue does not require prior antigenic stimulation for evaluation. Infants over one month of age will have many plasma cells in the lamina propria of the rectal mucosa [24]. This is a good screening test for evidence of antibody production in suspected humoral immune deficiency cases.

By a direct immunofluorescent method, the number of immuno-globulin-containing cells in the mucosa of the small intestine and rectum were counted in biopsy specimens from children [85]. In all biopsy specimens from healthy children, IgA-containing cells predominated and were numerous in children over 2 years of age; however, the number of IgM-containing cells did not change with age [85].

Examination of Circulating Lymphocytes for Surface Immunoglobulins

Immunoglobulin molecules (Ig) are easily detectable only on B-lympho-

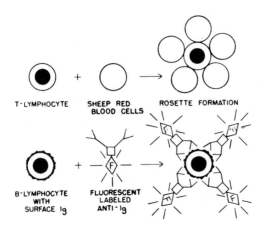

Figure 3-5
Detection of human thymus-derived (T) and antibody-producing (B) lymphocytes.

cytes (the antibody-forming type of lymphocytes). The number of immunoglobulin molecules on the surface of B-lymphocytes ranged from 50,000 to 150,000 [77], and appear to be receptors for antigens [99]. Lymphocytes (T-cells) which lack detectable Ig may have from 0 to 1000 molecules of detectable surface Ig per cell [77, 104].

The surface immunoglobulins on lymphocytes have been demonstrated by fluorescent-labeled antibody techniques [38, 46, 71, 72, 77, 78, 81, 91], radioisotope methods [64, 77, 107], fluorescent-labeled aggregated γ-globulin [27], immunocytoadherence test [21], and interaction with immune complexes [5].

The fluorescent-labeled antibody method is probably the most convenient to perform in the clinical laboratory for the specific detection of surface immunoglobulins on lymphocytes. It has been used for the detection of surface Ig on circulating lymphocytes in certain immune deficiency diseases [38, 72, 91]. Grey et al. [38] studied the distribution of surface Ig-containing peripheral blood lymphocytes with an immunofluorescence technique in normal patients as well as in cases of immune deficiency diseases and chronic lymphocytic leukemia.

Their findings were [38]:

A. Surface Ig was found on approximately 28% of peripheral blood lymphocytes. On an average, 15% of the lymphocytes contained IgG, 6% IgA, and 8% IgM; and the kappa:lambda ratio was 2:1.
B. Four patients with sex-linked agammaglobulinemia and one with acquired agammaglobulinemia had a decreased number of surface Ig-containing lymphocytes (0–4%).
C. Three patients with selective IgA deficiency and no detectable serum IgA had a normal number of cells (6–8%) with surface IgA.
D. Five patients with cellular immune deficiency states including the Wiskott-Aldrich syndrome had a normal or low percentage of lymphocytes with surface Ig.

E. Lymphocytes from 20 cases of chronic lymphocytic leukemia were monoclonal in nature, and cells from one person had a single associated Ig with some light and heavy chains. In three-quarters of the cases the heavy chain was IgM, and the remaining cases of chronic lymphocytic leukemia patients had no detectable heavy chain on the surface of the tumor lymphocyte but had light chains detectable by immunofluorescence. Thus, one can see that the demonstration of surface Ig on the lymphocytes will help in determining whether cells are thymus derived (T-cells) or bone marrow derived (B-cells).

TESTS FOR ASSESSMENT OF ANTIBODY FORMATION FOLLOWING ACTIVE IMMUNIZATION

Active Immunization with Diphtheria, Pertussis, and Tetanus
Extensive data on the response of infants at different ages is not available. Furthermore, most clinical laboratories are not geared to measure antibody response to diphtheria, pertussis, and tetanus. Following immunization with diphtheria toxin, one can administer a Schick test. A positive Schick test is seen in agammaglobulinemia. However, the test may be negative in agammaglobulinemic patients on therapy.

Active Immunization with Typhoid Vaccine
Typhoid immunizations can be given once a week for 3 weeks. The vaccine mixture of TAB should not be used. Infants can be immunized with a dose of 0.25 ml per injection [24]. Agglutinins can be easily determined in the clinical laboratory to typhoid O and H antigens. The anti-H titer after three injections will be 160 or greater, and patients with antibody deficiency may have a titer of less than 1:5 [24].

Lymph Node Biopsy
A biopsy can be performed 5–7 days after local antigenic stimulation. In children, diphtheria or tetanus toxoid antigens may be injected into the medial aspect of the thigh. Later, the inguinal node from the same thigh is removed for histologic examination. The node should be examined for lymphocytes in the paracortical areas and for numbers of plasma cells in the medullary portion and in the cortical germinal centers. A lymph node biopsy may not be essential for diagnosis in cases of combined immune deficiency demonstrated by other means; in

Figure 3-6
Positive Schick test
to diphtheria toxin.

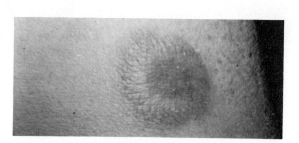

such cases of severe immune deficiency, a lymph node biopsy procedure would increase the hazard of infection. The histologic findings in the various immune deficiency diseases have been reported in detail [7, 9, 10, 23, 28, 36].

Tests for Evaluation of Cellular Immunity

Absolute Lymphocyte Count

The counts in normal children are usually above $2,000/mm^3$ during the first 4 years of life, being considerably higher up to age 8–10 months with a maximum of $7,600/mm^3$ (63% of WBC). The lymphocyte count declines during maturation to an average of 2,500 with a lower limit of $1,000/mm^3$ [39]. Normal infants should show a count·of greater than 1,500 small lymphocytes/mm^3. Children with cellular deficiency may have normal numbers of lymphocytes but still have a small number of small lymphocytes even though the majority are of medium and large size [43].

Delayed Type Skin Reactions

Many different antigens may be employed. However, the 5 following antigens are recommended as follows: trichophytin, *Candida* antigens, streptokinase-streptodornase, mumps, and purified protein derivative (PPD). Most normal persons show a positive response to one or more antigens. The most consistently positive antigen is *Candida,* which shows a positive delayed skin reaction in 80–95% of normal persons 7 months of age or older [34].

If skin reactions to the above panel of delayed hypersensitivity antigens are negative, then sensitivity to 2–4 dinitrochlorobenzene may be attempted. This procedure may result in unpleasant burn reactions. The World Health Organization Committee recommended that 2–4 dinitro-

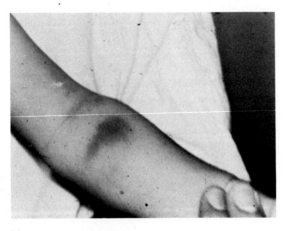

Figure 3-7
Positive skin test to intermediate strength PPD tuberculin.

fluorobenzene should be avoided [34]. Newborn infants sensitized with DNCB will demonstrate a specific delayed response to challenge within 2–3 weeks of age [92].

In the interpretation of skin tests, a *negative* skin test may result from abnormalities in the inflammatory response as well as from specific impairment of cellular sensitivity [45]. Therefore, both cellular sensitivity and the various other factors involved in the inflammatory response must be evaluated.

Bonforte et al. [14] recently reported on the use of an in vivo phytohemagglutinin (PHA) skin test to assess delayed hypersensitivity. The test, still in the period of evaluation, may be of value since most skin tests require the subject to have a previous exposure to the antigen. The response of PHA intradermal injection is a perivascular mononuclear cell accumulation similar to delayed hypersensitivity. However, there is evidence of dissociation between the in vivo PHA response and in vitro lymphocyte transformation to PHA in the same patient. It may be that only a small number of responsive lymphocytes are necessary to show a delayed skin reaction [63] while an in vitro technique measures total response of the cells. It can be concluded that PHA skin testing is of limited value in evaluating immune deficiency diseases.

Lymphocyte Stimulation Test [70, 89, 106]

This test is an in vitro test useful in the diagnosis of thymic dysplasia cases in infants whose absolute lymphocyte count appears within the normal range. In this test a pure lymphocyte fraction obtained from peripheral blood is cultured with phytohemagglutinin (PHA). Lymphocytes from normal persons will show 50 to 98% conversion to blast forms, while cells from individuals with thymic abnormalities demonstrate little or no transformation of lymphocytes in culture [39]. Also the

Figure 3-8
Positive skin test to test dose of dinitro-chlorobenzene.

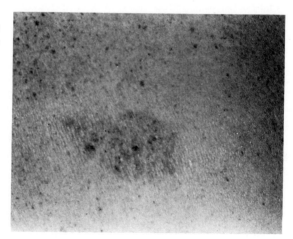

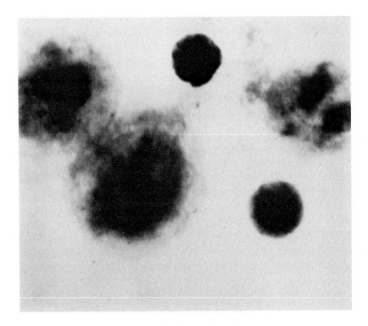

Figure 3-9
Positive blast transformation of lymphocytes after PHA stimulation. Note large blastoid lymphocytes along the left edge. (Wright's stain; 1,000×.)

lymphocytes may be cultured with specific antigen to study in vitro cell-mediated immunity [106].

Migration Inhibitory Factor Test
Then sensitized thymus-derived T-lymphocytes in the presence of antigen release a number of factors, one of which inhibits the migration of guinea pig macrophages from capillary tubes [80]. Also, the sensitized lymphocyte under the influence of antigen probably produces a soluble material which induces changes in macrophages with vacuolation increase in cytoplasmic granules [84].

The migration inhibition test may be performed in two ways. (a) Human blood lymphocytes are cultured with the specific antigen or mitogen as phytohemagglutinin and the MIF produced and released is assayed. The cell-free media is then tested for its ability to inhibit the migration of guinea pig macrophages [79, 80]. (b) A direct test of the inhibition of human leukocyte migration is more convenient to perform in the clinical laboratory [82, 93].

The lymphocytes of patients with a cellular immune defect will not produce a macrophage inhibitory factor (MIF) and show a negative reaction to a wide variety of antigens [79]. A 23-year-old female patient has been reported with a lymphocyte-monocyte defect in which the cells were unresponsive to autologous MIF and to homologous MIF from two of three healthy adults. The patient had a clinical history of recurrent infections [58].

Examination of Circulating Lymphocytes for T-Cell Markers
Sheep red blood cells (SRBC) were first noted to adhere to human lymphocytes with "rosette formation." The exact significance is not well known, but the normal rosette formation was found to be a sensitive index of the immunosuppressive properties of various antilymphocyte globulin preparations [3]. Recently, several investigators [15, 22, 46, 54, 110] have observed that SRBC formed spontaneous rosettes with human lymphocytes in very high percentage—too high to be explained as being caused by the binding of immunocompetent cells reacting against SRBC. These human lymphocytes which form spontaneous rosettes are now known to be thymus-derived or T-lymphocytes. Thus, the human rosette-forming cell can be used as a marker for T-lymphocytes and can identify the origin of circulating lymphocytes [46, 110].

Biopsy of Lymphoid Tissue
Various tissues may be examined to determine the extent of depletion of the thymus-dependent areas. Convenient tissues to examine are tonsils, adenoids, and inguinal lymph nodes.

Summary of Important Features in the Diagnosis of Immune Deficiency Diseases

Humoral Immune Deficiency Syndrome
HISTORY AND PHYSICAL EXAMINATION
A. Recurrent serum bacterial infections, i.e., pneumococcal and meningococcal organisms
B. Family history of similar disease in other males (primary disorders)
C. Poor growth
D. Very small lymph nodes and tonsils
E. Eczema

LABORATORY TESTS
A. Very low or absent serum immunoglobulins
B. Very low or absent isohemagglutinins
C. Positive Schick test after diphtheria-pertussis-tetanus (DPT) immunization
D. Poor antibody response to antigen as typhoid
E. Bone marrow, lymph nodes, and lamina propria of rectal mucosa show absence of plasma cells
F. Lymph node biopsy shows poorly developed follicles and germinal centers

Cellular Immune Deficiency Syndrome

HISTORY AND PHYSICAL EXAMINATION
A. Severe viral and fungal infections, i.e., generalized vaccinia after immunization for smallpox, generalized moniliasis
B. Family history of infant deaths
C. Very small lymph nodes and tonsils
D. Debilitation and wasting similar to graft vs. host reaction after fresh blood transfusions

LABORATORY AND SKIN TESTS
A. Lymphopenia
B. Skin tests negative to (*Candida* antigen, PPD, streptokinase-streptodornase)
C. Tests negative for dinitrochlorobenzene sensitization
D. Thymic shadow not seen on lateral chest x-ray
E. In vitro tests for response to PHA is poor as well as deficiency in migration inhibitory factor
F. Lymph nodes—depletion of lymphocytes from paracortical areas

Suggested Work-Up of Patients Suspected of Immune Deficiency Disease

INITIAL EVALUATION FOR HUMORAL IMMUNITY SHOULD INCLUDE
A. Serum protein electrophoresis (cannot be used as only test for screening)
B. Quantitation of IgG, IgM, IgA immunoglobulins
C. Schick test for diphtheria toxin
D. Blood type and isohemagglutinin titers

HISTORY.   In cases of a positive family history or a history of repeated bacterial infections as pneumonias, otitis media, and/or meningitis:
A. Antibody response to typhoid antigen should be evaluated
B. Rectal biopsy examination for the presence of plasma cells in the lamina propria of the mucosa. This procedure is helpful in children under 2 years of age when immunoglobulin and isohemagglutinin levels can be normally low [24]

FURTHER EVALUATION FOR CELLULAR SENSITIVITY
A. Skin tests to common antigens
B. Sensitization to DNCB
C. Lymphocyte transformation test
D. Migratory inhibitory factor production

BIOPSY OF LYMPHOID TISSUE CAN EVALUATE BOTH HUMORAL AND CELLULAR IMMUNITY
OTHER TESTS.   NBT, chemotaxis, and complement level tests may be helpful and ordered as indicated by the history and physical examination of the patient.

Procedures

General Methods

Standard methods are available in the clinical laboratory for these procedures:

A. Serum protein electrophoresis
B. Immunoelectrophoresis
C. Quantitation of immunoglobulins
D. Qualitative assay of humoral immunity by saline isohemagglutinin titers
E. Agglutination titers to typhoid O and H antigens

Determination of Salivary IgA

1. Collect saliva from patient stimulated with paraffin chewing. Special collection devices may be used to collect salivary secretions in order to measure volume and quantitate the immunoglobulins [13].
2. Homogenize mucus and centrifuge at 10,000 rpm for 60 min at 4° C to remove the thick mucus and debris.
3. Place 10 ml salivary secretions in a Schleicher and Schuell colloidion bag apparatus for concentration by vacuum dialysis against 0.15 M phosphate-buffered saline solution at pH 7.2.
4. Concentrate to final volume of 1.0 to 1.5 ml in cold room or ice bath.
5. Remove concentrated saliva and place in double-diffusion gel plate and react against anti-IgA and incubate 24 hours in a moist chamber. The test may be used on a qualitative and semiquantitative basis, and is useful to detect presence of secretory IgA in alimentary secretions in which the patient may show absence of IgA immunoglobulin present in the serum [2].

Schick Test with Diphtheria Toxin

1. Clean volar surface of the forearm with alcohol and allow to dry.
2. Inject 0.1 ml diphtheria Schick test toxin preparation containing 1/50 MLD/0.1 ml (Wyeth), intracutaneously.
3. A control test may be performed by heating the Schick test toxin for 25 min between 70° to 85° C.
4. A positive test shows a beginning reaction at 24 to 48 hours and reaches a maximum on day 4 and gradually subsides. The skin reaction begins with an erythema and progresses with induration and may result in necrosis. Usually the positive skin test results in pigmentation and scaling.
5. A test without a control should not be evaluated before day 5 as pseudoreactions to bacterial proteins may occur within one or two days and disappear by day 4, not followed by pigmentation or scaling.
6. A negative test is considered as immunity to diphtheria.
7. A positive test in previously immunized patients is presumptive for

the possible diagnosis of hypogammaglobulinemia. If the patient is receiving immunoglobulin therapy, the Schick test may be negative.

Procedures for Delayed Sensitivity Skin Tests

For skin testing, it is recommended that the following materials be injected intradermally.

1. PPD, stabilized, 0.1 ml of intermediate strength. If negative, repeat at second strength.
2. *Candida* antigen, 0.1 ml of a 1:10 dilution for infants or of a 1:100 dilution for older children and adults.
3. Trichophytin, as for *Candida* antigen.
4. Streptococcal antigens, 0.1 ml. Streptokinase-streptodornase, at a concentration of 4 units of streptokinase per 0.1 ml. If negative, repeat at a concentration of 40 units streptokinase per 0.1 ml.
5. Mumps skin testing antigen, 0.1 mg. Reactions are read at 4 hours to assess a possible Arthus reaction, and at 24 and 48 hours for delayed hypersensitivity. The diameter of swelling and redness should be recorded.

ANTIGENS AND TESTING TECHNIQUES.   Two preparations of *Candida* antigens are available from Hollister-Stier Laboratories (see Table 3–1). One is the monilia antigen, and it is usually used for testing for immediate hypersensitivity. The second preparation, a culture filtrate called Dermatophytin O, is recommended for delayed sensitivity tests.

1. Intradermal skin tests are given using a tuberculin type syringe with attached 27-gauge needle. It is convenient to give injections on the volar surface of the forearm.
2. The injection sites are circled with an indelible marking pencil and labeled with the initial of the antigen.
3. The diameter of the induration and erythema are carefully recorded at 24 and 48 hours.
4. Negative tests are repeated with the second strength antigen. If the initial test does not show 5 mm of erythema and induration at 24 or 48 hours, then it is recommended to repeat the test with the second strength antigen dose.

COMPLICATIONS OF SKIN TESTING.   Complications of skin tests may be severe local reactions with pain, induration, blister formation, and tissue necrosis. The occurrence of severe reactions may be reduced by using an intermediate or lower strength initial test antigen, if the patient has a history that he may strongly react. The initial test, if negative, is then followed by a second strength test.

INTERPRETATION OF RESULTS.   Normal subjects will usually react to one or more of the antigens. If a patient fails to show a positive test to any one of the five antigens, *Candida,* trichophytin, streptokinase-streptodornase, mumps, and PPD, this is strong evidence that a cellular immune defect is probably present. Such patients can be further evaluated by sensitization with dinitrochlorobenzene (DNCB) and with in vitro tests such as lymphocyte stimulation and production of migration inhibitory factor.

The incidence of skin reactivity to *Candida* antigen is low prior to 7 or 8 months of age [14, 24], and the incidence of skin reactivity to SK-SD is also low prior to 2 years of age in normal infants [14]. As previously stated, newborn infants sensitized to DNCB will demonstrate a positive reaction to a challenge test dose within 2 to 3 weeks of age [92].

INTERPRETATION OF TUBERCULIN REACTIONS.   There has been much controversy as to the type of tuberculin to be used for testing [33, 41, 47, 60]. An aqueous stabilized preparation of PPD, which is a PPD sus-

Table 3-1. List of Antigens for Evaluation of Delayed Hypersensitivity.

Antigen (Source)	Trade Name	Concentration		Amount (Route)
		Initial	Final	
1. Candida albicans (Hollister-Stier)	Dermato-phytin O	1:100	1:10	0.1 ml (ID)
2. Trichophytin (Hollister-Stier)	Dermato-phytin	1:100	1:10	0.1 ml (ID)
3. Streptokinase-Streptodornase (Lederle Labs.)	Varidase	4 units SK/ 0.1 ml	40 units SK/ 0.1 ml	0.1 ml (ID)
4. Mumps (Lilly)	Mumps	(2 complement fixing units/0.1 ml)		0.1 ml (ID)
5. PPD (Stabilized) (Panray Div., Ormont) or CDC stabilized PPD (Communicable Disease Center, Atlanta, Ga.)	PPD-Mantoux	Intermediate strength	Second strength	0.1 ml (ID)
(The antigens are relatively stable in solution and can be kept in the refrigerator for 6 months to one year)				
6. 1-Chloro,2,4-Dinitrobenzene (DNCB) (K & K)		2,000 μg/ 0.1 ml in acetone (sensitizing dose)	50 μg/0.1 ml in acetone (test dose)	0.1 ml

pension stabilized with the detergent Tween 80, is now available from the following sources: (a) CDC-PPD, Communicable Disease Center, Atlanta, Ga., and (b) PPD-soluble, Panray Division, Ormont Drug & Chemical Co., Englewood, N.J.

The supply of the CDC preparation is limited, but it has been made available to various public health departments. The Panray preparation has been made by Connaught Medical Research Laboratories in Canada.

In our experience, the CDC preparation is convenient for skin testing and appears to be well standardized. The Connaught preparations from Panray have been found to be satisfactory and standardized similar to the CDC preparation when tested in 1973.

The unstabilized preparations of PPD must be dissolved before use, may have adsorption loss on the bottle and syringe, and may result in a doubtful intermediate strength test in cases known to have active tuberculosis [41].

Several investigators agree that a stabilized preparation of PPD is preferable; however, there is controversy in the interpretation of the skin test reactions to PPD [41, 47]. Recommendations for the interpretations of the PPD test by the National Tuberculosis and Respiratory Disease Association in 1969 are as follows [26]:

A. Negative test—0–4 mm, skin induration and erythema
B. Doubtful test—5–9 mm, skin induration
C. Positive test—10 mm or more induration

On the other hand, Jones et al. [47] have presented evidence that the size of the skin test response does not correlate with in vitro lymphocyte transformation studies to PPD on the same patient. They found that the lymphocyte stimulation index correlated with the skin test strength that gave first evidence of erythema or induration. Some patients had small (1–4 mm) reactions to first strength PPD or intermediate strength PPD, and others reacted to only second strength PPD, but in each case the lymphocyte stimulation index was definitely greater than in the group of second strength nonreactors (no visible response).

Jones et al.'s conclusions [47] are that (a) any skin test reaction to any strength of PPD, including reactions to second strength PPD, should be considered as immunologic reactions; and (b) the current concept that reactions up to 4 mm or 9 mm represent nonspecific irritant or toxic reactions should be revised.

METHOD FOR DINITROCHLOROBENZENE CONTACT SENSITIZATION. There are numerous published procedures, but the procedure of Catalona et al. [19] is recommended since they have performed an excellent study and the test helps provide a semiquantitative measure of cellular immunity.

PROCEDURE

1. DNCB (see Table 3-1) is dissolved in acetone to form a stock solution of 2,000 μg/0.1 ml. From the stock solution, a test solution of

50 μg/0.1 ml is made up in acetone. Solutions are stored in amber bottles and refrigerated and made up fresh every two weeks.

2. The volar aspect of the arm is cleansed with acetone and allowed to dry.
3. A stainless steel ring, 2 cm in diameter (3 cm^3) with an affixed handle, is placed on the inner aspect of the upper arm and held in such a position that the enclosed circle of the skin is horizontal.
4. With the use of a 0.1 ml Biopette and a disposable polyethylene tip (Schwartz-Mann), the sensitizing dose of 2000 μg DNCB is applied.
5. The solvent is dried rapidly under an air stream with a portable hair dryer.
6. A weaker challenge test dose of 50 μg DNCB is applied to the volar surface of the forearm at the time of sensitization.
7. The sites are covered with bandages and the patients instructed not to wash the area for 24 hours.
8. Examine the sites at 24 hours for irritative reaction and at 7 and 14 days for a spontaneous flare. Subsequently, erythema and induration will begin to develop in normally responsive persons.
9. In the absence of this spontaneous flare at either site by 14 days, a challenge dose is reapplied and the site reexamined at 24 and 48 hours for a delayed hypersensitivity reaction. This reaction is well circumscribed and indurated with marked erythema and frequently with vesiculation in normal persons.

INTERPRETATION OF SKIN REACTIONS IN DNCB SENSITIZATION. The response is graded as follows:

A. A 4+ reaction is present if an unequivocal spontaneous flare occurs at both the sensitizing and challenging dose sites.
B. 3+ reaction is when a spontaneous flare is seen only at the sensitizing dose site.
C. 2+ reaction if, in the absence of spontaneous flare, reapplication of a challenge dose elicits an unequivocal delayed hypersensitivity skin reaction.
D. Any site with a doubtful reaction is biopsied with a 2 mm skin punch and submitted for histologic examination and if positive is graded 1+.

The lesions are scored as histologically positive if lymphocyte and macrophage cell infiltration are seen at the epidermal-dermal junction with extension into the epidermis.

Immunization for Normal Children

Fluid tetanus toxoid is administered at the time of injury. For clean wounds, a fully immunized child does not need a booster dose of tetanus toxoid unless more than 10 years have elapsed since the last immunization. For a contaminated case, a booster dose of tetanus toxoid is not necessary unless 5 years have elapsed since the last dose.

Table 3-2. Active Immunization and Tuberculin Testing Schedule for Normal Children. (Recommended by the Committee on Infectious Diseases, American Academy of Pediatrics, Oct. 17, 1971 [96].)

Age	Immunization	Test
2 months	DPT Polio (trivalent oral vaccine)	—
4 months	DPT Polio (trivalent oral vaccine)	—
6 months	DPT Polio (trivalent oral vaccine)	—
12 months	Measles (a, b)	Tuberculin test (c)
1–12 years	Rubella (a, b)	
18 months	Mumps (a, b) DPT Polio (trivalent oral vaccine)	
4–6 years	DPT Polio (trivalent oral vaccine)	
14–16 years	Diphtheria (adult type) (d) and tetanus	

(a) Measles vaccine may be given at 1 year as measles-rubella or measles-mumps-rubella combined vaccines.
(b) For single vaccines of measles, rubella or mumps, administration at one-month intervals is recommended.
(c) Tuberculin test is administered as clinically indicated and risk of exposure. The tuberculin test should be given prior to administration of measles vaccine.
(d) Combined tetanus and diphtheria (adult type) for those over 6 years of age in contrast to diphtheria and tetanus (DT) containing a larger amount of diphtheria antigen.

Tuberculin testing prior to the administration of attenuated measles vaccine is recommended since measles is known to suppress cell-mediated reactions [48, 57]. However, there is some controversy as to whether live attenuated mumps virus suppresses tuberculin-delayed hypersensitivity [8, 52]. The two studies, which reached opposite conclusions, had the problem of lack of parallel control groups in which children were tested with PPD prior to simultaneous vaccination of mumps virus [57].

In regard to smallpox vaccination, the Committee on Control of Contagious Diseases of the American Academy of Pediatrics [49] and the Advisory Committee on Immunization Practices of the Public Health Service [74] have made the following recommendations:

A. Routine vaccination against smallpox should be discontinued.
B. Vaccination is required only for individuals with special risks: (a) travelers to and from endemic areas and (b) health service personnel who contact patients. Such persons should be revaccinated every 3 years.
C. Continued monitoring of travelers entering the United States from endemic areas.
D. Strict observance of contraindication to smallpox vaccination, such as eczema, pregnancy, altered immune diseases, and infants under 1 year of age.
E. Continued active support to smallpox surveillance and eradication programs around the world.

NBT Test with and without Endotoxin Stimulation
(Method of M. Anderson and R. M. Nakamura, University of California at Irvine, adapted from Park et al. [66, 67])

Neutrophils which have been involved in active in vivo phagocytosis at the time the specimen is taken will activate enzymes capable of in vitro reduction of nitroblue tetrazolium dye test (NBT) to form blue-black formazan crystals. Monocytes from normal persons will be positive for NBT dye reduction. The test is helpful to differentiate active bacterial from viral infections, and for the diagnosis of chronic granulomatous disease.

Normal neutrophil cells which are negative to the NBT dye reduction test will become positive after stimulation with endotoxin stimulation to avoid false negative reactions [67]. A negative NBT test with and without endotoxin is characteristic of chronic granulomatous disease.

REAGENTS AND EQUIPMENT
Stock
A. Nitroblue tetrazolium chloride (Baker Chemical)—100 mg
B. *E. coli* endotoxin 0.55:B_5 (Difco)—100 mg
C. 37° C heating block
D. 0.15 M phosphate buffer pH 7.2 (Harleco)
Working solutions
A. Nitroblue tetrazolium chloride
0.2% in saline solution and 20 mg NBT in 10 ml physiologic saline solution; mix an equal volume of the above with an equal volume of phosphate buffer.
B. 0.15 M phosphate buffer pH 7.2
0.225 gm in 10 ml of saline solution (225 mg)
C. *E coli* endotoxin 10 mg diluted in 50 ml saline solution.

PROCEDURE
1. Venous blood is drawn into a plastic syringe and transferred to a disposable plastic tube, and 75–100 units heparin per ml blood is

added. Use heparin-drawn blood only. Heparinized Vacutainers
(Becton-Dickinson) may be used. EDTA interferes with the endo-
toxin stimulation test which appears to be complement dependent.
In a small disposable plastic tube

2. Mix 0.1 ml heparinized blood with 0.1 ml NBT solution.
3. Incubate 15 min in a constant temperature heating block at 37° C.
   Cover tubes with parafilm.
4. Leave at room temperature for 10 min.
5. Make smears and stain with Wright's stain.
6. Examine for black deposits only in neutrophils. Count 100 neutrophils and report results in percent of positive neutrophils.
   Results without endotoxin stimulation
   negative = 5–10%
   positive = 29% or greater (29% is the mean value for common
   acute bacterial infections. Some investigators believe that greater
   than 10% is significant to differentiate bacterial from viral and other
   diseases [59]).
7. If negative, mix 0.05 ml *E. coli* endotoxin with 0.5 ml heparinized
   blood and incubate at room temperature for 15 min.
8. Repeat the above procedures 1 through 5.
   Results with endotoxin stimulation
   negative = 5 to 10%
   positive = 29% or greater

READING OF RESULTS.   Monocytes are usually positive for formazan
granules. Park has stated [66] that only neutrophils with large dense
granules should be counted. However, Matula and Patterson [59] have
included neutrophils with a stippled cytoplasmic distribution of formazan
as "positive" cells. Formazan inclusions are differentiated from toxin
granulation in the neutrophils by their larger size and by their refractile
borders, which may be distinguished by rapidly focusing up and down.
   Since monocytes may be confused with certain fragmented cells, the
equivocal and doubtful cells should be counted separately. If the number
of equivocal cells raises the positive cells into a positive NBT response,
another 100 cells are counted to evaluate the response properly.

PERTINENT COMMENTS
A. Set up stimulated and unstimulated tests and run them together, to
   save time and unnecessary repetition.
B. Pediatric heparinized Vacutainers containing 2 ml are available (2 ml
   is more than sufficient for the test).
C. Eppendorf pipettes are useful for diluting.
D. The tubes should be covered with parafilm during incubation or the
   cells will become extremely fragile.
E. The test should be performed within 2 hours after collection of blood
   since neutrophils are fragile to endotoxin.
F. Endotoxin stimulation does not need to be performed if the test re-

sults without endotoxin are positive. When the neutrophils are unresponsive to endotoxin, then the test is helpful for the diagnosis of
chronic granulomatous disease.
G. We have tried three different techniques, including (a) siliconized
concave slides described by Park [66]; (b) fibrometer cups; and
(c) disposable plastic tubes. The concave slide preparations were
placed in petri dishes and placed on a support in a 37° C water bath
to make sure of a proper incubation temperature. The fibrometer
cups and disposable tubes were covered with parafilm and placed
in 37° C incubator blocks. Results are shown in Table 3-3. There
were no significant differences observed in the three different techniques. There is present a normal variability in differential counts
on blood smears [83].
H. Temperatures and incubation times are very important to control or
results will be variable [20]. The original procedure of Park [66] included a 15 min period of incubation at 37° C. Matula and Patterson
had increased the incubation time to 25 min [59]. Charette and
Komp [20] reported a marked discrepancy in the NBT test by the

Table 3-3. Comparison of Different Reaction Containers in the NBT Test.

Patient No.	% NBT Positive in Unstimulated Neutrophils		
	Concave Slides	Disposable Tubes	Fibrometer Cups
1	40	38	52
2	6	0	0
3	27	21	28
4	25	24	30
5	10	8	12
6	30	38	38
7	98	98	79
8	36	36	26
9	28	58	32
10	20	44	46
11	25	33	46
12	12	8	8
13	22	28	22
14	22	18	17
15	30	30	42
16	64	58	54

slide test placed in 37° C air incubator and fibrometer cup placed in a 37° C heating block. They have determined that the time taken for the blood NBT mixture to reach 37° C by the thermal heating block was 4 min, the water bath required 8 min, and the air incubator required 22 min [20].

LYMPHOCYTE TRANSFORMATION TESTS

Simple Lymphocyte Transformation Test with the Use of Wright's Stain and/or Acridine Orange (5–7 days)
(Modified from the method of Dukes et al. [37])

Normal lymphocytes can be stimulated by a mitogen such as phytohemagglutinin (PHA) to undergo blastogenesis. The transformed "blast" cells may be quantitated and visualized by Wright's stain or acridine orange, which is fluorochrome dye with cytochemical specificity for RNA–DNA.

EQUIPMENT
A. Sterile heparin tube
B. Equipment for removal of buffy coat cell and plasma suspension by aspiration
C. 5 ml sterile tubes—4
D. Racks to allow sedimentation
E. 37° C incubator
F. Slides and coverslips for blood smears
G. Slide sealant (clear nail polish)
H. Fluorescence microscope equipped with an Osram HB 200 mercury lamp with a UG 5 filter, darkfield condenser, and Wratten 2B secondary filter [31]

REAGENTS
A. Heparin containing benzyl alcohol only (NOT phenol) as preservative
B. Chromosome medium 1A with PHA (Difco), with PHA, 2–4 ml; 4–5 sterile tubes; chromosome medium 1A without PHA (Difco) 2–5 ml sterile tubes
C. Regular Wright's stain
D. Acridine orange (0.1% stock aqueous solution containing 0.2% Tween 80 wetting agent) (Harleco)
E. 2% acetic acid in isotonic saline
F. Isotonic saline solution
G. 2% ethanol in isotonic saline

PROCEDURE
1. Venous blood is collected in a sterile heparin tube.
2. The heparinized blood is allowed to sediment gently, and the buffy coat and plasma cells are removed by aspiration.

3. 0.1 or 0.2 ml buffy coat cell and plasma suspension with PHA are added to each of four 5-ml sterile tubes; and without PHA to 2 additional sterile tubes.
4. Place tubes containing blood in a 37° C incubator.
5. After 5 days remove 2 tubes containing PHA and 1 tube without PHA.
6. Aspirate medium from cells and make at least two blood smears of cells from each tube.
7. Stain one slide of each pair with regular Wright's stain and the other slide of each pair may be stained with acridine orange.
8. Steps 5, 6, and 7 are repeated after 7 days' incubation on the remaining tubes.

STAINING OF SMEARS WITH ACRIDINE ORANGE
1. Stain one set of slides with acridine orange 0.1%, diluted 1:10 with 2% acetic acid in isotonic saline solution, for 5 sec.
2. Excess acridine orange stain is removed by immersion into 2% ethanol in isotonic saline solution for 12 sec.
3. The slides are then rinsed in isotonic saline solution for 5 sec and a coverslip is placed on the slide and sealed.
4. The slides are examined with a fluorescence microscope equipped as noted above.

INTERPRETATION.   Blast cells are recognized by an enlarged cell with an increase in nuclear to cytoplasmic ratio with reticulated and prominent nuclei. These cells are contrasted to the small lymphocytes, which do not show nucleoli. A minimum of 1,000 lymphocytes are counted per slide; other disintegrating cells, neutrophils, and monocytes are not included in the counting.

The acridine orange stain will stain so that the nuclei (DNA) will have a greenish fluorescence, and the nucleoli (RNA) a red fluorescence. Cytoplasmic staining varies with cells, and lymphocytes are identified by the intense red cytoplasm rich in RNA, whereas the neutrophils show very little cytoplasmic staining. Monocytes have a reddish-brown color.

$$\frac{\text{no. transformed lymphocytes}}{\text{no. lymphocytes counted}} \times 100 = \% \text{ transformed lymphocytes}$$

Normal value is approximately 50% or greater transformation of lymphocytes.

Lymphocyte Transformation Test with Phytohemagglutinin and Tritiated Thymidine (4 days)
(Method of S. D. Deodhar and B. Barna, Dept. of Immunopathology, Cleveland Clinic and Research Foundation, Cleveland, Ohio, adapted from various reported procedures [12, 50, 86])

Normally, lymphocytes can be cultured and stimulated to proliferate, divide, and form blastoid cells with a nonspecific mitogen phytohemagglutinin (PHA). The response to PHA provides some measure of overall relevant T-cells. The response to PHA is evaluated in terms of the morphologic change and incorporation of tritiated thymidine measured by the direct counting of radioactivity. Cultures are set up in which the lymphocyte concentration is 10^6 cells/ml.

EQUIPMENT AND MATERIALS

A. Refrigerated centrifuge (International model PR–2)
B. Vortex mixer for resuspension of cell pellets
C. Hemocytometer and microscope
D. 37° C incubator with humidified 5% CO_2/95% air
E. Filtering flask
F. Scintillation counter (Beckman model LS–100)
G. Disposable glass culture tubes, 16 × 100 mm (Bellco, cat. no. 1711)
H. Plastic disposable sterile culture tubes, 16 × 125 mm, with screw cap (Falcon, cat. no. 3033)
 I. Pipettes, serologic with plug, plastic, sterile, individually wrapped. Falcon,
      1 ml cat. no. 7520—1000/case
      5 ml cat. no. 7543—200/case
      10 ml cat. no. 7551—200/case
J. Fenwal scrub nylon fiber (Fenwal, cat. no. FT 242)—6 pkg/case

REAGENTS

A. Spinner Modified Minimal Essential Medium, without glutamine (Gibco, cat. no. 138)
B. Fetal calf serum, heat inactivated (Gibco, cat. no. 614 HI)
C. 1-glutamine (Gibco, cat. no. 503)
D. Penicillin-streptomycin solution (Gibco cat. no. 514). 10,000 units/ml penicillin and 10,000 mcg/ml streptomycin
E. Phytohemagglutinin–M (Difco, cat. no. 0528–57)
F. Hank's balanced salt solution (Gibco, cat. no. 402)
G. Hank's balanced salt solution, calcium and magnesium free (Gibco, cat. no. 417)
H. Tritiated thymidine, 1 mCi in 1 ml (Nuclear Chicago, TRA 120)
 I. Thymidine (Nutritional Biochemicals)
J. Heparin—sodium heparin, 1,000 units/ml (Riker)
K. Trichloroacetic acid (Baker), anal. reagent, ACS crystals—1 lb. bottle
L. Tetraethylammonium hydroxide (10% in H_2O), (Eastman Chemicals, cat. no. 2078)—100 gm bottle
M. Toluene (Fisher, cat. no. T324)—1 gallon
N. Liquifluor (Nuclear Chicago, cat. no. 190100)—500 ml bottle

O. Scintillation fluid
    Liquifluor—42 ml
    Ethanol—380 ml
    Make up 1 liter with toluene.

REAGENTS AND MATERIALS FOR EACH CULTURE, DAY 1
A. Heparin
B. 20 ml syringe—2
C. 22 guage needles—2
D. 20 guage needles—2
E. 18 gauge needles—3
F. 15 ml graduated centrifuge tube—1
G. Alcohol swabs
H. Sterile towel—1
 I. Gauze pads
 J. 2½ ml syringe—1
K. 1 ml tuberculin syringes—2
L. 5 ml nylon fiber-filled syringe—1
M. Package plastic culture tubes—1
N. Package 6 silicone stoppers—1
O. Glass foil-covered tubes—6
P. 5 ml pipettes—1
Q. 10 ml pipettes—2
R. Diluting pipettes and diluting tubes—2
S. Hemocytometer and coverslip—1
T. Labels
U. 100 ml bottle—1
V. Bottle Hank's balanced salt solution (HBSS), calcium and magnesium free (Gibco)—1
W. Bottle $SMEM_{85}$, FCS_{15}, PSG (Spinner modified minimum essential medium with 15% fetal calf serum, penicillin 100 units/ml, streptomycin 100 mcg/ml, glutamine 292 mcg/ml) (Gibco)—1
X. Diluting fluid (1% HCl)
Y. Phytohemagglutinin (Bacto PHA–M, Difco)
NOTE: All reagents and materials are sterile. All procedures require aseptic techniques. Do NOT leave tubes or bottles uncapped. Do NOT lay sterile materials on workbench. Flame mouths of glass bottles and tubes. Do NOT flame plastic tubes or instruments.

PROCEDURES FOR DAY 1.   Note that step 18 must be performed between 5:00 and 5:30 P.M. to permit completion of Day 4 portion in one day.
 1. Draw 0.2 ml heparin into each of 2 sterile 20 ml syringes, coat walls of syringes with heparin. Do NOT discard heparin.
 2. Draw 35 ml blood into heparin-treated syringes.
 3. Allow syringes to stand, needle end up, for 2 hours in 37° C incubator.

4. Place 0.1 ml heparin in 15 ml graduated centrifuge tube. Remove syringe from incubator and attach sterile 20 gauge needle. Bend needle and allow a few drops of plasma to drip out, to remove any RBCs at top of syringe. Decant plasma into centrifuge tube.
5. Centrifuge at 1,500 rpm for 10 min.
6. With a spinal needle on a 2½ ml syringe, draw up 2 ml HBSS and resuspend cell pellet, then draw into syringe.
7. Change to a 22 gauge needle and transfer cell suspension to a 5 ml plastic syringe filled with nylon fiber.
8. Change to an 18 gauge needle; remove 1 ml HBSS.
9. Change back to spinal needle and rinse centrifuge tube, drawing rinse up into syringe.
10. Change back to 22 gauge needle and transfer rinse to nylon-filled syringe.
11. Incubate nylon "filter" syringe at 37° C for 20 min.
12. Draw 20–22 ml HBSS into 20 ml syringe and with 22 gauge needle attached, flush "filter" syringe to free mononuclear cells. Flush "filter" syringe with 20 ml air. (Polymorphonuclear cells should remain in nylon fiber.)
13. Centrifuge at 1,500 rpm for 10 min.
14. Decant supernatant and resuspend pellets in 5 ml medium ($SMEM_{85}$, FCS_{15}, PSG), using 5 ml pipette. Save pipette with residual cell suspension in tip.
15. Using residual cell suspension as source, draw cells into diluting pipette to 0.5 mark. Draw diluting fluid to 11 mark. Invert pipette several times, let out 3 drops, and place one drop in each of 2 hemocytometer chambers. Do NOT overfill chambers.
16. Count number of mononuclear cells in all 4 squares in each chamber. To compute:

$$\frac{\text{no. monos in 4 squares}}{0.4} \times 20{,}000 = \text{no. monos per ml of cell suspension}$$

17. Set up the following culture tubes on the basis of 1×10^6 mononuclear cells per ml of medium and 3 ml of this cell suspension per tube. Calculate cells needed and medium needed and pipette both into a bottle. Using a 10 ml pipette, mix and dispense 3 ml aliquots to the following tubes:
    a. 4 plastic tubes
       Label: number on each tube
             2 tubes—control
             2 tubes—PHA
    b. 6 glass foil covered tubes. Carefully remove foil caps and replace with silicone stoppers.
       Label: number on each tube
             3 tubes—control
             3 tubes—PHA

18. Using 1 ml plastic tuberculin syringe, with 18 gauge needle, add 4 drops of phytohemagglutinin to each *PHA* tube.
    NOTE TIME: PHA *must* be added between 5:00 and 5:30 P.M. This timing is critical since it affects pulsing with tritiated thymidine at 63 hours.
19. Place all tubes at 37° C.

REAGENTS AND MATERIALS FOR DAY 4, MORNING
A. Tritiated thymidine
B. HBSS
C. Fixative (3 parts menthanol + 1 part acetic acid)
D. Glass slides—6
E. Slide racks, permount, and coverslips
F. Diamond marker pencil
G. Pasteur pipette and bulb
H. Staining dishes—8
 I. Stains: filtered May-Grünwald and Giemsa stains
J. Distilled H_2O
   acetone:xylene 1:1—about 300 ml each
   acetone:xylene—about 600 ml each

PROCEDURES FOR DAY 4, MORNING
 1. Before 8:00–8:30 A.M., dilute tritiated thymidine in HBSS to a concentration of 20 μCi/ml.
 2. At 63 hours after initial addition of phytohemagglutinin (8:00–8:30 A.M.), the diluted tritiated thymidine is added. With the automatic pipette set to deliver 0.1 ml, dispense this amount into each *glass* culture tube (2 μCi per tube). Vortex tube briefly and return *immediately* to 37° C incubator.
    NOTE: Do not drop 0.1 ml on sides of tube, drop directly into medium. Pulse time is 6 hours (63–69 hours).
 3. Remove *plastic* tubes from incubator and centrifuge at 1,500 rpm for 10 min.
 4. Discard supernatant and drain tubes briefly on paper towel.
 5. Vortex pellets to resuspend and add 5 ml. fixative per tube. Let sit 30 minutes. (Fixative = 3 parts methanol + 1 part acetic acid.)
 6. Label one glass slide per tube and wipe slides free of any glass dust. Use diamond marker pencil.
 7. Centrifuge fixed tubes at 1,500 rpm for 10 min.
 8. Discard supernatant, leaving a few drops at bottom of tube.
 9. Using Pasteur pipette and bulb, resuspend pellets in the few remaining drops of fixative and drop on slide. Allow slide to air dry.
10. Slides should be placed in racks and are ready to be stained.
11. Prepare staining dishes in sequence as follows (dishes hold about 300 ml reagent to cover slides):
    a. May-Grünwald (filter stain first)
    b. Giemsa (dilute stock 1:15 in distilled H_2O)

     c. Distilled H_2O
     d. Acetone
     e. Acetone
     f. Acetone : Xylene 1 : 1
     g. Xylene
     h. Xylene
12. Stain slides following times:

May-Grünwald	5 minutes
Giemsa	5 minutes
Distilled H_2O	A few quick dips
Acetone	30 seconds
Acetone	30 seconds
Acetone/Xylene	2 minutes
Xylene	3 minutes
Xylene	3 minutes

13. Add drop of permount and coverslip.
14. Count blast cells and small lymphocytes for a total of 500 cells per slide.

$$\% \text{ blast transformation} = \frac{\text{\# blast cells}}{\text{total cells}}$$

Normal range—50% or greater
   slightly decreased   —30–45%
   markedly decreased—5–29%
   absent   —less than 5%

The morphologic change does not always occur in parallel with the thymidine uptake, especially in cases of variable immune deficiency [34]. Different values have been given for the normal range with various procedures and may be due to variability in the cultured cell survival.

Nonresponsiveness to PHA-stimulated peripheral blood lymphocytes has been observed in a wide variety of conditions, such as Swiss type agammaglobulinemia, ataxia-telangiectasia, Hodgkin's disease, and chronic lymphatic leukemia. Usually in cases of significant defects of function, less than 5% blastlike cells are seen.

REAGENTS AND MATERIALS NEEDED FOR DAY 4, AFTERNOON
A. 1 M thymidine, unlabeled, cold—0.6 ml
B. Ice bath for reagents and culture tubes
C. Reagents: normal saline solution; 5% TCA; 6.7% TCA; 0.1 N NaOH; scintillation fluid; TEAH (tetraethylammonium hydroxide)
D. Pasteur pipette

PROCEDURES—DAY 4, AFTERNOON
1. After 69 hours of culture (at 2:00–2:30 P.M.), add 0.1 ml unlabeled, cold 1 M thymidine to each glass culture tube to terminate pulsing.

2. Centrifuge at 2,000 rpm for 10 min.
3. All reagents and culture tubes should now be kept chilled in an ice bath during the following steps.
4. Decant culture tubes. Vortex pellet and wash with 5 ml saline solution. Centrifuge 2,000 rpm for 10 min.
5. Repeat saline wash. (NOTE: At this point tubes can be stored frozen if necessary.)
6. Vortex pellet. Add 5 ml 5% TCA. Mix again. Let stand in cold for 10 min.
7. Centrifuge at 2,000 rpm for 10 min.
8. Decant. Mix pellet. Add 1 ml 0.1 N NaOH and mix until cells are completely dissolved.
9. Add 4.5 ml of 6.7% TCA. Mix again. Let stand in cold for 10 min.
10. Centrifuge at 2,000 rpm for 10 min.
11. Decant and repeat steps 8, 9, and 10.
12. Label scintillation vial caps to correspond with tubes. (DO NOT label glass vial.)
13. Decant. Mix pellet. Add 0.1 ml TEAH (2 to 3 drops from Pasteur pipette). Vortex again. If pellet has not cleared, add one more drop of TEAH.
14. Mix until pellet is completely dissolved and clear.
15. Add 5 ml scintillation fluid. Mix and add to same vial.
16. Add 5 ml more to tube. Mix and add to same vial.
17. Vials should be tightly capped and kept at 40° C or placed immediately in counter.

Control values of unstimulated cultures may be high in certain diseases, and data should be given on stimulated and unstimulated cultures. Also, because of numerous variations in technique, culture media, phytohemagglutinin (PHA) preparations, and specific activity of different thymidine preparations, the PHA response to at least two to three normal donors should be included in each run.

Lymphocyte Transformation Test with Specific
Antigen and Tritiated Thymidine (6–7 days)
(Method of S. D. Deodhar and B. Barna, Dept. of Immunopathology, Cleveland Clinic, Cleveland, Ohio. Assay by morphological blast transformation and tritiated thymidine incorporation)

NOTES ON TECHNIQUE
A. All reagents and equipment are sterile, except for the final acid wash technique.
B. The assay can be used to test a drug suspected of causing hypersensitivity. The concentration of drug to be used in vitro may be estimated by the patient's previous dosage, if known. If this information is not available, consult the *Physician's Desk Reference* for dosages. Divide dosage by 5,000 ml (blood volume) to obtain

a workable concentration per milliliter. A range of three drug dilutions may be prepared representing (a) 10 × dosage per milliliter;
(b) dosage per milliliter; and (c) 1/10 dosage per milliliter.

REAGENTS.   See Lymphocyte Transformation Test with PHA.

EQUIPMENT.   See Lymphocyte Transformation Test with PHA, equipment items A–F.

MATERIALS
A. Sterile plastic syringe (50 ml)
B. Heparinized centrifuge tube
C. Hank's BSS
D. Culture medium SMEM (Spinner modified minimum essential
   medium supplemented with 15% fetal calf serum; 100 μ/ml peni-
   cillin; 100 mcg/ml streptomycin; and 292 mcg/ml 1-glutamine)
   Morphologic assay
E. Culture tubes—16 per patient
F. Pasteur pipette
G. Fixative (3 parts methanol + 1 part acetic acid)
H. Slides
 I. Slide rack, permount, and cover slips
J. Stains: filtered May-Grünwald; Giemsa
   Tritiated thymidine assay
K. Glass culture tubes—12 per patient
L. Tritiated thymidine (2 μCi in 0.1 ml; specific activity 500–5,000
   mCi/mM)
M. Saline solution (normal cold)
N. Materials for acid wash

PROCEDURE
1. Draw 40 ml heparinized blood in a sterile plastic syringe.
2. Allow syringe to stand, needle end up, at 37° C until a well-defined
   plasma layer appears.
3. Aspirate plasma into a heparinized centrifuge tube.
4. Centrifuge at 1,500 rpm for 10 min.
5. Decant supernatant and add 5 ml Hank's BSS to resuspend cells.
6. Centrifuge at 1,500 rpm for 10 min.
7. Decant supernatant and resuspend cells in 5 ml culture medium.
   NOTE: Before exposing cells to this medium, one must determine if
   the patient has any allergies to penicillin or streptomycin. If so,
   these reagents should be eliminated from the medium.
8. Count leukocytes in a hemocytometer. Adjust concentration to 1 ×
   10^6 cells per ml culture medium. Dispense 3 ml suspension per 16
   × 100 culture tube.
9. *Morphologic Assay* (continue with Steps 9, 10, and 11)
   Set up 4 culture tubes as controls (medium only), and 4 culture

tubes per antigen dilutions. A range of three antigen dilutions is usually tested, giving a total of 16 culture tubes per patient. Antigen solutions are added to tubes in volumes of not more than 0.3 ml/ tube. Entire culture is incubated at 37° C for 6 days, at which time half of the tubes are harvested (i.e., 2 tubes from control group and 2 tubes from each antigen dilution group). The remainder of the tubes are harvested on Day 7.

10. *Harvesting Procedure:* Centrifuge tubes, decant supernatant, re-suspend cell button by Vortexing, and add 5 ml fixative. Cells are fixed for a minimum of 30 minutes, centrifuged, fixative decanted, and the pellets resuspended with Pasteur pipettes and dropped onto slides. After the slides have air-dried, they are stained with May-Grünwald and Giemsa stains as described in the methods for Lymphocyte Transformation Test with Phytohemagglutinin (PHA).

11. Count blast cells and lymphs for a total of 500 cells per slide. Determine percent blast cells in control and antigen cultures. If antigen cultures have at least twice the percent blast cells appearing in controls, the test may be considered positive.

9a. *Tritiated Thymidine Assay* (Begin with Steps 1 through 8)
Set up 3 culture tubes as controls and 3 tubes per antigen dilution. It is best to use glass tubes since the final steps in this procedure involve reagents which deteriorate plastic.

10a. Add antigen solutions in volumes of not more than 0.3 ml/tube.

11a. Incubate at 37° C for 120 hours. Add tritiated thymidine (2 μCi in 0.1 ml). (Specific activity 500–5,000 mCi/mM) to each tube. Vortex tubes after addition of isotope. Reincubate for 18 hours.

12a. Terminate by two washes in cold normal saline solution, followed by the acid wash technique as given in the methods for Lymphocyte Transformation Test with PHA.

13a. Count samples in a beta scintillation counter.

Quantitative Lymphocyte Transformation Test
Applicable to Adults and Children
(Method by P. E. Runge, Susie W. Fong, and G. A. Granger, Departments of Molecular Biology and Pediatrics, University of California at Irvine)

A quantitative and semimicromethod is available to study the phytohemagglutinin (PHA) responsiveness of lymphocytes in different clinical conditions associated with deficiencies in cellular immunity. The standardization of existing culture conditions for maximal response and reproducibility has permitted valid comparison of PHA lymphocyte transformation as determined by the uptake of tritiated thymidine in serial studies of individuals and between patients and normal controls. Changes in PHA responsiveness of lymphocytes in patients may be used to evaluate the course of disease and the effectiveness of immunosuppressants, and to predict the risk of infections. In patients with cancer, it may be useful in formulating the criteria to proceed with immunotherapy, such as BCG immunization.

MATERIALS
A. Syringes, needles
B. Pipettes: graduated, Pasteur, lambda
C. Screw-cap culture tubes: 50 ml (20 × 150 mm.); 15 ml (16 × 125 mm)
D. Refrigerated centrifuge (International Model PR–2)
E. Vortex mixer for resuspension of cell pellets
F. Hemocytometer and microscope
G. Special racks to hold culture tubes on their sides at a 5° angle
H. 37° C incubator with humidified 5% CO_2/95% air
I. Filtering flask
J. Scintillation counter (Beckman model LS–100)
K. Nylon column (Hyland Lymphocyte Transport-Storage System)
L. Fiberglass filters (Whatman GS/A, 2.4 cm diam.)

ANTIGENS AVAILABLE
A. Phytohemagglutinin 20–30 μg 0.5 ml (PHA–P, Difco)
B. Pokeweed mitogen 0.01 ml/0.5 ml (Gibco)
C. Concanavalin A 25 μg/0.5 ml (Calbiochem)

REAGENTS
A. Heparin 1,000 units/ml (Riker Labs)
B. Culture media: RPMI 1640 (Flow Labs.)—83 ml; human serum (inactivated 56° C, 30 min)—15 ml; glutamine 29 mg/ml. (Gibco)
C. Antibiotics: penicillin 10,000 units (Sigma); streptomycin 10 mg (Lilly); Mycostatin 2,500 units (Squibb); Garamycin 3.2 mg (Schering)—1 ml each
D. Plasmagel (Labs. Roger Bellon)
E. Iron-Ficoll (Pharmacia)
F. Tritiated thymidine 2 μCi/ml in RPMI 1640 (Gibco) culture medium (tritiated methyl, 6.0 Ci/mM, Schwarz-Mann)
G. 2% acetic acid for white blood count (WBC)
H. 0.05% eosin for viability test
I. 0.15 M NaCl
J. 10% trichloracetic acid
K. NCS tissue solubilizer (Amersham/Searle)
L. Omnifluor scintillation fluid (New England Nuclear)
M. Wright's stain for blood smears (Fisher)

PROCEDURE
Isolation of leukocytes from peripheral blood
1. Five to 10 ml blood is drawn into a syringe containing 50–100 units heparin.

2. The heparinized blood is transferred to a 50 ml culture tube and mixed gently with a volume of Plasmagel equal to one-third the the blood volume.
3. After sedimentation of the erythrocytes at room temperature for approximately 40 min, the leukocyte layer is transferred to a new 50 ml culture tube.
4. After centrifugation at 450 g for 5 min in 4° C, the supernatant is carefully decanted.
5. The leukocyte pellet is resuspended with one ml RPMI 1640 with moderate agitation.
6. A white blood count (WBC), smear, and viability test with 0.05% eosin are performed.
7. The cell suspension is adjusted with RPMI 1640 culture medium to contain $1-2 \times 10^6$ cells/ml.

Isolation of lymphocytes from peripheral blood
1. Ten to 20 ml blood is drawn into a syringe containing 100–200 units heparin and transferred to a 50 ml culture tube.
2. A volume of Plasmagel equaling one-third the blood volume is mixed gently with the blood.
3. After sedimentation of the erythrocytes at room temperature for approximately 40 min, the leukocyte layer is passed slowly through a nylon column into a new 50 ml culture tube.
4. The effluent containing 90–95% lymphocytes is centrifuged at 450 g for 5 min in 4° C.
5. The supernatant is carefully decanted and the cell pellet is resuspended with 1 ml of RPMI 1640 with moderate agitation.
6. After smears, a viability test with 0.05% eosin, and the cell count are done, the cell suspension is diluted with culture medium to give a cell concentration of $0.5-1 \times 10^6$ cell/ml.

Quantitation of DNA synthesis in peripheral blood as determined by the uptake of tritiated thymidine
1. Leukocyte and lymphocyte suspensions of test and normal subjects are adjusted with culture media to contain $1-2 \times 10^6$ cells/ml and $0.5-1 \times 10^6$ cells/ml, respectively.
2. Triplicate or duplicate 1 ml cultures in screw cap tubes (15 ml) are set up with and without mitogens.
3. PHA is reconstituted with culture media at an optimal dose of 20–30 $\mu g/0.5$ ml.
4. Final cultures will be composed of 0.5 ml cell suspension and 0.5 ml mitogen.
5. Control culture tubes for test and normal subjects are set up without the addition of mitogens, but 0.5 ml medium is added to make a final culture volume of 1 ml.
6. The culture tubes are instilled with 5% CO_2/95% air, stoppered, and then placed on their sides at a 5° slant in special racks for 3 days at 37° C. Alternatively, the culture tubes, loosely stoppered,

may be placed in a 37° C incubator equipped with 5% CO_2, but the tubes may still require daily examination for pH changes and regassing with 5% CO_2 as required.

7. If the supernatants are required for further testing, culture tubes are centrifuged at 4° C for 5 min at 450 g to obtain a tight pellet.

8. The supernatant from each culture is decanted immediately and may be saved for lymphotoxin and migration inhibitory factor assays.

9. A cell count is performed after resuspension of the cell pellet with one ml RPMI 1640 medium warmed to 37° C. This recovered cell count is used in the final calculations (cpm/1 × 10^6 cells).

10. The cell suspension is recentrifuged to obtain a cell pellet.

11. After the medium is carefully decanted from each culture, 1 ml tritiated thymidine (2 μCi/ml in culture medium) is added to the dispersed cells. If the supernatants are not required for further studies after the 3 day incubation period, then the cell counts may be performed directly on the original culture. One-tenth ml is removed for cell count and replaced with 0.1 ml culture medium containing 2 μCi tritiated thymidine. Thus, steps 7–10 are eliminated.

12. After a 4-hour incubation period at 37° C, culture tubes are centrifuged at 4° C for 5 min at 900 g to obtain a cell pellet.

Two methods of harvesting the labeled cells are used: trichloracetic acid (TCA) precipitation with and without fiberglass filters.

TCA precipitation without fiberglass filters

1. After the supernatant is decanted, the cell pellet is dispersed with the Vortex mixer, washed one time with 5 ml *cold* 0.15 M NaCl by centrifugation at 4° C for 5 min at 900 g.

2. After the 0.15 M NaCl is decanted, the cells are dispersed by the Vortex mixer and resuspended with one ml *cold* 0.15 M NaCl.

3. Then 5 ml *cold* 10% TCA is added to precipitate the proteins and nucleic acids.

4. After centrifugation for 10 min at 900 g in 4° C, the 10% TCA is decanted and the culture tubes containing the precipitate are drained by standing them upside down in a rack.

5. 0.5 ml NCS solubilizer is added to each tube and then the tubes are placed at 37° C for 30 min.

6. The contents of each tube are carefully transferred into counting vials after the addition of 5 ml Omnifluor and thorough mixing with the Vortex apparatus.

7. The tubes are rinsed once with 10 ml Omnifluor and the washes are also transferred to the counting vials.

TCA precipitation with fiberglass filters

1. After the 4-hour labeling period at 37° C, the culture tubes are centrifuged at 4° C for 10 min at 900 g to obtain a cell pellet.

2. The supernatant is decanted and the cells are resuspended in 1 ml *cold* 0.15 M NaCl, using the Vortex mixer.

3. Then 5 ml *cold* 10% TCA is added to the cell suspension to precipitate the proteins and nucleic acids.
4. A fiberglass filter is placed in the holder of a filtering flask attached to a vacuum.
5. After the filter is moistened with cold 10% TCA, the precipitate is poured onto the filter from the culture tube.
6. The culture tube is rinsed twice with *cold* 10% TCA (5 ml) and the washes are added to the filter.
7. After a final rinse with *cold* 10% TCA, the filter is then transferred to a counting vial.
8. One-half ml NCS solubilizer is added to each counting vial and then the vials are placed at 37° C for 30 min.
9. Prior to counting the vials, 15 ml Omnifluor is added to each sample.

RESULTS.   In order to compare the PHA lymphocyte response of a patient on a longitudinal basis, attempts were made to study the same normal subject concurrently. To evaluate quantitatively the level of responsiveness induced by a mitogen, the $cpm/1 \times 10^6$ recovered cells of three replicate cultures were first averaged and then divided by the average of corresponding negative controls. This ratio

$$\frac{cpm/10^6 \text{ cells } + \text{ mitogen}}{cpm/10^6 \text{ cells } - \text{ mitogen}}$$

is called the *stimulation index* or SI.

Reproducibility among replicate cultures was increased by incorporating the recovered cell counts into the final calculations. In PHA positive cultures, the cell counts may be higher than the original number of cells applied, and in some instances there may be a loss of cells prior to labeling with tritiated thymidine.

To eliminate any variation in PHA response due to unexpected alteration in culture conditions, the SI of the patient with acute lymphoblastic leukemia (ALL) was compared to the SI of the normal control studied at the same time (Table 3-4). Over a long period of study, the SI of normal subjects can vary (range 6–200, average 87) but tended to be greater than 50. The actual $cpm/10^6$ recovered cells from PHA plus cultures are given in Table 3-4 to demonstrate the high number of counts incorporated by the lymphocytes under optimal culture conditions. In comparison, the actual $cpm/10^6$ cells from PHA minus cultures ranged from 500 to 3,000. In patients with ALL, particularly during the blastic phase, the uptake of tritiated thymidine in PHA minus cultures may be higher than normally expected due to the presence of dividing leukemic lymphocytes.

The SI was calculated for each subject studied to provide a basis of comparison. However, the most pertinent clinical information was derived from comparing the SI of the patient to that of the normal control during the course of disease (see Table 3-4). The ratios of patient

Table 3-4. Sequential Studies in a Patient with Acute Lymphatic Leukemia with Quantitative PHA Lymphocyte Transformation Test.

Time Interval Months	Donor	PHA + (25 µg/ml) cpm/10⁶ cells	PHA − cpm/10⁶ cells	SI $\frac{PHA +}{PHA -}$	$\frac{Pt\ SI}{N\ SI}$	Course
0	ALL	53,705	291	184	1.3	Remission
	Control 1	108,590	757	143		
1	ALL	11,700	514	23	1.0	Remission
	Control 1	5,272	221	24		
4	ALL	101,833	1,025	99	1.1	Remission
	Control 2	158,546	175	90		
6	ALL	59,348	3,677	16	1.0	Remission
	Control 1	55,590	3,193	17		
8	ALL	315,783	1,288	158	1.1	Remission
	Control 2	173,513	1,169	148		
	Control 3	188,501	941	200	0.8	
10	ALL	291,625	10,858	27	0.2	Early relapse
	Control 1	349,550	3,176	110		
10.5	ALL	2,594	2,401	1	0.2	Intensive therapy
	Control 3	18,508	1,781	6		
11	ALL	681,172	16,565	41	0.9	Partial remission
	Control 3	210,944	4,322	48		

SI/normal SI approximated 1.0 when the patient was in remission, but the ratios decreased markedly prior to a blastic crisis and during intensive induction chemotherapy. From our studies, the SI ratio comparing the patient to the normal control may be predictive of bone marrow relapse. Generally, the ALL patients in bone marrow remission appear to have normal cellular immunity while being treated with high dose maintenance chemotherapy (Table 3-5).

COLLECTION OF BLOOD AND ISOLATION OF LEUKOCYTES AND LYMPHO-
CYTES FROM PERIPHERAL BLOOD.   To reiterate, it is imperative to maintain sterile technique and equipment throughout the procedure. For maximal recovery of leukocytes, heparinized blood is preferred to the defibrination procedure employing glass beads. The blood specimen is generally processed soon after drawing. However, when there is an unavoidable delay up to 24 hours, the leukocytes are placed in culture media and stored at room temperature rather than at 4° C. To improve the recovery of leukocytes and to remove excessive erythrocyte contamination of the buffy coat, a sedimenting agent such as Plasmagel or iron-Ficoll is mixed with the blood and allowed to settle.

CULTURE MEDIA AND SUPPLEMENTATION WITH SERUM.   Studies were performed in our laboratory to determine the effect of different culture media and varying concentration of human serum on lymphocyte responsiveness to PHA. RPMI 1640 and MEM media containing 15% normal human serum gave optimal responsiveness compared to Waymouth media supplemented with the same serum concentration. Studies employing 5–35% human serum indicated that 5% was the minimum serum concentration required for a good response. Serum of different ABO blood group did not seem to alter the cellular response. However, group AB or pooled group O sera absorbed with A and B red cells were employed in our studies, in the event that isoagglutinins did react with leukocytes of test subjects. Supplementation of culture media with autologous serum was not employed perchance the serum contained unforeseen cytotoxic factors. Subsequently, pooled human serum pretested for cytotoxic activity was used to supplement our culture media.
    Fetal calf serum absorbed with human erythrocytes suppressed the PHA response fourfold when compared to human serum. Furthermore, fetal calf serum stimulated the uptake of tritiated thymidine in PHA minus cultures. Thus, the stimulation index may be erroneously low.

CELL DENSITY AND MORPHOLOGY.   By varying the cell density of leukocytes between 0.1 and 2.5 $\times$ 10^6 cells/ml in culture, maximal uptake of tritiated thymidine after PHA stimulation was obtained with 0.5 $\times$ 10^6 cells/ml. Moderately good response was discerned with cell densities as low as 0.25 $\times$ 10^6/ml and as high as 1.0 $\times$ 10^6/ml.
    The leukocyte/lymphocyte composition did not appear to correlate

Table 3-5. PHA Lymphocyte Transformation Tests in Various Patients.

Lymphocytes Source	Peripheral Blood				Bone Marrow			
	No.		(PHA + / PHA −)		No.		(PHA + / PHA −)	
	Pts.	Tests	Range	Av.	Pts.	Tests	Range	Av.
Acute lymphocytic leukemia								
Remission	4	12	16–914	193	4	12	1–93	34
Relapse	4	6	0.5–9	2.5				
Chronic lymphocytic leukemia	2	2	76–83	80				
Neuroblastoma	2	6	69–314	140	2	2	7–45	26
Normal patients	3	11	17–596	166				

with the level of response. Initial studies comparing purified lymphocytes and leukocytes with the usual composition of 70% polymorphonuclear cells and 30% lymphocytes did not indicate any difference in the uptake of tritiated thymidine after PHA stimulation. However, when specific antigens, such as PPD, are tested, glass adherent cells will be required for maximal lymphocyte response.

The optimal concentration of different mitogens was determined: PHA-P 25–30 μg/ml; pokeweed mitogen 0.01 ml/ml; Concanalvin A 25 μg/ml; lipopolysaccharide (*E. coli*) no response between 5 and 500 μg/ml. Optimal concentration of PHA–P was determined with each new lot of mitogen prior to tests. PHA-P in dosages of 15–20 μg/ml may be used in lieu of higher concentration to avoid agglutination of leukocytes and to facilitate the recovered cell counts. Pokeweed mitogen (PWM), which is a presumed stimulator of T and B lymphocytes, tended to parallel the lymphocyte response to PHA–P but to a much lesser extent. The stimulation indices of normal control subjects were only 5–10 times above the PWM negative control cultures in contrast to PHA stimulation indices of 100–200. The level of lymphocyte response to Concanavalin A (25 μg/ml) tended to approximate the lymphocyte response to PWM. Lipopolysaccharide, which has been considered a specific B-cell stimulator in animals, did not stimulate human lymphocytes from varying sources.

CULTURE CONDITION. Maximal uptake of tritiated thymidine and DNA synthetic activity occurred between 40 and 60 hours after PHA stimulation (25 μg/ml). Between 72 and 96 hours, the incorporation of tritiated thymidine gradually decreased to 50% below the peak response. The labeling of lymphocytes with tritiated thymidine was determined to be adequate at 4 hours.

The conditions standardized for maximal response of peripheral blood lymphocytes were found to be equally applicable to the study of lymphocytes derived from bone marrow, lymph nodes, adenoids, and spleen. These same culture conditions have also been applied to mixed lymphocyte cultures with good results.

Micromethod for Evaluation of Lymphocyte Response to Phytohemagglutinin

Park and Good [70] have developed a new microtechnique for evaluation of lymphocyte response to phytohemagglutinin. The method utilizes 50 μl peripheral blood and can be briefly outlined as follows:
1. 50 μl heparinized peripheral blood is incubated at 37° C, directly with 50 μl tissue culture medium and 50 μg PHA, for 24 hours.
2. Then 0.5 μCi of tritiated thymidine in 50 μl tissue culture medium is added and incubated for an additional 16 hours.
3. After incubation, red cells are selectively typed in distilled water and the white cells are trapped on a millipore filter.

4. The radioactivity in the cells on the filter is measured with a scintillation counter.

Migration Inhibition Assay of Human Leukocytes
(Method of J. Shirley and R. M. Nakamura, Department of Pathology, University of California at Irvine, adapted from [52, 83, 93])

MATERIALS
A. RPMI—1640 tissue culture medium (Gibco). (a) Add bovine calf serum so that the final concentration is 10%. (b) Add penicillin-streptomycin solution (10,000 units penicillin and 10,000 mcg streptomycin per ml), 1 ml/100 ml tissue culture medium (Gibco). (c) pH must be maintained between 7.3 and 7.4.
B. 6% Gentran 75 in 0.9% saline solution (Travenol).
C. Mackaness type chambers (Lexy Culture Chamber, Mini Lab Co.). These chambers are approximately 15 mm in diameter and 3 mm deep, and hold approximately 0.85 ml.
D. Sterile 20 μl Micro Disposable Pipets (Dade)
E. Lipo-Hepin (Riker) (1,000 U.P.S. units/ml)
F. Sterile syringes and needles for blood collection and tissue culture medium chamber injection
G. Hemocytometer
H. Critoseal
 I. Silicone grease, autoclaved in a 2.5 ml glass syringe
 J. Sterile plastic test tubes
K. Sterile Pasteur pipettes
L. Microhematocrit centrifuge
M. 37° C incubator
N. Round cover glass, No. 1 (Corning)

PROCEDURE
1. Collect blood in a heparinized syringe (usually 8–15 ml from rabbits and 30 ml from humans).
2. Add one-third volume Gentran 75 to two-thirds volume whole blood. Mix and allow to settle out at 37° C for 45–90 min.
3. Collect leukocyte-rich plasma and wash once in RPMI–1640 by centrifuging at 150 g for 10 min.
4. Decant the tissue culture medium and count leukocytes on the hemocytometer, adjusting the volume with RPMI–1640 so that the cell concentration equals 1×10^7 cells/ml.
5. Partially assemble Mackaness chambers by securing bottom cover glass onto the chamber using silicone grease. On the inside of this cover glass place 2 dabs of silicone grease.
6. Fill capillaries to 20 μl mark. Seal with critoseal and spin 5 min at 600 g in a microhematocrit centrifuge.
7. Cut capillary tubes at the cell-fluid interface and mount cell-filled

capillaries onto the silicone dabs in the chamber. Seal top coverslip into place and fill chamber with tissue culture medium via injection ports. Avoid air bubbles. Seal injection ports with silicone grease.
8. Incubate in an ordinary incubator at 37° C for 24 hours.
9. After 24 hours of incubation, the migration area of leukocytes is mapped by projection microscopy and measured by planimetry. Migration patterns are easily compared by weighing their enlargement on paper at the same magnification. The evaluation of leukocyte migration is expressed by the following formula:

$$\text{\% migration in presence of antigen} = \frac{\text{average area of migration with antigen}}{\text{average area of migration without antigen}} \times 100$$

If emphasis is placed on the inhibitory effect of migration, the following formula is preferred:

$$\text{\% inhibition in presence of antigen} = \left(1 - \frac{\text{average area of migration with antigen}}{\text{average area of migration without antigen}}\right) \times 100$$

COMMENTS
A. Cells may be centrifuged either at room temperature or at 4° C.
B. With the addition of antibiotics to the tissue culture medium and with an incubation time of 24 hours, it is not necessary to maintain strict sterility during chamber assembly. The tissue culture medium and leukocyte-filled fluid must be kept sterile.
C. Antigen should be added to the tissue culture medium in the chamber and not to the media inside the capillary tubes. In this way, one population of cells can be assayed against several antigens.
D. The dose of antigen used depends on the particular antigen under study. Most proteins can be used easily at a concentration of 100 μg/ml without producing toxicity. Before using new antigens, various doses of antigen should be assayed on normal cells to determine the nontoxic effective dose.
E. Assays should be run in duplicate—two chambers with two capillaries per each antigen concentration to be tested.
F. When using peripheral leukocytes for migration inhibition assays it may be necessary to add an indicator population of macrophages to assure good migration. Guinea pig macrophages can be collected and 1×10^7 cells may then be added to 0.5×10^6 peripheral leukocytes in 0.5 ml of tissue culture medium.
G. Viability of leukocytes can be checked during all phases of the assay by staining the cells with Trypan Blue stain.

PROCEDURE FOR THE DETECTION OF HUMAN T-LYMPHOCYTES
(Method of Jondal et al. [46])
    Isolation of lymphocytes
1. Blood is collected in a heparinized syringe (Lipo-Hepin[Riker])
2. Lymphocytes were separated on a Ficoll-Isopaque gradient. The

composition is as follows: 9 gm Ficoll (Pharmacia) are dissolved in 100 ml distilled water, 20 ml Isopaque (Gallard-Schlesinger Chemical Corp.) are mixed with 25 ml distilled water. 96 parts of Ficoll are mixed with 40 parts of Isopaque.
3. 3 ml gradient were overlaid with 6–8 ml whole blood in plastic tubes and spun at 850 g for 30 min at 4° C.
4. The cells were removed from the interphase and washed 3 times with Hank's balanced salt solution (BSS) (centrifuged 10 min at 260 g).
5. The lymphocytes adjusted to a concentration of 4×10^6 cells/ml in Hank's BSS.

SHEEP RED BLOOD CELLS.   Sheep red blood cells were stored at 4° C in Alsever's solution, 1:1 and used until hemolysis occurred. The cells were washed twice and adjusted to a 0.5% suspension which is approximately 80×10^6 cells/ml in Hank's BSS. The cells were centrifuged 10 min at 260 g.

PROCEDURE FOR THE DETECTION OF ROSETTES
1. Mix 0.25 ml lymphocyte suspension with 0.25 ml of 0.5% sheep red blood cells and incubate at 37° C for 5 min.
2. Spin the mixed cell suspension at 200 g for 5 min and then incubate in ice for 1 to 2 hours, at 0 to 4° C.
3. Remove the supernatant and resuspend the top layer of the pellet gently by shaking.
4. Mount one drop of the suspension on the glass slide, cover with coverslip, and seal with clear nail polish or paraffin. Count the cells under the microscope until 200 lymphocytes are counted. All lymphocytes binding more than 3 sheep red cells (SRBC) are considered positive.
5. The suspension may be placed in a hemocytometer chamber and counted as above at $100 \times$ magnification.

INTERPRETATION.   The percentage of rosette-forming cells from peripheral blood in human cases varied from 52 to 81%.

DISCUSSION OF TECHNICAL ASPECTS
1. The incubation temperature and the ratio of lymphoid cells to red blood cells are found to be important factors.
2. Centrifugation should be carried out at 4° C. Care must be taken to keep the temperature at 4° C till counting and to resuspend the cells gently in order not to break the rosettes.
3. Incubation at 37° C for 1 hour will give rosette formation by antibody-secreting cells, which are the B-type lymphocytes.

The B-cells form rosettes composed of several layers of erythrocytes agglutinated by secreted antibodies. Clumping of nucleated cells that may hamper the rosette test can be prevented by using buffer without calcium and magnesium ions.

Detection of Rosette-Forming Human T Lymphocytes
(Method of Wybran et al. [110])

ISOLATION OF CIRCULATING LYMPHOCYTES
1. Peripheral circulating blood is collected in syringes coated with Lipo-Hepin (Riker)
2. Lymphocytes are separated on a gradient method described by R. Harris and E. O. Ukaejiofo [40]. The composition of the gradient is as follows: 24 parts 9% Ficoll (Pharmacia) 10 parts 34% Hypaque (sodium metrezoate, Winthrop)
3. 0.25 ml heparinized capillary blood or a 0.25 ml aliquot of defibrinated venous blood diluted 1 part in 3 parts phosphate-buffered saline solution (pH 7.3) is layered onto 2 ml of a mixture of 9% Ficoll-34% Hypaque gradient and centrifuged at 400 g for 40 min at 18° C. A clean suspension of lymphocytes should appear as a thin white layer immediately below the supernatant Ficoll-Hypaque interface.
4. The lymphocytes are washed 3 times with 10 ml phosphate-buffered saline solution, pH 7.3, and the concentration is adjusted to 5×10^6 cells/ml. Cells are centrifuged at 260 g for 10 min.

SHEEP RED CELLS.   Sheep red cells are stored in Alsever's solution 1:1. Before use, the cells are washed three times with phosphate-buffered saline solution (pH 7.3) and adjusted to a concentration of 4×10^7 cells/ml.

PROCEDURE
1. 0.05 ml sheep red cells is added to 0.05 ml of lymphocyte suspension. The final ratio desired is 8 sheep red cells for each lymphocyte.
2. The mixture is centrifuged at 200 g for 5 min, at room temperature.
3. The cells are gently resuspended and placed in a hemocytometer chamber. 500 lymphocytes are examined and the number of rosettes are counted.

INTERPRETATION.   A rosette-forming cell (RFC) is defined as a lymphocyte which has 3 or more sheep red blood cells adhering to its surface. The number of RFC is expressed per 100 lymphocytes. If no RFC are found after viewing 500 lymphocytes, at least 3,500 more lymphocytes are evaluated. Only cells with a morphology of lymphocytes were found to form rosettes. Results: Rosette-forming cells in 50 normal persons ranged from 4 to 40% with peripheral blood lymphocytes [110]. Updated methods and results have been published by Wybran et al. [111, 112].

Detection of Immunoglobulins on the Surface of B-Lymphocytes
(Method of Grey et al. [38])
Sedimentation of Lymphocyte-Rich Fraction
1. Blood is collected in a heparinized syringe (Lipo-Hepin [Riker]).
2. For a cleaner preparation of lymphocytes, blood is allowed to sediment in Dextran; red cells may be sedimented by the addition of ¼ volume of 5% Dextran M.W. 180,000 (Pharmacia), according to the procedure described by Schellekins et al. [86].
3. The lymphocyte-rich plasma is removed and centrifuged for 10 min at 400 g.
4. The cells are washed twice with Hank's balanced salt solution (BSS) and the cells are centrifuged for 10 min at 260 g.
5. Alternatively, blood may be sedimented with Plasmagel (Roger Bellon Lab.) which contains 3% soluble gelatin. Plasmagel is mixed with the heparinized blood 1:2.5 and blood is sedimented at 37° C for 30 min [90]. Plasma with white cells and gelatin is pipetted off and centrifuged at 750 g for 4 min. The cells are washed with Hank's BSS and centrifuged for 10 min at 260 g.

GRADIENT SEPARATION OF LYMPHOCYTES
1. A 1 ml suspension of lymphocytes in Hank's BSS is placed in 2 ml of 9% Ficoll-34% Hypaque gradient. The gradient consists of 24 parts 9% Ficoll (Pharmacia) and 10 parts Hypaque (Winthrop).
2. The gradient suspension is centrifuged at 400 g, for 20 min, at 18° C.
3. The lymphocytes are found at the white layer interface immediately below the supernatant Ficoll-Hypaque interface.
4. The lymphocytes are washed 3 times with 10 ml Hank's BSS and the concentration is adjusted to 5×10^6 cells. Cells are centrifuged at 260 g for 5 minutes.

IMMUNOFLUORESCENT STAINING PROCEDURE
1. To 0.1 ml suspension of $1-10 \times 10^6$ cells and 0.1 ml fluoresceinated antisera (anti-IgG, IgM, IgA or polyvalent antisera in a concentration of 1–3 mg/ml) are mixed.
2. The reaction mixture is incubated at room temperature for 30 min with occasional gentle shaking.
3. Cells are then washed 3 times in Hank's BSS and resuspended in 0.5 ml the same buffer.
4. A drop of the cell suspension is then placed on a slide, overlayered with a coverslip, and the edges sealed with melted paraffin or clear nail polish.
5. The preparation is examined with a fluorescence microscope.

Results: Approximately 28% of peripheral blood lymphocytes from normal individuals contained surface Ig and about 15% contained IgG, 6% IgA, and 8% IgM immunoglobulins [38].

TECHNICAL PRECAUTIONS. The procedures for the detection of surface immunoglobulins may seem simple, but certain precautions must be taken as follows.

A. The cells must be processed on a gradient so that live lymphocytes are separated from dead cells and debris. This is done by gradient separation [64, 105] and is helpful since dead lymphocytes will non-specifically absorb fluorescein or radioactive-labeled antibody [64, 71].

B. The fluorescein-labeled antibody should have a high antibody titer and the conjugate should not result in nonspecific staining.

C. The temperature of the reaction should be controlled in the procedure. Several investigators have performed the immunofluorescent staining of lymphocytes at 2 to 4° C [71, 105], and the reactions were viewed immediately after washing the cells at 4° C. The movement of anti Ig–Ig complex on the lymphocyte cell membrane depends on the amount of anti-Ig reacted with the surface Ig [105]. When cells are examined immediately after 4° C incubation and after exposure to fluorescein-labeled anti-Ig, an irregular fluorescence all around the cell membrane is seen. If the temperature is increased, the fluorescent reaction becomes concentrated in one pole of the cell [105].

References

1. Allansmith, M., McClellan, B. H., Butterworth, M., and Maloney, J. R. The development of immunoglobulin levels in man. *J. Pediatr.* 72:276, 1968.
2. Ammann, A. J., and Hong, R. Selective IgA deficiency: Presentation of 30 cases and a review of the literature. *Medicine* 50:223, 1971.
3. Bach, J. F., Dormont, J., Dardenne, M., and Balner, H. In vitro rosette inhibition by antihuman antilymphocyte serum. Correlation with skin graft prolongation in subhuman primates. *Transplantation* 8:265, 1969.
4. Baehner, R. L., and Nathan, D. G. Quantitative Nitroblue-Tetrazolium test in chronic granulomatous disease. *N. Engl. J. Med.* 278:971, 1968.
5. Basten, A., Sprent, J., and Miller, J. F. A. P. Receptor for antigen-antibody complexes used to separate T cells from B cells. *Nature [New Biol.]* 235:178, 1972.
6. Bellanti, J. A., and Schlegel, R. J. The diagnosis of immune deficiency diseases. *Pediatr. Clin. North Am.* 18:49, 1971.
7. Bergsma, D., and Good, R. A. *Immunologic Deficiency Diseases in Man.* New York: National Foundation, 1968.
8. Berkovich, S., Firkig, S., Brunell, P. A., Portugalaza, C., and Steiner, M. Effect of live attentuated mumps vaccine virus on the expression of tuberculin sensitivity. *J. Pediatr.* 80:84, 1972.
9. Berry, C. L., and Thompson, E. M. Clinico-pathological study of thymic dysplasia. *Arch. Dis. Child.* 43:579, 1968.
10. Berry, C. L. Histopathological findings in the combined immunity-deficiency syndrome. *J. Clin. Pathol.* 23:193, 1970.

98   I: Diagnostic Patterns of Immunologic Disorders

11. Bienenstock, J., and Perey, D. Y. E.   Immune mechanisms of mucosal resistance. *Med. Clin. North Am.* 56:391, 1972.
12. Bloom, B. R., and Glade, P. R.   *In Vitro Methods of Cell Mediated Immunity.* New York: Academic, 1971.
13. Bluestone, R., Gumpel, J. M., Goldberg, L. S., and Holborow, E. J. Salivary immunoglobulins in Sjögren's syndrome. *Int. Arch. Allergy Appl. Immunol.* 42:686, 1972.
14. Bonforte, R. J., Topilsky, M., Siltzbach, L. E., and Glade, P. R.   Phytohemagglutinin skin test: A possible in vivo measure of cell mediated immunity. *J. Pediatr.* 81:775, 1972.
15. Brain, P., Gordon, J., and Willetts, W. A.   Rosette formation by peripheral lymphocytes. *Clin. Exp. Immunol.* 6:681, 1970.
16. Brandtzaeg, P., Fjellanger, I., and Gjeruldsen, S. T.   Human secretory immunoglobulins: I. Salivary secretions from individuals with normal or low levels of serum immunoglobulins. *Scand. J. Haematol.* Suppl. No. 12:83, 1970.
17. Buckley, C. E., III, and Dorsey, F. C.   Serum immunoglobulin levels throughout the life span of the healthy man. *Ann. Intern. Med.* 75:653, 1971.
18. Buckley, R. H., Dees, S. C., and O'Fallon, W. M.   Serum immunoglobulins: I. Levels in normal children and in uncomplicated childhood allergy. *Pediatrics* 41:600, 1968.
19. Catalona, W. J., Taylor, P. T., Rabson, A. S., and Chretien, P. B.   A method for dinitrochlorobenzene contact sensitization—a clinicopathologic study. *N. Engl. J. Med.* 286:399, 1972.
20. Charette, R., and Komp, D. M.   NBT test and incubation temperature. *N. Engl. J. Med.* 287:991, 1972.
21. Coombs, R. R. A., Gurner, B. W., Janeway, C. A., Wilson, A. B., Gell, P. G. H., and Kelus, A. S.   Immunoglobulin determinants on the lymphocytes of normal rabbits: I. Demonstration by the mixed antiglobulin reaction of determinants recognized by anti-γ, anti-μ, anti-Fab and anti-allotype sera, anti-As4 and anti-As6. *Immunology* 18:417, 1970.
22. Coombs, R. R. A., Gurner, A. B. W., Wilson, A. B., Holm, G., and Lindgren, B.   Rosette formation between human lymphocytes and sheep red cells not involving immunoglobulin receptors. *Int. Arch. Allergy Appl. Immunol.* 39:658, 1970.
23. Cooper, M. D., Gabrielson, A. E., and Good, R. A.   Central and peripheral lymphoid tissue in immunologic processes and human disease. In S. H. Meyerson (ed.), *Lymph and the Lymphatic System.* Springfield, Ill.: Thomas, 1968, p. 276.
24. Davis, S. D., Schaller, J., and Wedgewood, R. J.   Antibody deficiency syndromes. In B. M. Kagen and E. R. Stiehm (eds.), *Immunologic Incompetence.* Chicago: Year Book, 1971, p. 179.
25. De Meo, A., and Anderson, B. R.   Defective chemotaxis associated with a serum inhibitor in cirrhotic patients. *N. Engl. J. Med.* 286:735, 1972.
26. *Diagnostic Standards and Classification of Tuberculosis.* New York: National Tuberculosis and Respiratory Disease Association, 1969, 12th ed.
27. Dickler, H. B., and Kunkel, H. G.   Interaction of aggregated γ-globulin with B lymphocytes. *J. Exp. Med.* 136:191, 1972.
28. Dische, M. R.   Lymphoid tissue and associated congenital malformations in thymic agenesis. *Arch. Pathol.* 86:312, 1968.

29. Douglas, S. D., and Fudenberg, H. H.   Host defense failure: The role of phagocytic dysfunction. *Hosp. Practice* 4:29, 1969.
30. Douwes, F. R.   Clinical value of NBT test. *N. Engl. J. Med.* 287:822, 1972.
31. Dukes, C. D., Parsons, J. L., and Stephens, C. A. L., Jr.   Use of acridine orange in lymphocyte transformation test. *Proc. Soc. Exp. Biol. Med.* 131:1168, 1969.
32. Edelson, P. J.   Diagnosis of immunologic deficiency in children. *Calif. Med.* 116:19, 1972.
33. Freedman, S. O.   Tuberculin testing and screening: A critical evaluation. *Hosp. Practice* 7:63, 1972.
34. Fudenberg, H. H., et al.   Primary immunodeficiencies. Report of a World Health Organization Committee. *Pediatrics* 47:927, 1971.
35. Gartner, O. T., Gilbert, R., Jr., and McDermott, M.   Anti A and Anti B antibodies in children. *J.A.M.A.* 201:206, 1967.
36. Gatti, R. A., and Good, R. A.   The immunological deficiency diseases. *Med. Clin. North Am.* 54:281, 1970.
37. Good, R. A., Biggar, W. D., and Park, B. H.   Immunodeficiency diseases in man. In B. Amos (ed.), *Progress in Immunology.* 1st International Congress of Immunology. New York: Academic, 1971, p. 699.
38. Grey, H. M., Rabellino, E., and Pirofsky, B.   Immunoglobulins on the surface of lymphocytes: IV. Distribution in hypogammaglobulinemia, cellular immune deficiency, and chronic lymphatic leukemia. *J. Clin. Invest.* 50:2368, 1971.
39. Gustafson, S. R., and Coursin, D. B.   Immunologic deficiency states. In S. R. Gustafson and D. B. Coursin (eds.), *Pediatric Patient.* Philadelphia: Lippincott, 1969, pp. 13–66, 262–271.
40. Harris, R., and Ukaejiofo, E. O.   Rapid preparation of lymphocytes for tissue typing. *Lancet* 2:327, 1969.
41. Holden, M., Dubin, M. R., and Diamond, P. H.   Frequency of negative intermediate strength tuberculin sensitivity in patients with active tuberculosis. *N. Engl. J. Med.* 285:1506, 1971.
42. Holmes, B., Page, A. R., and Good, R. A.   Studies of the metabolic activity of leucocytes from patients with a genetic abnormality of phagocytic function. *J. Clin. Invest.* 46:1422, 1967.
43. Hong, R.   Diseases of delayed hypersensitivity. In B. M. Kagen and E. R. Stiehm (eds.), *Immunologic Incompetence.* Chicago: Year Book, 1971.
44. Johansson, G. S. O., and Berg, T.   Immunoglobulin levels in healthy children. *Acta Paediatr. Scand.* 56:572, 1967.
45. Johnson, M. W., Maibach, H. I., and Salmon, S. E.   Skin reactivity in patients with cancer: Impaired delayed hypersensitivity or faulty inflammatory response? *N. Engl. J. Med.* 284:1255, 1971.
46. Jondal, M., Holm, G., and Wigzell, H.   Surface markers on human T and B lymphocytes: I. A large population of lymphocytes forming nonimmune rosettes with sheep red blood cells. *J. Exp. Med.* 136:207, 1972.
47. Jones, H. E., Miller, S. D., and Greenberg, J. H.   Measurement of tuberculin reactions. *N. Engl. J. Med.* 287:721, 1972.
48. Kadowaki, J., Nihira, M., and Nako, T.   Reduction of phytohemagglutinin-induced lymphocyte transformation in patients with measles. *Pediatrics* 45:508, 1970.

49. Karzon, D. T.   Smallpox vaccination in the United States: The end of an era. *J. Pediatr.* 81:601, 1972.
50. Kolb, W. P., Williams, T. W., and Granger, G. A.   Lymphocyte activation and lymphotoxin production. In B. R. Bloom and P. R. Glade (eds.), *In Vitro Methods of Cell Mediated Immunity.* New York: Academic, 1971.
51. Krivit, W., and Good, R. A.   Aldrich's syndrome (thrombocytopenia, eczema, and infection in infants). *A.M.A. J. Dis. Child.* 97:137, 1959.
52. Kupers, T. A., Petrich, J. M., Holloway, A. W., and St. Geme, J. W., Jr.   Depression of tuberculin delayed hypersensitivity by live attenuated mumps virus. *J. Pediatr.* 76:716, 1970.
53. Lamelin, J. P.   Inhibition of macrophage migration. In J. P. Revillard (ed.), *Cell Mediated Immunity—In Vitro Correlates.* Baltimore: University Park Press, 1971.
54. Lay, W. H., Mendes, N. F., Bianco, C., and Nussenzweig, V.   Binding of sheep red blood cells to a large population of human lymphocytes. *Nature* 230:531, 1971.
55. Lehrer, R. I.   The role of phagocytes in resistance to infection. *Calif. Med.* 114:17, 1971.
56. Levine, L., Wyman, L., Broderick, E. J., and Ipsen, J., Jr.   Field study in triple immunizations (diphtheria, pertussis, tetanus): Estimation of 3 antibodies in infant sera from single heel puncture using agglutination techniques. *J. Pediatr.* 57:836, 1960.
57. Lischer, H. W.   Viral suppression of delayed hypersensitivity. *J. Pediatr.* 80:174, 1972.
58. Louie, J. S., and Goldberg, L. S.   Lymphocyte-monocyte defect. *Clin. Exp. Immunol.* 11:469, 1972.
59. Matula, G., and Paterson, P. Y.   Spontaneous in vitro reduction of Nitroblue-Tetrazolium by neutrophils of adult patients with bacterial infection. *N. Engl. J. Med.* 285:311, 1971.
60. McClement, J. H.   The tuberculin test. *Hosp. Practice* 7:12, 1972.
61. Miller, D. R., and Kaplan, H. G.   Decreased nitrotetrazolium dye reduction in the phagocytes of patients receiving prednisone. *Pediatrics* 45:861, 1970.
62. Mims, J. W.   Mechanism of NBT test. *N. Engl. J. Med.* 287:49, 1972.
63. Najarian, J. S., and Feldman, J. D.   Passive transfer of tuberculin sensitivity by tritiated thymidine-labelled lymphoid cells. *J. Exp. Med.* 114:779, 1961.
64. Nossal, G. J. V., Warner, N. L., Lewis, H., and Sprent, J.   Quantitative features of a sandwich radioimmunolabeling technique for lymphocyte surface receptors. *J. Exp. Med.* 135:405, 1972.
65. Olson, G. B., South, M. A., Rawls, W. E., et al.   Phytohemagglutinin unresponsiveness of lymphocytes from babies with congenital rubella. *Nature* 214:695, 1967.
66. Park, B. H., Fikrig, S. M., and Smithwick, E. M.   Infection and Nitroblue-Tetrazolium reduction by neutrophils. *Lancet* 2:532, 1968.
67. Park, B. H., and Good, R. A.   NBT test stimulated. *Lancet* 2:616, 1970.
68. Park, B. H., South, M. A., Barrett, F. F., Montgomery, J. R., Heim, L. and Good, R. A.   The use of Nitroblue-Tetrazolium reduction (NBT) test in diagnosis and treatment of bacterial endocarditis. *Pediatr. Res.* 4:463, 1970.

69. Park, B. H.   The use and limitations of the Nitroblue-Tetrazolium test as an aid in the differential diagnosis of febrile disorders. *J. Pediatr.* 78:230, 1971.
70. Park, B. H., and Good, R. A.   A new micromethod for evaluating lymphocyte responses to phytohemagglutinin: Quantitative analysis of the function of thymus dependent cells. *Proc. Natl. Acad. Sci. U.S.A.* 69:371, 1972.
71. Pernis, B., Forni, L., and Amante, L.   Immunoglobulin spots on the surface of rabbit lymphocytes. *J. Exp. Med.* 132:1001, 1970.
72. Pernis, B., Forni, L., and Amante, L.   Immunoglobulins as cell receptors. *Ann. N.Y. Acad. Sci.* 190:420, 1971.
73. Perper, R. J., Zee, T. W., and Michelson, M. M.   Purification of lymphocytes and platelets by gradient centrifugation. *J. Lab. Clin. Med.* 72:842, 1968.
74. Public Health Service Recommendation on Smallpox Vaccination. *Morbidity and Mortality, Center for Disease Control* 20:339, 1971.
75. Quie, P. G., White, J. G., Holmes, B., and Good, R. A.   In vitro bacteriocidal capacity of human polymorphonuclear leukocytes: Diminished activity in chronic granulomatous diseases of childhood. *J. Clin. Invest.* 46:668, 1967.
76. Quie, P. G.   Chronic granulomatous disease of childhood. *Adv. Pediatr.* 16:287, 1969.
77. Rabellino, E. S., Colon, S., Grey, H. M., and Unanue, E. R.   Immunoglobulins on the surface of lymphocytes: I. Distribution and quantitation. *J. Exp. Med.* 133:156, 1971.
78. Rabellino, E., and Grey, H. M.   Immunoglobulins on the surface of lymphocytes: III. Bursal origin of surface immunoglobulins on chicken lymphocytes. *J. Immunol.* 106:1418, 1971.
79. Rocklin, R. E., Rosen, F. S., and David, J. R.   In vitro lymphocyte response of patients with immunologic deficiency diseases. *N. Engl. J. Med.* 282:1340, 1970.
80. Rocklin, R. E., and David, J. R.   Method for the production of MIF by human blood lymphocytes. In B. R. Bloom and P. R. Glade (eds.), *In Vitro Methods of Cell Mediated Immunity.* New York: Academic, 1971, p. 281.
81. Roff, M. C., Sternberg, M., and Taylor, R. B.   Immunoglobulin determinants on the surface of mouse lymphoid cells. *Nature* 225:553, 1970.
82. Rosenberg, S. A., and David, J. R.   In vitro assay for inhibition of migration of human blood leukocytes. In B. R. Bloom and P. R. Glade (eds.), *In Vitro Methods of Cell Mediated Immunity.* New York: Academic, 1971, p. 297.
83. Rümke, C. L.   Variability of results in differential counts on blood smears. *Triangle* 4:156, 1960.
84. Salvin, S. B., Nishio, J., and Gribick, M.   Lymphoid cells in delayed hypersensitivity: I. In vitro vs. in vivo responses. *Cell. Immunol.* 1:62, 1970.
85. Savilahte, E.   Immunoglobulin containing cells in the intestinal mucosa and immunoglobulins in the intestinal juice. *Clin. Exp. Immunol.* 11:415, 1972.
86. Schellekens, P. T. A., and Eijsvoogel, V. P.   Lymphocyte transformation in vitro: I. Tissue culture conditions and quantitative measurements. *Clin. Exp. Immunol.* 3:571, 1968.

87. Schur, P. H., Borel, H., Gelfand, E. W., Alper, C. A., and Rosen, F. Selective gamma-G globulin deficiencies in patients with recurrent pyogenic infection. *N. Engl. J. Med.* 283:631, 1970.
88. Schur, P. H.   Human gamma-G subclasses. In R. S. Schwartz (ed.), *Progress in Clinical Immunology.* New York: Grune & Stratton, 1972, vol. 1, p. 71.
89. Sell, S., and Gell, P. G. H.   Studies on rabbit lymphocytes in vitro: I. Stimulation of blast transformation with an antiallotype serum. *J. Exp. Med.* 122:425, 1965.
90. Shannon, D. C., Johnson, G., Rosen, F. S., and Austen, K. F.   Cellular reactivity to *Candida albicans* antigen. *N. Engl. J. Med.* 275:690, 1966.
91. Siegel, F. P., Pernis, P., and Kunkel, H. G.   Lymphocytes in human immunodeficiency states: A study of membrane associated immunoglobulin. *Eur. J. Immunol.* 1:482, 1972.
92. Smith, R. T., and Robbins, J. B.   Developmental aspects of immunity. In R. E. Cooke (ed.), *The Biologic Basis of Pediatric Practice.* New York: McGraw-Hill, 1968, p. 525.
93. Søborg, M.   The leukocyte migration technique for in vitro detection of cellular hypersensitivity in man. In B. R. Bloom and P. R. Glade (eds.), *In Vitro Methods of Cell Mediated Immunity.* New York: Academic, 1971, p. 289.
94. Southam, C. M., and Levin, A. G.   A quantitative Rebuck technique. *Blood* 27:734, 1966.
95. Stiehm, E. R., and Fudenberg, H. H.   Serum levels of immune globulins in health and disease: A survey. *Pediatrics* 37:715, 1966.
96. Stokes, J., Jr.   Pediatrics immunization and the new academy schedule. *Hosp. Practice* 7:127, 1972.
97. Stoop, J. W., Zegers, B. J. M., Sander, P. C., and Ballieux, R. E. Serum immunoglobulin levels in healthy children and adults. *Clin. Exp. Immunol.* 4:101, 1969.
98. Straus, R. R., Paul, B. B., and Sharra, A. J.   Effect of phenylbutazone on phagocytosis and intracellular killing of guinea pig polymorphonuclear leukocytes. *J. Bacteriol.* 96:1982, 1968.
99. Sultizeanu, D.   Antibody-like receptors on immunocompetent cells. *Curr. Top. Microbiol. Immunol.* 54:1, 1971.
100. Taylor, W. F., Qaqundah, B. Y., Fong, S. W., and Wharton, E. B. Qualitative assay of humoral immunity by saline isohemagglutinin titers. *Ann. Allergy* 29:377, 1971.
101. Tomasi, T. B., Jr., and Bienenstock, J.   Secretory immunoglobulins. In F. J. Dixon, Jr., and H. G. Kunkel (eds.), *Advances in Immunology.* New York: Academic, 1968.
102. Tomasi, T. B., Jr.   Secretory immunoglobulins. *N. Engl. J. Med.* 287: 500, 1971.
103. Uffelman, J. A., Engelhard, W. E., and Jotliff, C. R.   Quantitation of immunoglobulin in normal children. *Clin. Chim. Acta* 28:185, 1970.
104. Unanue, E. R., Grey, H. M., Rabellino, E., Campbell, P., and Schmidtke, J.   Immunoglobulins on the surface of lymphocytes: II. The bone marrow as the main source of lymphocytes with detectable surface bound immunoglobulin. *J. Exp. Med.* 133:1188, 1971.
105. Unanue, E. R., Perkins, W. D., and Karnovsky, M. J.   Ligand-induced movement of lymphocyte membrane macromolecules: I. Analysis by

immunofluorescence and ultrastructural radioautography. *J. Exp. Med.* 136:885, 1972.
106. Valentine, F.   Lymphocytic transformation: The proliferation of human blood lymphocytes stimulated by antigen in vitro. In B. R. Bloom and P. R. Glade (eds.), *In Vitro Methods of Cell Mediated Immunity.* New York: Academic, 1971, p. 445.
107. Vitetta, E., Baur, A. S., and Uhr, J. W.   Cell surface immunoglobulin: II. Isolation and characterization of immunoglobulin from mouse splenic lymphocytes. *J. Exp. Med.* 134:224, 1971.
108. Waldmann, T. A., Strober, W., and Blaese, R. M.   Immunodeficiency and malignancy—various immunologic deficiencies of man and the role of immune processes in the control of malignant disease. *Ann. Intern. Med.* 77:605, 1972.
109. Windhorst, D. B.   Functional defects of neutrophils. *Adv. Intern. Med.* 16:329, 1970.
110. Wybran, J., Carr, M. C., and Fudenberg, H. H.   The human rosette forming cell as a marker of a population of thymus derived cells. *J. Clin. Invest.* 51:2537, 1972.
111. Wybran, J., and Fudenberg, H. H.   Tymus derived rosette-forming cells in various human disease states: cancer, lymphoma, bacterial and viral infections and other diseases. *J. Clin. Invest.* 52:1026, 1973.
112. Wybran, J., Levin, A. S., Spitler, L. E., and Fudenberg, H. H.   Rosette-forming cells, immunologic deficiency diseases and transfer factor, *N. Engl. J. Med.* 288:710, 1973.

4

The Role of Complement and Other Biochemical Mediators in Immunologic Disease

Ernest S. Tucker, III

The Importance of Biochemical Mediators in the Pathogenesis of Immune Injury

Our current understanding of the important factors in the pathogenesis of immunologic tissue injury is based on knowledge of biochemical mediators which are activated by those reactions. These biochemical factors may originate as cleavage products of parent molecules in the circulation, or they may be released from the storage vacuoles of cells. They produce a variety of physiologic effects. The varied effects may be constriction of smooth muscle, increase in vascular permeability, hydrolytic digestion of tissues, intense pain, or cellular infiltrates of tissue.

In the discussion of reaginic hypersensitivity in Chapter 5, mediators such as histamine, slow-reacting substance of anaphylaxis, and eosinophil chemotactic factor are discussed. These substances are released because of the immune reaction of the atopic or reaginic type. In this chapter, the varied factors which are generated in the course of complement activation and their physiologic effects will be described. A recurring theme will be that activation of biochemical mediators is the principal means by which immune reactions cause tissue injury and disease. As a corollary theme, it will be apparent that when these mediators can be blocked with inhibitors or pharmacologic antagonists, much of the potential tissue injury can be avoided.

It is appropriate to divide the discussion of biochemical mediators into two categories. One category deals with those mediators which provoke the immediate type of immune reaction, or the so-called *acute allergic* reactions, and the other category is concerned with those factors which play an important role in the pathogenesis of delayed or cellular hypersensitivity. The basis of this division seems appropriate since the

104

acute reactions are those which are initiated by the reaction of circulating antibody with antigen, while the immune reaction of delayed sensitivity is triggered by the interaction between sensitized lymphocytes and antigen. The acuteness of the immediate type reaction is a consequence of the potent physiologic effects of biochemical substances which are activated or released, while delayed reactions exhibit a more prolonged time course for cell recruitment before full development of the reaction.

In general, it can be noted that intense vascular changes are characteristic of the acute allergic reactions. These changes produce the findings which have long been associated with inflammation, notably erythema or rubor, increase in local temperature or calor, pain or dolor, and swelling or tumor due to changes in vascular permeability. In addition, the development of tissue necrosis occurs rapidly in certain acute reactions following intravascular thrombosis and influx of polymorphonuclear leukocytes which release their destructive hydrolytic enzymes. Permeability changes and necrosis may also develop in the delayed type (cellular sensitivity) reactions, but the period of onset is prolonged and the degree of change is much less striking in its time course of development.

Biochemical Factors Important in Acute Immunologic Reactions

There are four categories of biochemical factors which are important in the pathogenesis of acute immunologic reactions: (a) vasoactive factors, (b) chemoattractants, (c) hydrolytic enzymes, and (d) activators of proteolytic enzyme systems. These factors may be either found in the plasma or released from cells as a consequence of the immune reaction. These acute reactions can be further divided into two groups: those that are dependent on the serum complement system for their pathologic effects, and those that are not. Each of these reactions is characterized by a certain class of antibody which is involved in the tissue response. In those where antibody of the IgE class is important, the reactions are not complement dependent [46a] and appear to be on the basis of the physiologic effects of factors released from mast cells or basophil leukocytes (reaginic reactions). Where the antibody is of the IgG or IgM class, activation of the complement system appears to play a central role in the pathogenesis of the immune injury [46, 47, 74]. Indeed, in many instances, the pleomorphic nature of the immune response to a given antigen is such that both types of acute allergic reaction may be encountered in a given disease. In other situations, the singular nature of the reaction may be outstanding and involve only one of these two types of processes. Since Chapter 5 deals with the pathogenesis of those disorders due to antibody of the IgE type, the discussions of acute reactions in this chapter will focus on the complement-dependent types of immune injury.

Serum Complement as an Immunologic Mediator System

The serum complement system of man and higher vertebrates is composed of 11 separate components [10, 72]. Each of these components exhibits activity in a pattern of sequential interaction similar to the "cascade" system which has been described in blood coagulation [71]. Following initial activation, each component exerts limited proteolytic activity in a sequential fashion on a subsequent component until there has been activation of the entire system. Most of these components have been isolated and characterized in terms of their physicochemical characteristics as well as of their biochemical and biological activities. Table 4-1 summarizes some of the physicochemical data for the various components of the complement system. It has been found that a variety of biologic activities are associated with activation of the complement system. These activities have been associated with either individual components or fragments cleaved from these components as the result of limited proteolysis. It is because of their biologic or physiologic effects that the complement system assumes such importance in the pathogenesis of certain forms of acute immunologic tissue injury. Before proceeding to a discussion of the biologic activities of complement components, it is necessary to discuss the sequence of activation of the components with regard to the initiating factors, interactions, and biochemistry of cleavage products produced.

Sequential Activation of Complement Components by the Intrinsic (Classic) Mode of Activation

The system which has been used to determine complement activity, following its discovery by Bordet in 1898, has been the phenomenon of immune hemolysis [8]. Since the description of a "complement fixation test" in 1901 by Bordet and Gengou, the amount of complement has been estimated by a dilution of serum to a point where the capacity for immune hemolysis is abolished. In this way, a crude estimate of complement activity could be gained and comparisons could be made among sera.

The hemolytic system which is commonly used today utilizes sheep red blood cells which are washed and coated with an antibody called a *hemolysin*. The hemolysin is prepared in rabbits by injection with sheep red cells. The sheep cells which are treated with hemolysin are referred to as *sensitized cells*. Since the hemolysin is of the appropriate class (IgG or IgM), it will "fix" complement when mixed with serum [46, 73]. If there is sufficient complement, hemolysis of the cells will occur and release of hemoglobin will ensue. In our current understanding of complement activation, it is known that all 11 components of

Table 4-1. Physical and Chemical Characteristics of the Molecular Components of the Human Serum Complement System.

Component		Synonym	Mol. Wt.	Sed. Coefficient	Electrophoretic Mobility	Serum Conc. μg/ml
C1	C1q	—	4×10^5	11	γ-2	100– 200
	C1r	—		7	β	
	C1s	C1 esterase	8×10^4	4	α-2	20
C4 ⎫		β 1E globulin	2.29×10^5	10	β-1	430
C2 ⎬-----C3 convertase			1.15×10^3	6	β-2	5
C3		β 1C globulin	1.85×10^5	9.5	β-1	800–1,500
C5		β 1F globulin		8.7	β-1	75
C6		Trimolecular				
		complex		5.6	β-2	10
C7				6.7	β-2	
C8		—	1.5×10^5	8	γ-1	
C9		—	7.9×10^4	4.5	α-2	1–2

complement are required to produce this immune hemolysis [72, 85]. Indeed, this hemolytic system can be adapted as a method for analysis of individual complement components by preparation of so-called cellular intermediates containing components from purified preparations but omitting the one under analysis.

Experimental work in the past two decades has produced considerable data which has clarified much of the complexity of the immune hemolytic reaction. From these studies, it has become apparent that the cell membrane surface is an important steric factor in the process of complement fixation or activation. The cell membrane appears to act as a nidus upon which the interaction of complement components can take place. Its discovery, therefore, as a system for demonstrating complement activity appears to have been quite fortuitous.

In the initial reaction of complement in the classic mode, the antibody is fixed to sites on the cell membrane and appears to sustain a distortion of the Fc portion of the molecule so that binding of the subunit C1q takes place. C1q becomes activated and, in turn, binds another subunit C1r [33]. These two components together, in tandem with the antibody, activate a third subunit of the first component of complement known as C1s. C1s is then bound together with C1q and C1r in the presence of calcium to form a trimolecular complex which is known as C1a or C$\overline{\text{I}}$* [41]. This active first component of complement

* Bar above designated complement component indicates actuation of the molecule (*Bull. W.H.O.* 39:935–938, 1968).

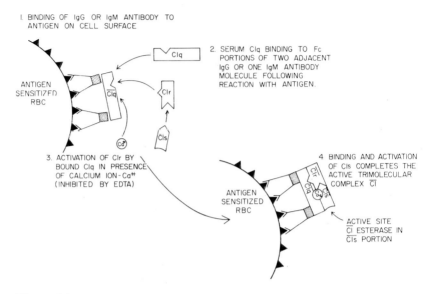

Figure 4-1
Initial activation of C1 of the classic pathway of complement.

exhibits esterolytic activity which is associated with the C1s subunit [41, 58]. This sequence of activation of C1 is demonstrated in Fig. 4-1. The active C1 then proceeds to produce a cleavage of C4 from plasma which generates two fragments known as C4a and C4b. C4b binds the cell surface to a limited extent [76]. The remaining C4b and the C4a fragment decay to an inactive state in the serum. This activation sequence of C4 by C̄1 is demonstrated in Fig. 4–2.

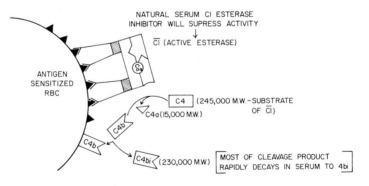

Figure 4-2
Activation of C4 by C1 in the classic complement pathway.

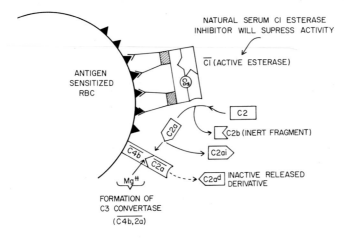

Figure 4-3
C2 activation to form C3 convertase of the classic complement pathway.

Almost at the same time as it exhibits activity on C4, C1 esterase (C$\overline{1}$) also produces a cleavage of C2 from the plasma [84]. This results in the production of two fragments, one known as C2a, and the other as C2b. C2a becomes bound in a bimolecular complex with C4b in the presence of magnesium (Mg^{++}) and results in the generation of a new enzyme activity referred to as C3 convertase [77]. This convertase will act upon C3 to produce cleavage of that component from the plasma. The activation of C2 and formation of the C3 convertase is diagrammatically demonstrated in Fig. 4-3.

The complex known as C3 convertase formed by C4b and C2a has a short half-life under in vitro conditions of about 12 to 15 min at 37° C, and presumably a similar short half-life in vivo [83]. While this enzyme is active, it produces cleavage of C3 yielding two fragments known as C3a and C3b [74]. In this instance, the small fragment C3a is found to exhibit biologic activities referred to as chemotactic and anaphylatoxic [6, 15, 96]. These activities will be discussed in more detail later. The C3b becomes fixed to the cell surface and it also participates in a variety of biologic activities, including immune adherence, conglutinin reaction, phagocytosis, and adherence to antigen-antibody complexes [18, 43, 79]. Most importantly, however, for the subsequent activation of other components, the C3b, in concert with C$\overline{4b,2a}$, produces cleavage of C5, which begins the subsequent activation of the remainder of the complement components. The schematic diagram of C3 activation is shown in Fig. 4-4.

The cleavage of C5 by the C$\overline{3b}$ produces two fragments known as C5b and C5a. The C5a fragment, as will be discussed later, also ex-

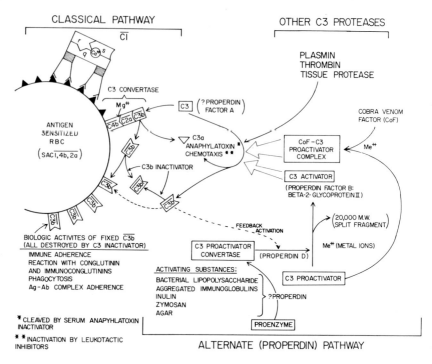

Figure 4-4
Modes of C3 activation and biologic activities.

hibits anaphylatoxic and chemotactic activities [6, 15]. The C5b fragment is fixed to the cell membrane and appears to be important in promoting phagocytosis in addition to activation of C6. However, it rapidly decays from the surface to an inactive C5i fragment that is released into the plasma. The C5b, while fixed to the cell surface, prepares a site for addition of C6 from the plasma, and C6 in turn allows for fixation of C7. It should be noted that there is a serum inactivator which can neutralize the C6 which has become bound [88]. The trimolecular complex of $\overline{C5,6,7}$ may dissociate as a trimolecular unit from the surface and exhibit chemotactic activity [97]. This will be discussed later.

With the addition of C7, the attachment of C8 to the cell membrane follows, and at this point a limited degree of lysis begins [65]. This lysis appears to be due to an attack on the integrity of the phospholipid structure of the cell membrane which is markedly enhanced by the attachment of C9 [54, 65]. A similar enhancement can be induced by chelating agents such as phenanthroline. At this point, the attack on the cell membrane is substantial and marked disruption occurs with leakage of cell contents so that the osmotic balance of the cell is distorted and

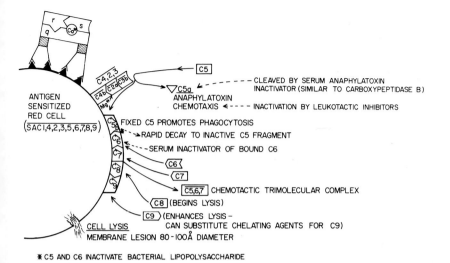

Figure 4-5
Activation of the terminal complement components and their biologic activities.

rupture of the cell occurs. The sequence of activation of the terminal components leading to cell lysis is schematically depicted in Fig. 4-5.

Fig. 4-4 emphasizes C3 as a molecule of central importance which is activated by another system in the serum distinct from the early reacting complement components. This system was initially called the alternate pathway of complement activation, but it is now known to contain factors which had previously been identified as part of the properdin system, so that the two now appear to be synonymous [37].

Activation of Complement by the Extrinsic (Alternate) Mode or Properdin System

The phenomenon of cell lysis unrelated to immune phenomena was recognized for some time, both in the experimental laboratory and in instances of the human disease known as paroxysmal nocturnal hemoglobinuria (PNH) [40]. It was noted that individuals with the disease PNH exhibited a defect in the integrity of their red cell membranes which caused an increased degree of fragility. In the experimental laboratory, the spontaneous lysis of guinea pig red cells had been noted in the presence of certain materials such as agar, zymosan, and a factor from the venom of the cobra, *Naja naja* [5, 38]. This phenomenon did not appear to be related to an immune reaction, but because of strong suspicion of complement contributing to the cell lysis, studies were undertaken to determine its role in those reactions. These studies led to the observation that the terminal components of complement had been activated in much the same way as occurred in the classic system of immune hemolysis. There was, however, no evidence of activation of the early-reacting complement components. A similar activation of terminal components was found to occur in the human disease PNH [40, 103]. The convergence of these findings clearly indicated that a system in the fluid phase of plasma or serum was capable of initiating activation of the terminal complement components. It has now been clearly demonstrated that this plasma system, called the alternate system of complement activation, resulted in the cleavage of native C3 with production of two fragments, C3a and C3b, identical with those fragments produced by C3 convertase cleavage [39]. The C3a fragment produced shows anaphylatoxic and chemotactic activity, while the C3b factor exhibits an affinity for fixation to cellular membranes and can cause lysis of nonsensitized red blood cells under appropriate conditions.

It was thus apparent that the interdigitation of the classic and alternate systems came at the point of C3 activation. In a recent flurry of experimental work, many factors of the alternate system have been isolated and their sequence of interaction determined, so that currently there is a rather clear understanding of the workings of this system [39, 59, 75, 78]. As mentioned, the components of the alternate pathway are identical with many of the individual properdin factors, and it now appears that the alternate pathway is essentially the properdin system [37, 75, 78].

This extrinsic system appears to be activated by various substances which include endotoxin (bacterial lipopolysaccharide), aggregated immunoglobulins, especially of the IgA class, inulin, zymosan, and agar [30, 39]. The mechanism of initial activation is unknown, but there is some evidence that it proceeds by activation of the molecule properdin itself. Properdin, then, causes conversion of a proenzyme into an active molecule which is known as C3 proactivator convertase. This convertase is thought to be the molecule properdin factor D [86]. This molecule then converts another proenzyme which is known as C3 proactivator into the active enzyme C3 activator as a result of cleaving a fragment of approximately 20,000 molecular weight from the C3 proactivator [75]. This C3 activator is known to be identical with properdin factor B and also identical with the beta-2-glycoprotein II previously purified by Heidi and Haupt [39]. Studies of this system have now revealed that the C3 activator is increased in quantity as a result of feedback effect by the C3b cleavage product on the properdin D enzyme [75, 86]. In addition, it has also been determined that the C3 proactivator may combine with the cobra venom factor (Cof) in the presence of metal ions to produce a complex which exerts a proteolytic action on C3 which is also identical to that of the C3 activator [39, 75]. Once there has been cleavage of C3, with release of the C3a fragment and C3b fragment, the terminal complement sequence can then be activated by the same terminal reactions that occur in the classic system. The interactions of molecules in the alternate pathway and classic system are demonstrated in the diagram in Fig. 4-4.

It should be mentioned that, in addition to activation by the alternate pathway, cleavage of C3 may also follow release and activation of enzymes from tissues and plasma [98], including plasmin, thrombin, and various tissue proteases which are released from injured cells. As a result of this C3 cleavage, products identical to C3a and C3b are produced. This affords another point of interrelationship between the complex and varied proteolytic systems in the plasma and tissues of vertebrates.

Biologic Activities of Activated Components of Complement

There are diverse biologic activities associated with the activated complement components which are depicted in Fig. 4-6. The first of these to be considered is virus inactivation, demonstrated in vitro, in which the importance of antiviral antibody, as well as complement components C1 and C4, has been demonstrated [80]. The mechanism proposed has been that antibody produces binding of the early reacting components of

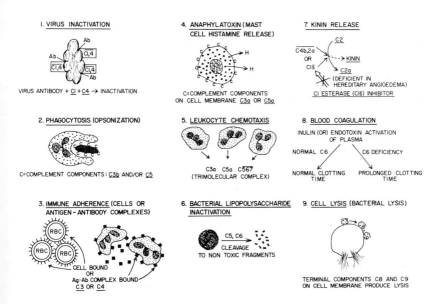

Figure 4-6
Biologic activities of complement components.

complement to the virus surface protein and renders it incapable of cellular invasion through the plasma membrane.

Another activity of substantial importance in host defense associated with active components is that of phagocytosis or opsonization. The complement components C3b and C5 have demonstrated activity in this function in studies of phagocytosis in vitro. In cases where inherited defects in C3 and C5 have been found, the problem of severe and recurrent infection has clearly suggested a defect of phagocytosis in vivo [70, 86]. The mechanism involved in phagocytosis appears to be fixation of complement components to the surface of the particle either as a result of immune reaction on the particle surface, or as a fluid phase reaction producing the activated component, which then attaches to the particle surface. Once the components are on the particle surface and encounter a phagocyte, there are receptor areas on the plasma membrane of the cell which react with the components and apparently induce engulfment of the particle [34, 43, 69].

Another complement reaction which has been utilized in assays in vitro and which may be of great significance in vivo is that of immune adherence. This can be demonstrated where complement components C3 and C4 are on a cell surface or bound to antigen-antibody complexes [43, 79]. For example, when the C3b component is "fixed" on the red cell surface, a close contact of such coated red cells causes them to adhere through interaction with the specific receptor areas on the cell membranes. Under similar conditions, the binding of antigen-antibody complexes containing C3 or C4 occurs on the surfaces of different cells such as platelets and polymorphonuclear leukocytes. A similar type of adherence can be demonstrated where there is immobilization of the immune reactants on a particulate surface. In these situations, there is adherence between the cells and the particulate surface containing the bound immune reactants and complement components.

A fourth complement activity of potential biologic significance is that which produces histamine release from mast cells or basophils. This activity is associated with the fragments C3a and C5a [15, 24]. The activity has been called anaphylatoxic since it was initially thought to be of importance in systemic anaphylaxis; however, in view of recent studies, it does not now appear important in that reaction [31].

Perhaps one of the most important activities relates to the production of immune tissue injury. This activity is that which causes emigration of neutrophils to tissue sites where the immune reactants are localized. This chemotactic activity is exhibited by the fragments C3a, C5a, and the trimolecular complex $\overline{C5,6,7}$, all of which may be generated as a consequence of activation of complement by either the classic or the alternate pathways [6, 29, 86, 96]. The tissue damage in these reactions develops after the leukocytes arrive and discharge their granules containing various hydrolytic enzymes, which digest and destroy the tissue. The granule release from neutrophils appears to involve a reaction similar to immune adherence where there is membrane stimulation by complement components fixed to the immune reactants [43].

The experimental findings of protection afforded the normal animal injected with bacterial endotoxin have been contrasted with the lethal effect of endotoxin in C5-deficient mice and in rabbits deficient in C6. It appears that the complement components afford protection by their breakdown of endotoxin similar to the action of a detergent, and thus they detoxify the endotoxic lipopolysaccharide [48]. This detoxification has been demonstrated in vitro and seems to explain the action of C5 and C6 in vivo.

In addition to the activated complement components, various inhibitors of the complement system also occur in plasma [1, 10, 22, 86, 88, 91, 99]. The total number and the spectrum of these inhibitors has yet to be discerned. In one instance, such an inhibitor has been recognized primarily because of its deficiency in a particular disease state. This inhibitor, known as C1 esterase inhibitor, is deficient in the disease known as hereditary angioneurotic edema [26]. From the previous discussion it can be recalled that C1 esterase produces cleavage of C2, giving rise to the products C2a and an inert fragment C2b. There also appears a polypeptide which exhibits physiologic activity similar to that of bradykinin [57]. Because of the normal presence of C1 esterase inhibitor, this reaction apparently is limited in extent and no physiologic changes are produced. However, in the absence of this inhibitor, large amounts of the kinin are generated, and in those tissue sites where reactivity occurs, considerable vascular permeability ensues, resulting in marked edema. The edema may produce airway obstruction if it occurs in the larynx and trachea. Under such circumstances, it can cause a life-threatening situation. The circumstances which trigger such a reaction are not known, but the lack of this inhibitor of C1 esterase is a definite finding in those cases.

Recent studies in experimental animals have demonstrated a role for complement in blood coagulation involving a pathway which can be activated by either inulin or endotoxin [104]. The findings to date indicate that the complement component C6 participates in release of platelet factor III in blood coagulation. Discovery of the importance of complement in blood coagulation was made when comparing clotting time in normal rabbits versus those who were C6 deficient. In these experiments, when the activating substance was inulin or endotoxin, a prolonged clotting time was observed in the C6-deficient rabbits in contrast to the normal. Clotting times using kaolin, glass, or diatomaceous earth as activators, however, gave normal clotting times in both normal and C6-deficient rabbits. These differences in clotting time with different activators indicate that the role in complement in blood coagulation involved a system different from the known intrinsic coagulation system of plasma.

The last activity of complement to be discussed is that of cell lysis. It has been pointed out that, in studies of the sequence of activation of complement components, cell lysis serves as the prime indicator of complement activity and depends on the addition of the terminal components C8 and C9, which attack the cell membrane, producing disruption. Under certain conditions, the phenomenon may result in intravascular destruction of erythrocytes because of immune hemolysis. In other instances, it may serve a protective effect when causing lysis of bacterial cells in the host. Bacterial lysis occurs when there has been reaction of the bacteria with antibody and fixation of complement. The probability also exists that the alternate pathway produces sufficient active C3 to cause lysis of bacteria as a means of natural nonimmune protection [20].

In summary, it can be said that the biologic activities of complement are of sufficient diversity not only to account for its role as a mediator of disease in the immune destruction of tissue, but also as an important part of host defense in infections and inflammatory processes.

Participation of Complement in Experimental Immunologic Tissue Injury

There are two forms of experimental acute immunologic tissue injury which have been well studied as regards the role of complement: the Arthus reaction and acute immunologic glomerulonephritis. In both situations, the immune reactants have been defined, the sites of their reaction localized to certain areas of tissue, and the time course of the reaction measured, along with morphologic studies of the cellular changes in the tissues [12, 16, 42, 93]. Most of these studies have been carried out in animals which were either deficient in certain complement components or which had been experimentally depleted of certain components. A method of depleting the third component of complement by treatment of experimental animals with cobra venom factor (Cof) has allowed the definitive assessment of the role of complement in these immune reactions [5, 23, 72]. By this treatment, the complement hemolytic activity of the animal can be abolished due to the marked reduction in the level of plasma C3. This depletion can be accomplished for periods of time of a few days without apparent harm or injury to the animal. Under various conditions of study, the control animals exhibit extensive lesions of tissue necrosis and cellular infiltrates. Those animals which are depleted of complement fail to show significant tissue injury in spite of clear evidence that the immune reaction is taking place. In the Arthus reaction, the depleted animals show no evidence of vasculitis, edema, or necrosis in the skin, and in the examples of immunologic glomerulonephritis there is marked reduction of proteinuria and no evidence of glomerular destruction in the presence of immunofluorescent localization of antibody in the glomerular basement membrane [12, 13, 42].

The contribution of neutrophils to the tissue injury has also been evaluated in a similar fashion. Instead of complement depletion, animals are subjected to depletion of their circulating neutrophils by prior treatment with alkylating agents such as nitrogen mustard (HN_3). This drug effectively reduces the total of circulating neutrophils when given 3 to 4 days before instituting immunologic injury. In animals whose neutrophil counts are reduced to levels less than 50 per cubic millimeter, no evidence of tissue necrosis can be observed in either the Arthus or glomerulonephritic lesions [12, 16, 42]. However, moderate edema and proteinuria are often observed, apparently due to a permeability reaction. The hemorrhagic necrosis normally seen in the Arthus lesion is prevented in the absence of the polymorphonuclear leukocytes. These findings correlate well with the complement studies and have confirmed the importance of the lack of neutrophil emigration in the complement depletion studies. In these studies, chemotaxis failed to occur.

These studies serve to clarify the participation of the complement and neutrophils in these forms of acute immune injury. They provide a basis for our understanding of pathogenic factors in certain human diseases. As models, they allow critical studies on human disease to be carried out and interpreted in accord with the experimental data. Recent studies of human disease, especially glomerulonephritis, have revealed findings parallel to those of the experimental models [60, 62]. These studies have included immunofluorescence of renal biopsies to detect deposits of antibody and complement, evaluation of complement components in the serum, and evaluation of the morphology of the tissue injury [45, 53]. They have given considerable insight into the pathogenesis of human renal diseases when interpreted within the context of the data from experimental animal studies. It is through this twofold approach of experiment in the laboratory and observation in the clinic that a better understanding of these immunologic diseases in man has been produced. This understanding is being extended to the study of many human diseases that are suspected to be due to immunologic injury. The appreciation of the role of mediators in the diseases rather than a singular focus on the immune reaction itself has considerably enhanced the outlook for control of these diseases through inhibitors and antagonists of these mediators.

Role of the Complement System in the Lesions of Human Immunologic Disease

The varied biologic effects of the complement system suggest that they are important in the pathogenesis of immunologic disease. As described above, this can be demonstrated experimentally. It can also be shown on a comparative basis in animals and in man.

There are three major types of disease where complement bears a relationship to the development of the tissue injury. These are immune hemolytic anemia, immune vasculitis, and different forms of immunologic glomerulonephritis.

Hemolytic Anemia

The pathogenesis of immune hemolytic anemia parallels the in vitro phenomenon of immune lysis of red blood cells [61]. A commonly encountered type of immune hemolytic anemia in man is the hemolytic disease of the newborn due to fetal-maternal blood incompatibility [100]. The most common antigens involved are those of the Rh system and the ABO system. The basis for the development of an immune reaction is due to the fact that the fetus possesses antigens on its red cells which provoke an antibody response in the mother. A prior episode of sensitization during a previous pregnancy is an important factor in subsequent development of high titers of antibody against the Rh and ABO antigens.

The stimulus for increased antibody production is due to placental microhemorrhages which allow mixing of the fetal and maternal blood. Once exposure has occurred, an increased antibody response on reexposure may be sufficient to cause severe hemolytic anemia. Because the second response is of the anamnestic type, the antibody produced is of the IgG class and of a molecular size which will cross the placenta and enter the fetal circulation. Once the antibody enters the circulation of the fetus, it reacts with the antigens of the red cell membrane, and complement fixation ensues with lysis of the cells. Because of the hemolysis, the infant becomes severely anemic and accumulates bilirubin pigment from the red cell breakdown which can cause damage of the central nervous system.

The blood of infants with hemolytic anemia characteristically exhibits a positive direct and often a seropositive indirect Coombs' antiglobulin reaction. This occurs with antiglobulin reagents reacting primarily with immunoglobulins as well as with complement components on the cell surface. Indeed, the presence of a positive Coombs' test in the presence of a rising serum bilirubin should lead one to suspect this as a possible diagnosis. In other situations, the development of hemolytic anemia is less clearly defined. Often they may be related to drug therapy where the drug functions as a hapten and becomes attached to the red cell surface [61]. It may provoke an antibody response in the host, causing production of complement fixing antibodies that react with the drug [61, 81]. In other situations, the cause may be more obscure. Hemolytic anemia may be encountered as a result of immune complex formation in the circulation which produces activated complement components that become attached to the red cells and produce hemolysis. This has been referred to as an "innocent bystander" type of reaction [103].

Vasculitis

The contribution of complement to the development of immune vasculitis has been well studied in experimental animals [11]. Observations on the pathogenesis of vasculitis in humans appear to correlate well with data derived from experimental studies [35, 36, 89]. The initial event in the development of vasculitis appears to be a localization of immune reactants within or surrounding the walls of the blood vessels. This localization can be produced in an animal which has been actively or passively sensitized to various antigens.

The prototype of this form of injury has been exemplified in the Arthus reaction. In the Arthus reaction, the sensitive animal is injected with antigen into the subcutaneous tissue and, on diffusion from the injection site, the antigen will encounter antibody within the vessel wall as it contacts the blood plasma [12]. At optimal concentrations of antigen and antibody, a precipitate will form and complement fixation will occur. As a consequence of complement fixation, chemotactic factors are produced and cause a heavy influx of leukocytes [16] into the blood vessel wall to the site of the antigen-antibody precipitate. On arrival, these leukocytes, mostly neutrophils, release their granules containing a variety of hydrolytic enzymes. These enzymes cause marked destruction of the tissue.

Histologically the lesion exhibits extensive necrosis of the vessel wall and surrounding tissue. Disseminated vasculitis can be induced experimentally following induction of circulating immune complex formation [25]. This may be achieved by an injection into the circulating blood of antigens which stimulate a substantial antibody response. Approximately 4 to 7 days following injection, the antibody appears in the circulation, and when it combines with circulating antigen, immune complexes will form. Usually, the antibody is of the IgM class and exhibits considerable complement fixing activity. These circulating complexes are of varied molecular size. Some of the complexes may be much heavier than 23 S, while others may be only slightly more than 7 S in terms of their sedimentation coefficient. It has been found that a certain size of complex is optimum for localization of the complexes within the intima of blood vessels beneath the endothelium [14]. This critical size is in the range of 16 to 19 S.

Important in localization of these complexes are other factors such as those that affect the permeability of the endothelium [44, 50]. Factors such as histamine appear important in this connection. The local increase of blood pressure on the endothelial surface also accounts for localization of complexes. Because of this, more deposition occurs at points of bifurcation and at points of constriction where the pressures are the greatest [50]. Once localization of the complex has occurred, it appears to be stationary and provides a focus for chemotactic attraction of leukocytes (PMN). Leukocytes enter the vessel wall and release their hydrolytic enzymes, causing tissue destruction. When there has been widespread deposition of such complexes in many blood vessels through-out the body, there is also an accompanying widespread vasculitis. When such deposits localize within the glomerular tuft, this leads to one of the forms of acute glomerulonephritis [13].

Glomerulonephritis

The various forms of glomerulonephritis all appear to be complement dependent [62, 93]. As mentioned in the above section, the localization of immune complexes capable of fixing complement may occur within the glomerular tuft along the basement membrane and cause one form of acute glomerulonephritis. The tissue destruction is produced by neu-trophils emigrating to the glomerular basement and releasing their de-structive enzymes [13]. In another form of glomerulonephritis, the event of neutrophil emigration, with release of hydrolases, remains the same but the initiating reaction is different. In this type the antigen is an intrinsic part of the tissue of the glomerular tuft (basement mem-brane), and the antibody reacts wherever the appropriate tissue is en-countered [42]. These sites are usually along the basement membrane in the glomerulus, where complement fixation occurs and provides the focus for neutrophilic chemotaxis and glomerular destruction.

In humans, both forms of glomerulonephritis have been recognized [62]. The acute nephritis which accompanies lupus erythematosus ap-pears to be on the basis of deposition of immune complexes formed by antinuclear antibody with DNA or DNA-nucleoprotein antigens. Such complexes have been shown to be potent in their ability to fix comple-ment [82]. In other instances where immune reaction with the basement membrane is the initiating factor, the human disease known as Good-pasture's syndrome exhibits a form of glomerulonephritis [60] re-sembling that due to antibasement membrane antibody. Recently there have been case reports of individuals with antibasement membrane nephritis following exposure to hydrocarbon solvents [7]. There are many instances of glomerulonephritis which exhibit the presence of a granular deposition of γ-globulin and complement along the glomerular basement membrane. These findings suggest an etiology of immune complex deposition. These granular deposit patterns outnumber those of the smooth linear deposition which is characteristic of antibasement membrane glomerulonephritis.

Forms of glomerulonephritis have recently been described where deposition of immunoglobulin is not a conspicuous feature but where the presence of complement, especially C3, and deposition of properdin factors are notable features [94]. Some of these types of cases have been referred to as hypocomplementemic nephritis due to a marked lowering of complement activity in the blood of the patients with this form of acute glomerulonephritis. In these cases, activity of the extrinsic system (alternate pathway) of complement activation has been found increased and is apparently important in the pathogenesis of this nephritis [94]. The factor (or factors) stimulating the activation of the alternate system has been identified as a serum β-globulin.

Other Diseases
There has been considerable experimental work to establish a role of complement in the pathogenesis of acute arthritis and an attempt to relate complement activation to the morbidity of arthritis in humans. It has been possible to induce experimentally acute monoarticular arthritis by direct injection of antigen into joint spaces [23], but acute arthritis as a feature of experimental disseminated immune complex disease appears to occur infrequently. The participation of complement in human arthritis remains an open question, although the finding of cleavage products of complement components in the joint fluid of arthritics points to the likelihood of some role of complement [105].

Not all reactions which activate complement components are due to a triggering by immune reactions. It has been shown that the release of proteases from damaged tissues and activation of the fibrinolytic system is sufficient to produce active proteolytic enzymes which can cleave complement components to produce the biologically active fragments which have been discussed [96]. In this connection, it appears that complement may have an ubiquitous role in the inflammatory process due to a variety of nonimmune mechanisms. It is thus important to keep in mind the possible overlap and confusion of assigning complement a definite role in the pathogenesis of disease unless it can be clearly shown that the activation of the complement system is a necessary prerequisite to the tissue injury. Otherwise, complement activation may be only a secondary consequence of the tissue damage due to other causes.

Inherited Deficiencies of Complement Components and Inhibitors

The previous discussions emphasized the role of complement in the development of the tissue injury. In addition to its destructive potential, complement serves an important role in host defense, especially in the inactivation and the destruction of invasive microorganisms. This important role is clearly demonstrated in instances of those individuals who have inherited deficiencies of certain critical factors of the complement sequence.

Recently a case was reported which exemplified the protective functions of complement [86]. The patient had severe recurrent infections. In studies of the complement system, marked lowering of the third component (C3) was found and most was in the form of inactive C3b. When the catabolism of C3 was studied by injection of radio-labeled C3, it was found to be rapidly converted to the inactive C3b fragment. In addition, this patient's serum was shown to lack the ability to produce chemotactic factors, and it did not enhance phagocytosis or give rise to bacteriolysis when compared to plasma of other normal individuals. In addition, it was also found that this patient's serum was deficient in the properdin factor B, or C3 activator, which has been discussed previously. It appears that this case represents one of an unusual instance where there is intense in vivo activity of the C3b inactivator [86].

Other types of complement deficiency have reinforced the importance of the complement system in host defense. A defect in the fifth component of complement (C5) has been identified in a family [70]. The discovery was initially prompted by examination of a young infant in the family who had recurrent infections with gram negative organisms but who improved substantially after receiving transfusions of plasma. A deficiency of C2 [2] and deficiency of C1r [21] have been described, but neither exhibited a clinical problem of recurrent infection, although these patients appeared to have a markedly increased incidence of auto-immune hypersensitivity disease. Some observers have speculated that these deficiencies of the early reacting components interfere with the ability of the host to neutralize viruses and consequently allow for growth with dissemination of virus that might account for the apparent hypersensitivity diseases noted in these patients. The properties of complement components important in the in vitro inactivation of viruses has been discussed in the preceding section of this chapter.

There have been described other abnormalities of the complement system which are indirectly related to impairment of host defense. In the immune deficiency syndrome, such as the classic form of sex-linked recessive agammaglobulinemia, the levels of C1q are often substantially below normal [52]. In these situations, the assessment of the importance of C1q is limited by the associated immunologic deficiency.

Electrophoretic variants of both C4 and C3 have received attention, but their significance remains unclear [3].

As mentioned previously, a disease known as paroxysmal nocturnal hemoglobinuria is associated with an abnormality of the complement system [40]. On laboratory testing, the individuals who manifest this disease show increased fragility of red blood cells with a tendency to spontaneous lysis. The defect appears due to activation of the extrinsic (or by-pass) system of complement activation with subsequent attachment of the terminal complement components to cause red cell lysis.

The disease hereditary angioneurotic edema (HANE), which was mentioned briefly in an earlier section of this chapter, concerned a deficiency of the inhibitor of C1 esterase. It is another disorder of the complement system which is inherited and which produces a functional problem [26]. Because of lack of this inhibitor, the affected individual will exhibit episodes of angioedema which may be life threatening if it occurs in the larynx and trachea. This disease is inherited as an auto-somal dominant. The heterozyote appears to have a substantial decrease in the level of C1 esterase inhibitor (CINH). Utilization of C4 and C2 as natural substrate of C1 esterase causes the levels of these complement components to be markedly reduced during acute attacks. The trigger mechanisms of the reaction are unknown but seem to be due to activation of C1 esterase by either a proteolytic enzyme or allosteric mechanism. The mediator of the edematous reaction, shown in Fig. 4-6, is a polypeptide which exhibits activity of a kinin. It has been shown to be different from bradykinin [57].

The occurrence of chemotactic inhibitors has been described. In one instance, the presence of a chemotactic inhibitor has been described in a number of patients with alcoholic cirrhosis [22], and in another instance a young child who manifested frequent skin and respiratory infections was found to have a serum inhibitor of chemotactic activity [99]. Other deficiencies of chemotaxis have been described in relation to some of the abnormalities of the complement system already mentioned, especially those involving C3, but these have been due not to an inhibitor but rather to depletion or lack of a component [53, 86].

Complement Levels in Disease

Methods are now available for determination of complement components and complement activity on a routine basis in the clinical laboratory. Because of this, there is increasing information in the medical literature relating the levels of various components of complement and total hemolytic activity of complement to various diseases. Much of the interest in complement has centered on diseases which are presumed to be on an immunologic basis. These include the so-called collagen diseases, rheumatoid arthritis, acute and chronic glomerulonephritis, and certain infectious diseases.

The information relating to serum complement levels in disease often appears conflicting [92]. In clinical reports of the same or similar diseases, complement levels may be reported decreased, normal, or increased. They often appear not to represent a uniform change in direction with the disease process. Much of this variation occurs because of the time of sampling during the activity of the disease process. During periods where the disease process is active and complement activation is presumably at maximum, the levels of complement components would be expected at a low level in contrast to quiescent periods when normal levels might be encountered, or during a recovery phase where there might be increase in a particular component [53]. Because of this time course variation, there also appears to be confusion as to the merit of complement determinations in the clinical evaluation of various diseases. However, if one is sufficiently aware of this limitation and takes into account the time course variation, complement levels can be useful in monitoring the activity of particular diseases, especially those due to immune reactions.

From the earlier discussion in this chapter on activation of the complement system, it is apparent that the activities of both the intrinsic and extrinsic pathways of complement activation may be monitored by selective determination of individual components [45]. Activity of the intrinsic pathway can be determined by measuring the levels of C3 and C4. Activation of the complement system by this pathway would result in the lowering of the levels of these components. The activity of the extrinsic pathway, on the other hand, can be monitored by determination of levels of C3 and C3 proactivator since, with activity in the extrinsic pathway, the levels of these two factors will decrease substantially. There are currently available methods and materials for determining levels of each of these factors by means of the radial immunodiffusion technique of Mancini. In those situations where tissue biopsy material may be available, an assessment of complement fixation by means of the fluorescent antibody technique can be carried out on frozen sections of the biopsied tissue [56]. Studies of this type would add confirmatory data to the determination of serum levels of the components.

It should always be remembered that a decrease in complement activity or a decrease in individual component does not necessarily imply the existence of an immunologic disease or disorder. It is well recognized that proteolytic enzymes which are released from various tissues as a result of nonimmune injury, such as ischemia with coagulation necrosis and toxic necrosis, will produce cleavage of complement components similar to that which is produced by immune activation of the complement sequence [96]. As the result of this nonimmune cleavage, the levels of hemolytic activity of complement and those of individual components may decrease. In this connection it is important, if possible, to differentiate the onset of decreased complement levels in relation to the progress of disease. If the decrease follows tissue destruction due to trauma, ischemia, or toxins, it is probable that the decrease is related to the release of tissue proteases. In contrast, low complement levels preceding the onset of tissue damage points more directly to an immunologic etiology. This decrease may develop as a consequence of the activation of either the intrinsic or extrinsic complement pathway. In those infectious diseases where complement levels are decreased, the explanation could be related to release of tissue proteases as a result of damage by toxins from the organisms, or by complement fixation as a result of an immune response to the infectious organism itself. In a severe infection, it is not always possible to differentiate between these two possibilities for an explanation as to the decrease in complement activity.

In the following paragraphs the general aspects of complement activity in relation to certain diseases will be covered briefly.

Arthritis

Reports in the literature are varied regarding complement levels in rheumatoid arthritis. Generally, it appears that complement levels are normal or possibly elevated with the exception of some rheumatoid factor positive patients who show low levels of total hemolytic complement [28]. The low complement levels appear to be associated with severe active disease and often indicate the development of vasculitis as a complication. In the synovial fluid, during active disease, decrease in complement components has been reported. The presence of cleavage products of complement components has been identified in synovial fluid, indicating complement depletion in relation to the inflammatory synovitis [105].

Hemolytic Anemias

Hemolytic anemias due to immune reactions are usually associated with evidence of binding of complement components to the red cells [61, 100]. The presence of antibody and complement on the surface of red cells gives a positive direct Coombs' reaction. The complement components are most abundant on the red cell surface when the antibody is of the IgM class, in contrast to those hemolytic anemias which involve antibody of IgG type; then only small amounts of complement components are usually identified on the red cell [61]. Most characteristically, the hemolytic anemia associated with cold agglutinins are due to antibody of the IgM [61] class.

Rheumatic Fever

During episodes of activity in rheumatic fever, both hemolytic and levels of individual complement components tend to be reduced. Presumably the reduction is related to the inflammation in the tissues; it does not seem to bear a primary pathogenic relationship to the disease process [98]. By means of fluorescent antibody, complement components have been identified in lesions of fibrinoid necrosis in rheumatic fever, but not in the giant cell reactions known as Aschoff bodies.

Infectious Disease

Complement activity and levels of various components may vary widely in infectious diseases. Decreased levels are frequently noted in bacterial endocarditis, where there are complications of glomerulonephritis [102]; in bacteremia [66]; and in acute viral hepatitis [4].

Hypersensitivity and Autoimmune Disease

In diseases such as lupus erythematosus [51], scleroderma [90], serum sickness [13], and acute vasculitis [36], complement levels are reported ranging from low to normal, and in rare instances, increased. The decreased levels appear correlated with active phases of the diseases. In lupus erythematosus with active nephritis, low levels of C3 and low levels of other components, in addition to a decrease in total hemolytic activity, have been reported [87]. Presumably the mechanism which accounts for the decrease is fixation of complement by immune complexes of nuclear factors and antinuclear antibody. In serum sickness a similar mechanism seems to be operative [13]. In addition to low levels of complement components, a decrease in levels of components of the alternate or extrinsic pathway has also been reported in certain hypersensitivity diseases as lupus erythematosus [87].

The basis for decreased levels in other hypersensitivity diseases is less clear. Possibly the decreases are related to the inflammatory tissue destruction, but the possibility of decrease in the complement level bearing a pathogenetic relationship cannot be dismissed. There have been studies which suggest a role of complement in the development of these hypersensitivity diseases, but the evidence is indirect and mainly related to decreased serum levels and evidence of complement deposition in the tissue lesions by fluorescent antibody techniques.

Glomerulonephritis

The study of complement levels in glomerulonephritis has resulted in numerous clinical reports and studies attributing significance to these findings. In general, acute glomerulonephritis and active phases of chronic glomerulonephritis are associated with low serum complement levels and, in some instances, with low levels of components of the extrinsic pathway [45]. In addition, renal biopsy material which has been studied by fluorescent antibody technique has demonstrated deposition of complement components and components of the properdin system in the glomeruli in glomerulonephritis [45].

The serum levels may return to normal after the acute phase subsides, but in some cases of chronic glomerulonephritis a persistent decrease in levels of C3 has been noted. In fact, one form of chronic glomerulonephritis (hypocomplementemic nephritis) is persistently associated with low levels of C3 [94]. In this disease normal levels of early reacting components are encountered with decreased C3 and later reacting components with an associated decrease in properdin activity indicated by decrease in the level of C3 activator. The renal biopsy material in these cases has failed to show deposition of immunoglobulins, but has demonstrated deposition of C3 and properdin. A so-called "nephritic factor" has been identified in the serum of patients with this disease. This nephritic factor appears to be important in the activation of the alternate pathway and is presumably responsible for the decreased levels of the terminal complement components.

In the glomerulonephritis associated with lupus erythematosus, there are decreases in the levels of both early and late complement components as well as decreases in levels of properdin factor B [87]. Renal biopsies provide evidence of deposition of properdin and complement in the glomeruli. These findings indicate that both the intrinsic and extrinsic pathways are important in this disease. It is of interest to note that the morphologic form of lupus glomerulonephritis varies from membranous to diffuse proliferation and does not correlate with the pattern of deposition of immune reactants, complement components, or properdin factors.

In other reports, the sera of patients with membranoproliferative glomerulonephritis or acute poststreptococcal glomerulonephritis have exhibited normal levels of the early reacting complement components with decrease in the late reacting components and properdin factors [101]. On biopsy, deposition of properdin and C3 were identified in the glomeruli, but immunoglobulins and early reacting complement components were not found. These findings suggest that some mechanism other than immunologic activation of complement is important in the pathogenesis of these types of glomerulonephritis.

The Role of Immune Reactants in the Activation of Other Biochemical Factors

In the past few years, there has been considerable speculation and preliminary data regarding the role of the plasma kinin system in acute immunologic injury. Various observers have reported in vitro experiments where activation of the kinin-generating system appeared to occur as a consequence of antigen-antibody reactions [27, 49, 67, 68]. For the most part, these studies were performed with crude preparations, some of which were contaminated with bacterial products, while others were apparently active with various proteolytic enzymes from the blood plasma. The basis for the activation of the kinin system was believed to arise from the activation of the initial component of that system, the Hageman factor or factor XII of the intrinsic pathway of blood coagulation. More recently there have been elegant studies with purified preparations of Hageman factor which have failed to demonstrate any activation by antigen-antibody reactants or activation by aggregated immunoglobulins of different types [17]. These studies were carried out with known activators as controls and have effectively eliminated the possibility that antigen-antibody reactions exhibit a primary effect on the kinin-generating system through activation of Hageman factor [17]. Studies which would indicate that immune reactants could activate the plasma kinin system through a mechanism not involving Hageman factor have not yet been reported. Presumably such mechanisms, if they exist, would explain the previously mentioned findings of investigators who have noted kinin generation initiated by immune reactions.

The discussions in Chapter 5 on the pathogenesis of reaginic reactions delineate the mechanisms of release of biochemical mediators from mast cells as a result of immune reactions involving IgE antibody. In the chapters on immune deficiency disease (2 and 3) and on autoimmunity (7 and 8), the pathogenesis of biochemical factors in delayed hypersensitivity or cellular immunity is discussed. The underlying mechanisms of these reactions are predicated on the release of soluble factors from sensitized lymphocytes (T-cells) following antigen contact [19]. These factors exhibit various activities ranging from monocyte chemotaxis and inhibition of macrophage migration to cytotoxicity. They appear to account for the varied cellular events observed in the evolution of the delayed sensitivity reaction [63]. Each of the major types of immune reaction demonstrates a dependence on certain biochemical factors for the development of its tissue reactions. These reactions in turn produce the lesions that characterize the different forms of immunologic injury ranging from edema and congestion to necrosis and granuloma formation.

It can be expected that increasing knowledge of the biochemical intricacies of diverse immunologic diseases will abound from research in the coming years. This offers our best hope for a therapeutic approach to these diseases—to isolate and attack those critical biochemical factors at important stages in the pathogenesis of the disease process.

Assays for Complement Activity

Various methods for assaying activity of the complement system have been described. The most useful are those which allow quantitation of individual components by means of a radial immunodiffusion technique based on the method of immunochemical determination originally described by Mancini et al. [64]. For determination of functional complement activity, a hemolytic assay utilizing a sheep red blood cell system and rabbit antibody as the sensitizing hemolysin is recommended [85]. This total hemolytic assay affords a general screening test to determine activity of the entire complement sequence and the presence of inhibitor activity. While total hemolytic activity is best suited for screening for a complement abnormality, individual component determinations are more applicable to precise definition of the defect.

By the use of selective measurements of complement components C3 and C4, along with quantitation of C3 activator (properdin factor B), one can estimate the contribution of the intrinsic and extrinsic pathways of complement activation in a given disease process. These assays are carried out by means of a radial immunodiffusion as described in the following section on procedures. Specialized assays for complement components and activities would include hemolytic titrations for specific complement components, measurements of peptidase and esterase activity of components, and biologic tests including phagocytosis, chemotaxis, generation of anaphylatoxin, and tests for inhibitor activity such as C1 esterase inhibitor.

The approach to determining complement abnormalities associated with varied clinical disorders is suggested as follows:
1. Measure total hemolytic activity on fresh or fresh frozen ($-40°$ C) serum. If low, proceed to 2.
2. Determine serum C3 level by radial immunodiffusion. Proceed to 3 if value abnormal.
3. Determine serum C4 and C3 activator (properdin factor B; Beta-II glycoprotein II) by radial immunodiffusion to differentiate intrinsic and extrinsic complement pathway activation. If these values are normal and hemolytic activity is low, proceed to step 4.

4. Determine levels of other complement components, either by radial immunodiffusion or specific component hemolytic titrations, on fresh or serum rapidly frozen and preserved at $-40°$ C. For these assays consult with special reference laboratories such as Scripps Clinic and Research Foundation, La Jolla, Calif. 92037; or Cordis Laboratories, Miami, Fla. 33137; or the immunology laboratory of the nearest medical school.

Tissue Studies

The evaluation of complement in tissue lesions is aided by the technique of fluorescent antibody reaction with cryostat sections of fresh tissue biopsies such as percutaneous renal biopsy. In addition to determining the pattern of immunoglobulin deposition in the glomeruli (granular versus smooth linear), the degree of complement (C3) fixation in those deposits can be determined. This information contributes to understanding the pathogenesis of the disease process. In addition to C3, the amount of C3 activator can also be determined by this technique using fluorescent-labeled anti-C3 activator, which is available from the sources mentioned in the following section on the immunofluorescence procedure.

Hemolytic Assay for Total Complement Activity (CH_{50} Units)

PROCEDURE
1. Prepare VB^{++} diluent
   a. Weigh the following:

83.8 gm	NaCl
2.52 gm	$NaHCO_3$
3.0 gm	Na 5–5 diethyl barbiturate
4.6 gm	5–5 diethyl barbituric acid
1.0 gm	$MgCl \cdot 6 H_2O$
0.14 gm	$CaCl_2$ (anhydrous) or 0.20 g$CaCl_2 \cdot 2H_2O$

   b. Dissolve the last three components in 500 ml hot distilled water.
   c. Dissolve other components in 500–1,000 ml distilled water.
   d. Combine above solution and bring to a total volume of *2,000* ml with distilled water. This solution is five times isotonicity. Store at 1–4° C. Label stock solution.
   e. For use, dilute stock solution by addition of exactly four volumes of distilled water.
2. Collect serum (either fresh or stored below $-40°$ C).
3. Prepare sensitized sheep (EA) erythrocytes (also available from Cordis) and standardize cell suspension to give optical density of 0.680 at 541 nanometers (0.5 cm light path) (O.D. 0.680 = 1 × 10^9 cell/ml). When sensitizing cells add appropriate dilution of hemolysin to washed erythrocytes and incubate for 30 minutes at 37° C.
4. Prepare protocol for complement titration
   a. 0.5 ml EA per test tube.

   b. Dilute human serum 1/40 and add amounts to each tube increasing by 0.1 ml to 1.0 ml.

   c. Add VB^{++} diluent as appropriate to each tube to a volume of 1.5 ml; prepare appropriate controls.

   d. Incubate tubes with gentle shaking at 37° C for one hour.

   e. Add VB^{++} diluent to a final total volume of 5.0 ml.

   f. Centrifuge at 1,800 rpm for 15 min.

   g. Decant supernatant and read at 412 mm.

   h. Calculate Y value:

$$Y = \frac{\text{color-corrected O.D. of tube}}{\text{O.D. 100\% lysis}}$$

   i. Using log paper, plot curve of Y vs. ml serum (complement) for each tube.

   j. Determine CH$_{50}$ by calculation:

$$CH_{50} = \frac{\text{original serum (C) dilution}}{\text{vol. serum (C) at } Y = 0.5}$$

Hemolytic Assays for Specific Complement Components
These assays are based on the addition of a specific component to a reaction mixture containing all the other intermediates in the hemolytic sequence. Such intermediates are commercially available (Cordis) or can be prepared.

Immunoprecipitin Assays for β–1–C Globulin (C3) and C3 Activator (Properdin Factor B)

IMMUNOELECTROPHORESIS
1. Fresh serum is electrophoresed at pH 7.4–8.0 at 1–4° C in 2.5% buffered agar according to standard technique for immunoelectrophoresis.
2. The antisera trough is filled with anti-human β–1–C globulin, C4, or C3 activator, then diffusion is allowed to proceed at 25° C for 5 hours, then for 8 to 10 hours at 1–4° C. Precipitin arcs form indicating the presence of β–1–C globulin and/or the conversion product β–1–A globulin. (Assay materials are available from various commercial sources: Custom Reagent Laboratory (C3 activator plates); Behringwerke (C3 activator antiserum); Hyland; Meloy.)

RADIAL IMMUNODIFFUSION
1. Buffered agar plates containing antisera to β–1–C globulin, C4, or C3 activator can be prepared or purchased.
2. Neat and diluted serum are added to wells in the agar and diffusion time allowed 12 to 18 hours.
3. Diameters of the precipitin circles formed are measured and compared to a plot of known amounts of complement or C3 proactivator

for quantitation. (This method does not distinguish β–1–C from the conversion product β–1–A globulin.)

Immunofluorescence Technique for Tissue Fixation
of β–1–C Globulin (C3)

1. Tissue obtained by biopsy or dissection is rapidly frozen and sectioned in a cryostat at -15 to $20°$ C.
2. Tissue sections are placed on glass slide and thawed. They are washed in 2 changes of phosphate-buffered saline solution (PBS) for 5 min each, then briefly fixed for 10 min in a mixture of equal volumes of absolute alcohol and dry ether (all at $4°$ C).
3. Slides are then placed in 95% ethanol for 10 min at room temperature.
4. Wash slides in 2 changes of PBS for a total of 10 min. Remove slides and allow to drain dry for staining.
5. Place slide on staining rack in moist chamber and apply 1 to 2 drops of fluorescein-labeled antisera to β–1–C globulin (C3) or C3 activator (see Immunoelectrophoresis, step 2) over the tissue and leave for 20 to 30 min.
6. Wash slides in PBS for three (3) changes for a total of 15 min. Dry around tissue and coverslip using a 9 parts glycerine and 1 part PBS mixture.
7. Observe with either darkfield or brightfield fluorescence microscope with an ultraviolet blue exciter filter (Zeiss UG–2, Corning 5–58, or Corning 5840). Sites of Beta–1–C fixation are shown by bright yellow-green fluorescence.

References

1. Abramson, N., Alper, C. A., and Lachmann, P. J.   Deficiency of C3 inactivator in man. *J. Immunol.* 107:19, 1971.
2. Agnello, V., de Bracco, M. M. E., and Kunkel, H. G.   Hereditary C2 deficiency with some manifestations of systemic lupus erythematosus. *J. Immunol.* 108:837, 1972.
3. Alper, C. A., and Rose, F. S.   Genetic considerations. In D. G. Ingram (ed.), *Biological Activities of Complement.* Basel: Karger, 1972.
4. Alpert, E., Isselbacher, K. J., and Schur, P. H.   The pathogenesis of arthritis associated with viral hepatitis: Complement-component studies. *N. Engl. J. Med.* 285:185, 1971.
5. Ballow, M., and Cochrane, C. G.   Two anticomplementary factors in cobra venom: Hemolysis of guinea erythrocytes by one of them. *J. Immunol.* 103:944, 1969.
6. Becker, E. L.   The relationship of the chemotactic behavior of the complement derived factors, C3a, C5a, and C5,6,7, and a bacterial chemotactic factor to their ability to activate the proesterase 1 of rabbit polymorphonuclear leukocytes. *J. Exp. Med.* 135:376, 1972.
7. Beirne, G. J., and Brennan, J. T.   Glomerulonephritis associated with

exposure to hydrocarbons: Mediated by antibodies to glomerular basement membrane. *Arch. Environ. Health* 25:365, 1972.

8. Bordet, J.   Sur l'agglutination et la dissolution des globules rouges par le serum d'animaux injectiés de sang defibriné. *Ann. Inst. Pasteur* (Paris) 12:688, 1898.

9. Borsos, T., and Rapp, H. J.   Hemolysin titration based on fixation of the activated first component of complement. Evidence that one molecule of hemolysin suffices to sensitize an erythrocyte. *J. Immunol.* 95: 559, 1965.

10. Broom, D. H., Schultz, D. R., and Zarco, R. M.   The separation of nine components and two inactivators of components of complement in human serum. *Immunochemistry.* 7:43, 1970.

11. Cochrane, C. G.   Immunologic factors in peripheral vascular disease. In J. L. Orbison and D. E. Smith (eds.), *The Peripheral Blood Vessels.* International Academy of Pathology IV. Baltimore: Williams & Wilkins, 1963.

12. Cochrane, C. G.   Mediators of the Arthus and related reactions. In P. Kallos and B. H. Waksmann (eds.), *Progress in Allergy.* Basel: Karger, 1967, vol. 11.

13. Cochrane, C. G., and Dixon, F. J.   Cell and tissue damage through antigen-antibody complexes. In P. A. Miescher and H. J. Müller-Eberhard (eds.), *Textbook of Immunopathology.* New York: Grune & Stratton, 1969, vol. 1.

14. Cochrane, C. G., and Hawkins, D.   Studies on circulating immune complexes: III. Factors governing the ability of circulating complexes to localize in blood vessels. *J. Exp. Med.* 127:137, 1968.

15. Cochrane, C. G., and Müller-Eberhard, H. J.   The derivation of two distinct anaphylatoxin activities from the third and fifth components of human complement. *J. Exp. Med.* 127:371, 1968.

16. Cochrane, C. G., Weigle, W. O., and Dixon, F. J.   The role of polymorphonuclear leukocytes in the initiation and cessation of the Arthus vasculitis. *J. Exp. Med.* 100:481, 1959.

17. Cochrane, C. G., Wuepper, K. D., Aiken, B. S., Revak, S. D., and Spiegelberg, H. L.   The interaction of Hageman factor and immune complexes. *J. Clin. Invest.* 51:2736, 1972.

18. Cooper, N. R., and Becker, E. L.   Complement associated peptidase activity of guinea pig serum. *J. Immunol.* 98:119, 1967.

19. David, J. R.   Lymphocytic factors in cellular hypersensitivity. In R. A. Good and D. W. Fisher (eds.), *Immunobiology.* Stamford: Sinaur, 1971.

20. Davis, S. D., Iannetta, A., and Wedgwood, R. J.   Bactericidal reactions of serum. In D. G. Ingram (ed.), *Biological Activities of Complement.* Basel: Karger, 1972.

21. Day, N. K., Geiger, H., and Stroud, R.   C1r deficiency: An inborn error associated with cutaneous and renal disease. *J. Clin. Invest.* 51:1102, 1972.

22. DeMeo, A. N., and Andersen, B. R.   Defective chemotaxis associated with a serum inhibitor in cirrhotic patients. *N. Engl. J. Med.* 286:735, 1972.

23. De Shazo, C. D., Henson, P. M., and Cochrane, C. G.   Acute immunologic arthritis in rabbits. *J. Clin. Invest.* 51:50, 1972.

24. Dias da Silva, W., Eisele, J. W., and Lepow, I. H.   Complement as mediator of inflammation: III. Purification of the activity with anaphylatoxin properties generated by interaction of the first four components of the complement and its identification as a cleavage product of C'3. *J. Exp. Med.* 126:1027, 1967.
25. Dixon, F. J., Vazquez, J. J., Weigle, W. O., and Cochrane, C. G.: Pathogenesis of serum sickness. *A.M.A. Arch. Pathol.* 65:18, 1958.
26. Donaldson, U. H., and Evans, R. R.   A biochemical abnormality in hereditary angioneurotic edema: Absence of serum inhibitor of C'1 esterase. *Am. J. Med.* 35:37, 1963.
27. Eisen, V., and Smith, H. G.   Plasma kinin formation by complexes of aggregated gammaglobulin and serum proteins. *Br. J. Exp. Pathol.* 51: 328, 1970.
28. Franco, A. E., and Schur, P. H.   Hypocomplementemia in rheumatoid arthritis. *Arthritis Rheum.* 14:231, 1971.
29. Gewurz, H.   Alternate pathways to activation of the complement system. In D. G. Ingram (ed.), *Biological Activities of Complement.* Basel: Karger, 1972.
30. Gewurz, H., Shin, H. S., and Mergenhagen, S. E.   Interactions of the complement system with endotoxic lipopolysaccharide: Consumption of each of the six terminal complement components. *J. Exp. Med.* 128: 1049, 1968.
31. Giertz, H.   Pharmacology of anaphylatoxin. In H. Z. Movat (ed.), *Cellular and Humoral Mechanism in Anaphylaxis and Allergy.* Basel: Karger, 1969.
32. Gigli, I., and Austen, K. F.   Fluid phase destruction of C2hu by C1hu: II. Unmasking by C4hu of C1hu specificity for C2hu. *J. Exp. Med.* 130:833, 1969.
33. Gigli, I., Kaplan, A. C., and Austen, K. F.   Modulation of function of the activated first component of complement by a fragment derived from serum. *J. Exp. Med.* 134:1466, 1971.
34. Gigli, I., and Nelson, R. A.   Complement dependent immune phagocytosis: I. Requirements for C'1, C'4, C'2, C'3. *Exp. Cell Res.* 51:45, 1968.
35. Gocke, D. J., Hsu, K., Morgan, C., Bombardieri, S., Lockshin, M., and Christian, C. L.   Vasculitis in association with Australia antigen. *J. Exp. Med.* 134:330s, 1971.
36. Gocke, D. J., Hsu, K., and Morgan, C.   Association between polyarteritis and Australia antigen. *Lancet* 2:1149, 1970.
37. Goodkofsky, I., and Lepow, I. H.   Functional relationship of factor B in the properdin system to C3 proactivator of human serum. *J. Immunol.* 107:1200, 1971.
38. Gotze, O., and Müller-Eberhard, H. J.   Lysis of erythrocytes by complement in the absence of antibody. *J. Exp. Med.* 132:898, 1970.
39. Gotze, O., and Müller-Eberhard, H. J.   The C3 activator system: An alternate pathway of complement activation. *J. Exp. Med.* 134:90s, 1971.
40. Gotze, O., and Müller-Eberhard, H. J.   Paroxysmal nocturnal hemoglobinuria: Hemolysis initiated by the C3 activator system. *N. Engl. J. Med.* 286:180, 1972.
41. Haines, A. L., and Lepow, L. H.   Studies on human C'1–esterase: I. Purification and enzymatic properties. *J. Immunol.* 92:456, 1964.

42. Hawkins, D., and Cochrane, C. G.   Glomerular basement membrane damage in immunological glomerulonephritis. *Immunology* 14:665, 1968.
43. Henson, P. M.   Complement-dependent adherence to cells to antigen and antibody, mechanisms and consequences. In D. G. Ingram (ed.), *Biological Activities of Complement*. Basel: Karger, 1972.
44. Henson, P. N., and Cochrane, C. G.   Immunological induction of increased vascular permeability: I. A rabbit passive cutaneous anaphylactic reaction requiring complement, platelets and neutrophils. *J. Exp. Med.* 129:153, 1969.
45. Hunsicker, L. D., Ruddy, S., Carpenter, C. B., Schur, P. H., Merrill, J. P., Müller-Eberhard, H. J., and Austen, K. F.   Metabolism of third complement component (C3) in nephritis: Involvement of the classic and alternate (properdin) pathways for complement activation. *N. Engl. J. Med.* 287:835, 1972.
46. Ishizaka, T., Tada, T., and Ishizaka, K.   Fixation of C'1 and C'1a by rabbit gamma G and gamma M. Antibodies with particulate and soluble antigen. *J. Immunol.* 100:1145, 1968.
46a. Ishizaka, T., Ishizaka, K., Bennich, H., and Johansson, S. G. O.   Biologic activities of aggregated immunoglobulin E. *J. Immunol.* 104:854, 1970.
47. Isliker, H., Jacot-Guillarmod, H., Waldesduomalow, H. L., Fellenberg, N., Von, R, and Cerottini, J. C.   Complement fixation by different IgG preparations and fragments. In P. Meischer and T. Grabar (eds.), *Mechanisms of Inflammation Induced by Immune Injury*. 6th International Symposium of Immunopathology. Basel: Schawbe, 1967.
48. Johnson, K. J., Ward, P. A., Osborn, M. J., and Arroyave, C. M.   C5 as an inactivator of bacterial endotoxin. *Fed. Proc.* 31:736 (abstract), 1972.
49. Kaplan, A. O., Spragg, J., and Austen, K. F.   The immunologic activation of the bradykinin-forming system in man. In K. F. Austen and E. L. Becker (eds.), *Biochemistry of the Acute Allergic Reactions*. Oxford: Blackwell, 1971.
50. Kniker, W. T., and Cochrane, C. G.   The localization of circulating immune complexes in experimental serum sickness. The role of vasoactive amines and hydrodynamic forces. *J. Exp. Med.* 127:119, 1968.
51. Koffler, D., Agnello, V., Thoburn, R., and Kunkel, H. G.   Systemic lupus erythematosus: Prototype of immune complex nephritis in man. *J. Exp. Med.* 134:169s, 1971.
52. Kohler, P. F., and Müller-Eberhard, H. J.   Complement-immunoglobulin relations: Deficiency of C'1q associated with impaired immunoglobulin G synthesis. *Science* 163:474, 1969.
53. Kohler, P. F., and Ten Bensel, R.   Serial complement component alterations in acute glomerulonephritis and systemic lupus erythematosus. *Clin. Exp. Immunol.* 4:192, 1969.
54. Kolb, W. P., Haxby, J. A., Arroyave, C. M., and Müller-Eberhard, H. J.   Molecular analysis of the membrane attack mechanism of complement. *J. Exp. Med.* 135:549, 1972.
55. Lachmann, P. J., and Müller-Eberhard, H. J.   The demonstration in human serum of conglutinogen-activating factor and its effect on the third component of complement. *J. Immunol.* 100:691, 1968.
56. Lachmann, P. J., Müller-Eberhard, H. L., and Kunkel, H. G.   The lo-

calization of the in vivo bound complement in tissue sections. *J. Exp. Med.* 115:63, 1963.
57. Lepow, I. H.   Permeability-producing peptide by-product of the interaction of the first, fourth and second components of complement. In K. F. Austen and E. L. Becker (eds.), *Biochemistry of the Acute Allergic Reactions.* Oxford: Blackwell, 1971.
58. Lepow, I. H., Nass, G. S., Todd, E. W., Pensky, J., and Hinz, C. F., Jr. Chromatographic resolution of the first component of human complement into three activities. *J. Exp. Med.* 117:983, 1963.
59. Lepow, I. H., and Rosen, F. S.   Pathways to the complement system. *N. Engl. J. Med.* 286:942, 1972.
60. Lerner, R. A., Glassock, R. J., and Dixon, F. J.   The role of antiglomerular basement membrane antibody in the pathogenesis of human glomerulonephritis. *J. Exp. Med.* 126:989, 1967.
61. Levine, B. B., and Redmond, A. P.   Immunochemical mechanisms of penicillin-induced Coombs' positivity and hemolytic anemia in man. *Int. Arch. Allergy Appl. Immunol.* 31:594, 1967.
62. Lewis, E. J., and Couser, W. G.   The immunologic basis of human renal disease. *Pediatr. Clin. North Am.* 18:467, 1971.
63. MacKaness, G. B., and Blanden, R. V.   Cellular immunity. *Prog. Allergy* 11:89, 1967.
64. Mancini, G., Vaermann, J. P., Carbonara, A. O., and Heremans, J. F. Single radial diffusion method for immunological quantitation of proteins. *Protides Biol. Fluids* 11:370, 1964.
65. Manni, J. A., and Müller-Eberhard, H. J.   The eighth component of human complement (C8): Isolation, characterization and hemolytic efficiency. *J. Exp. Med.* 130:1145, 1969.
66. McCabe, W. R.   Serum complement levels in bacteremia due to gram negative organisms. *N. Engl. J. Med.* 288:21, 1973.
67. Movat, H. Z.   Activation of the kinin system by antigen-antibody complexes. In R. E. Silva and A. M. Rothschild (eds.), *International Symposium on Vasoactive Polypeptides.* São Paulo, Brazil: Edart Livaria Editora Ltd., 1967.
68. Movat, H. S., and DiLorenzo, N. L.   Activation of the plasma kinin system by antigen-antibody aggregates: I. Generation of permeability factor in guinea pig serum. *Lab. Invest.* 19:187, 1968.
69. Miller, M. E.   Demonstration of a major role in the fifth component of complement (C5) in the enhancement of phagocytosis. *Fed. Proc.* 29:433 (abstract), 1970.
70. Miller, M. E., and Nilsson, U. R.   A familial deficiency of the phagocytosis-enhancing activity of serum related to a dysfunction of the fifth component of complement (C5). *N. Engl. J. Med.* 282:354, 1970.
71. Müller-Eberhard, H. J.   Chemistry and reaction mechanisms of the complement system. *Adv. Immunol.* 8:1, 1968.
72. Müller-Eberhard, H. J.   Complement. *Annu. Rev. Biochem.* 38:389, 1969.
73. Müller-Eberhard, H. J., and Calcott, M. A.   Interaction between C'1q and gamma G globulin. *Immunochemistry* 3:500, 1966.
74. Müller-Eberhard, H. J., Dalmasso, A. P., and Calcott, M. A.   The reaction mechanism of beta 1C-globulin (C'3) in immune hemolysis. *J. Exp. Med.* 123:33, 1966.

75. Müller-Eberhard, H. J., and Gotze, O.   C3 proactivator convertase and its mode of action. *J. Exp. Med.* 135:1003, 1972.
76. Müller-Eberhard, H. J., and Lepow, I. H.   C'1 esterase effect on activities and physico-chemical properties of the fourth component of complement. *J. Exp. Med.* 121:819, 1965.
77. Müller-Eberhard, H. J., Polley, M. J., and Calcott, M. A.   Formation and functional significance of a molecular complex derived from the second and the fourth component of human complement. *J. Exp. Med.* 125:359, 1967.
78. Naff, G. B, Properdin—its biologic importance. *N. Engl. J. Med.* 287:716, 1972.
79. Nelson, D. S.   Immune adherence. *Adv. Immunol.* 3:131, 1963.
80. Notkins, A. L.   Infectious virus—antibody complexes: Interaction with anti-immunoglobulins, complement and rheumatoid factor. *J. Exp. Med.* 134:415, 1971.
81. Petz, L. D., and Fundenberg, H. H.   Coombs-positive hemolytic anemia caused by penicillin administration. *N. Engl. J. Med.* 274:171, 1966.
82. Petz, L. D., Sharp, G. C., Cooper, N. R., and Irvin, W. S.   Serum and cerebral spinal fluid complement and serum autoantibodies in systemic lupus erythematosus. *Medicine* (Baltimore) 50:259, 1971.
83. Polley, M. J., and Müller-Eberhard, H. J.   Enhancement of the hemolytic activity of the second component of human complement by oxidation. *J. Exp. Med.* 126:1013, 1967.
84. Polley, M. J., and Müller-Eberhard, H. J.   The second component of human complement: Its isolation fragmentation by C'1 esterase and incorporation into C'3 convertase. *J. Exp. Med.* 128:533, 1968.
85. Rapp, H. J., and Borsos, T.   *Molecular Basis of Complement Action.* New York: Appleton-Century-Crofts, 1970.
86. Rosen, F. S., and Alper, C. A.   An enzyme in the alternate pathway to C3 activation (the properdin system) and its inhibition by a protein in normal serum. *J. Clin. Invest.* 51:80A, 1972.
87. Rothfield, N., Ross, A., Minta, J. O., and Lepow, I. H.   Glomerular and dermal deposition of properdin in systemic lupus erythematosus. *N. Engl. J. Med.* 287:681, 1972.
88. Ruddy, S., and Austen, K. F.   Natural control mechanisms of the complement system. In D. G. Ingram (ed.), *Biological Activities of Complement.* Basel: Karger, 1972.
89. Schroeter, A. L., Copeman, P. W. M., Jordan, R. E., Sams, W. M., Jr., and Winkelmann, R. K.   Immunofluorescence of cutaneous vasculitis. *J. Clin. Invest.* (Abstract, *Am. Soc. Clin. Invest.*) 48:75A, 1969.
90. Schur, P. H., and Austen, K. F.   Complement in human disease. *Annu. Rev. Med.* 19:124, 1968.
91. Tamura, N., and Nelson, R. A.   Three naturally occurring inhibitors of components of complement in guinea pig and rabbit serum. *J. Immunol.* 99:582, 1967.
92. Townes, A. S.   Complement levels in disease. *Johns Hopkins Med. J.* 120:337, 1967.
93. Unanue, E., and Dixon, F. J.   Experimental glomerulonephritis: IV. Participation of complement in nephrotoxic nephritis. *J. Exp. Med.* 119:964, 1964.
94. Vallota, E. H., Forristal, J., Davis, N. C., and West, C. D.   The C3

nephritic factor and membranoproliferative nephritis: Correlation of serum levels of the nephritic factor with C3 levels, with therapy and with progression of the disease. *J. Pediatr.* 80:947, 1972.
95. Ward, P. A.   Biological activities of the complement system. *Ann. Allergy* 30:307, 1972.
96. Ward, P. A.   Complement derived chemotactic factors and their interactions with neutrophilic granulocytes. In D. G. Ingram (ed.), *Biological Activities of Complement.* Basel: Karger, 1972.
97. Ward, P. A., Cochrane, C. G., and Müller-Eberhard, H. J.   Further studies on the chemotactic factor of complement and its formation in vivo. *Immunology* 11:141, 1966.
98. Ward, P. A., and Hill, J. H.   Role of complement in the generation of leukotactic mediators in immunologic and nonspecific tissue injuries. In B. K. Forscher and J. C. Houck (eds.), *Immunopathology of Inflammation.* Amsterdam: Excerpta Medica, 1971.
99. Ward, P. A., and Schlegel, R. J.   Impaired leucotactic responsiveness in a child with recurrent infections. *Lancet* 2:344, 1969.
100. Weiner, W.   Hemolytic disease of the newborn and other conditions following iso-immunization. In B. G. H. Gell and R. R. A. Coombs (eds.), *Clinical Aspects of Immunology.* Philadelphia: Davis, 1968, 2nd ed.
101. Westberg, N. G., Naff, D. B., and Boyer, J. T.   Glomerular deposition of properdin in acute and chronic glomerulonephritis with hypocomplementemia. *J. Clin. Invest.* 50:642, 1971.
102. Williams, R. C., Jr., and Kunkel, H. G.   Rheumatoid factor complement and conglutinin aberrations in patients with subacute bacterial endocarditis. *J. Clin. Invest.* 41:666, 1962.
103. Yachnin, S.   Further studies on the hemolysis of human red cells by late acting complement components. *Immunochemistry* 3:505, 1965.
104. Zimmerman, T. S., and Arroyave, C. M.   Participation of complement in initiation of blood coagulation and in the normal coagulation process. In K. F. Austen and E. L. Becker (eds.), *Biochemistry of the Acute Allergic Reactions.* Oxford: Blackwell, 1971.
105. Zvaifler, N. J.   Breakdown products of C′3 in human synovial fluids. *J. Clin. Invest.* 48:1532, 1969.

5

Laboratory Tests for the Evaluation of Atopic or Reaginic Disorders

Ernest S. Tucker, III

C ertain types of acute allergic reactions are called *atopic* or *reaginic disorders*. These reactions are associated with signs and symptoms of sudden onset due to the release of pharmacologically active mediators [10]. These mediators, such as histamine, produce vasodilatation, increased vascular permeability, mucous secretion, and constriction of smooth muscles. Such mediator release is due to an immune reaction in various target tissues. The symptoms that result are due to the physiologic effects of the mediators on those tissues. In the skin, the immune reaction produces vasodilatation and edema causing a wheal and flare reaction resembling the triple response of inflammation first described by Lewis [34]. In other tissues, similar vascular effects are noted, in addition to events such as increased mucous secretion and smooth muscle contraction causing bronchoconstriction in the respiratory tract or increased motility in the intestines.

Atopic disorders develop in sensitized host tissues on contact with allergens. Diverse clinical manifestations result from varied exposure of different tissues to many allergens. Inhalant allergens produce respiratory symptoms, while ingested antigens may provoke intestinal or systemic symptoms. The approach to the diagnosis of these disorders necessitates a history that documents episodes of recurrent symptoms on exposure to the same or similar agents. Once suspected, these disorders can be definitively identified by appropriate testing. These tests are based on the release of mediators by antigen exposure in vivo and in vitro. This chapter will delineate the pathophysiology of reaginic disorders and an approach to be followed in reaching a clinical diagnosis.

Pathophysiology of Reaginic Reactions

Progress in our current understanding of reaginic disorders dates to the work of various investigators since 1900. Much of the early experimental work dealt with the phenomenon of anaphylaxis where it could be shown that an animal made sensitive by injection of a foreign substance would exhibit a profound systemic response on reinjection of the same substance [43]. In some species, the severe reactions lead to death of the animal through the effects of the cardiovascular and respiratory systems. The conditions of anaphylaxis have been extensively explored, and today the phenomenon provides an excellent model for the study of reaginic reactions [9, 16].

Among the factors necessary for the production of anaphylaxis, certain are of prime importance. These are:

1. sensitization of the animal by prior exposure to the antigen (or immunogen).
2. production by the sensitized animal of a specific type of antibody (reaginic): immunoglobulin E (IgE) in man and fast-migrating IgG and/or IgE in other animal species (homocytotropic antibody).
3. widespread fixation of reaginic antibody to certain cells throughout the animal's tissues. Mast cells, basophils, and possibly platelets which contain abundant pharmacologic substances are important sites of fixation.
4. re-exposure of the animal to the antigen by any route which allows dissemination throughout the animal's tissues (shock dose).
5. interaction of the antigen with reaginic antibody fixed to cell surfaces leading to release of the biochemical mediators such as histamine, serotonin, slow reacting substance of anaphylaxis (SRS–A), and eosinophil chemotactic factor (ECF–A).
6. tissue response to the released mediators resulting in major physiologic effects such as vascular dilatation, increased vascular permeability, mucous secretion, and smooth muscle constriction. Widespread effects may produce shock and respiratory insufficiency, causing death. Local effects may be limited and innocuous.

It is apparent from studies of these pathogenic mechanisms in anaphylaxis that the release of biochemical mediators such as histamine and probably SRS–A from mast cells or basophils accounts for the pathology of reaginic reactions [23]. This common pathway is activated by many different antigens by combining with specific reaginic (also called anaphylactic, homocytotropic, or IgE) antibody attached to the plasma membranes of the cells [23] (Fig. 5-1). The mediator release does not occur in the absence of specific reaginic antibody, and there are no physiologic effects even from massive exposure to a diversity of antigens. However, in the sensitive host who has abundant specific reaginic antibody throughout the tissues, a small amount of antigen may cause a severe and even lethal reaction due to release of the potent physiologic mediators (Fig. 5-2).

The key to understanding reaginic disorders is based on an appreciation of the importance of this pathogenic sequence of antigen-induced release of potent pharmacologic substances. This understanding can be

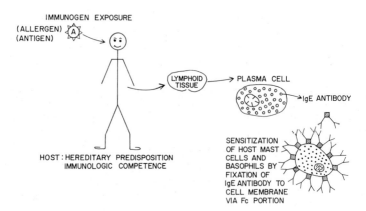

Figure 5-1
Development of atopic sensitivity (IgE-mediated hypersensitivity).

applied to the diagnosis of atopic disorders. One can easily recognize the similarities between the profound shock and respiratory distress of systemic anaphylaxis and the localized vasodilatation and edema of a urticarial wheal.

The pathogenesis of reaginic disorders is quite different from that of the other major type of acute allergic reaction which is produced by complement-fixing antigen-antibody complexes (Fig. 5-3). As discussed elsewhere in this book (chapter 4), these immune complexes produce tissue injury by activation of the complement system, which

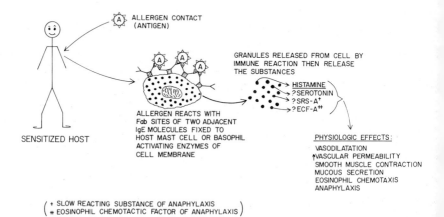

Figure 5-2
Pathogenesis of atopic reactivity (reaginic sensitivity—IgE-mediated reaction).

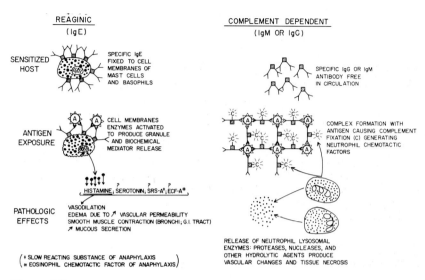

Figure 5-3
Comparison of reaginic reactivity and complement-mediated reactions.

in turn promotes chemotaxis of cells such as neutrophils to tissue foci of the complexes, where they release their lysosomal contents of different hydrolytic enzymes [12]. The difference in pathogenic sequence accounts for the longer time period required in the onset of the complement-dependent tissue reactions. These reactions can seldom be observed to begin in less than one hour due to the time required for neutrophil emigration (as in the Arthus reaction). Reaginic or atopic reactions, on the other hand, characteristically begin within a few minutes and develop peak reactivity in less than one hour, the time largely depending on the rapidity of antigen diffusion in the tissues to sites of antibody fixation.

These differences in pathogenesis and time course are due to the differences in the types of antibodies responsible for each of these two acute allergic reactions. In humans, the antibody responsible for reaginic disorders belongs to the class designated immunoglobulin E (IgE), while those which produce complement dependent reactions belong to either the immunoglobulin G (IgG) or M (IgM) class (Table 5-1). IgE is a fast-migrating γ-globulin with a high content of carbohydrate (11% w/w) of about 200,000 molecular weight [22]. Its molecular structure consists of two light chains that may be either κ or λ specificity and two heavy chains designated as ε (epsilon) specificity. Attachment to mast cell membranes is a function of the Fc portion of the heavy chains of the molecule, leaving the Fab portions free to combine with antigen [8] (see Fig. 5-1).

Table 5-1. Comparison of Characteristics of Reaginic and Complement-Fixing Antibodies.

Characteristics	Reaginic IgE	Complement Fixing	
		IgG	IgM
Molecular weight	200,000 (8 S)	150,000 (7 S)	900,000 (19 S)
Heat lability (56° C for 30 min)	+	−	−
Destroyed by disulphide bond-reducing agents	+	−	− (dissociated to 5–7 S units)
Form precipitates with antigen	+ (with sufficient concentration)	−	−
Fixation to basophils or mast cells	+	−	−
Form-circulating complexes	+	+	+
L chain types	κ, λ	κ, λ	κ, λ
H chain types	ε	γ	μ
Normal serum concentration	250–350 ng/ml	7–16 mg/ml	0.5–2 mg/ml

Activation of cell membranes for the release of biochemical mediators requires antigen binding to two adjacent molecules of IgE fixed to the cell membrane [22] (see Fig. 5-2). IgE will not fix complement and is not responsible for complement dependent reactions. The ability of IgE to fix to cell membranes is destroyed by heating for 4 hours at 56° C and also by reduction and alkylation of the molecule [22]. There is narrow species specificity for IgE in that it can passively sensitize primates such as monkeys and chimpanzees, but it does not sensitize the cells of unrelated species such as guinea pig, rat, and mouse [8, 23]. Because of this affinity for sensitization of only closely related species, IgE has been called *homocytotropic,* in contrast to other immunoglobulins of IgG subclasses in man that will passively sensitize tissues of distantly related species such as guinea pig and which are called *heterocytotropic antibodies* [8]. These heterocytotropic antibodies do not sensitize the tissues of the host animal or related species, and because of this fact they do not appear to be of pathogenic significance in intrinsic reaginic or atopic diseases. Only reaginic (or homocytotropic, IgE) antibodies seem to be primarily responsible for such disorders in man. Occasional reports have suggested that immune reactants formed with

IgG in man could produce cellular release of biochemical mediators, but they have not yet been well confirmed [41, 42]. In animals, the occurrence of IgG antibodies that produce mediator release has been well documented [8].

Aside from the uniqueness of the IgE antibody with its selective affinity for fixation to certain cell membranes, other aspects of the molecular and cellular mechanisms of reaginic reactions should be emphasized. The antigens which sensitize and provoke the host reaction are not unique but may be derived from a variety of animal, plant, or synthetic sources. The major requirement for sensitization is that the antigen be immunogenic, that is, capable of eliciting antibody response in the host. Simple haptens are not effective. Production of reaginic antibody is often enhanced in animals by administering the antigen with adjuvants such as *Hemophilus pertussis* vaccine, alum, or complete Freund's adjuvant [35, 36]. Antigens which provoke the tissue reactions, however, need not be of immunogenic size. Molecules possessing a minimum of two antigenic determinants are all that is needed to induce release of vasoactive substances from the sensitized cells [15, 21, 30]. Univalent haptens have proved effective in blocking the release reactions if given to sensitized animals prior to antigenic challenge [29].

The pharmacologic mediators appear to be released from sensitized mast cells or basophils as a consequence of antigen challenge. These mediators include histamine [23] and probably SRS–A [23] and ECF–A [28]. They exhibit potent biologic effects such as smooth muscle contraction, vascular permeability, vasodilatation, mucous secretion, and emigration of eosinophils to the sites of tissue reactivity. These effects account for much of the altered physiology characteristic of reaginic or atopic reactions.

Clinical Patterns of Atopic Disorders

The different types of atopic disorders occur principally because of various modes of antigen exposure and variation in the susceptibility of individuals to these disorders. Such variation has been noted among families where siblings and their parents may all exhibit notable difficulty with recurrent allergic disorders [3, 19, 40, 47]. Experiments in animals have ascertained that the ability to produce high levels of reaginic antibody is transmitted as a polygenic dominant trait [32]. Because of the familial pattern it is important to note in the clinical history any atopic disorders in relatives and family members.

A third factor of importance which determines the clinical pattern of an atopic disease is the shock organ or tissue primarily affected. The shock organ characteristically exhibits the most severe reaction in a sensitive person who has been exposed to antigen [45]. Often, these reactions are observed in tissues at the site of exposure or entry of the antigen. However, they do frequently occur in remote tissues such as in a case where food ingestion produces an urticarial reaction in the skin. This remote selectivity of organs and tissues is not clearly understood, but it may be due to a differential affinity of the tissue for larger amounts of reaginic antibody (IgE).

The tissues most commonly involved in atopic disorders are those of the respiratory tract, skin, and intestine.

Respiratory Tract

Allergic Rhinitis, Nasal Polyps, and Sinusitis

Reaginic reactions of the nasal and sinus mucosa occur when a sensitive person inhales an allergen that produces increased production of mucus, edema, and vascular engorgement [36]. These effects are due to the local release of biochemical mediators discussed earlier in this chapter. The allergen or allergens are usually those ubiquitous in the environment and are often found to be pollens of various plants, fungal spores, insect parts, animal danders, and various dusts from either synthetic or natural materials. Recurrent episodes may be frequent and produce a chronic edematous reaction of the mucosa that becomes polypoid, eventually forming distinct polyps that project from the surface. The symptoms of watery rhinorrhea, frequent sneezing, and blocked nasal passages are all characteristically associated with these disorders, which are commonly called "hay fever." Smears of the nasal secretions usually exhibit large numbers of eosinophils because of the release from the local cell reservoirs of eosinophil chemotactic factor that specifically attracts the eosinophils to the immune reaction site in the mucosa.

Asthma

Bronchial asthma presents a complex of symptoms due to inadequate breathing which results from bronchospasm and excessive secretions. In the sensitive individual there are "attacks" which are precipitated by exposure to antigen. Such exposure can be either by inhalation, a common mode, or by ingestion or injection of antigenic substances. The pathogenesis of the "attack" is similar to other atopic reactions wherein the release of pharmacologically active materials from sensitized cells occurs rapidly following antigen exposure [14]. These pharmacologic substances constrict the bronchial smooth muscle, promote mucous secretion from the glands and epithelium, and alter vascular flow, producing mucosal edema (Fig. 5-4). These physiologic changes obstruct airflow and cause wheezing along with the sensation of dyspnea. Eosinophils are noted in abundance in smears of the bronchial secretions, probably because of their chemotactic attraction. Antihistamines only partially suppress these reactions [14, 18], indicating the importance of the other biochemical mediators in the pathogenesis of the disorder. Corticosteroids often produce dramatic suppression. The episodic recurrence of "attacks" distinguishes asthma from other conditions that

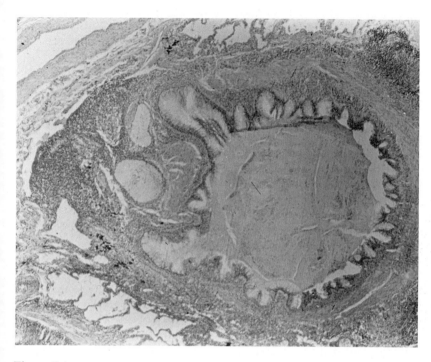

Figure 5-4
Bronchus from fatal case of asthma. The mucous plugging, smooth muscle
hypertrophy, and chronic inflammation are characteristic histologic findings
in this disease.

may provoke similar reactions. Such recurrences are often seasonal and
are associated with other allergic reactions such as rhinitis or eczema.
The classic distinction between so-called extrinsic and intrinsic asthma
pertains more to the clinical aspects of the disorders than to the pathophysiology of the reactions, which appear similar in the release of
pharmacologic mediators.

Atopic Skin Disorders

Urticaria
The occurrence of pruritic edematous wheals involving the skin and
subcutaneous tissue, which are called urticaria or hives, may be due to
an allergic reaction [14]. In fact, atopic reactions are the most common
cause of urticarial lesions, although it may be difficult to establish firmly
a cause-effect relationship with a particular antigen. Urticarial reactions
characteristically develop rapidly following antigen exposure (usually
in less than 30 min) and subside within a few hours. The mode of anti-

gen exposure is usually by ingestion or injection. Rarely is there a reaction due to skin contact because of the barrier afforded by the epithelium and basement membrane of the skin. Only when there are cuts or breaks in the skin can a reaction be provoked by this route. (Skin testing for atopic sensitivity, which will be discussed below, utilizes this approach.)

The pathogenesis of urticaria is similar to that of other atopic disorders [14]. Release of mediators follows antigen exposure in the sensitive person. These mediators cause marked changes in vascular permeability which result in the edematous wheals (Fig. 5-5). The wheals may vary in size and distribution depending on many factors including amount of antigen exposure, degree of individual sensitivity, and "shock organ" selectivity. In some individuals, the reactions may be described as giant size and involve whole body areas such as the face, trunk, or an extremity. The antigens most frequently causing these reactions are nuts, fish and egg foods, and various drugs such as penicillin.

Eczema and Dermatitis

Certain forms of chronic dermatitis which occur mostly in young children and infrequently in adults are regarded as atopic, although there is little direct evidence to support this pathogenesis of these disorders. Most of the evidence is indirect, and the allergic basis for these reactions is surmised by their association with other forms of atopic reactivity, elevated serum IgE levels [6, 19, 27], and the clearing of lesions following withdrawal and avoidance of presumed antigens, especially certain foods such as eggs [14]. The skin lesions only remotely resemble those characteristically found in atopic disorders such as urticaria. The lesions are chronic and eruptive with vesicle formation and exudation. Antihistamines have no effect on the development or

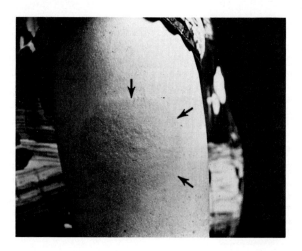

Figure 5-5
Urticarial wheal of upper arm in a case of penicillin hypersensitivity which developed rapidly following injection of the drug.

regression of the lesions, in contrast to those of urticaria. The histopathology of the lesions exhibits chronic inflammation and minimal edema, also in contrast to the predominance of marked edema in urticaria. Eosinophilia is commonly noted in the peripheral smear but not in the lesions. Positive skin tests for atopic reactivity to a variety of test antigens are also common. Their pathologic significance is unclear, however, since removal of the reactive antigens and desensitization often does not result in clearing of the lesions.

Other Atopic Disorders

Gastrointestinal Allergy

Atopic reactions of the gastrointestinal tract are also more suspect than proved. As indicated in the discussions above, atopic reactions of the skin and respiratory tract may follow ingestion of various foods [45]. These reactions are not regarded as primary atopic gastrointestinal reactions unless they are also associated with symptoms of vomiting, diarrhea, bloating, pain, and flatulence indicative of a primary effect. Often, however, such symptoms will occur without any associated evidence of an atopic reaction in other tissues. In these cases the differential diagnosis will encompass many possibilities aside from atopic disorders. Deficiencies of digestive enzymes, fibrocystic disease, galactose intolerance, sprue and coeliac disease, and various inflammatory diseases may produce symptoms identical to those described for atopic diseases of the gastrointestinal tract. The differential diagnosis of these disorders necessitates a careful history to determine the disease pattern and its relationship to precipitating factors, especially certain foods.

In this connection, it is of importance to establish the presence of IgE antibody to a suspected food antigen and to demonstrate sensitivity by skin tests or basophil histamine release tests, to be described later in this chapter. Relief of the gastrointestinal symptoms should occur on withdrawal of the suspected food antigen, and avoidance of the food should prevent their recurrence. This relief of symptoms on removal and avoidance does not demonstrate or prove an immunologic basis for the disorder. Proof of immunologic etiology is difficult and is only indirectly confirmed by association of the gastrointestinal reaction with other atopic disorders, demonstration of sensitivity by skin tests, and precipitation of symptoms on ingestion of the antigen.

Anaphylaxis

The profound systemic response of anaphylaxis mentioned earlier in this chapter may rarely occur in man. The circumstances of occurrence are usually following injection of a drug or parenteral administration of immune animal serum for passive immunization. The sudden onset of hypotension, respiratory difficulty, and collapse appear to be due to the widespread release of biochemical mediators from circulating basophils and tissue mast cells [24]. Epinephrine, a potent beta-adrenergic agent, will rapidly antagonize the physiologic effects of these mediators when given in a 0.3 ml dose of 1:1000 dilution. Where the clinical history indicated previous atopic reactions, especially to a drug or serum to be injected, appropriate skin tests or other testing should be done prior to administration to determine the individual's state of sensitivity [31]. In those sensitive individuals who must receive the drug or serum, premedication with large doses of antihistamines should be carried out, and the drug or serum should be given slowly with epinephrine available for immediate use in case of anaphylactic response.

Laboratory Tests and Procedures in the Evaluation of Atopic Disorders

There are currently five types of tests and procedures that are useful in the diagnosis of atopic disorders. These are (a) direct and passive transfer skin tests; (b) leukocyte (basophil) histamine release: direct and passively sensitized cells; (c) antigen-specific serum IgE determinations by radioimmunoassay (RAST); (d) serum IgE determinations by radioimmunoassay; and (e) Schultz-Dale reactions for determination of biochemical mediators. In addition to these, other less specific but useful tests are absolute eosinophil counts in the peripheral blood, nasal and sputum smears for eosinophils, and quantitation of serum immunoglobulins.

Skin Tests

Cutaneous reactivity to antigens may be observed in sensitive individuals, and this reactivity may be passively transferred by an injection of serum from a sensitive person into the skin of a nonsensitive individual (Prausnitz-Küstner reaction). In order to provoke the reaction, antigen must reach the dermal connective tissue either by injection or by a scratch or prick which breaks through the epithelium and basement membrane. The characteristic reaction which develops rapidly (in less than 20 min) is due to the sudden release of vasoactive factors from the IgE-sensitized mast cells in the subcutis. The reaction appears as an erythematous wheal surrounded by a zone of blanching. The usual reaction size is a wheal of about 2 cm (20 mm) diameter. Much larger wheals surrounded by an erythematous zone may develop in the markedly sensitive individual.

Since other types of immune reactions can also produce skin reactions, it is important to differentiate atopic sensitivity by the rapid onset of the erythema and edema. An Arthus type reaction seldom begins in less than one hour due to the time required for neutrophil migration into the tissue site. The skin reactions of delayed hypersensitivity require 8–10 hours before they are observable, due to the delay in monocyte recruitment and macrophage activation. Both of these latter reactions frequently exhibit necrosis with induration in addition to edematous changes.

The procedures for skin testing are described here in outline.

Scratch or Prick Tests
1. Patient in prone position with back exposed.
2. Cleanse skin with alcohol and let sites air dry.
3. Apply drops of test antigens* in aqueous or glycerolsaline medium according to a predetermined pattern for identification. Use controls with glycerolsaline medium alone and with histamine acid phosphate 1:1000 in 50% glycerine. (NOTE: allow about 4 cm between test sites.)
4. After application of the test antigen, lightly prick or scratch so as to abrade the skin for approximately 2 mm. (NOTE: have 1:1000 epinephrine available to treat immediately anaphylaxis in unsuspected cases of marked sensitivity.)
5. After 20 min, examine the sites and record positive reactions according to degree of reactivity on a scale of 1+ to 4+, ranging from erythema of 2 cm or less to a wheal with pseudopods and surrounding erythema greater than 2 cm in diameter.

Intradermal Tests
These tests are usually performed in the skin of the upper arm since greater reactivity may be expected with injection of antigen than with diffusion in the scratch test. In the case of marked reaction and/or anaphylaxis, a tourniquet can be applied to the arm to reduce dissemination of the antigen, along with the administration of epinephrine and antihistamines. The intradermal test should not be performed with antigens giving a reaction of 2+ or greater in the scratch or prick test because of the possibility of a severe local or systemic reaction. Also because of the risk of increased reactivity, the antigens used in intradermal testing should be more dilute than those used in scratch tests.

1. Cleanse with alcohol and mark the test sites.
2. Give intradermal injections of antigen in a volume of 0.02 ml using a tuberculin syringe with a 26 gauge needle. (Epinephrine 1:1000 and a tourniquet should be available in case of an anaphylactic reaction.) Use glycerolsaline medium controls.
3. Observe reactions at 20 min and carefully compare to the controls, since nonspecific irritant effects of the test agents may cause reactivity. A positive area of erythema or wheal reaction will be 1½ to

* Available commercially in combinations and individually.

2 times the diameter of the control reaction or greater. The positive reactions can be graded on a scale from 1+ to 4+.

Passive Transfer Test (Prausnitz-Küstner Reaction) [2, 45]
The serum of sensitive individuals usually contains sufficient IgE antibody to the reactive antigens so that intracutaneous injection of such serum into a nonsensitive person produces passive sensitization of the tissue. A period of 18–24 hours is required for the passively transferred IgE antibody to become fixed to the cell membranes of the local mast cells. After this period, challenge with the appropriate antigen by intradermal injection of the transfer site causes release of vasoactive factors and the ensuing wheal and flare reaction. This method affords an indirect way of determining the presence of reaginic antibody, but it has been replaced by more direct measurements afforded by the radioisotope antigen absorbent technique. Also, the risk of transfer of the agent of hepatitis has substantially reduced the use of this test among humans. Passive transfer to animals is effective only in homologous or closely related species such as monkeys and chimpanzees; it does not sensitize the tissues of distant species such as guinea pigs, rabbits, mice, or rats.

Certain IgG antibodies of man do sensitize mast cells and tissues of rats and guinea pigs for release of vasoactive factors on exposure to antigen, but these IgG antibodies (heterocytotropic antibodies) do not exhibit this reactivity in man or homologous species. Only IgE (or reaginic or atopic) antibodies show this reactivity in man.

Leukocyte Histamine Release Tests

An in vitro approach to the detection of reaginic sensitivity is afforded by the technique of leukocyte histamine release [38]. The presence of blocking antibody can also be detected by this method. The detection of sensitizing serum antibody (IgE) by passive sensitization of leukocytes in vitro followed by antigen challenge and measurement of histamine release is another useful application of this technique [33]. The amount of histamine released correlates with the amount of antigen exposure and thus provides a somewhat quantitative measure of the degree of atopic sensitivity. This sensitivity is usually expressed in terms of the amount of antigen required to release 50% of the available histamine from a standardized leukocyte preparation.

A general outline of the procedure is as follows (modified from Campbell et al. [11]). Use plastic tubes and pipettes or siliconized glassware.

EQUIPMENT
A. 2 each 50 ml plastic syringes
B. 10 ml and 25 ml test tubes

C. Plastic or siliconized glassware (adequate for 1 set of test determina-
   ation)
   a. 10 each *50 and 100 lambda* pipettes
   b. 50 each 5 ml test tube
   c. 150 each 10 ml test tube
   d. 150 each 25 ml test tubes (conical)
   e. 5 each 250 ml beakers
   f. 5 each 500 ml beakers
   g. 5 each 2 x 70 mm stirring rods
D. Centrifuge—refrigerated
E. Agitator—mechanical
F. Heating plate (temp adjustable) and glass beads
G. 37° C incubator water bath (temp regulated)
H. Ice bath
I. Instruments for fluorometric assay
J. Hemocytometer WBC counting chamber
K. Light microscope
L. Rubber bulb pipette aspirator
M. Test tube racks

REAGENTS
A. 1 liter dextran-EDTA-saline solution (see Appendix to Chapter 5)
B. 1 liter Tris buffer (see Appendix to Chapter 5)
C. 1 liter cation Tris buffer (see Appendix to Chapter 5)
D. 500 ml 10% perchloric acid
E. 1 liter butanol
F. 1 kgm NaCL
G. 500 ml 3 N NaOH
H. 1 liter 1 N NaOH
I. 1 liter 0.1 N HCl
J. 2 liters Heptane
K. 100 ml 0.1% orthophthaldialdehyde
L. 250 ml 6 N H_3PO_4

1. A volume of whole blood is collected (approximately 50 ml) in a
   plastic syringe and mixed with a dextran-EDTA-saline solution to
   sediment the red cells.
2. After sedimentation of the red cells, the plasma layer containing
   the leukocytes is removed by careful pipetting and centrifuged at
   350 g and at 4° C to sediment the leukocytes. Pour off the supernatant and save.
3. The sedimented cells are washed by gently resuspending in a
   special Tris buffer at 4° C by agitation with 1–2 ml volume initially,
   then to a final volume of 20 ml. Centrifuge as above and discard
   the supernatant.

4. Repeat the wash above and resuspend the cells in a final volume of 15 ml cation Tris buffer at 4° C. Perform a hemocytometer cell count to determine numbers of leukocytes which may vary from 10 to 20 million/ml. (Platelets are largely lost in the initial centrifugation and are of no consequence since they contain little histamine.)

5. Prepare a protocol for dilutions of antigen to be tested with aliquots of the washed cell suspension. The antigen dilutions are usually calculated on the basis of amounts comparable to those producing skin reactivity and will range from 10 μg N/ml to 10^{-5} μg N/ml. Reaction volumes of 3 to 5 ml may be selected with addition of 1 ml aliquots of the cell suspension. All dilutions, additions, and mixing are carried out at 4° C.

6. After adding the cell suspension, tubes are transferred to a 37° C bath for one hour with constant surveillance to keep the cells evenly suspended. The cation Tris buffer is used as diluent and appropriate blanks without antigen are always included to determine background histamine release. Duplicates to determine 100% histamine release are also included and treated by heating for 15 min in boiling water or by addition of 20 drops of 10% perchloric acid.

7. After incubation at 37° C for one hour, the tubes are centrifuged to bring down all the cells into a button (approximately 600 g). The supernatant is poured off and mixed with 1 ml 10% perchloric acid and analyzed for histamine content by fluorometric assay. The histamine is stable under these conditions. If assay for histamine is carried out on a Schultz-Dale apparatus, perchloric acid is omitted and the solutions cooled to 4° C until analyzed, which should be immediately.

Histamine is most easily determined by fluorometric assay based on the fluorescence of a condensation product formed by histamine with orthophthaldialdehyde [46]. Proceed with analysis of the above tubes with the added perchloric acid as follows:

8. Centrifuge to remove precipitated protein (600 g).

9. Add a 5 ml aliquot of supernatant from each sample to 10 ml butanol and 1.5 gm NaCl in a 25 ml test tube. Then add 1.0 ml 3 N NaOH to each sample with vigorous agitating in a mechanical agitator for 5–10 min.

10. Centrifuge to separate organic and aqueous phases at 200 g for 3–5 min. Aspirate the top layer containing organic extract and add to 3.0 ml 0.1 N HCl and 15 ml heptane. Agitate vigorously and centrifuge again at 200 g for 5 min. Aspirate and discard the upper layer. Place tubes in an ice bath.

11. Remove 2 ml from the bottom of each tube and add to iced tubes containing 0.5 ml 1 N NaOH with agitation for thorough mixing. (Prepare histamine standards and treat in same way with NaOH— 0.25, 0.15, 0.08, 0.04, and 0.02 μg histamine base/ml.) Use 0.1 N HCl as blank.

12. After mixing the above tubes, add 0.1 ml 0.1% orthophthaldialde-hyde to each tube and mix well. Allow to react for 1 hour at 4° C in an ice bath, then add 0.2 5 ml 6 N H_3PO_4. After the samples are at room temperature, measure fluorescence at 450 nm with activation at 350 nm. Do not delay measurements since the condensation product is unstable after 30 min.

13. The percent of histamine released by the various quantities of antigen is then calculated by comparing the histamine values for each dilution to those prepared for 100% release. (Care should be taken to subtract the background histamine release from each determination, as well as any intrinsic fluorescence of the blanks.) Determination of the reference standards provides a control as to accuracy of the measurements. A variation of less than 5% among the duplicate blank tubes and duplicate 100% release tubes provides adequate control of precision of the analysis. On completion of the analysis, the amount of antigen producing 50% histamine release can be determined.

Histamine can also be assayed by the Schultz-Dale technique, which will be outlined later. The principle is based on the fact that a segment of guinea pig ileum will contract when exposed to histamine. The amount of contraction is roughly proportional to the amount of histamine so that, by comparison to preparations yielding 100% release, the relative percent of histamine in a given sample can be determined. The method is more cumbersome and subjective than the fluorometric assay, which is preferred.

In addition to its use in the direct measurement of reaginic sensitivity, the technique of leukocyte histamine release can be applied to the detection of blocking antibody and as an indirect method for measuring reaginic antibody by passive sensitization of the cells. In the procedure to detect blocking antibody, various dilutions of serum are mixed with a predetermined amount of antigen that will ordinarily cause release of 50% of the histamine from a standardized cell suspension. The inhibition of release due to serum factors can then be determined by measuring the percent histamine release and calculation of the 50% release amount of antigen. This newly determined 50% release figure will exceed that found without pretreatment with serum in the event that blocking antibody is present. If no blocking antibody is present, the 50% release figures will be comparable.

The technique of passive sensitization of leukocytes for detecting reaginic antibody is somewhat more complex than that of the direct determination of sensitized cells [33]. It is necessary that susceptible cells from a nonsensitive donor be available. Such donors can be selected from those who have negative skin tests to the antigens under study. The cells of these donors can be checked for histamine release on exposure to the antigen, and if negative, they should be suitable for use in passive sensitization. Since EDTA and heparin are known to enhance passive sensitization, these agents are included in the sensitizing mixture [38]. The additional details of the passive sensitization technique are as follows:

1. Donor cells are prepared and washed twice as in the direct method given above. They are suspended in 10 ml of special Tris buffer at 37° C.
2. 2 ml aliquots of the cell suspension are then added to tubes containing two-fold serial dilutions of the test serum in EDTA-heparin Tris buffer solution. Mix by gentle swirling at intervals for 1 hour at 37° C. After this sensitization, the cells are washed twice by centrifuging at 400 g and resuspending in 10 ml cation Tris buffer at 4° C. The final volume of the suspension should be 3.5 ml in each of the tubes.
3. Aliquot duplicate volumes of 1 ml to tubes containing an amount of antigen adequate to produce maximum histamine release. Prepare blanks for each set of tubes from the remaining cell suspension. Incubate with antigen for 1 hour at 37° C. Centrifuge and complete the analysis for histamine determinations as in the direct method. The activity of the test serum for reaginic antibody is proportional to the reciprocal of the serum dilution which produces 50% histamine release from the sensitized cells.

Antigen Specific Serum IgE Determinations
by Radioimmunoassay (RAST) (3 days)
Since the advent of methods for the determination of IgE and the studies which have confirmed the importance of this immunoglobulin as the mediating antibody in atopic reactions, the measurement of specific IgE antibodies has added a major dimension in the clinical evaluation of reaginic disorders. The method of the radioallergosorbent test described by Wide et al. [48] is based on the formation of an insoluble polymeric complex of antigen (allergen) by coupling the allergen to Sephadex® or cellulose activated by cyanogen bromide. During incubation with atopic serum, the specific IgE antibody is adsorbed out by reaction with the insoluble allergen. The amount of IgE is then determined by reacting anti-IgE radiolabeled with ^{125}I with the insoluble material followed by washing and counting of the radioactivity. The amount of IgE specific for the antigen (allergen) is thus directly determined. The results of this method correlate well with the detection of reaginic sensitivity by other sensitive methods such as provocation. Indeed, the RAST procedure appears to be equally accurate in some instances with in vivo testing by provocation with allergens.

The overall range of agreement between provocation and RAST testing methods is generally 70–75% [7]. In the 25% where correlation is poor, the cause is probably due to various factors such as differences in patient states of responsiveness, variation in potency of test antigen extracts, differences in seasonal amounts of circulating reagins, and variation in the response of specific tissues to provocation with certain antigens. As additional data accumulate, it is expected that the RAST test will prove to be quite useful as a screening test for reaginic disorders. The details of the method are as follows (modified from Wide et al. [48]):

EQUIPMENT
A. Closed vessel (glass flask)
B. Refrigerator (4° C)

REAGENTS
A. Sephadex or cellulose particles (Pharmacia)
B. Cyanogen bromide
C. 0.6 M HCl
D. 0.02 M phosphate buffer, pH 7.8
E. 100 ml acidified silver nitrate
F. Allergen extract as appropriate

PREPARATION OF ALLERGEN PARTICLE COMPLEX
1. Sephadex or cellulose particles are activated by treatment with cyanogen bromide in a closed vessel at a concentration of 15 mg/ml in 0.6 M HCl for 4 hours followed by repeated washing in phosphate buffer of 0.02 M, pH 7.8 until effluent is negative for bromide ion when tested with acidified silver nitrate.
2. The activated particle solution is then mixed with allergen extract for 4 hours at room temperature at an adjusted concentration of allergen ranging from 5 to 10 mg/ml followed by washing to remove excess allergen in phosphate buffer.
3. The allergen particle complex is then stored at 4° C for use.

RAST TEST PROCEDURE
1. In a typical test, 0.5 ml allergen particle complex (conc. 1 mg/ml) is added to 50 microliters test serum and incubated at room temperature overnight, followed by washing and subsequent addition the next day of anti-IgE [125]I (about 50,000–60,000 cpm in 0.5 mg/ml normal rabbit γ-globulin). The mixture is again incubated overnight at room temperature and washed to remove any excess IgE [125]I. Counts are determined by counting in a gamma spectrometer and compared to a control which is run in parallel using normal serum and a buffer control.
2. Maximum uptake ranges about 60% of the total contrasted to control uptake of 0.2–0.3%. Uptake of more than 1.5 times the background control is to be considered as positive. Positive samples are usually repeated at two serum dilutions. If known positive sera are available as reference standards, the amount of specific IgE for each antigen tested can be calculated as a relative percentage.

SERUM IGE DETERMINATIONS BY RADIOIMMUNOASSAY

The significance of the serum IgE level in relation to the diagnosis of reaginic disease remains an open subject [20]. The levels reported as normal are in the range of 250 to 350 ng/ml. In patients with asthma and various allergic disorders, the values reported have ranged from 400 to levels above 1,600 ng/ml [1, 20, 25]. Recently, this relationship has been viewed in a way that attaches a different meaning to an elevated serum IgE level [5]. Individuals with helminth infestations and other disorders exhibiting markedly elevated IgE levels have been examined for their responsiveness as recipients in P-K (Prausnitz-Küstner) testing with a test serum from a single donor who was sensitive to an extract of guinea pig dander. Those individuals with IgE levels above 2,000 units/ml did not respond in P-K testing even at 16 times the reagin concentration which produced a response in those individuals with levels below 200 units/ml. These data were interpreted to indicate diminished reaginic reactivity in the presence of elevated IgE because of saturation of mast cell binding sites by the excessive amount of IgE, thus preventing any additional sensitization. The elevated levels of IgE then appeared to protect against reaginic sensitivity to specific allergens. It seems that the measurement of IgE levels thus may be of most value when determined in conjunction with the RAST procedure for specific allergens. Various methods for determining serum concentrations of IgE have been published. Two of the methods that may be used in the clinical laboratory are described below.

EQUIPMENT

A. 37° C incubator
B. Gamma spectrometer
C. 5 × 7 glass slide or large petri dish
D. Moist chamber
E. Kodak NS-54-T x-ray film
F. Equipment to develop film
G. Log-log paper

REAGENTS

A. Purified IgE radio-labeled with [125]I
B. Water bath
C. Aragose gel in barbital buffer (pH 8.2, ionic strength 0.05) containing 0.01 % merthiolate (Pharmacia; Schwarz-Mann)
D. Radio-labeled anti-IgE (exclusion fraction from DEAE at 0.01 M sodium phosphate buffer pH 8.0)
E. 1% BSA
F. Phosphate-buffered saline solution
G. Buffered saline solution (pH 8.0)
H. Distilled water
 I. Sephadex (Pharmacia)

Sephadex Coupled Antibody Method (after Johansson [26]) (2 days)
1. Activated Sephadex® similar to that used in the RAST procedure above is prepared as an immunoabsorbent by coupling anti-IgE to the particles.
2. Purified IgE radio-labeled with ^{125}I is then mixed with an aliquot of test serum in a ratio of 1:1 (total volume 100 μl/0.5 ml anti-IgE Sephadex®). Standards* are prepared at dilutions of the IgE–[125]I and added to separate aliquots of the anti-IgE Sephadex®.
3. The mixtures are incubated for 18 hours (overnight) and then washed to remove excess unreacted serum or IgE–[125]I. The washed particles are counted in a gamma spectrometer.
4. A curve is prepared from the counting data on the standards at selected dilutions and the inhibition of binding by the test serum is calculated by comparison of the difference between the comparable cpm of IgE–[125]I in the standard versus the test serum.

Radial Radioimmunodiffusion (after Arbesman et al. [1]) (6 days)
1. 0.85% agarose gel in barbital buffer is heated and allowed to cool to 56° C in a water bath. Radio-labeled anti-IgE in 1% BSA in phosphate-buffered saline solution is mixed thoroughly with agarose solution, avoiding bubble formation, and left for 30 min at 56° C. The agarose is then poured on a glass slide (5 × 7″) or large petri dish and allowed to cool and form a gel. Wells of 5 mm diameter are then cut in the agarose gel (spaced at 1 cm from each other).
2. The wells are filled according to an outlined protocol with 30 μl of each test serum, and appropriate dilutions of a reference serum, in each well. The reference serum will provide measurements for plotting a standard curve.
3. Incubate plate or petri dish in a moist chamber at 37° C for 48 hours, then remove and wash in buffered saline solution (pH 8.0) for 48 hours followed by an hour rinse in distilled water. Dry the plates and expose to x-ray film (Kodak NS–54–T) for 24 hours.
4. Develop film and measure the outer diameters of the rings formed. On log-log paper plot the square of the diameters of the various dilutions of the reference serum along the X axis and the IgE levels of the reference samples in ng/ml along the Y axis. The values of IgE in the test sera can be determined from the standard curve by locating their position on the curve from the value of the squares of the diameter of their respective circles.

This method compares well in accuracy and precision with other published methods and has the advantage of not being based on the availability of purified IgE.

* WHO Reference Standard 68–341 contain 2.42 ng per unit relative to purified myeloma IgE [4].

Schultz-Dale Reactions

The physiologic action of biochemical mediators released in atopic reactions can be utilized as the basis for a modified type of biologic assay. The assay is based on the contraction of smooth muscle due to the action of the mediator. Tissues such as intestine and bronchi from sensitized animals are found to contract on exposure to antigen in vitro. Such reactions were first described independently by Schultz [44] and later by Dale [13], and their usefulness in the detection of reaginic reactivity has not been surpassed. Not only do such reactions stimulated by antigen provide a useful in vitro counterpart of reaginic sensitivity, but the contractile responsiveness of these tissues from unsensitized animals can be employed in a general method for assay of various biochemical mediators which cannot be determined satisfactorily by other means. Passive sensitization of these tissues by homocytotropic and heterocytotropic antibodies also allows a means for detecting those reactants [17]. By measure of inhibition of the reactions with certain antagonists of biochemical mediators, highly specific assays can be achieved with this technique.

The apparatus requirements are for a glass chamber of special design which allows tissue to be suspended in a physiologic solution under constant oxygenation at 37° C and which will also allow addition of reactants to the medium and a means of emptying and refilling the chamber with solution for each determination. In addition, a physiologic recorder is needed with a point of attachment for the tissue and a transducer connected to a continuous writing recorder that can be easily switched on and off for each determination (recorder no. 350 available from Harvard Apparatus). See Fig. 5-6 for diagram of glass chamber, volume approximately 150 ml, 40 mm diameter by 180 mm length.

ADDITIONAL MATERIALS

A. Animal tissue (monkey bronchus; fresh human appendix if available; guinea pig ileum)
B. 1 ml syringe with long needle (24–26 gauge)
C. 37° C incubator

REAGENTS

A. Antigen extracts
B. Physiologic solution of Tyrode's stock prepared as follows, and prewarmed immediately before use:
   1. Anhyd. KCl   1.950 gm/liter
   2. Anhyd. $CaCl_2$ 1.454 gm/liter
   3. $MgCl_2 \cdot 6 H_2O$ 2.130 gm/liter
   4. NaCl   80.00 gm/liter
   5. $NaHCO_3$ 10.15 gm/liter

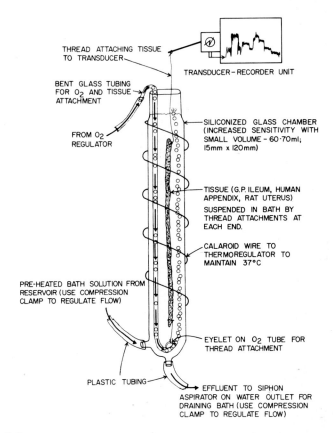

THREAD ATTACHING TISSUE
TO TRANSDUCER

TRANSDUCER-RECORDER UNIT

BENT GLASS TUBING
FOR O₂ AND TISSUE
ATTACHMENT

SILICONIZED GLASS CHAMBER
(INCREASED SENSITIVITY WITH
SMALL VOLUME - 60-70ml;
15mm x 120mm)

FROM O₂
REGULATOR

TISSUE (G.P. ILEUM, HUMAN
APPENDIX, RAT UTERUS)
SUSPENDED IN BATH BY
THREAD ATTACHMENTS AT
EACH END.

CALAROID WIRE TO
THERMOREGULATOR TO
MAINTAIN 37°C

PRE-HEATED BATH SOLUTION FROM
RESERVOIR (USE COMPRESSION
CLAMP TO REGULATE FLOW)

EYELET ON O₂ TUBE FOR
THREAD ATTACHMENT

PLASTIC TUBING

EFFLUENT TO SIPHON
ASPIRATOR ON WATER OUTLET FOR
DRAINING BATH (USE COMPRESSION
CLAMP TO REGULATE FLOW)

Figure 5-6
Schematic diagram of Schultz-Dale tissue bath.

Mix in above order of 100 ml aliquots of each to avoid formation of precipitate (add $NaHCO_3$ last) and add distilled H_2O to
make 1 liter. Add 1.0 gm dextrose. Adjust pH to 7.5–7.8 (critical
to avoid irritation of tissue). Solution is stored at 4° C and diluted
1:10 for use. Keep solution iced while using.

C. Atropine sulfate conc. 10^{-6} M (if necessary to suppress spontaneous contraction of tissue)

D. Chymotrypsin or carboxypeptidase B (to inactivate bradykinin)

DIRECT ASSAY

1. Select animal tissue appropriate to the determination desired. For
passive sensitization to detect homocytotropic antibody of humans,
use fresh tissue from either monkey bronchus or human surgical
specimens of fresh appendix if available. For general determination

of histamine or other mediators use guinea pig ileum. (See Table 5-2 for other tissues that may be used.)

2. In preparation of the tissue, the animal is sacrificed and the tissue is taken rapidly and thoroughly washed in physiologic solution of Tyrode's stock.
3. After thorough washing, the tissue is cut into segments appropriate for the chamber size (about 200 mg) and a selected segment is attached in the chamber to the recorder while moist (do not allow drying to occur). Immediately before use, prewarm diluted Tyrode's solution to 37° C. Be sure that oxygen flow through the chamber is uniform and not disruptive so as to avoid artefacts in the recording. When the suspended tissue appears stabilized (atropine sulfate can be added to the working Tyrode's solution in a concentration of 10^{-6} M to suppress spontaneous contractions) begin recording to establish a base line. Each tissue should be standardized for its response to the biochemical mediator under study. In the case of histamine standards of 1, 10, and 100 μg/ml are added in sequence to determine the amount of tissue contraction.
4. Add samples using a long needle (24–26 gauge) with a 1 ml syringe. Reaction is usually immediate; if no reaction occurs allow 30 sec before flushing bath chamber and replenishing the bathing solution.
5. If the assay involves use of an inhibitor to determine the presence of certain reactants (e.g. antihistamines to antagonize histamine) the inhibitor is first added to the bath at an appropriate concentration followed by addition of the test sample after 30 sec. In the case of assay for bradykinin, chymotrypsin or carboxypeptidase B will inactivate bradykinin by cleavage and should be mixed for 30–60 sec with the test sample prior to application to the bath in order to measure inactivation of that mediator.

PASSIVE SENSITIZATION

1. In assays to determine the presence of reaginic antibody by passive sensitization, tissues from the same or homologous species are washed free of blood and other materials with Tyrode's solution.
2. Section into appropriate segments for testing (about 200 mg). These segments are then passively sensitized by suspending them in 1.0 ml test serum diluted 1:3 in Tyrode's solution and incubated at 37° C for one hour.
3. After incubation, the segments are washed 3 times in Tyrode's solution and suspended in the apparatus for testing by addition of antigen extracts. Responsiveness to histamine is determined by calibration with histamine standards as above.

Table 5-2 summarizes the various biochemical mediators which can be detected by the Schultz-Dale technique along with the appropriate test tissue and antagonists to be used in their identification.

Table 5-2. Tissues and Antagonists Used in the Biological Assay of Biochemical Mediators.

Mediator	Responsive Tissue	Antagonist/Inhibitor
Histamine	Guinea pig ileum	Antihistamines (mepyramine at 0.1 μg/ml)
Slow-Reacting Substance of Anaphylaxis	Guinea pig ileum	None
Serotonin	Estrus rat uterus	Bromolysergic acid diethylamide (1 μg/ml)
Bradykinin	Estrus rat uterus	Carboxypeptidase (5 mg/ml) Chymotrypsin (5 mg/ml)
Prostaglandins	Gerbil colon	Polyphloretin phosphate (PPP) (200 μg/ml)

Establishing the Diagnosis of Atopic Disease

The prevalence of allergic disease is estimated to be very high in the U.S. population. A figure of 31 million people having one or more allergic disorders is the estimate given in recent data from the National Center for Health Statistics [37]. Hay fever, asthma, and other allergic conditions are reported at a prevalence of 1 in 10 among children under 17 years of age. Because of this high incidence, the possibility of an underlying allergic disorder should always be considered in the differential diagnosis of many chronic or recurrent conditions, especially those affecting the respiratory tract, skin, and gastrointestinal tract. Once considered, the possibility should not be relinquished until it has been adequately excluded. The approach to the diagnosis is taken largely on the tack of attempting to exclude an allergic disorder, since often there are no direct ways to definitely ascertain such a diagnosis.

The information that can be gained from a probing history may uncover a pattern that will strongly suggest the possibility of an allergic disorder. Characteristically the history may reveal a pattern of recurrent episodes which tend to involve mainly one organ or tissue. Such episodes may also be found related to environmental factors and seasonal occurrences when pollens and other allergens are abundant. Certain foods may be known to precipitate episodes, and certain activities such as housecleaning or cooking with flour may precede the onset of symptoms. The history will often reveal that the parents, grandparents, or siblings have an allergic disorder. The familial occurrence of such allergic disorders is a notable feature of atopic disease. The physical examination may contribute information on the extent and severity of the disorder and may serve to pinpoint the "shock organ."

During acute episodes, the physical findings will reflect the pathophysiologic effects of the released biochemical mediators. Abundant mucous exudation from the nose, along with edema and hyperemia of the nasal mucosa, wheezing, urticarial lesions of the skin, or evidence of gastrointestinal hypermotility may be observed. Laboratory studies often reveal eosinophilia both in the peripheral blood smear and in smears of nasal mucous secretions. A hypochromic anemia is not uncommon in chronic disorders. Skin tests with a variety of common allergens will usually exhibit some positive reactions. Certain positive skin reactions of intensity may be significant when related to the history. When the skin test results are not considered by the physician in relation to the history, a definitive diagnosis may be elusive. The significance of a positive skin test can be determined only within the context of the clinical history.

Measurement of serum IgE levels usually shows an elevation in atopic disorders, but as previously indicated the significance of these increased IgE levels is often unclear. Essentially, the elevated level of IgE can be interpreted only to mean that one has responded to certain antigens with an increased production of IgE antibodies. The measurement of specific IgE antibodies by the RAST procedure may aid in defining the importance of certain allergens in a given reaginic disorder. High levels of specific IgE previously noted correlate well with provocative tests. Demonstration of leukocyte histamine release in response to certain allergens can provide supportive correlation, but it does not appear to be more definitive than the RAST procedure, and it is somewhat more complex to perform.

Reaginic disorders may mimic symptoms of other diseases, especially certain diseases in children such as fibrocystic disease, certain immune deficiency syndromes, and chronic granulomatous disease. Laboratory tests to rule out the presence of those disorders should be included in the diagnostic work-up of a suspected atopic patient. Pilocarpine iontophoresis of sweat to determine sodium and chloride is an excellent screening test for fibrocystic disease. Quantitation of serum immunoglobulins and skin tests for delayed sensitivity to monilia and mumps antigens are useful in excluding immune deficiency disease (see Chapter 3). The nitroblue tetrazolium test will determine the presence of chronic granulomatous disease.

Summary

The possibility of an atopic disorder should always be of prime consideration in acute recurrent and chronic diseases of the nose, sinuses, respiratory tract, skin, and gastrointestinal tract. The clues will be provided by the history and physical exam. These clues should prompt the pertinent laboratory tests to provide the data needed for definitive diagnosis by a process akin to the triangulation method (Fig. 5-7) used by navigators to locate their position in calm or stormy seas.

History ─────────────────────── *Physical Examination*

Episodic seasonal, environmental, or post ingestion symptoms

Rhinitis, sinusitis, otitis, skin rash, wheezing and cough, gastrointestinal disorders

Onset usually in childhood

Complaints often refer to a single "shock organ" such as nose, sinuses, skin, respiratory, or G.I. tract

Frequent family history of allergy

Asthenic body build; often development delayed during childhood

Specific findings related to "shock organ" such as rhinorrhea, congestion of mucous membranes, cough with mucous production, wheezing, skin rash, diarrhea and hyperactive bowel sounds

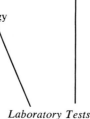

Laboratory Tests

Eosinophilia of blood and mucous secretions

Hypochromic anemia is frequent

Positive skin test reactivity to groups of various allergens

Elevation of serum IgE level

RAST test positive for specific allergens

Normal C4 levels in serum during acute attacks rules out hereditary angioedema

Figure 5-7
Triangulation in the diagnosis of atopic disease.

Appendix

*Dextran—*EDTA*—Saline Solution*
(Mix in 100 ml polycarbonate tube just before use)
1. 375 mg dextrose
2. 5.0 mg 0.1 M EDTA
3. 12.5 ml 6% dextran in saline solution

Special Tris Buffer
(Prepare just prior to use)
1. 10 ml Tris stock—Trizma, pH 7.7   37.50 gm
    NaCl   70.15 gm
    KCl   3.73 gm
    Distilled H_2O q.s. ad 1000 ml
    pH = 7.7
2. 1.0 ml 3% human serum albumin
    Distilled H_2O q.s. ad 100 ml

Cation Tris Buffer
1. 10 ml Tris stock (see above)
2. 80 ml distilled H_2O
3. 1 ml 3% human serum albumin
4. 1 ml cation stock—80 ml 0.075 M $CaCl_2$
                        20 ml 0.5 M $MgCl_2$
5. Distilled H_2O q.s. ad 100 ml

Serum Dilutions in EDTA—*Heparin Tris Buffer*
(Prepare by mixing volumes in steps)
1. Use 4 50-ml polycarbonate tubes containing 2.5 ml special Tris buffer
2. Prepare two-fold dilutions of test serum by adding 2.5 ml serum to tube No. 1 above, and after mixing, serially transfer 2.5 ml successively from each tube to the next after mixing (final dilutions 1:2, 1:4, 1:8, 1:16)
3. Add 2.0 ml isotonic EDTA-heparin to each of the above dilutions. Prepare by mixing 2 ml 0.1 M EDTA
                500 μg heparin in 1 ml
                1 ml special Tris buffer
                6 ml distilled H_2O

Antigen Dilutions for Leukocyte Histamine Release
Antigen dilutions are made in cation Tris buffer according to PN/ml (1 μg PN = 100 Protein Nitrogen Units)
1. Dilute 0.5 ml antigen solution (100 μg/ml) in 4.5 ml cation Tris buffer to give final concentration of 10 μg PN/ml.
2. Prepare sequential dilutions to 5.0 ml final volumes containing the following antigen concentrations in μg PN/ml: 1.0, 0.3, 0.1, 0.03, 0.01, 0.003, 0.001, 0.0003, 0.0001, 0.00003, 0.00001. Dilute only to 0.03 μg PN/ml for the passive sensitization technique.

References

1. Arbesman, C. E., Ito, K., Wypysch, J. I., and Wicher, K.   Measurement of serum IgE by a one-step single radial radiodiffusion method. *J. Allergy Clin. Immunol.* 49:72, 1972.
2. Augustin, R.   Demonstration of reagins in the serum of allergic subjects. In D. M. Weir (ed), *Handbook of Experimental Immunology*. Philadelphia: Davis, 1967.
3. Bazaral, M., Orgel, H. A., and Hamburger, R. N.   IgE levels in normal infants and mothers and an inheritance hypothesis. *J. Immunol.* 107: 794, 1971.
4. Bazaral, M., and Hamburger, R. N.   Standardization and stability of immunoglobulin E (IgE). *J. Allergy* 49:189, 1972.
5. Bazaral, M., Orgel, H. A., and Hamburger, R. N.   The influence of

serum IgE levels of selected recipients, including patients with allergy, helminthiasis and tuberculosis on the apparent P-K titer of a reaginic serum. *Clin. Exp. Immunol.* 14:117, 1973.

6. Berg, T., and Johansson, S. G. O.   IgE concentration in children with atopic diseases. *Int. Arch. Allergy Appl. Immunol.* 36:219, 1969.

7. Berg, T., Bennich, H., and Johansson, S. G. O.   In vitro diagnosis of atopic allergy: I. A comparison between provocation tests and the radioallergosorbent test. *Int. Arch. Allergy Appl. Immunol.* 40:770, 1971.

8. Bloch, K. J.   Immunoglobulin heterogeneity and anaphylactic sensitization. In K. F. Austen and E. L. Becker, *Biochemistry of the Acute Allergic Reactions.* 1st International Symposium. Philadelphia: Davis, 1968.

9. Bloch, K. J.   The antibody in anaphylaxis. In H. Z. Movat (ed.), *Cellular and Humoral Mechanisms in Anaphylaxis and Allergy.* Basel: Karger, 1969.

10. Brockelhurst, W. E.   The probable role of known mediators in hypersensitivity reactions. In H. O. Schild (ed.), *Immunopharmacology.* Oxford: Pergamon, 1968, 1st ed.

11. Campbell, D. H., Garvey, J. S., Cremer, N. E., and Sussdorf, D. H. *Methods in Immunology.* New York: Benjamin, 1970, 2nd ed.

12. Cochrane, C. G.   Immunologic tissue injury mediated by neutrophilic leukocytes. In F. J. Dixon, Jr., and H. G. Kunkel (eds.), *Advances in Immunology.* New York: Academic, 1968, vol. 9.

13. Dale, H. H.   The anaphylactic reaction of plain muscle in the guinea pig. *J. Pharmacol. Exp. Ther.* 4:167, 1913.

14. Frankland, A. W.   The pathogenesis of asthma, hay fever and atopic diseases. In P. G. H. Gell and R. R. A. Coombs, *Clinical Aspects of Immunology.* Philadelphia: Davis, 1968, 2nd ed.

15. Frick, O. L., Nye, W., and Raffel, S.   Anaphylactic reaction to univalent haptens. *Immunology* 14:563, 1968.

16. Greaves, M. W., and Mongar, J. L.   Mechanism of the anaphylactic reaction. In H. O. Schild (ed.), *Immunopharmacology.* Oxford: Pergamon, 1968, 1st ed.

17. Halpern, B. N., Liacopoulos, P., Liacopoulos-Broit, N., Binaghi, L. R., and Van Neer, F.   Patterns of in vitro sensitization of isolated smooth muscle tissues with antibody. *Immunology* 2:351, 1969.

18. Halpern, B.   Antihistaminics in immunopathologic reactions. In P. A. Miescher and H. J. Müller-Eberhard (eds.), *Textbook of Immunopathology.* New York: Grune & Stratton, 1968, vol. 1.

19. Hamburger, R. N., Orgel, H. A., and Bazaral, M.   Genetics of human serum IgE levels. In Laurence Goodfriend (ed.), *Control Mechanisms in Reagin-Mediated Hypersensitivity.* New York: Marcel-Dekker, 1974.

20. Henderson, L. L., Swedlund, H. A., Van Dellen, R. G.   Evaluation of IgE tests in an allergy practice. *J. Allergy Clin. Immunol.* 48:361, 1971.

21. Ishizaka, K., Ishizaka, T., and Banovitz, J.   Biologic activity of soluble antigen-antibody complexes: IX. Soluble complexes of rabbit antibody with univalent and divalent haptens. *J. Immunol.* 93:1001, 1964.

22. Ishizaka, K.   Characterization of human reaginic antibodies and immunoglobulin E. In H. Z. Movat (ed.), *Cellular and Humoral Mechanics in Anaphylaxis and Allergy.* Basel: Kargar, 1969.

23. Ishizaka, K., and Ishizaka, T.   IgE immunoglobulins of human and monkey. In K. F. Austen and E. L. Becker (eds.), *Biochemistry of the*

Acute Allergic Reactions. 2nd International Symposium. Oxford: Blackwell, 1971.

24. James, L. P., Jr., and Austen, K. F.   Fatal systemic anaphylaxis in man. *N. Engl. J. Med.* 270:597, 1964.

25. Johansson, S. G. O.   Raised levels of a new immunoglobulin class (IgND) in asthma. *Lancet* 2:951, 1967.

26. Johansson, S. G. O.   Serum IgND levels in healthy children and adults. *Int. Arch. Allergy Appl. Immunol.* 34:1, 1968.

27. Juhlin, L., Johannson, S. G. O., Bennich, H., Hogman, C. F., and Thyresson, N.   Immunoglobulin E in dermatoses. *Arch. Dermatol.* 100:12, 1969.

28. Kay, A. B., and Austen, K. F.   The IgE mediated release of an eosinophil leukocyte chemotactic factor of anaphylaxis from human lung. *J. Immunol.* 107:899, 1971.

29. Landsteiner, K., and Van der Scheer, J.   Anaphylactic shock by dyes: II. *J. Exp. Med.* 67:97, 1938.

30. Levine, B. B.   The nature of antigen-antibody complexes which initiate anaphylactic reactions. *J. Immunol.* 94:111, 1965.

31. Levine, B. B.   Immunologic mechanisms of penicillin allergy, a haptenic model system for the study of allergic diseases of man. *N. Engl. J. Med.* 275:1115, 1966.

32. Levine, B. B.   Genetic factors in reagin production in mice. In K. F. Austen and E. L. Becker (eds.), *Biochemistry of the Acute Allergic Reactions.* 2nd International Symposium. Oxford: Blackwell, 1971.

33. Levy, D. A., and Osler, A. G.   Studies on the mechanism of hypersensitivity phenomena: XIV. Passive sensitization in vitro of human leukocytes to ragweed pollen antigen. *J. Immunol.* 97:203, 1966.

34. Lewis, T.   *The Blood Vessels of the Human Skin and Their Responses.* London: Shaw, 1927.

35. Malkiel, S., and Hargis, B. J.   Anaphylactic shock in the pertussis-vaccinated mouse. *J. Allergy* 23:352, 1952.

36. Mendelson, L. M., Nyhan, W. L., and Hamburger, R. N.   Allergic rhinitis-pediatric grand rounds, University of California, University of San Diego (Specialty Conferences). *Calif. Med.* 117:37, 1972.

37. National Center for Health Statistics.   *Chronic Conditions and Limitations of Activity and Morbidity in the United States, July 1965–June 1967.* Vital and Health Statistics, Publication No. 1000, Series 10, No. 61, Jan. 1971. Washington, D.C.: Government Printing Office.

38. Osler, A. G., Lichtenstein, L. M., and Levy, D. A.   In vitro studies of human reaginic allergy. In F. J. Dixon, Jr. and H. G. Kunkel (eds.), *Advances in Immunology.* New York: Academic, 1968, vol. 8.

39. Ovary, Z., Benacerraf, B., and Bloch, K. J.   Properties of guinea pig 7S antibodies: II. Identification of antibodies involved in passive cutaneous and systemic anaphylaxis. *J. Exp. Med.* 117:951, 1963.

40. Penrose, L. S.   Genetic background of common diseases. *Acta Genet. Med. Gemellol.* (Roma) 4:257, 1953.

41. Reid, R. T., Minden, P., and Farr, R. S.   Reaginic activity associated with IgG immunoglobulin. *J. Exp. Med.* 123:845, 1966.

42. Reid, R. T.   Reaginic activity associated with immunoglobulins other than IgE. *J. Immunol.* 104:935, 1970.

43. Richet, C.   *Anaphylaxis* (J. M. Bligh, trans.). London: Constable, 1913.

44. Schultz, W. H.   Physiological studies in anaphylaxis: I. The reaction of smooth muscle of the guinea pig sensitized with horse serum. *J. Pharmacol. Exp. Ther.* 1:549, 1910.

45. Sheldon, J. M., Lovell, R. G., and Mathews, K. P.   *A Manual of Clinical Allergy.* Philadelphia: Saunders, 1967, 2nd ed.

46. Shore, P. A., Burkhalter, A., and Cohn, V. H.   A method for the fluorometric assay of histamine in tissues. *J. Pharmacol. Exp. Ther.* 127:182, 1959.

47. Weiner, A., Zieve, I., and Fries, J.   The inheritance of allergic disease. *Ann. Eugenics* 7:141, 1936.

48. Wide, L., Bennich, H., and Johansson, S. G. O.   Diagnosis of allergy by an in vitro test for allergen antibodies. *Lancet* 2:1105, 1967.

6

Immune Complexes and Cryoglobulins in Human Diseases

The role of antigen-antibody complexes in the pathogenesis of vasculitis and glomerulonephritis in human disease has been well established [17, 23, 95]. During the past several years, evidence has been presented that antigen-antibody complexes unrelated to the specific tissue may mediate pathologic mechanisms with injury. The glomerulonephritis seen in serum sickness, poststreptococcal infection, systemic lupus erythematosus, and certain infectious diseases are believed to be mediated by immune complexes [15, 42, 44, 77, 89]. Australia antigen-antibody complexes have been found to be localized in the vascular lesions of human cases of polyarteritis nodosa [31]. Also, immune complexes probably play a significant role in the pathogenesis of lesions in rheumatoid arthritis [10].

Cryoglobulins are serum proteins that are insoluble at 4° C and redissolve on heating to 37° C. These reversibly cold-precipitable globulins have been described in many clinical conditions including lymphoproliferative disorders, collagen diseases, and viral infections [6]. The patients with cryoglobulinemia have a wide variety of conditions such as glomerulonephritis, vasculitis, and purpura, which suggests that many of these patients demonstrate an immune complex type of autoimmune disorder.

When Does One Suspect Immune Complex Disease and/or Cryoglobulinemia?

Findings on History and Physical Examination

Immune complexes or cryoglobulins may be suspected to play a role in the pathogenesis of diseases which show clinical signs and symptoms of
A. Glomerulonephritis
B. Vasculitis with multisystem involvement
C. Synovitis with joint swelling and pain
D. Serositis—pleural effusion and pain

E. Purpura
F. Raynaud's syndrome
G. Anemia
H. Deficient exocrine function—i.e., Sjögren's syndrome
I. Lymphoproliferative disorders, e.g., leukemia, lymphoma
J. Certain bacterial or viral diseases, e.g., (a) subacute bacterial endo-
   carditis, (b) infectious mononucleosis, (c) cytomegalic inclusion dis-
   ease, (d) syphilis, and (e) leprosy
K. Malignant tumors
L. Cirrhosis

Findings on Common Laboratory Tests
A. Urinalysis—proteinuria and hematuria may indicate glomerulonephritis.
B. Complete blood count—findings may show evidence of hemolytic
   anemia, pancytopenia, lymphoproliferative disorder, or infectious
   mononucleosis.
C. Protein electrophoresis—abnormal globulins may indicate the presence of monoclonal proteins.

Laboratory Tests in the Work-Up of Suspected
Immune Complex Diseases
The following tests are helpful in the evaluation of an immune complex
disorder.
A. Serum protein analyses including electrophoresis and immunoelectrophoresis [13, 58, 75]
B. Semiquantitative serum cryoglobulins, formation of cryoprecipitate
   at 4° C [13, 66]
C. Test for immune complexes in serum, joint fluid with (a) C1q component of complement [1, 2]; (b) monoclonal rheumatoid factor
   [99]; and (c) the platelet aggregation test [63, 68]
D. Biopsy of kidney, muscle, or synovium for routine histology, electron microscopy, and immunofluorescent studies
E. Measurement of complement levels in serum and/or joint fluid [9, 28,
   78]

Recommended Laboratory Tests in Cases of Cryoglobulinemia
If the serum is positive for cryoglobulins, further tests should indicate if
it is a pure cryoglobulin or a mixed cryoglobulin. The studies would
include
A. Serum protein immunoelectrophoretic studies
B. Quantitation of immunoglobulin
C. Quantitation of cryoglobulins
D. Analysis of serum for presence of (a) rheumatoid factor, (b) anti-
   nuclear factor activity, (c) cold agglutinin activity, and (d) auto-
   immune antibody by Coombs' test

Immune Complexes in the Pathogenesis of the Arthus Reaction and Serum Sickness

Arthus Reaction and Insoluble Immune Complexes [16, 23, 95]

Immune complexes may be soluble or insoluble depending upon the ratio of antibody to antigen. An example of tissue injury resulting from insoluble immune complexes is the Arthus reaction. A local Arthus reaction with vasculitis is produced when antigen is injected into a sensitized host. Insoluble immune complexes are formed which precipitate and localize along the vascular basement membrane. The complexes fix complement with chemotaxis of polymorphonuclear leukocytes, phagocytosis of immune precipitates, destruction of lysosomes, release of proteolytic enzymes, and resultant tissue injury. In the pathogenesis of the reaction, fixation of complement with polymorphonuclear leucocyte infiltration is necessary for tissue injury.

Serum Sickness and Soluble Immune Complexes [17, 23, 95]

An example of soluble immune complexes is observed in serum sickness. When a large amount of foreign serum protein is injected, there

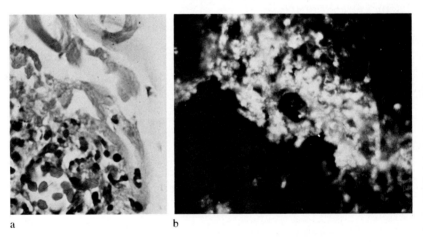

a   b

Figure 6-1

Experimental arthus reaction. (a) Microscopic sections of a rabbit skin blood vessel. Lesion was produced by local injection of bovine serum albumin (BSA) into a previously immunized animal. A neutrophilic inflammatory reaction occurs within a few hours. (H&E section; about 100× before 35% reduction.) (b) BSA was found to be localized around blood vessels in experimental Arthus reaction, by the reaction of a frozen section with fluorescein isothiocyanate-labeled rabbit anti-BSA. Similarly, rabbit γ-globulin was found to be localized in a similar area as BSA when the tissue section was reacted with fluorescein isothiocyanate-labeled guinea pig anti-rabbit IgG. (About 100× before 35% reduction.)

is an initial induction period before production of antibodies to the injected foreign protein. The antibody which is produced combines with antigen in serum, and at first there is an extreme excess of antigen with formation of soluble antigen-antibody complexes. With the appearance of antigen-antibody complexes, there is a simultaneous lowering of serum complement and appearance of inflammatory lesions in the kidneys, heart, arteries, and joints similar to lesions found in acute glomerulonephritis, systemic lupus erythematosus, polyarteritis nodosa, and rheumatoid arthritis. Immunofluorescence studies have provided evidence for deposition of circulating complexes with localization of IgG and C3 in the affected organs [17, 23, 53] (Fig. 6-4).

The soluble antigen-antibody complexes may initiate tissue damage by reacting with various serum components. They can activate part of the C1q component of complement to an active esterase. In addition, they will cause the formation of fibrinolysin, anaphylatoxin, and active vasoactive peptides. On a cellular level, the following reactions may be seen [17, 18, 19, 23, 95]:

A. Degranulation of mast cells with liberation of various amines
B. Attachment of complexes to leukocytes and platelets with agglutination
C. Contraction of smooth muscle
D. Increase of vascular permeability
E. Endothelial proliferation
F. Chemotactic attraction of mature granulocytes, in the presence of complement (Fig. 6-2).
G. Production of degenerative, hyaline change in various tissues

Immune complexes, especially the smaller sizes, may equilibrate be-

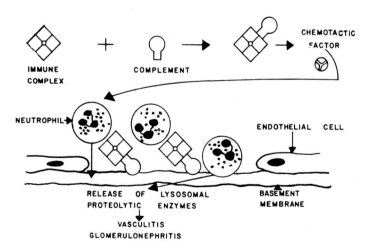

Figure 6-2
Immune complex injury.

tween the intravascular and extravascular fluid compartments similar to serum proteins [64]. The amount of protein in the extravascular fluid spaces after equilibration correlated exponentially with the effective hydrodynamic diffusion radius of the protein molecules or complex [64].

The larger size complexes localize along vascular and glomerular basement membranes. The localization of the complexes is dependent on the size of the complexes as well as the presence of vascular permeability factors as vasoactive amines [11]. The following steps are involved in the deposition of immune complexes [19]:

1. Immune complexes of varying size are in circulation.
2. In the presence of basophilic leukocytes with adherent IgE immunoglobulin antibody, the antigen reaction with cell-fixed IgE induces the release of a soluble intermediate platelet agglutinating factor (PAF).
3. The PAF activates platelets to clump and release serotonin and vasoactive amines (Fig. 6-3).
4. The amines cause an increased permeability of blood vessels, mainly in areas of platelet agglutination along the blood vessel wall.
5. With the increased permeability, immune complexes of greater than 19S become lodged along the basement membrane. The fixation of complement with the release of chemotactic factors and attraction of polymorphonuclear leukocytes will result in injury to the basement membrane.

The vascular injury results from complement activation with release of proteolytic enzymes from polymorphonuclear leukocytes. Soluble

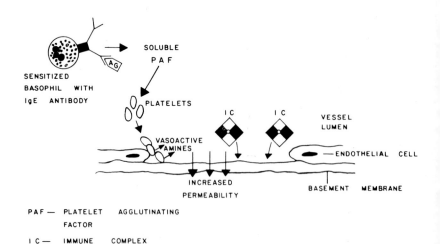

Figure 6-3
Mechanism of immune complex deposition (observed in rabbits).

Figure 6-4
Immune complex glomeru-
lonephritis. By the direct
fluorescent antibody test,
there is evidence of localization of IgG in an irregular
pattern along the basement
membrane. A similar fluo-
rescent staining pattern was
seen when the section was
reacted with fluorescein-
labeled anti-C3. The patient
showed a clinical picture of
progressive glomerulonephritis and the nature of the
antigen is unknown. (Ap-
proximately 400× before
30% reduction.)

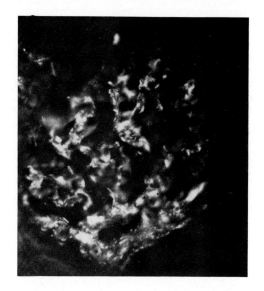

immune complex disease, such as serum sickness, may be inhibited with
the use of antihistamines and serotonin antagonists [18].

More recently, evidence has been accumulating that glomerulonephritis may result without significant participation by complement factors [40, 97]. Henson has described four immunologic reactions which
cause in vitro release of histamine and serotonin from rabbit platelets
[39]. They are as follows:

A. Complement dependent lytic release—(antigen + antibody + complement + platelets)
B. Complement dependent nonlytic release—(particulate antigen +
   antibody + complement to C3 + platelets)
C. Neutrophil dependent release—(antigen + antibody + complement
   to C3 + neutrophils + platelets)
D. Leukocyte dependent release—(sensitized blood leukocytes + antigen + platelets)

The fourth reaction involves sensitized leukocytes and causes release
of vasoactive amines without complement from platelets. In a study
of experimental immune complex disease in rabbits [40], a correlation
was obtained between (a) the presence of a complement independent
reaction which required blood leukocytes, antigen, and platelets, and
(b) the deposition of immune complexes with induction of glomerulonephritis. Experimental depletion of C3 did *not* decrease the severity of
the glomerulonephritis but significantly reduced the extent of arteritis
[40].

Very little is known about the relationship of immune complexes to the kinin-forming and intrinsic clotting systems in inflammatory injury [20]. The Hageman factor has been found to be involved in the pathway of activation of the clotting system and the kinin-forming system [78]. Extensive laboratory in vitro studies did not show any evidence of inter-action between the Hageman factor and immune complexes [20]. The immunoglobulins did not activate the Hageman factor; however, bac-terial contaminants did activate the Hageman factor and initiated the intrinsic clotting system [20].

Systemic Lupus Erythematosus (SLE)—Primary Model of Immune Complex Disease in Humans

Role of Immune Complexes in the Pathogenesis of SLE

Great progress has been made on the understanding of pathogenic events during the disease course of lupus erythematosus; however, as in many of the autoimmune diseases, the exact etiology is unknown [25]. Systemic lupus erythematosus may be classified under the category of non-organ specific autoimmune disease along with rheumatoid arthritis and other collagen diseases. In the general theories of autoimmunity, lupus erythe-matosus may come under the category of abnormal immune mecha-nisms in which there is some disturbed tolerance or failure of self recog-nition. There is production of antibodies to many cellular constituents and native DNA. Specific antibody reactive to native DNA has not been induced experimentally, although experimental animals such as mice [11] and dogs [46] have been shown to demonstrate a spontane-ous lupus-like disease similar to the human disease.

There is a wide spectrum of overlap between pure discoid and classic systemic lupus, and a small percentage of discoid lupus may eventually develop systemic lupus erythematosus. The clinical manifestations of systemic lupus involve multiple organ systems. The disease may be diagnosed when multisystem involvement with glomerulonephritis is seen in the presence of LE cells or antinuclear antibodies [24]. It has been well known that when a lupus patient is exposed to excessive sun-light, there may be an exacerbation of symptoms. The patient will de-velop fever, skin lesions, pleuritis, anemia, and antibodies to DNA.

The alteration of nuclear DNA by ultraviolet light has been well docu-mented recently [29, 90, 91, 92]. Tan and co-workers have demonstrated that, during the exacerbation of a clinical case of lupus, DNA appears in the circulation [89]. DNA in serum was detected by the agar gel double diffusion technique. With the appearance of DNA in the serum, there is elevation of fever with proteinuria, and prednisone treatment results in a gradual disappearance of the free DNA or DNA-anti-DNA immune complexes. Free serum DNA is only rarely seen in other disease condi-tions. In the pathogenesis of lupus, it is felt that the antigen-antibody complexes of DNA and anti-DNA are the important toxic immune complexes which cause diffuse membranous and proliferative glomerulonephritis or focal glomerulonephritis (Fig. 6-5).

The distribution of C3 and IgG in an irregular lumpy-bumpy pattern is in marked contrast to the linear type of fluorescent pattern seen in Goodpasture's syndrome, which shows basement membrane antibodies. The evidence for the role of antigen-antibody complexes in nephritis of systemic lupus may be listed as follows [5]: (a) The deposition of immunoglobulins and complement within the membrane of glomeruli is similar to the findings of serum sickness. (b) Antinuclear antibodies can be specifically eluted from glomeruli in greater concentrations than in serum. (c) Serum complement levels are depressed during periods of active nephritis. (d) DNA and other nuclear antigens have been demonstrated in glomeruli by immunofluorescence.

The cutaneous manifestations of systemic lupus are varied. Fluorescence studies of the skin have demonstrated fixation of immunoglobulins and complement along the basement membrane. Also, immune complexes of DNA in the upper part of the dermis have been observed. In addition, antibodies have been seen in the nuclei of squamous epithelial cells [69, 88]. Ultraviolet rays have been shown to cause alteration of the DNA or human skin in vivo [91]. The in vivo changes were demonstrated by immunofluorescence using antibodies specific for DNA

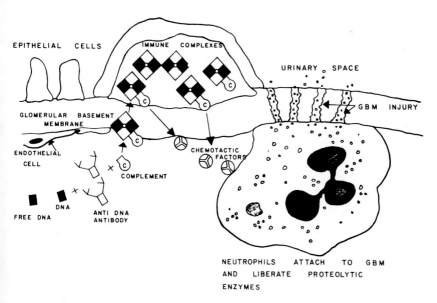

Figure 6-5
DNA-antibody complex glomerulonephritis in systemic lupus erythematosus.

altered by exposure to ultraviolet light. Therefore, the skin of systemic lupus patients may be a potential source of nuclear antigens released into the circulation during tissue damage which combine with circulating antinuclear antibodies to form immune complexes potentially harmful to other organs.

In systemic lupus erythematosus, circulating cold-insoluble complexes were observed in a significant number of patients. The cryoglobulins in systemic lupus may possess biologic properties similar to immune complexes and were observed along with other circulating immune complexes in active cases of lupus nephritis [85].

Recent evidence has been obtained that a high molecular weight immune complex (greater than 19S) independent of the DNA-anti-DNA system may play a role in the nephritis process of SLE [1, 2]. In SLE patients, this system is mediated by the in vivo interaction of rheumatoid factor and the C1q component of complement with circulating complexes. Such patients demonstrate serum cryoglobulins [2, 44]. The rheumatoid factor has been detected in the cryoprecipitates from patients with SLE, and in addition fluorescent localization studies with fluorescein-labeled aggregated γ-globulin demonstrated the presence of rheumatoid factor in the glomeruli of SLE patients. Thus, rheumatoid factor containing cryoglobulin complexes may play a role in the pathogenesis of the renal injury in SLE. In addition to large cryoglobulin complexes which can react with rheumatoid factor and C1q in lupus patients, Agnello et al. [2] have demonstrated low molecular weight (approximately 7S) C1q reactants in the sera of SLE patients. Both the large complexes and unidentified low molecular weight reactants are associated with the active state of the disease. Glomerulonephritis, depression of complement, and cryoglobulinemia are seen.

Cellular Sensitivity and Lymphocytotoxic Antibodies in SLE

There have been conflicting reports as to the status of cellular sensitivity in systemic lupus erythematosus [32, 41]. One group of investigators observed that cellular immunity is depressed during the early stages prior to treatment [7]. A recent report indicates that, in many cases of SLE patients, the cellular immune mechanisms are not depressed when studied by conventional skin test antigens and lymphocyte transformation techniques [32]. Delayed cellular sensitivity to nuclear antigens has been observed in certain cases of SLE [32]. The SLE patients have a high incidence of lymphocytotoxic antibodies [93]. The presence of cytotoxic antibodies was definitely related to the presence of clinical symptoms and correlated inversely with the white blood count and serum C3 levels [12]. The action of lymphocytotoxic antibodies on cell membranes may lead to complement-mediated cell injury, which in turn results in the release of nuclear antigens and other intracellular antigens [12].

Role of Complement and Properdin in SLE

Total serum complement levels are decreased in active cases of SLE largely due to the action of immune complexes and cytotoxic antibodies. Properdin [67] is a distinct protein involved in the alternate pathway of complement activation which is nonantibody-mediated [62, 78]. Properdin was demonstrated by indirect immunofluorescence in the kidneys of SLE patients [42, 76]. One patient showed localization of properdin in both the kidney and skin [76]. The presence of properdin suggests that the alternate pathway of complement activation is involved in the pathogenesis of SLE [42, 76]. The low C3 levels observed in cases of SLE were found to be due largely to the decreased synthesis of C3 [84]. Perhaps the cytotoxic antibodies may be partly responsible for the decreased synthesis of C3.

Evidence for Genetic and Etiologic Factors in SLE

For a long time, many investigators have thought about the genetic predisposition to systemic lupus erythematosus. Grumet and co-workers [37] have shown that patients with systemic lupus have a high frequency association with human leukocyte antigens HL–A8 (33%) and W15 (40%), compared to control population frequencies of 11% and 10%, respectively. The association of histocompatibility linked immune response genes similar to the association seen above are observed in mice [47, 54].

More recently in the various kidney biopsies associated with lupus, investigators have demonstrated viral-like bodies which are tubuloreticular structures that were first believed to have a superficial resemblance to a myxovirus [3, 34, 36, 43]. Also noted in SLE cases were particles resembling degenerating C type viral particles [3]. These so-called viral-like structures have been demonstrated in the cytoplasm of endothelial cells of many cases of SLE. A thorough electron microscopic study incorporating blind controls demonstrated the viral-like tubuloreticular structures (TRS) in the buffy coat of lymphocytes of patients with systemic lupus erythematosus, discoid lupus erythematosus, and other connective tissue diseases [36].

The clinical evaluation of SLE patients demonstrated no significant differences between those with TRS positive or TRS negative lymphocytes. There was some evidence that patients with TRS positive lymphocytes had indications of greater disease activity [36]. The possible etiology of systemic lupus may be compared to an explanation of autoimmunity and malignancy in the spontaneous disease of New Zealand mice (counterpart in mice of human lupus). The mouse disease probably results from a genetic defect in which there may be a lysogenic or defective virus which may initiate immunologic imbalance. The immunologic imbalance is manifested by (a) an abnormal antibody response with production of autoantibodies to nuclear antigens and immune complex disease; and (b) cellular immunity which may be depressed with impaired immune surveillance, resulting in a malignancy [87].

Systemic lupus erythematosus also occurs in dogs, and like its counterpart in man it is a multisystem disease which usually affects young adult females [24]. The results of genetic analysis of an established breeding colony were consistent with the concept that canine systemic lupus can be explained by vertical transmission of an infectious agent in a genetically susceptible individual [46]. However, the etiology of SLE in humans is still largely unknown. The role of viruses in the mediation of immunologic mechanisms in genetically prone individuals still remains to be investigated.

Role of Immune Complexes in Rheumatoid Arthritis

Pathogenesis of Joint Lesions

Polyarthritis with pannus formation and destruction of the joint spaces is the hallmark of rheumatoid arthritis. Other features include vasculitis, but glomerulonephritis is absent in rheumatoid arthritis. Glomerulitis is the hallmark of most immune complex diseases. There is abundant evidence that γ-globulin complexes are involved in the immunopathologic mechanisms in the synovial lesions of rheumatoid arthritis [10, 27, 99, 100]. Some of the findings may be listed as follows [9, 10, 28, 99, 100]: (a) depression of complement in the synovial fluid; (b) high concentration of γ-globulin complexes; (c) deposition of immunoglobulin and complement in the synovium (detected by immunofluorescence studies); (d) deposition of immunoglobulins and complement in leukocytes; and (e) synthesis of immunoglobulins in the synovium.

In addition, cryoprecipitable complexes with varying amounts of IgG, IgM, and DNA have been found in the joint fluid of patients who have detectable rheumatoid factor in their serum [49, 100]. The cryoproteins found in the joint were not seen in the companion serum samples [49].

Role of Rheumatoid Factor (RF)

The rheumatoid factor (RF) includes both 7S and 19S immunoglobulins with antibody specificity to certain determinants on the γ-globulin molecule. The determinants are exposed by physical aggregation of γ-globulin or by immune complex formation. Thus, rheumatoid factor may be an antibody directed against γ-globulin determinant ordinarily hidden in the intact molecule but exposed after an antigen-antibody reaction. The RF is detected in the serum of 80% of cases of rheumatoid arthritis [10].

What causes production of the RF factor? The exact mechanism of production of the RF factor in rheumatoid arthritis is unknown. The RF factor in rheumatoid arthritis is usually polyclonal in nature and may be produced as an antibody to an antigen-antibody complex. The γ-globulin is altered in the reaction with a specific antigen, such as bacteria or a virus, and may initiate production of RF. The presence of RF is found in a wide variety of diseases [30, 45]. The RF may be produced by the host in an attempt to inactivate the "so-called viral-antibody complex" with subsequent complement fixation.

There is some evidence to support the latter possibility. Notkins and co-workers [4, 65] have reported some interesting experiments with viral-antibody complexes and RF. They demonstrated that interaction of antiviral antibody with virus can still result in the formation of infectious viral-antibody complexes. Such complexes may be recovered from chronically infected animals. In vitro experiments have shown that RF itself failed to induce neutralization of the herpes simplex viral-antibody complexes, but increased the susceptibility of the complexes to neutralization by complement [65].

The RF factor is found in diseases other than rheumatoid arthritis, and conversely cases of rheumatoid arthritis may be negative for RF. However, the presence of high titers of RF correlates with the more active severe cases [30]. In rheumatoid arthritis, the RF will interact with antigen-antibody complexes as well as aggregates of γ-globulin with the capability to fix complement and initiate a destructive Arthus type of inflammatory reaction in the joint space (see Fig. 6-6). The attracted polymorphonuclear cells will release the lysosomal enzymes with pro-

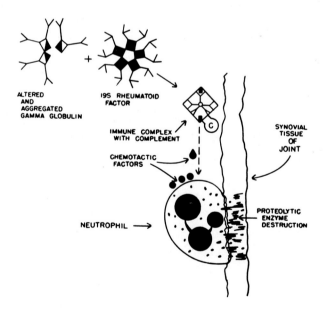

Figure 6-6
Role of rheumatoid factor in the pathogenesis of joint lesions in rheumatoid arthritis.

teolytic destruction of tissues [14]. The complexes can, in turn, activate plasma kallikrein and lead to kinin formation and initiate synovitis. Immunoconglutinins were observed to be bound to rheumatic synovial tissue and increased complement fixation [59]. The rheumatoid synovial fluid characteristically demonstrates low total hemolytic complement during the active stages [9, 28].

Currently, viruses have been suspected in the etiology of a wide variety of collagen vascular diseases. Viruses are known to induce the alteration of host tissue with the formation of neoantigens. An immune reaction can occur against the altered host tissue with formation of auto-antibodies and immune complexes. The concept that rheumatoid arthritis is due to a virus has been investigated. So far in a study of 187 specimens from 142 subjects with rheumatoid arthritis, there is no definitive evidence of virus infection by a variety of sensitive methods [70].

Reactivity of γ-Globulin Complexes
Rheumatoid arthritis patients have γ-globulin complexes in both sera and joint fluid. The rheumatoid factor involved is usually *polyclonal* and combines with γ-globulin to form immune complexes. The complexes found in the serum and joint fluid differ in their immunochemical properties. The γ-globulin complexes from the joint fluid of patients react readily in vitro with C1q and with polyclonal or monoclonal RF to form a precipitate. The joint fluid complexes are pathogenic and contribute to the inflammatory destruction of the joint space.

Winchester et al. [99] demonstrated that the γ-globulin complexes in the sera and joint fluid of rheumatoid arthritis differed in their reactivity to C1q and monoclonal RF. Serum complexes from patients with rheumatoid arthritis consisted mainly of high molecular weight but acid-dissociable 7S γ-globulin molecules. The exact nature of the complex is unknown, although 7S γ-globulin rheumatoid factors play a role in the formation of the complex. The serum complexes do not precipitate with C1q but are able to demonstrate an in vitro precipitin in gel diffusion with monoclonal RF. The serum complexes in rheumatoid arthritis are not associated with an in vivo depression of serum complement, and their different properties help explain the low incidence of glomerulonephritis in patients with rheumatoid arthritis.

Methods for Detection of Immune Complexes

Common Clinical Laboratory Tests for Suspected
Cases of Immune Complex Disease
These tests are presumptive and may be of value if positive results are obtained. Other tests elaborated below should be performed if the patient has clinical evidence of immune complex disease. The common laboratory tests are (a) immunoelectrophoresis (IEP) and (b) test for cryoglobulins.

Often one may suspect immune complex disease on the basis of the results obtained from a serum immunoelectrophoresis performed in the laboratory. The immune complexes may show a marked trailing from the antigen well usually within the IgG area toward the cathode and are indicated by an opaque diffuse oblong spot [75]. The spot is connected to the antigen well but appears to show a narrowing just to the left of the antigen well (Fig. 6-7). The opaque spots confined closely to the cathodal side of the antigen well indicate the possible presence of an abnormal immunoglobulin (monoclonal gammopathy) [75]. Such spots do not show the constriction on the cathodal side of the antigen well (Fig. 6-8).

IEP patterns of certain sera may show arcs close to the antigen well but usually demonstrates definite crescent-shaped precipitate arcs on the cathodic side. The precipitate may be due to lipoproteins and euglobulins [58] (Fig. 6-9).

Figure 6-7
Immunoelectrophoretic pattern of patient with serum immune complexes. The immunoelectrophoretic pattern was developed with specific anti-IgG antiserum. Top well—normal patient's serum; lower well—serum from patient with SLE with serum cryoglobulins and DNA–anti-DNA immune complexes. Note the IgG precipitin arcs and trailing phenomenon extending toward the cathode from the lower well.

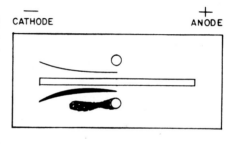

CATHODE   ANODE

Figure 6-8
Immunoelectrophoretic pattern of patient with monoclonal macroglobulinemia. Immunoelectrophoretic pattern was developed with specific anti-IgM antiserum. Top well—normal serum; lower well—patient with monoclonal macroglobulinemia. Note scooped monoclonal type of IgM arc near lower well. The large diffuse protein precipitate adjacent to the lower well differs from the trailing effect with the constriction seen produced by certain serum immune complexes as shown in Figure 6-7.

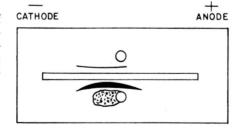

CATHODE   ANODE

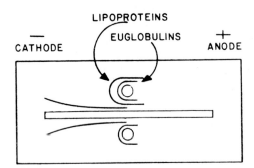

Figure 6-9
Immunoelectrophoretic pattern
of different sera reacted with
specific anti-IgG antiserum.
Note pattern of euglobulin and
lipoproteins produced adjacent
to antigen well.

Although the IEP patterns described above are not diagnostic, since certain immune complexes do not give a cathodal trailing effect, they are extremely helpful. A positive result is one more piece of evidence for confirmation of suspected immune complex disease. Conversely, a negative IEP does not rule out the possibility of immune complexes. The sera of patients with suspected immune complex disease also should be tested for cryoglobulins. Many mixed cryoglobulins behave biologically as immune complexes and are capable of inducing tissue injury.

The more precise laboratory methods to detect immune complexes in biological fluids of patients with immune complex disease involve (a) physicochemical techniques of ultracentrifugation and column chromatography, (b) immunochemical methods with biologic reagents as C1q and monoclonal rheumatoid factor (RF), and (c) platelets.

Immune complexes may be detected in biopsy tissues such as kidney, synovium, and blood vessels by immunofluorescence studies or by enzyme-labeled antibody reagents.

Physicochemical Methods [83]
The physicochemical methods for studying immune complexes are (a) analytical ultracentrifugation, (b) preparative ultracentrifugation, and (c) column chromatography.

Analytical ultracentrifugation is the quantitative application of centrifugal force to a solution of particles. The centrifugal force causes molecules or particles of varying size to sediment at different rates in a standard solution. The sedimentation coefficient is calculated from the observed velocity of sedimentation divided by the strength of the centrifugal force. Various immunoglobulins such as IgG and IgM have been found to have different sedimentation rates. The IgG and IgM immunoglobulins are 7S and 19S, respectively. The immune complexes can be detected in sera by analytical ultracentrifugation.

The preparative ultracentrifugation method often employs a sucrose density gradient as a medium to separate molecules of different size. The contents of the tube are analyzed after the centrifugation cycle, and the denser molecules or particles will migrate to the bottom of the tube.

The various particles are fractionated by punching a hole in the bottom of the tube and collecting sequential fractions. By the use of known markers as specific antibody or radio-labeled IgM, immune complexes may be fractionated from a serum sample.

Column chromatography by gel filtration is based on the separation of molecules on the basis of size. Gel columns with gel beads of different pore size are used.

Immunochemical Reactions with Biologic Reagents

Biologic reagents which are useful in the laboratory which can detect immune complexes are (a) C1q component of complement [1, 2, 99], (b) monoclonal rheumatoid factor [2, 99], and (c) platelets for the platelet aggregation test [63, 68].

Recent studies have shown that circulating immune complexes in serum, synovial, and other body fluids may be detected by reaction with C1q [1, 2] and rheumatoid factors [99]. The ability for the demonstration of in vitro precipitation of immune complexes is dependent not only on the size and nature of the immune complexes, but also on their immunochemical properties.

C1q is one of the 11 components of complement. It has a molecular weight of about 400,000 and is the first component of complement to attach to immunoglobulin in an antigen-antibody reaction. The C1q may be isolated from normal serum by precipitation with calf thymus deoxyribonucleic acid (DNA) [1]. Agnello and co-workers [1] have described a gel diffusion method for demonstrating precipitin reactions of C1q with aggregated γ-globulin and immune complexes. Optimal reactions were observed with 0.6% agarose in 0.01 M EDTA at pH 7.2 and ionic strength 0.09. Precipitation with C1q usually occurs with γ-globulin aggregate greater than 19S and with other soluble immune complexes found in 2 to 20 times antigen excess. Generally, C1q reacts with large γ-globulin and immune complexes. However, as previously described, there are low molecular weight C1q reactants in sera of certain patients with SLE.

The classic rheumatoid factor (RF) found in sera of patients with rheumatoid arthritis is polyclonal in nature and has the ability to react with large aggregates of γ-globulin and large immune complexes. Monoclonal rheumatoid factor (RF) is found in certain lymphoproliferative disorders. The monoclonal RF can be isolated and is ideal for use in the clinical laboratory to detect the presence of both small and large immune complexes.

The monoclonal 19S rheumatoid factor is often associated with mixed cryoglobulins and found in lymphoproliferative disorders, infectious mononucleosis, and other diseases. The reactivity of the monoclonal RF is enhanced in the cold. The C1q component of complement and polyclonal RF will both react and precipitate large complexes and large aggregates of γ-globulin in the joint fluid of patients with rheumatoid arthritis. The C1q does not precipitate the smaller immune complexes in the serum of patients with rheumatoid arthritis. In contrast, the immune complexes from both the joint fluid and sera of rheumatoid arthritis patients will show an in vitro precipitin reaction with monoclonal RF. A platelet aggregation test may be used to detect circulating immune complexes [63, 68]. A standardized suspension of washed fresh human platelets is incubated overnight at 5 to 8° C with dilutions of the serum or joint fluid (previously heat inactivated at 56° C for 30 min). The sedimentation patterns are read with a dark background illumination; a smooth white button and a dark even pattern on the bottom of the well indicate negative and positive reactions, respectively. The validity of the procedure to detect immune complexes was confirmed with ultracentrifugal sedimentation analyses [63].

Detection of Immune Complexes by Immunofluorescent Study of Tissue Biopsy Material

Glomerulonephritis is often noted in immune complexes and is the hallmark of immune complex disease [15, 53, 77]. Glomerulonephritis is not often seen in rheumatoid arthritis.

Immune complexes play an important role in the pathogenesis of the joint lesions. As discussed below, the serum of rheumatoid arthritis usually contains small immune complexes while the joint fluid may contain large γ-globulin aggregates. Further, the immune complexes in serum and synovial fluid from these patients possess different reactive properties, which may explain the low incidence of glomerulonephritis, as seen in rheumatoid arthritis.

The glomerulonephritis in systemic lupus erythematosus, poststreptococcal glomerulonephritis, and other diseases is most likely due to immune complexes. Fluorescent antibody studies with the demonstration of IgG, IgM, and C3 in an irregular lumpy-bumpy pattern along the epithelial side of the basement membrane is strong evidence for the pathogenic role of immune complexes in the kidney lesions [15, 42, 53, 77].

Similarly, immunofluorescence studies of joint synovial tissue may provide indirect evidence of γ-globulin immune complexes with the demonstration of fixation of immunoglobulin and complement in the synovial tissue and cells. Biopsy of tissue from patients with polyarteritis nodosa and chronic Australia antigenemia showed localized IgM, Australia antigen, and complement in the blood vessel walls [31].

Cryoglobulins and Relationship to Various Diseases

The cryoglobulins consist of complexes of immunoglobulins or single immunoglobulins which may have been altered by some unknown process. They are insoluble at 4° C but may possess the ability to aggregate at temperatures as high as 30° C [66, 74]. Such a temperature can be reached in peripheral capillaries [86]. Many of the cryoglobulins have the ability to fix complement and initiate an inflammatory reaction similar to classic antigen-antibody complexes and thus probably play a significant role in the pathogenesis of viral diseases with the production of lesions of vasculitis and glomerulonephritis [6, 60, 96].

Classification of Cryoglobulins
The cryoglobulins may be classified as follows (Table 6-1):

PURE CRYOGLOBULINS.   These are found in patients with lymphomas or myelomas and are usually a monoclonal IgM or monoclonal IgG. The classic example is Waldenström's macroglobulinemia with an IgM cryoglobulinemia.

ESSENTIAL CRYOGLOBULINS.   These are similar to the pure cryoglobulins. Either monoclonal IgM or IgG, they are found in conditions with benign gammapathy. Some of these cases may eventually develop a malignant lymphoma later in the course of the disease.

MIXED CRYOGLOBULINS.   Many contain rheumatoid factor activity with an IgM, IgA, or IgG monoclonal protein. Mixed cryoglobulins are seen in collagen vascular diseases and certain viral infections. In such conditions, the patients have associated autoantibodies. The cryoglobulins may fix complement in vitro and in vivo. Besides precipitating in the cold in vitro, the cryoglobulin complexes may precipitate in the vessels and kidney glomeruli in vivo and produce syndromes of purpura, arthritis, and glomerulonephritis.

Macroglobulinemia and Associated Cryoglobulins
and Pyroglobulins
Many patients with lymphoproliferative disorders have IgM monoclonal protein. The abnormal IgM in patients with macroglobulinemia often exhibit unusual temperature dependent properties. Cryoglobulins in one series have been found in 30% of 48 patients with macroglobulinemia [74]. Pyroglobulins, which are monoclonal proteins and form irreversibly precipitate gel at 56° C, were noted in 4 of 40 patients [74]. The clinical significance of pyroglobulinemia is not known [49].
    Other patients with macroglobulinemia have an abnormal IgM with antibody activity and show evidence of mixed cryoglobulins. The IgM protein often have (a) rheumatoid factor activity and/or (b) cold agglutinin activity with usually anti-I specificity [50]. The formation of IgM-IgG complexes often leads to hyperviscosity and cryoglobulinemia. The abnormal macroglobulin with the antibody activity may arise from a unique IgM cell clone with resultant manifestation of mono-

Table 6-1. Classification of Cryoglobulins.

Cryoglobulin	Disease	Constituents
Pure cryoglobulin	Lymphoma or myeloma	IgM monoclonal or IgG monoclonal
Essential cryoglobulin	Benign gammopathy	IgM monoclonal or IgG monoclonal
Mixed cryoglobulin	Rheumatoid arthritis Systemic lupus erythematosus Sjögren's disease Malignancy (epithelial) Viral infections as cytomegalic	IgM + IgG IgA + IgG IgG + IgG (often one immunoglobulin is monoclonal with antibody activity as rheumatoid factor)

Constituents Identified in Cryoglobulins.
(Modified after Barnett et al. [6].)
1. IgG monoclonal
2. IgM monoclonal
3. Mixed cryoglobulins (one of the components
   may be monoclonal)
   IgG, IgM
   IgG + IgM
   IgG + IgA + IgM
   IgG + IgM + C3 complement
   IgG + C3 + fibrinogen
   IgG + IgM + α2M
   Lipoproteins + immunoglobulin

clonal rheumatoid factor or monoclonal cold agglutinin [73]. These are in contrast to the rheumatoid factor (RF) from patients with rheumatoid arthritis, in which the RF is polyclonal in nature. Also, the cold agglutinins seen in mycoplasma pneumonic infections are polyclonal in nature [22].

The cold agglutinins associated with macroglobulinemia often show maximal agglutination of red cells at $0°$ C with some activity at higher temperatures and no agglutinating activity above $30°$ C [81]. After low temperature agglutination, the reaction is reversible at higher temperatures. Maximal hemolysis occurs at $22°$ C in the presence of complement [81]. The usual cold agglutinin is monothermic in behavior, with agglutination and hemolysis occurring at the same temperature. On the other hand, the "bithermic" Donath-Landsteiner cold hemolysis from cases of paroxysmal hemoglobulinuria demonstrates a two-temperature stepwise pattern. In paroxysmal hemoglobinuria, the cold agglutinin antibody fixation occurs at low temperatures, above $30°$ C [22, 81]. The reaction can proceed in the absence of antibody immunoglobulin and has been explained by an alternate pathway of complement activation [33, 62].

Autoimmune hemolytic anemia unrelated to cold agglutinin may also occur in macroglobulinemia [74]. The presence of two or more M proteins, biclonal and triclonal gammopathy, has been reported [79]. A biclonal gammopathy may be related with the presence of identical structure of the light chains.

Hyperviscosity Syndrome Associated with Abnormal
Macroglobulins and Cryoglobulins
Twenty-five to 30% of patients with abnormal macroglobulins show evidence of gel formation upon cooling [74]. Such cryoglobulins may contribute to a hyperviscosity syndrome without evidence of aggregation in vivo.

The hyperviscosity syndrome may be seen in a wide variety of disorders of immunoglobulin metabolism [74]. The serum viscosity is often expressed as relative viscosity and is usually determined in vitro with an Ostwald viscometer [26, 72]:

$$\text{serum viscosity } \eta \text{ rel}^{37°C} = \frac{\text{flow time for serum (sec)}}{\text{flow time for saline (sec)}}$$

Normal η rel$^{37°C}$ is usually 1.6 to 1.9. When η rel reaches a critical level, which may be 7 or 8 η rel$^{37°C}$, and the patient demonstrates symptoms, the treatment is plasmaphoresis reduction of the serum viscosity to 5 η rel$^{37°C}$ or less [74].

Although macroglobulinemia alone without evidence of cryoglobulins may cause a hyperviscosity syndrome, the presence of cryoglobulin, especially of the mixed type, will enhance the viscosity of the serum.

Thus, patients with evidence of cryoglobulins are more susceptible to develop symptoms of the hyperviscosity syndrome. In addition, the macroglobulins and cryoglobulins may interfere with platelet function and such patients may develop blood clotting complications.

*Mixed Cryoglobulins and Their Similarity
to Immune Complexes*

Many of the mixed cryoglobulins have been studied and found to contain specific antigens, antibodies, and complement. Cryoglobulins are often associated with some unusual infections as viruses [94] and lepromatous leprosy [8]. Wager et al. [94] have studied cryoglobulins in cases of cytomegalovirus infection and infectious mononucleosis and have detected the following antibodies in the cryoprecipitates: (a) antiglobulin rheumatoid factor; (b) antinuclear antibodies; (c) heterophile antibody; and (d) cold agglutinins.

In cases of mixed cryoglobulinemia, the complexes of IgM–IgG appear to contain desoxyribonucleic acid (DNA) tightly bound to the immunoglobulins [6]. The DNA bound to the cryoglobulins was not susceptible to DNase at a neutral pH; it was sensitive only to DNase at pH 3.0. Such complexes of cryoglobulins bound to DNA may play a role in the development of nephritis and vasculitis in cases of cryoglobulinemia. The DNA to cryoglobulins was observed in cases of essential mixed cryoglobulinemia [6]. Stastny and Ziff [85], in their study of cold insoluble complexes associated with systemic lupus erythematosus, found the cold complexes consisted of the IgG and C1q components of complement and did not contain DNA or selective amounts of antinuclear antibody.

Role of Cryoglobulins in Glomerulonephritis

Cryoglobulins have been found in patients with poststreptococcal and nonpoststreptococcal glomerulonephritis [6, 55]. IgG, IgM, and C3 globulins were observed in the cryoprecipitates in several of the patients, and the proteins were observed to be localized in the glomerular basement membrane upon immunofluorescence studies. No evidence of streptococcal antigen was found in the cryoprecipitates, and attempts to localize the streptococcal antigen on the glomeruli of the patients were negative [55]. In one case of glomerulonephritis, fibrinogen was noted with immunoglobulin and complement in the cryoprecipitate [55].

Cryoglobulins with glomerulonephritis have been noted in cytomegalovirus infection [6] and infectious mononucleosis. Such cryoproteins have been demonstrated to possess biologic properties similar to immune complexes [57]. The cryoprotein complex is able to fix complement components and initiate the inflammatory reaction with basement membrane damage and possible deposition of fibrinogen products. The cryocomplexes may aggregate at temperatures as high as 30° C [66], and there is evidence that this temperature is regularly reached in peripheral capillaries and may cause vasculitis [86].

Role of Cryoglobulins in Systemic Lupus Erythematosus

In a study of SLE patients, cryoprecipitates were observed with circulating complexes; in such cases, an active nephritic process was usually present [2, 44, 85]. Circulating cold insoluble complexes of cryoglobulins were observed in one-third of the cases of systemic lupus erythematosus and consisted mainly of IgG and C1q components of complement without evidence of DNA or significant amounts of anti-DNA antibody [85]. The presence of the cryoglobulins was associated with a decrease of C3 in 90% of the cases, while in SLE without cryoproteins, only 12% demonstrated a decrease in serum C3 concentration. The isolated cryoprotein, containing IgG and C1q, produced a significant reduction in in vitro hemolytic activity of human complement.

Hanauer and Christian first demonstrated that serum from SLE patients contains cryoprecipitates with C1q and rheumatoid factor [38]. Rheumatoid factors have been detected in the cryoprecipitates of the patient with SLE, and kidney biopsies of cases of nephritis have shown deposits of IgM and rheumatoid factor which have been localized in the glomeruli by fluorescence-labeled aggregated γ-globulin [44]. This is strong evidence that rheumatoid factors are present in cryoprecipitates and are also deposited in the kidney in vivo [2, 44]. This mechanism is independent of the DNA-anti-DNA and is mediated by the interaction in vivo of rheumatoid factor and the C1q component of complement with circulating complexes. The interaction is manifested by cryoglobulinemia. Other noncryoglobulin complexes are present in serum which are precipitable by both C1q and rheumatoid factor when examined in vitro [2]. Rheumatoid factors, isolated from the SLE patients with cryoprecipitates, were able to combine with the serum residual complexes at warm temperatures. This indicates that the interaction of these substances and their subsequent deposition in the kidney in vivo are possible.

The monoclonal rheumatoid factor was found to react with low molecular weight complexes in a small number of systemic lupus patients, as well as in a few cases of nonrheumatic diseases [2]. However, monoclonal rheumatoid factor did not react with complexes in some hyperglobulinemic purpura patients [99] in which the complexes had a 7S IgG rheumatoid factor component.

Cryoglobulins and Rheumatoid Arthritis

Cryoprecipitates have been observed in the synovial fluid of patients with rheumatoid arthritis [6, 49]; however, such patients had no detectable cryoglobulin in their sera. In one study, the synovial fluid of all 21 patients with rheumatoid arthritis studied showed evidence of cryoprecipitates. Twelve of the 21 patients had a mixed cryoglobulin with

IgG–IgM, and both κ and λ light chains. Ten of the 12 mixed synovial cryoprecipitates had antiglobulin RF activity. Three contained antinuclear antibody activity of the IgG class, and IgM antinuclear antibody was found in two. One patient with Reiter's syndrome had synovial cryoglobulin with the presence of denatured DNA and RF activity.

Summary

The pathogenic role of antigen-antibody complexes in autoimmune disorders is unquestioned. Cryoglobulins are seen in a wide variety of conditions (glomerulonephritis, vasculitis, and purpura) which suggest that many of these patients demonstrate an immune complex type of autoimmune disorder. Many autoantibodies have been found in the cryoprecipitates and support the theory that cryoglobulins represent antibodies formed to specific antigen-antibody complexes, which lead to new complexes with cryoprecipitable properties. The mixed cryoglobulins can fix complement and have been shown to possess biological properties similar to specific antigen-antibody complexes. Significant evidence over the last few years indicates that mixed cryoglobulins play an in vivo pathogenic role in lesions of glomerulonephritis and vasculitis.

Methods

Common Laboratory Procedures
Standard electrophoretic and immunoelectrophoretic procedures are well described elsewhere [13, 75].

Test for Serum Cryoglobulin (2 days)
(Method of Peetom [66] and Cawley [13])
This method quantitates and types the cryoglobulin.

EQUIPMENT AND REAGENTS
1. Equipment for serum immunoelectrophoresis
2. Cold saline solution
3. Refrigeration at 4° C
4. Wintrobe sedimentation tubes
5. Refrigerated centrifuge
6. 0.05 M phosphate buffers, pH 7.0
7. Barbital buffer, pH 8.6, 0.05 ionic strength

PROCEDURE
1. Two Wintrobe sedimentation tubes for each patient are filled with fresh serum to the top mark. A control sample should also be run concomitantly.
2. Place one sample of each tube erect in a 37° C water bath and the other tube erect in the refrigerator at 4° C.

3. Allow tubes to stand 24 hours.
4. Inspect tubes and compare 4° C tube with tube incubated at 37° C for relative cloudiness and precipitation.
5. Test is negative if no cloudiness or precipitation is seen.
6. If a precipitate is observed, centrifuge the 4° C tube at 2,500 g in a refrigerated centrifuge at 4° C for 30 min.
7. The amount of precipitate is quantitated with the Wintrobe tube; 1 mm precipitate would represent 1% cryoglobulin.
8. To type the precipitate, wash the precipitate four times with cold (4° C) 0.05 M phosphate buffer, pH 7.0 (higher salt concentration of buffer will tend to dissolve cryoprecipitate).
9. Suspend precipitate in 10 volumes of barbital buffer, pH 8.6, 0.05 ionic strength, and dissolve precipitate by placing the suspension in a 37° C water bath.
10. Perform the immunoelectrophoretic determination and react against various monospecific anti-IgG, IgM, IgA, κ and λ light chain antisera.

Quantitative Determination of Cryoglobulins (2 days)
(Modified from Agnello et al. [2])

MATERIALS
See test for serum cryoglobulin.
1. Let blood clot at 37° C, separate serum, and let stand for 24 hours at 4° C. Serum control is allowed to stand for 24 hours at 37° C.
2. Centrifuge control serum 30 min at 1,000 g, at warm temperature.
3. Centrifuge second serum containing cryoprecipitate at 4° C, 30 min, 1,000 g, and wash 3 times with ice cold 0.05 M phosphate buffer pH 7.0 (higher salt concentration of buffer will dissolve the cryoglobulin).
4. Dissolve precipitates of cryoglobulin, and control sample in phosphate-buffered saline solution 0.15 M, pH 7.0, and read O.D. at 280 nm (1 mg protein is equal to approximately 1.5 O.D. units). Normal values upper limit of normal is 80 μg/ml [21].
5. The precipitate may also be dissolved in 0.1 M NaOH and the protein can be determined by the Folin technique [48].

Preparation of one C1q Component of Complement
(Modified from method of Agnello et al. [1])

C1q is a 400,000 MW protein and is isolated from normal serum by precipitation with calf thymus deoxyribonucleic acid (DNA).

MATERIALS AND REAGENTS
A. Veronal buffer, pH 8.6, 0.025 M
B. EDTA buffer, 0.01 M
C. Refrigerated centrifuge

D. DNA (Worthington)
E. Agitator
F. Refrigeration at 4° C
G. Phosphate buffer, pH 6.9, 0.05 M; pH 5.3, 0.3 M; pH 7.2, ionic strength 0.09
H. Magnesium chloride 0.003 M
 I. DNase I (Worthington)
 J. Sephadex G 200 (Pharmacia)
K. 28% $(NH_4)_2 SO_4$

PROCEDURE

1. Pooled fresh serum is dialyzed overnight at 4° C against pH 8.6, 0.025 M veronal, 0.01 M EDTA buffer. The pH of the serum is checked to ensure completion of dialysis. The serum is then centrifuged at 1,000 g for 30 min at 4° C to remove the nonspecific precipitates.
2. A precipitin curve is made from the reaction of serum and DNA to determine maximal precipitation.
3. The optimal amount of DNA (usually $25 \mu g/ml$) is then added to the pooled serum, agitating gently at normal temperature for 1 hour and kept at 4° C for 24 hours. The solution is spun at 1,000 g for 30 min and the precipitate obtained is washed 4 times with pH 6.9, 0.05 M phosphate buffer.
4. The precipitate, which has a weak gel-like consistency, is then adjusted to 0.003 M magnesium chloride; 100 μg DNase I is added per milliliter of suspension. (The DNase I is dissolved at 4 mg/ml in pH 6.9, 0.05 M phosphate buffer, 0.003 M $MgCl_2$.)
5. The suspension is then agitated gently at room temperature for 3 hours and dialyzed against the suspending buffer (pH 6.9, 0.05 M phosphate, 0.003 M $MgCl_2$) until most of the precipitate is dissolved. The solution is then spun at 100,000 g for 30 min.
6. The supernatant contains approximately 70% C1q and is further purified by column chromatography with Sephadex G 200 in pH 5.3, 0.3 M phosphate buffer, according to the procedure of Müller-Eberhard [63]. This procedure removes the DNase and digestion products. The C1q protein will be found in the exclusion fraction.
7. Fractions containing C1q are pooled and precipitated by adding 28% $(NH_4)_2 SO_4$. The precipitate is allowed to stand at 4° C for 5 hours. The precipitate is then dissolved in phosphate buffer, pH 7.2, ionic strength 0.09, and 0.01 M EDTA, and dialyzed until most of the precipitate is in solution.

The isolated material should have greater than 90% C1q by radial immunodiffusion. The preparation is used at 0.2 mg/ml, for the detection of serum immune complexes. Phosphate buffer, pH 7.2, ionic strength 0.09, and 0.01 M EDTA are used as the buffer system.

Detection of Serum Immune Complexes with C1q
Precipitin Reaction (4 days)
(Method of Agnello et al. [1])

The optimal conditions for reaction of C1q, with aggregated γ-globulin in gel diffusion, were determined as 0.6% agarose gel, with pH 7.2 phosphate buffer, ionic strength 0.09, and 0.01 M EDTA.

MATERIALS
A. Agarose gel (Seakem)
B. Phosphate buffer, pH 7.2, ionic strength 0.09 M, 0.01 M EDTA, sodium azide 0.001%
C. No. 2 Whatman filter
D. Pipette
E. 9 cm plate
F. Hyaluronidase (Worthington)
G. Centrifuge
H. C1q
I. Refrigeration at 0° C
J. Heat-aggregated IgG (for positive control)

PROCEDURE
1. Agarose gel is prepared in phosphate buffer. The heated gel solution is filtered through No. 2 Whatman filter.
2. 22 ml of the gel is pipetted into a 9 cm plate to give a 5 mm thick gel. Wells are made 9 mm in diameter, with a center-to-center distance between wells of 12 mm.
3. Serum samples are diluted two-fold with agar buffer and placed in the wells. Joint fluid is allowed to clot and treated with hyaluronidase and centrifuged to remove debris.
4. C1q is added to the opposite wells at a concentrate of 0.2 mg/ml.
5. The reaction is allowed to proceed at room temperature for 48 hours and then 0° C for 72 hours. (Plates are examined daily.)
   NOTE: C1q will react with highly positively charged substances in serum or endotoxin. A faint precipitin line may be seen between C1q and the normal serum if an ionic strength of the buffer below 0.08 is used.
6. Heat-aggregated IgG may be used for a positive control at a concentration of 1 mg/ml.

Preparation of Aggregated IgG
(Method of Müller-Eberhard and Kunkel [61])

MATERIALS
A. F II IgG—1.5 gm
B. Physiologic saline solution—150 ml
C. Heat to 63° C
D. Na_2SO_4
E. Refrigeration at 4° C

F. Centrifuge
G. Distilled water—20 ml
H. Phosphate buffer, pH 7.2, ionic strength 0.09, 0.01 M EDTA

PROCEDURE
1. 1.5 gm of FII IgG is dissolved in 150 ml physiologic saline solution and heated at 63° C for 12 min.
2. The aggregates are precipitated by the addition of 10 gm Na_2SO_4. After 1 hour at 4° C, centrifuge 20 min at 2,000 g.
3. Suspend in 20 ml distilled water and dialyze against phosphate buffer, pH 7.2, 0.09 ionic strength, 0.01 M EDTA. The material should contain 12–15 mg protein/ml, S rate 90–110.
4. The protein, whose concentration can be determined by the Folin reaction [65], is used for immunodiffusion studies at a concentration of 1 mg/ml.

Isolation of Monoclonal Rheumatoid Factor
(Schrohenloher et al. [80])

MATERIALS
A. Distilled water, cold
B. Saline solution; phosphate buffered 0.05 M, 0.01 M EDTA
C. Sodium acetate buffer, pH 4.1, 0.1 M
D. Centrifuge
E. Sephadex G–200 (Pharmacia)
F. Heat to 56° C

PROCEDURE
1. The RF may be precipitated from sera with 15 volumes of cold distilled water. The precipitate is washed 2 times with small volumes of cold water and then dissolved in saline solution equal to the volume of serum utilized.
2. The euglobulin is dialyzed and equilibrated against 0.1 M sodium acetate buffer, pH 4.1, and insoluble materials are removed by centrifugation 30 min at 1,000 g.
3. The euglobulin is placed on Sephadex G–200 column equilibrated with 0.1 M sodium acetate buffer at pH 4.1.
4. The RF is in the void volume and the collected fractions are dialyzed against phosphate buffered saline solution 0.05 M, with EDTA 0.01, and concentrated to protein concentrations of 3–4 mg and heated at 56° C for 45 min to destroy C1q activity.

Detection of Immune Complexes by Monoclonal
Rheumatoid Factor (4 days)
(Winchester and Agnello et al. [99])

MATERIALS
A. 0.6% agarose gel (Seakem)
B. Phosphate-buffered saline solution, pH 7.2, sodium azide 0.001%

C. Heat to boiling
D. No. 2 Whatman filter
E. Pipette
F. 9 cm plate
G. Monoclonal RF
H. Heat-aggregated IgG (for positive control)

PROCEDURE

1. 0.6% agarose gel is prepared in phosphate buffered saline, pH 7.2, 0.001% sodium azide. The solution is brought to a boil and is filtered through a No. 2 Whatman filter.
2. 22 ml of the gel is pipetted into a 9 cm plate to give a gel of 5 mm thickness.
3. Wells are cut 9 mm in diameter, with a center-to-center distance between wells of 12 mm.
4. Serum samples are diluted twofold with buffer and placed in the wells.
5. Monoclonal RF is used at a concentration of 1 mg/ml.
6. The reaction is allowed to proceed at room temperature for 48 hours, then 0° C for 72 hours. (Plates are examined daily.)
7. Heat-aggregated IgG may be used for a positive control at a concentration of 1 mg/ml.

References

1. Angello, V., Winchester, R. J., and Kunkel, H. G.   Precipitin reactions of the C1q component of complement with aggregated γ-globulin and immune complexes in gel diffusion. *Immunology* 19:909, 1970.
2. Agnello, V., Koffler, D., Eisenberg, J. W., Winchester, R. J., and Kunkel, H. G.   C1q precipitins in the sera of patients with systemic lupus erythematosus and other hypocomplementemic states: Characterization of high and low molecular weight types. *J. Exp. Med.* 134:228s, 1971.
3. Andres, G. A., Spiele, H., and McClusky, R. T.   Virus-like structures in systemic lupus erythematosus. In R. S. Schwartz (ed.), *Progress in Clinical Immunology*. New York: Grune & Stratton, 1972, vol. 1, p. 23.
4. Ashe, W. K., Daniels, C. A., Scott, G. S., and Notkins, A. L.   Interaction of rheumatoid factor with infectious herpes simplex virus-antibody complexes. *Science* 172:176, 1971.
5. Barnett, E. V., Kantor, G., Bickel, Y. B., Forsen, R., and Gonick, H. C.   Systemic lupus erythematosus. *Calif. Med.* 11:467, 1969.
6. Barnett, E. V., Bluestone, R., Cracchiolo, A., Goldberg, L. S., Kantor, G. L., and McIntosh, R. M.   Cryoglobulinemia and disease. *Ann. Intern. Med.* 73:95, 1970.
7. Bitter, T., Bitter, R., Silberschmidt, R., and Dubois, E. L.   In vivo and in vitro study of cell mediated immunity (CMI) during the onset of systemic lupus erythematosus (SLE). *Arthritis Rheum.* 14:152, 1971 (Abstract).
8. Bonomo, L., and Dammacco, F.   Immune complex cryoglobulinemia in lepromatosus leprosy: A pathogenetic approach to some clinical features of leprosy. *Clin. Exp. Immunol.* 9:175, 1971.

196   I: Diagnostic Patterns of Immunologic Disorders

9. Britton, M. C., and Schur, P. H.   The complement system in rheumatoid synovitis: II. Intracytoplasmic inclusions of immunoglobulins and
complement. *Arthritis Rheum.* 14:87, 1971.
10. Broder, I., Urowitz, M. B., and Gordon, D. A.   Appraisal of rheumatoid arthritis as an immune complex disease. *Med. Clin. North Am.*
56:529, 1972.
11. Burnet, M.   Implications for autoimmune disease in man, studies on
NZB mice and their hybrids: II. Renal and thymic disease. *R. Inst.
Public Health Hyg. J.* 29:95, 1966.
12. Butler, W. T., Sharp, J. T., Rossen, R. D., Lidsky, M. D., Mittal, K. K.,
and Gard, D. A.   Relationship of the clinical course of systemic lupus
erythematosus to the presence of circulating lymphocytotoxic antibodies.
Arthritis Rheum. 15:231, 1972.
13. Cawley, L. P.   *Electrophoresis and Immunoelectrophoresis.* Boston:
Little, Brown, 1969.
14. Chayen, J., and Bitensky, L.   Lysomal enzymes in inflammation. *Ann.
Rheum. Dis.* 30:522, 1971.
15. Churg, J., and Grishman, E.   Ultrastructure of immune deposits in
renal disease. *Ann. Intern. Med.* 76:479, 1972.
16. Cochrane, C. G.   Mediators of the Arthus and related reactions. In
P. Kallos and B. H. Waksman (eds.), *Progress in Allergy.* Basel and
New York: Karger, 1967, vol. 11, pp. 11–35.
17. Cochrane, C. G., and Dixon, F. J.   Cell and tissue damage through
antigen-antibody complexes. In P. Mieshner and H. Müller-Eberhard
(eds.), *Textbook of Immunopathology.* New York: Grune & Stratton,
1969, vol. 1, p. 94.
18. Cochrane, C. G.   Mechanisms involved in the deposition of immune
complexes in tissues. *J. Exp. Med.* 134:75s, 1971.
19. Cochrane, C. G.   Initiating events in immune complex injury. In
B. Amos (ed.), *Progress in Immunology.* 1st International Congress of
Immunology. New York: Academic, 1971.
20. Cochrane, C. G., Wuepper, K. D., Aiken, B. S., Revak, S. D., and
Spiegelberg, H. L.   The interaction of Hageman factor and immune
complexes. *J. Clin. Invest.* 51:2736, 1972.
21. Cream, J. J.   Cryoglobulins in vasculitis. *Clin. Exp. Immunol.* 10:117,
1972.
22. Dacie, J. V.   *The Haemolytic Anaemias: Congenital and Acquired.
Part II. The Autoimmune Haemolytic Anaemias.* New York: Grune &
Stratton, 1962, 2nd ed., pp. 341–718.
23. Dixon, F. J.   The role of antigen-antibody complexes in disease. *Harvey
Lect.* 58:21, 1963.
24. Dubois, E. L.   *Lupus Erythematosus.* New York: Blakiston, 1966.
25. Estes, D., and Christian, C. L.   The natural history of systemic lupus
erythematosus by prospective analysis. *Medicine* (Baltimore) 50:85,
1971.
26. Fahey, J. L., Barth, W. F., and Solomon, A.   Serum hyperviscosity
syndrome. *J.A.M.A.* 192:464, 1965.
27. Ferguson, R. H., and Worthington, J. W.   Recent advances in rheumatic
diseases: 1967 through 1969. *Ann. Intern. Med.* 73:109, 1970.
28. Franco, A. E., and Schur, P. H.   Hypocomplementemia in rheumatoid
arthritis. *Arthritis Rheum.* 14:231, 1971.

29. Freeman, R. G., Knox, J. M., and Owens, D. W.   Cutaneous lesions of lupus erythematosus induced by monochromatic light. *Arch. Dermatol* 99:677, 1969.
30. Freyberg, R. H.   Differential diagnosis of arthritis. *Postgrad. Med.* 51:20, 1972.
31. Gocke, D. J., Hsu, K., Morgan, C., Bombardieri, S., Lockshin, M., and Christian, C. L.   Vasculitis in association with Australia antigen. *J. Exp. Med.* 134:330s, 1971.
32. Goldman, J. A., Litwen, A., Adams, L. E., Krueger, R. C., and Hess, E. V.   Cellular immunity to nuclear antigens in systemic lupus erythematosus. *J. Clin. Invest.* 51:2669, 1972.
33. Götze, O., and Müller-Eberhard, H. J.   Paroxysmal nocturnal hemoglobinuria-hemolysis initiated by the C3 activator system. *N. Engl. J. Med.* 286:180, 1972.
34. Grausz, H., Earley, L. E., Stephens, B. F., Stephens, B. G., Lee, J. C., and Hopper, J., Jr.   Diagnostic import of virus-like particles in the glomerular endothelium of patients with systemic lupus erythematosus. *N. Engl. J. Med.* 283:506, 1970.
35. Grayzel, A. I., and Beck, C.   Rubella infection of synovial cells and the resistance of cells derived from patients with rheumatoid arthritis. *J. Exp. Med.* 131:367, 1970.
36. Grimley, P. M., Frantz, M. M., Michelitch, H. J., and Decker, J. L.   Tubuloreticular structure of circulating lymphocytes in systemic lupus erythematosus (SLE). *Arthritis Rheum.* 15:112, 1972.
37. Grumet, F. C., Coukell, A., Bodmer, J. E., Bodmer, W. F., and McDevitt, H. O.   Histocompatibility (HL–A) antigens associated with systemic lupus erythematosus. *N. Engl. J. Med.* 285:193, 1971.
38. Hanauer, L. B., and Christian, C. L.   Studies of cryoprotein in systemic lupus erythematosus. *J. Clin. Invest.* 46:400, 1967.
39. Henson, P. M.   The role of complement and leucocytes in the immunologic release of vasoactive amines from platelets. *Fed. Proc.* 98:1721, 1969.
40. Henson, P. M., and Cochrane, C. G.   Acute immune complex disease in rabbits—the role of complement and a leucocyte dependent release of vasoactive amines from platelets. *J. Exp. Med.* 133:554, 1971.
41. Horwitz, D. A.   Impaired delayed hypersensitivity in systemic lupus erythematosus. *Arthritis Rheum.* 15:353, 1972.
42. Hunsicker, L. G., Ruddy, S., Carpenter, C. B., Schur, P. H., Merrill, J. P., Müller-Eberhard, H. J., and Austen, K. F.   Metabolism of third complement component (C3) in nephritis. *N. Engl. J. Med.* 287:835, 1972.
43. Kavano, K., Miller, L., and Kimmelstill, P.   Virus-like structures in lupus erythematosus. *N. Engl. J. Med.* 281:1228, 1969.
44. Koffler, D., Agnello, V., Thoburn, R., and Kunkel, H. G.   Systemic lupus erythematosus: Prototype of immune complex nephritis in man. *J. Exp. Med.* 134:169s, 1971.
45. Lawrence, J. S., Locke, G. B., and Ball, J.   Rheumatoid serum factor in population in the U.K.: I. Lung disease and rheumatoid serum factor. *Clin. Exp. Immunol.* 8:723, 1971.
46. Lewis, R. M., and Schwartz, R. S.   Canine systemic lupus erythematosus: Genetic analysis of an established breeding colony. *J. Exp. Med.* 134:417, 1971.

47. Lilly, F.   The effect of histocompatibility-Z type of response to the Friend leukemia virus in mice. *J. Exp. Med.* 127:465, 1968.
48. Lowry, O. A., Rosebrough, D. J., Farr, A. J., and Randell, R. J.   Protein measurement with the Folin and phenol reagent. *J. Biol. Chem.* 193:265, 1951.
49. Marcus, R. L., and Townes, A. S.   The occurrence of cryoproteins in synovial fluid: The association of a complement fixing activity in rheumatoid synovial fluid with the cold precipitable protein. *J. Clin. Invest.* 50:282, 1971.
50. Marsh, W. L.   Anti i: A cold antibody defining the I:i relationship in human red cells. *Br. J. Haematol.* 7:200, 1961.
51. Martin, W. J., Mathieson, D. R., and Eigler, J. O. C.   Pyroglobulinemia: Further observations and review of 20 cases. *Mayo Clin. Proc.* 34:95, 1959.
52. McCluskey, R. T.   Evidence for immunologic mechanisms in several forms of human glomerular diseases. *Bull. N.Y. Acad. Med.* 46:769, 1970.
53. McCluskey, R. T.   The value of immunofluorescence in the study of human renal disease. *J. Exp. Med.* 134:242s, 1971.
54. McDevitt, H. O., and Benacerraf, B.   Genetic control of specific immune responses. In F. J. Dixon, Jr., and H. G. Kunkel (eds.), *Advances in Immunology.* New York: Academic Press, 1969, vol. 11, p. 31.
55. McIntosh, R. M., Kaufman, D. B., and Kulvinskas, C.   Cryoglobulins: I. Studies on the nature, incidence, and clinical significance of serum cryoproteins in glomerulonephritis. *J. Lab. Clin. Med.* 75:566, 1970.
56. McIntosh, R. M., and Grossman, B.   IgG, B_1C fibrinogen cryoprotein in acute glomerulonephritis. *N. Engl. J. Med.* 235:1521, 1971.
57. McIntosh, R. M., Kulvinskas, C., and Kaufman, D. B.   Cryoglobulins: II. The biological and chemical properties of cryoproteins in acute poststreptococcal glomerulonephritis. *Int. Arch. Allergy Appl. Immunol.* 41:700, 1971.
58. McKay, G. G.   Practical applications of immunoelectrophoresis. In H. R. Dettelbach and S. E. Ritzmann (eds.), *Lab Synopsis.* Somerville, N.J.: Behring Diagnostics, Hoechst Pharmaceuticals, Inc., 1969, 2nd rev. ed., vol. 2.
59. Mellbye, O. J., and Munthe, E.   Specific binding of immunoconglutinin in tissue and synovial fluid from patients with rheumatoid arthritis. *Clin. Exp. Immunol.* 8:713, 1971.
60. Meltzer, M., Franklin, E. C., Elias, K., McCluskey, R. T., and Cooper, H.   Cryoglobulinemia—a clinical and laboratory study. *Am. J. Med.* 40:837, 1969.
61. Müller-Eberhard, H. J., and Kunkel, H. G.   Isolation of a thermolabile serum protein which precipitates γ-globulin aggregates and participates in immune hemolysis. *Proc. Soc. Exp. Biol. Med.* 106:291, 1961.
62. Müller-Eberhard, H. J.   Chemistry and reaction mechanisms of complement. In F. J. Dixon and H. G. Kunkel (eds.), *Advances in Immunology.* New York: Academic, 1968, vol. 8, p. 1.
63. Myllylä, G., Vaheri, A., and Penttinen, K.   Detection and characterization of immune complexes by the platelet aggregation test: II. Circulating complexes. *Clin. Exp. Immunol.* 8:399, 1971.
64. Nakamura, R. M., Spiegelberg, H. L., Lee, S., and Weigle, W. O.

Relationship between molecular size and intra- and extravascular distribution of protein antigens. *J. Immunol.* 100:376, 1968.

65. Notkins, A. L.   Infectious virus-antibody complexes. *J. Exp. Med.* 134:41s, 1971.

66. Peetoom, F., and Van Loghem-Langereis, E.   IgM-IgG (B_2M–7s-γ) cryoglobulinemia: An autoimmune phenomenon. *Vox Sang.* 10:281, 1965.

67. Pensky, J., Hinz, C. F., Todd, E. W., Wedgwood, R. J., Boyer, J. T., and Lepow, I. H.   Properties of highly purified human properdin. *J. Immunol.* 100:142, 1968.

68. Penttinen, K., Vaheri, A., and Myllylä, G.   Detection and characterization of immune complexes by the platelet aggregation test: I. Complexes formed in vitro. *Clin. Exp. Immunol.* 8:389, 1971.

69. Percy, J. S., and Smyth, C. J.   The immunofluorescent skin test in systemic lupus erythematosus. *J.A.M.A.* 208:485, 1969.

70. Phillips, P. F.   Virologic studies in rheumatoid arthritis and other connective tissue diseases. *J. Exp. Med.* 134:313s, 1971.

71. Pruzanski, W., and Ogryzlo, M. A.   The changing pattern of diseases associated with M components. *Med. Clin. North Am.* 56:371, 1972.

72. Ritzmann, S. E., Coleman, S. C., and Levin, W. C.   The effect of mercaptenes upon a macrocryoglobulin: Modifications induced by cysteamine, penicillamine, and penicillin. *J. Clin. Invest.* 39:1320, 1960.

73. Ritzmann, S. E., and Levin, W. C.   Cold agglutinin disease: A type of primary macroglobulinemia: A new concept. *Tex. Rep. Biol. Med.* 20:236, 1962.

74. Ritzmann, S. E., Daniels, J. C., and Levin, W. C.   Paralymphomatous disease: The syndrome of macroglobulinemia in leukemia and lymphoma. In *14th Clinical Conference on Cancer at M. D. Anderson Tumor Institute, Houston.* Chicago: Year Book, 1970, pp. 169–221.

75. Ritzmann, S. E., Lawrence, M. C., and Daniels, J. C.   Serum protein analysis—immunoelectrophoresis. In J. B. Fuller (ed.), *Selected Topics in Clinical Chemistry.* Chicago: American Society of Clinical Pathology Workshop Manual, 1972, p. 148.

76. Rothfield, N., Ross, H. A., Menta, J. O., and Lepow, I. H.   Glomerular and dermal deposition of properdin in systemic lupus erythematosus. *N. Engl. J. Med.* 287:681, 1972.

77. Roy, L. P., Fish, A. J., Michael, A. F., and Vernier, R. L.   Etiologic agents of immune deposit disease. In R. S. Schwartz (ed.), *Progress in Clinical Immunology.* New York: Grune & Stratton, 1972, vol. 1, p. 1.

78. Ruddy, S., Gigli, I., and Austen, K. F.   The complement system of man. *N. Engl. J. Med.* 287:489, 545, 591, and 641, 1972.

79. Sanders, J. H., Fahey, J. L., Finegold, I., Ein, D., Reisfeld, R., and Berard, C.   Multiple anomalous immunoglobulins: Clinical structural and cellular studies in three patients. *Am. J. Med.* 47:43, 1969.

80. Schrohenloher, R.E., Kunkel, H. G., and Tomasi, T.B.   Activity of dissociated and reassociated 19S anti-γ-globulin. *J. Exp. Med.* 120:1215, 1964.

81. Schubothe, H.   The cold hemagglutinin in disease. *Semin. Hematol.* 3:27, 1966.

82. Schur, P. H., and Austen, K. F.   Complement in the rheumatic diseases. *Bull. Rheum. Dis.* 22:666, 1971–72.

83. Schultze, H. E., and Heremans, J. F. *Molecular Biology of Human Proteins.* Amsterdam, London, and New York: Elsevier, 1966, vol. 1.
84. Slwinski, A. J., and Zvaifler, N. J. Decreased synthesis of the third component of complement (C3) in hypocomplementemic systemic lupus erythematosus. *Clin. Exp. Immunol.* 11:21, 1972.
85. Stastny, P., and Ziff, M. Cold-insoluble complexes in complement levels in systemic lupus erythematosus. *N. Engl. J. Med.* 280:1376, 1969.
86. Swisher, S.S., and Vaughan, J. H. Acquired hemolytic disease. In M. Samter (ed.), *Immunological Diseases.* Boston: Little, Brown, 1971, 2nd ed.
87. Talal, D. Immunologic and viral factors in the pathogenesis of systemic lupus erythematosus. *Arthritis Rheum.* 13:887, 1970.
88. Tan, E. M., and Kunkel, H. G. An immunofluorescent study of the skin lesions in systemic lupus erythematosus. *Arthritis Rheum.* 9:37, 1966.
89. Tan, E. M., Schur, P. H., Carr, R. I., and Kunkel, H. G. Deoxyribonucleic acid (DNA) and antibodies to DNA in the serum of patients with systemic lupus erythematosus. *J. Clin. Invest.* 45:1732, 1966.
90. Tan, E. M. Antibodies to deoxyribonucleic acid irradiated with ultraviolet light: Detection by precipitin and immunofluorescence. *Science* 161:1353, 1968.
91. Tan, E. M., and Stoughton, R. B. Ultraviolet light induced damage to desoxyribonucleic acid in human skin. *J. Invest. Dermatol.* 52:537, 1969.
92. Tan, E. M., Freeman, R. G., and Stoughton, R. B. Action spectrum of ultraviolet light induced damage to nuclear DNA in vivo. *J. Invest. Dermatol.* 55:439, 1970.
93. Terasaki, P. I., Mottironi, V. D., and Barnett, E. V. Cytotoxins in disease—autocytotoxins in lupus. *N. Engl. J. Med.* 283:724, 1970.
94. Wager, O., Räsänen, J. A., Hagman, A., and Klemola, E. Mixed cryoglobulinemia in infectious mononucleosis and cytomegalovirus mononucleosis. *Int. Arch. Allergy App. Immunol.* 34:345, 1968.
95. Weigle, W. O. Fate and biological action of antigen-antibody complexes. In W. H. Taliaferro and J. H. Humphrey (eds.), *Advances in Immunology.* New York: Academic, 1961, vol. 1, p. 283.
96. Whitsed, H. M., and Penny, R. IgA/IgG cryoglobulinemia with vasculitis. *Clin. Exp. Immunol.* 9:183, 1971.
97. Wilson, C. Immunological mechanisms of glomerulonephritis. Medical Staff Conference, University of California at San Francisco. *Calif. Med.* 116:47, 1972.
98. Winchester, R. J., Agnello, V., and Kunkel, H. G. Gamma globulin complexes in synovial fluids of patients with rheumatoid arthritis— partial characterization and relation to lowered complement levels. *Clin. Exp. Immunol.* 6:689, 1970.
99. Winchester, R. J., Kunkel, H. G., and Agnello, V. Occurrence of γ-globulin complexes in serum and joint fluid of rheumatoid arthritis patients: Use of monoclonal rheumatoid factors as reagents for their demonstration. *J. Exp. Med.* 134:286s, 1971.
100. Zvaifler, H. J. Immunoreactants in rheumatoid synovial lesions. *J. Exp. Med.* 134:276s, 1971.

7

Autoimmunity, Immunologic Unresponsiveness, and Interrelationships

Definitions

Autoimmunity is a concept—not a disease—that may help explain the pathogenesis of a number of diseases. Autoimmunity is the failure of an organism to recognize its own tissue, and includes any immune response to the host's own tissue, whether it is humoral (i.e., circulating antibodies) or cellular (i.e., delayed hypersensitivity). Normally, an individual's immune mechanisms recognize his own tissues and avoid reacting against them. In autoimmune states, the immune mechanisms may injure, or even destroy, specific tissues of the host individual.

Instead of autoimmune, the term *autoallergic* is often used. The term *allergy,* first originated by von Pirquet to mean altered reactivity due to previous exposure, now is often interpreted to mean harmful reactions secondary to immune mechanisms. Today, *allergy* is used to identify immune reactions as well as nonimmunologic reactions such as non-specific reactions to food substances. *Hypersensitivity* is a term often used interchangeably with the term *allergy,* but it should be used to describe nonimmunologic reactions.

From another viewpoint, autoimmunity may be considered a termination of the natural unresponsive state [65]. A definition of unresponsiveness is the inability to make a detectable immune response to an antigenic challenge, as distinguished from *tolerance,* which is the term commonly used in transplantation immunology in addition to nonimmunologic events to describe the endurance without ill effect of substances such as endotoxin or a drug.

In an autoimmune response, two types of responses may be evident, singly or both together: (a) the cell-mediated response and (b) humoral response with production of antibodies. Further, the cell-mediated response may be divided into (a) nonspecific response which includes phagocytic mechanisms of the cells; and (b) the specific response with cellular or delayed hypersensitivity. The humoral response can also be divided into (a) nonspecific response which includes complement, immunoconglutinins, and properdin; and (b) the specific response with the formation of immune type antibodies.

Development of the Natural Unresponsive State

Currently, it is believed that the development of the natural unresponsive state results from a direct contact between the self constituents and potential antibody-producing cells, a phenomenon first predicted by Burnet [6]. Since then, many investigators have artificially induced an unresponsive state to different antigens during the newborn period, when an immature immune system is present. Further evidence of this development was gained from the experiments by Tripplet [58], who demonstrated that the tree frog would reject its own pituitary gland when implanted into another animal and reimplanted into the original frog after maturation of the immune system. The pituitary gland was shown to be biologically functioning by secretion of the hormone which causes a color change in the frog. In addition, in certain strains of mice, there is a deficiency of the MuB_1 protein, and when these mice are injected with normal mouse sera, they give rise to an antibody to the MuB_1 protein. The MuB_1 protein is now recognized as a counterpart of the fifth component of human complement [14].

Thus, it can be stated that the mode of induction of the natural unresponsive state is probably by two mechanisms [10]: (a) the clones of immunocompetent cells capable of reacting to self antigens are eliminated by the mechanism of the clonal selection theory of Burnet; and (b) antibody-producing cells are made unresponsive by early exposure to self antigens.

Cellular Aspects of Unresponsiveness

Cells Involved in Induction of Immune Response
or Immunologic Unresponsiveness

The cells which are involved are (a) macrophages, (b) lymphoid cells from thymus or T-cells, and (c) antibody producing or B-cells from the bone marrow (analogous to cells derived from bursa of Fabricius of birds). The evidence for direct cooperation between T-lymphocytes and B-lymphocytes was initially provided by the observation of Claman and Chaperon [15]. When specific antigen sensitive cells interact for the production of antibody, specifically reactive cells from the thymus and bone marrow must both interact. The role of the macrophage appears to be nonspecific by providing the surface for the antigen to interact with the thymus and bone marrow cells [13, 69, 70]. No difference was found between macrophages studied in unresponsive and normal animals.

In many of the antigens, the T-cells and the B-cells interact with the macrophage which processes the antigen. The T-cells reduce the need for high dose of antigen for antibody formation by the B-cells [37]; also the T-cells release mitogenic factor which causes proliferation of the cells [21]. The T-cell independent antigens which can directly act on B-cells for antibody production are the carbohydrate containing antigens of polysaccharide and other bacterial antigens which have repeated antigenic determinants [38]. Thus, it appears that the T-cell serves a function of concentrating the antigen and decreases the requirement for a large dose of antigen to initiate an immune response.

Cellular Sites of Unresponsiveness

The cellular sites of immunologic responsiveness have been recently shown by Weigle, Chiller, and co-workers to be at the level of both the bone marrow and thymus cells [12, 13, 69, 70]. The total unresponsive state demonstrates tolerance at the level of thymus and bone marrow cells. The unresponsive state is specific for the antigen.

In the studies of Weigle, Chiller et al. [13, 69, 70], adult mice were made unresponsive to deaggregated human γ-globulin (specific tolerogen). A tolerogen is an antigen existing in a form or under conditions that induce a specific unresponsive state in the host. The following observations were made: (a) The thymus cells and bone marrow cells were both needed for immunologic reconstitution of lethally irradiated mice. (b) The thymus and bone marrow cells probably have specific receptor sites. (c) The bone marrow cells required a higher dose of the tolerogen than the thymus cells for the induction of unresponsiveness. (d) The induction of unresponsiveness is much slower in bone marrow cells than thymus cells, and the unresponsiveness is of longer duration. (e) The bone marrow cells maintain an unresponsive state of shorter duration than the thymus cells and also require higher levels of tolerogen for induction. (f) Unresponsiveness at the level of either the thymus or the bone marrow cells manifests itself in the condition of general unresponsiveness.

Termination of Unresponsiveness and Its Relation to Autoimmunity

It is apparent that the spontaneous loss of unresponsiveness to a specific antigen is more rapid in bone marrow cells than in thymus cells. The dose of tolerogen needed to induce unresponsiveness in bone marrow cells was considerably greater than that needed to induce unresponsiveness in thymus cells [13, 68, 70]. These observations lead to the speculation that, in certain autoimmune states, there may be selective unresponsiveness in the thymus or T-cells without concomitant tolerance in the B-cells.

In organs which are often involved in autoimmune diseases such as the thyroid, testes, adrenals, and brain, there is a very low concentration

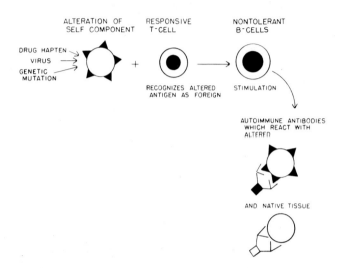

Figure 7-1
Postulated autoantibody formation in certain organ specific autoimmune
disorders.

of native antigens in circulation. The low antigen concentrations may be
sufficient to induce unresponsiveness to the thymus-derived cells but not
to the bone marrow cells. The unresponsive state would exist only at
the level of the thymus-derived cells and the animal would appear
normal. However, if a genetic mutation or viral transformation results
in an interaction between thymic cells and altered host antigen, then an
initiation of an immune response would occur. Such events probably
occur in the pathogenesis of thyroiditis (Fig. 7-1).

In cases of tissue components which are present in high concentrations in body fluids, such as serum proteins, immunologic unresponsiveness is probably present in both bone marrow and thymus cells and
protect against an autoimmune response.

Thymus-Derived Lymphocytes and Their Relation to Autoimmunity

A hypothesis has been advanced by Allison and co-workers [1] to
ascribe a regulatory function to the T-cells, besides the known cell-
mediated immune properties. They believe that (a) the T-cell participates in antibody formation against many antigens; and (b) the T-cells
can exert a specific feedback control on synthesis of antibody by B-cells
and play a key role in preventing autoimmunity.

Normally T-lymphocytes are unresponsive to self antigens so they
do not interact with the B-cells in the initiation of an immune response.
In line with the theory proposed above, unresponsiveness may not be

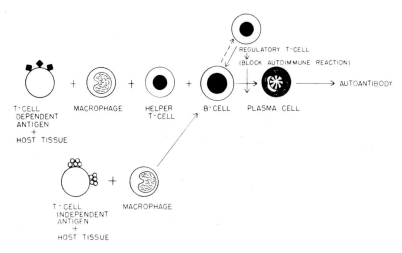

Figure 7-2
Postulated regulatory T-cells in prevention of autoimmune reactions.

present in the B-cells, and B-lymphocytes can produce autoantibodies in several situations.

The factors which favor autoantibody formation are conditions in which (a) the T-cells and B-cells are usually resistant to induction to unresponsiveness. Genetic factors may play a significant role; and (b) the T-cell functions decline with age as evidenced by the spontaneous increase in the incidence of autoantibodies in males and females with increase in age [55, 72].

In the various interactions of T-cells, the conditions which give rise to autoantibody are when T-cells are made responsive and interact with B-cells to produce antibody. The following conditions may favor the induction of autoantibody formation [1]: (a) interaction of virus with self tissue component; (b) Haptens or drug plus the self tissue component; and (c) nonspecific stimulation of T-cells by adjuvants or allogenic cells.

It is well known that the T-cells are involved in immunologic surveillance against malignant cells. However, a postulated regulatory function of T-cells will help explain the high incidence of autoimmune reactions associated with malignancy [26], aging [55, 72], and primary and secondary immune deficiency diseases [3, 23, 49] (Fig. 7-2).

General Theories of Autoimmunity

The following processes may possibly give rise to autoimmunization.

Abnormal Immune Mechanisms [9, 10]
Burnet proposed the existence of "forbidden clones" of immunologically competent cells which produce autoantibodies. The clones, which de-

velop as a result of mutations, successfully made the normal homeostatic mechanisms which can destroy them. Autoantibody production may be a normal process, usually suppressed by the presence of the corresponding autoantigens (immunoparalysis). Transformation or a quantitative decrease of the antigens may lead to an increased production of autoimmune antibodies.

Abnormal proliferation of the immunologically competent cells that produce small amounts of autoantibodies under physiologic conditions can occur in disease with malignant lymphoid proliferation, and in viral infections, which are often accompanied by an increased production of lymphoid cells. Disturbances of the thymus or peripheral lymphoid tissue may result in a deficiency of functions with failure of self-recognition by the immunologically competent cells. This is supported by the fact that patients with immune deficiency diseases are extremely susceptible to the development of autoimmune diseases [23]. Patients with secretory IgA deficiency lack protective antibodies in the alimentary tract and have a high incidence of autoimmune diseases [3, 4].

Sequestered Antigen

This theory assumes that a natural unresponsive state does not exist to certain antigens since they are sequestered within a tissue barrier and unable to contact potential antibody-producing cells. Previously, it was used to explain thyroiditis, uveitis, and allergic aspermatogenesis. This theory has been largely disproved in the case of thyroiditis. Thyroglobulin behaves similarly to a serum protein and can persist in circulation and equilibrate between the extravascular and intravascular fluid compartment and reach all potential lymphoid cells [39, 42]. Experimentally, an unresponsive state has been induced to heterologous bovine thyroglobulin in newborn [39, 40] and adult [44] rabbits. Native thyroglobulin has been detected in neck lymphatics of normal animals [18] and can be detected in the serum of newborn human infants [50].

Cross-Reacting Antigen

Foreign materials contain antigenic determinants with structural relationships to various host antigens. An example is the formation of autoantibodies after injections of heterologous beef insulin into humans. The heterologous insulin elicits antibodies which will cross react with native homologous insulin. Experimental autoimmune thyroiditis has been induced by the injection of soluble heterologous cross-reacting thyroglobulin [66].

Altered Body Constituents

This mechanism may be constantly operative. Modification of the cellular self antigen by inflammation, trauma, viruses, bacteria, drugs, etc. may initiate an immune reaction since the self-recognition system now considers them as foreign. Factors which prevent the initiation of an autoimmune reaction may be the nature and concentration of normal tissue antigen to prevent the termination of the natural unresponsive state [69, 70].

The mechanism of alteration of body constituents has been observed in many of the experimental autoimmune diseases. Experimental thyroiditis has been induced by the injection of soluble homologous thyroglobulin altered by the addition of hapten groups [64] and pepsin digestion [67]. Recent evidence indicates that mycobacteria in the adjuvant appears to attract polymorphonuclear leukocytes to the granuloma at the site of injection of the antigen [67]. Subsequently, the neutrophils will cause alteration of the homologous thyroglobulin and initiate thyroiditis.

Types of Human Autoimmune Disorders

Autoimmune diseases in man can be broadly classified into two main categories [5, 29]. A third category can include diseases which overlap the two main categories.

Organ Specific Autoimmune Disorders
These diseases are characterized by chronic inflammatory changes in a particular organ; the autoantibodies in this group of diseases are directed against the specific diseased organ and not against other tissues. The autoantibodies are often organ specific and demonstrate a narrow species specificity. There is a familial incidence and coincidence of diseases within the same organ-specific group. Examples in this category are (a) Hashimoto's thyroiditis; (b) primary hypothyroidism; (c) thyrotoxicosis (Graves' disease); (d) chronic atropic gastritis (pernicious anemia); (e) primary adrenal atrophy (Addison's disease); and (f) post-rabies vaccination encephalomyelitis.

It should be emphasized that the presence of an antibody or lymphoid cell sensitized to an autoantigen does not prove that the immune mechanism is the cause or etiology of the disease. Similar to Koch's postulates in the demonstration of acid fast bacilli as the etiologic agent in tuberculosis, Humphrey and White [29] proposed certain postulates to demonstrate a definite role of immunity in the pathogenesis of a disease. The organ specific autoimmune disease thyroiditis has been shown to fulfill these postulates: (a) immune response (humoral antibodies or cellular sensitivity to autoantigen) at some stage of the disease; (b) recognition of a specific antigen; (c) production of antibodies against the same antigen in experimental animals; (d) appearance of tissue lesions similar to human disease in actively sensitized animals; and (e) the reproduction of the disease of the experimental animal in a normal animal by transfer of antibody in serum or immunologically potent cells. Cell [41] and serum [43] transfer of experimental thyroiditis has been demonstrated with methods which minimized and ruled out the possibility of transfer of active antigen from the donor animal.

Non-Organ Specific Autoimmune Disorders
These diseases are characterized by widespread pathologic changes in many different organs and tissues throughout the body. Further characteristics may be enumerated as follows: (a) serum autoantibodies in these diseases lack organ and species specificity; (b) familial incidence and clinical overlap of the various "connective tissue disorders"; (c) experimental lesions not readily produced. Animal disease models arise spontaneously in the later life of animals of the appropriate genotype. Examples are (a) systemic lupus erythematosus; (b) rheumatoid arthritis; (c) hemolytic anemia; and (d) other "connective tissue disorders" such as systemic scleroderma.

Diseases with Non-Organ Specific Autoantibodies with
Lesions Concentrated in One or Few Organs
The diseases which can be interpreted as belonging to both the above categories are (a) Sjögren's disease, including Mikulicz disease; (b) chronic active or lupoid hepatitis; (c) primary biliary cirrhosis; and (d) certain cases of acquired hemolytic anemia often associated with connective tissue disorders.

The conditions included in the above categories tend to be associated with one another [5, 10]. Patients with autoimmune thyroid disease have a high incidence of gastric parietal cell autoantibodies. There is evidence of association between autoimmune thyroiditis and rheumatoid arthritis and systemic lupus erythematosus.

Antigen Source and Relationship to the Location of Autoimmune Lesions

The source of antigen is often sought in autoimmune disease and may be (a) outside the host—introduction of a foreign antigen or heterologous insulin, foreign protein serum sickness; (b) the combination of an exogenous source with a component of host tissue. A drug such as quinidine may adhere to the patient's red cells and function as haptens. The host forms antibody to the drug-erythrocyte complex and causes hemolytic anemia; or (c) no evidence of an exogenous antigen. In many non-organ specific autoimmune diseases no definite antigen can be demonstrated, and one can speculate on the possibility of a virus by vertical genetic transmission.

Relationship of the Location of Damage to the Origin of the Antigen Inciting Autoantibody Production [26]

A. Primary damage. The site of the damage is related to the specificity of the antibody, i.e., thyroid gland and antithyroid antibody.

B. Consequential damage. The site of damage is affected by the presence of a cross-reacting tissue antigen. If thyroid antigens were liberated during inflammation and absorbed onto other tissues, then the damage following interaction with specific antibody would be an example of consequential damage.
C. Coincidental damage. The site of the damage is unrelated to the specificity of the antibody. Immune complex disease with resultant damage to vessels and kidney is caused by chance deposition. Cases of glomerulonephritis resulting from thyroid-antithyroid immune complexes have been observed [31]. Thus, the distribution and characteristics of the autoimmune lesions may differ even though the same specific antigen-antibody reaction may be involved.

Observations Which Indicate Involvement of Autoimmune Mechanisms in a Given Disease

In recognition of possible autoimmune pathogenesis in disease, MacKay and Burnet [36] have listed the following characteristics which are often seen: (a) hypergammaglobulinemia with elevated serum γ-globulin levels; (b) the existence of serum autoantibodies; (c) the presence of amyloid, indicating deposition of denatured γ-globulin; (d) inflammatory tissue lesions with many lymphocytes and plasma cells; (e) coexistence of the disease with other lesions consistent with immunologic injury; and (f) improvement of disease with immunosuppressive therapy.

Classification of Disorders Believed To Have a Primary or Secondary Relationship to Autoimmunization (Modified from Pirofsky [49])

Hematologic Diseases
Autoimmune hemolytic anemia, idiopathic thrombocytopenic purpura, idiopathic neutropenia, idiopathic pancytopenia, cold hemagglutination disease, paroxysmal cold hemoglobinuria, acquired hemophilia, the leukemias, the lymphomas, pernicious anemia

Neuromuscular Diseases
Acute demyelinating encephalitis, multiple sclerosis, Landry's paralysis, Guillain-Barré syndrome, peripheral neuritis, myasthenia gravis

Collagen Diseases
Lupus erythematosus, polyarteritis nodosa, scleroderma, dermatomyositis, Sjögren's disease, rheumatoid arthritis, rheumatic fever, thrombotic thrombocytopenia, erythema nodosa, Stevens-Johnson syndrome

Endocrine Diseases
Thyroiditis, thyrotoxicosis, Addison's disease, aspermatogenesis

Gastrointestinal Diseases
Portal cirrhosis, acute hepatitis, chronic active hepatitis, lupoid hepatitis, biliary cirrhosis, ulcerative colitis, regional enteritis, adult coeliac disease, atropic gastritis

Skin Diseases
Pemphigus vulgaris, pemphigus foliaceus, bullous pemphigoid, cicatricial pemphigoid, dermatitis herpetiformis, Behçet's syndrome, exfoliative dermatitis

Kidney Diseases
Goodpasture's syndrome, immune complex glomerulonephritis, nephrotic syndrome and IgE immunoglobulin, nephropathy with mesangial IgG-IgA deposits, chronic membranoproliferative glomerulonephritis

Miscellaneous Diseases
Sympathetic ophthalmia, postcardiotomy syndrome, postinfarction syndrome

Immunopathologic Mechanisms in Autoimmune Disorders

The exact etiologic factors are often unknown in the various immunologic diseases. However, the various immune mechanisms are helpful in explaining the course of events and pathogenesis. The immunopathologic mechanisms may be classified according to Sell [52, 53] as follows: (a) neutralization or inactivation of biologically active molecules; (b) cytotoxic or cytolytic mechanisms; (c) anaphylactic or atopic mechanisms; (d) toxic immune complex mechanisms; (e) delayed or cellular sensitivity mechanisms; and (f) granulomatous sensitivity (Figs. 7-3–7-6).

Neutralization or Inactivation of Biologically Active Molecules

This is seen in clinical cases as follows:

A. Patients who have hemophilia with deficiency of this protein may develop an immune response to the injected antihemophiliac globulin.

B. Pernicious anemia with antibody to intrinsic factor would be an example of this category. Also, long-acting thyroid stimulator (LATS) in thyrotoxicosis would be another example.

C. The reaction is often seen following immune reactions to heterologous hormones such as antibodies to insulin.

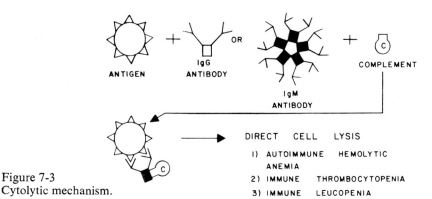

Figure 7-3
Cytolytic mechanism.

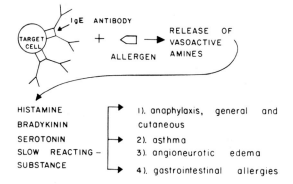

Figure 7-4
Anaphylactic mecha-
nism.

Figure 7-5
Toxic immune com-
plexes.

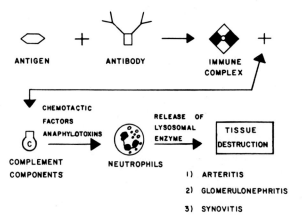

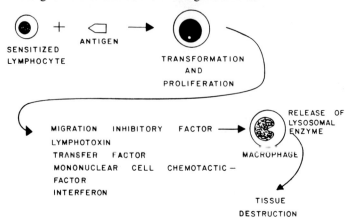

Figure 7-6
Cellular immunity.

Cytotoxic or Cytolytic Mechanisms
In this case, circulating antibodies react with an antigenic component of cells or antigen intimately associated with the cell. Often the complement system is activated with death or lysis of the target cells. Cytolytic or cytotoxic reactions often involve erythrocytes, leukocytes, platelets, and vascular endothelial cells. In the case of erythrocytes, transfusion reactions, erythroblastosis fetalis, acquired hemolytic anemia, and hemolytic reactions to various drugs such as quinidine are seen. Leukocytes become the target in cases of chronic agranulocytosis and acute agranulocytosis following sensitivity to drugs such as sulfapyridine. Platelet reactions are often seen in acute idiopathic thrombocytopenic purpura following viral infections such as rubella. An example of drug sensitivity is purpura caused by sensitivity to Sedormid.

Anaphylactic or Atopic Mechanisms
There is release of vasoactive amines by the reaction of allergen or antigen with cells sensitized by IgE antibody. The cell type most often involved is a mast cell or basophil which results in the release of histamine after the interaction of the antigen and IgE antibody. The acute reactions are called anaphylactic reactions, and the chronic reactions are referred to as atopic. The chemical mediators often associated with the immediate sensitivity are (a) histamine, which causes capillary vasodilatation, increased capillary permeability, and bronchial constriction; (b) slow-reacting substrate (SRS), a lipopolysaccharide derived from polymorphonuclear leukocytes which causes prolonged smooth muscle contraction [48]; (c) serotonin, which has similar physiologic properties to the slow-reacting substances; and (d) bradykinin, which causes in-

creased capillary permeability and smooth muscle contractions. The classic example of anaphylactic reaction is allergy to penicillin, which may give rise to urticaria or bronchial asthma.

Toxic Immune Complex Mechanisms

During the past several years, evidence has accumulated as to the toxic nature of immune complexes which can initiate activation of complement [19]. Examples of immune complex diseases are experimental serum sickness, immune complex glomerulonephritis, periarteritis nodosa, and lupus erythematosus.

The localization of immune complexes is enhanced by the reaction of antigen with basophilic leukocytes with adherent IgE antibody. The reaction causes a release of platelet agglutinating factor (PAF), which causes clumping of platelets along the vessel wall and subsequent release of vasoactive amines [16]. The vasoactive amines increase the permeability of the vascular basement membranes, and complexes which are greater than 19S become lodged. The immune complexes tend to localize against the basement membrane of vessels and kidney glomeruli or basement membrane. Following localization of the immune complexes, there is fixation of complement with release of chemotactic factor which in turn attracts polymorphonuclear leukocytes. Then the polymorphonuclear leukocytes release proteolytic enzymes with destruction of the basement membrane and the vascular wall. Experimentally, when the animal is depleted of polymorphs or complement, no inflammatory reaction or destructive reaction is seen, although the immune complexes may be detected by fluorescent antibody techniques. The kidney glomerular vessels have fenestrations along the endothelial cells, and the immune complexes may be trapped nonspecifically. A wide variety of immune complexes, including bacteria and viruses, may initiate glomerular injury [46]. Immunofluorescent studies of the kidney in immune complex disease show fixation of IgG and beta 1C in a lumpy-bumpy pattern along the epithelial side of the basement membrane. The classic illustration of immune complex nephritis in humans is the glomerulonephritis seen in systemic lupus erythematosus. More recently, Australia antigen, which is associated with long incubation serum hepatitis, has been localized in immune complexes along the vessel wall in clinical cases of periarteritis nodosa [24] and arthritis [2].

Delayed Cellular or Sensitivity Mechanisms [59]

These reactions are initiated by specific lymphocytes capable of reacting to allergens. Classically, no humoral antibodies are involved, and when the antigen is injected into or absorbed through the skin, a delayed skin reaction is seen in 24 to 48 hours with a typical mononuclear cellular infiltrate. The sensitized lymphocytes give rise to the chemotactic factor, macrophage inhibitory factor, and cytotoxic factors which are the biochemical mediators of the sensitized lymphoid cells.

Granulomatous Sensitivity [22]
Granulomatous sensitivity is characterized by a reticulum cell response. The onset of granulomatous reactions is more delayed than are the true cellular sensitivity reactions. Microscopic findings show a foreign body and granulomatous reaction to poorly soluble antigens. Tuberculosis may result in different types of immune response consisting of circulating antibody, classic delayed sensitivity, and granulomatous hypersensitivity. Other examples of granulomatous hypersensitivity are zirconium granuloma, sarcoidosis, and Wegener's granulomatosis, which is a triad of granulomatous arteritis, glomerulonephritis, and sinusitis.

Autoimmune Disorders and Immunologic Deficiency States

Fudenberg [23] has discussed the hypothesis that autoimmune disease is not necessarily a function of immunologic hyperactivity as postulated by the "forbidden clone" and "sequestered antigen" theories. On the other hand, autoimmunity diseases may result from either generalized or selective immune deficiency syndromes. Pathogenic mechanisms may be due to (a) mutation of lymphocytes with the formation of abnormal lymphocytes. An agammaglobulinemic person cannot destroy the many invading microorganisms which evoke tissue alteration with subsequent mutation of lymphocytes; and (b) genetic predisposition to a particular microorganism which can invade specific tissues and expose new antigenic sites. The host lymphocyte will interact with the newly exposed antigenic sites and produce sensitized cells and autoantibodies. This latter concept may explain the presence of autoimmune disease in persons who have normal levels of circulating immunoglobulins. Genetic factors may cause alteration of host antigen in the synthesis and degradation of the components.

Selective IgA deficiency patients show a high incidence of autoimmune disease, autoimmune phenomenon, or unusual antibody formation. IgA is the major immunoglobulin component of certain local secretions of the alimentary tract which has direct access to the external environment. Selective IgA deficiency has been defined as follows [4]: (a) less than 0.05 mg/ml serum IgA; (b) no deficiency of the immunoglobulin, e.g., IgG, IgM, IgD, or IgE; (c) normal cellular immunity; and (d) normal humoral antibody.

In a series of IgA deficiency cases reported by Ammann and Hong [3], 10 to 15 patients were positive for 1 or more autoantibodies. Three patients had thyroiditis, 1 cerebral vasculitis, 1 pulmonary hemosiderosis, 1 cystic fibrosis, and 9 had recurrent respiratory tract infections. All were under 16 years of age. There was high evidence of anti-IgA antibodies, and anti-milk precipitating antibodies.

The gastrointestinal tract serves as a selective absorption barrier, and in IgA deficient patients foreign material may cross the barrier in the absence of IgA and initiate an autoimmune response. Not all autoimmune diseases are related to selective IgA deficiency; however, in cases of IgA deficiency, one should investigate for autoimmune disorders. It is possible that IgA immunoglobulin may be involved in a feedback control mechanism for IgG and IgM antibody production [1].

Thymus and Autoimmunity

There is much evidence that the thymus is directly or indirectly involved in the origin of idiopathic autoimmune disease [55]. Thymic abnormalities have been observed in children with agammaglobulinemia, which is associated with a high frequency of autoimmune phenomena. Yunis et al. [72] have reported that involution of the thymus is related to autoimmunity, and that genetic factors are involved in the involution of the thymus dependent system. Thymectomy in mice accelerates the development of immune deficiency and autoimmunity. The autoimmune susceptible strains were likely to show decreased cell-mediated responses with aging. The stress of infections results in lymphoid depletion and production of autoimmunity in both neonatally thymectomized and aging animals. This link between immunodeficiency and autoimmunity does not have to be explained by cross-reacting exogenous antigens. Viruses, for example, may enter host tissue and initiate immunologic imbalances.

The above observations support the postulates that T-cells may play a specific regulatory feedback control on the production of antibodies by B-cells, and that alteration of the mechanism in aging and immunodeficiency states may be an important factor in autoimmune reactions [1].

Viral Infections and Autoimmune Disorders

Present concepts of autoimmune diseases include viral infections as playing an important role [20]. Autoimmune diseases of animals of known or suspected viral origin include (a) autoimmune hemolytic anemia of NZB mice; (b) Aleutian mink disease; (c) lymphocytic choriomeningitis of mice; (d) scrapie disease of sheep; and (e) equine infectious anemia.

The autoimmune diseases of man in which viruses are suspected to play a role in the pathogenesis are (a) systemic lupus erythematosus (virus-like particles have been reported in the glomerular endothelial and liver cells of patients. A causal relationship has not been established); (b) Hashimoto's and Graves' diseases of the thyroid; (c) certain autoimmune hemolytic anemias; (d) ulcerative colitis; (e) rheumatoid arthritis; (f) chronic demyelinizing diseases, e.g., kuru and Creutzfeldt-Jakob disease; and (g) vasculitis (caused by immune complexes of viruses such as Australia antigen-antibody complexes initiating periarteritis nodosa [24]).

Viral interaction with tissue may vary from latent symbiosis to cytotoxic injury. Often, viral agents may be transmitted vertically from parent to offspring, and the replicating viral antigen becomes a part of the host (self) tissue. Thus, if sometime later in life the host develops an immune response to the virus or viral antigens, then a state of "autoimmunity" is developed.

Hotchin [28] and Oldstone and Dixon [45] showed that when lymphocytic choriomeningitis virus (LCM) was inoculated into newborn mice, the mice did not die but later were found to be partially tolerant to the virus. Later in life, the mice developed extensive viral immune complex disease with glomerulonephritis and a wasting syndrome. Inoculation of LCM virus into adult mice causes immediate infection and death secondary to the intense inflammatory host immune response to the offending viral agent. The results of these experiments suggest that a state of initial immunologic nonreactivity of the newborn may later develop an autoimmune syndrome to a particular virus, as the LCM virus.

The hereditary character of idiopathic autoimmune disease could be explained by the passive transfer of virus during pregnancy or by a genetic predisposition of a newborn to certain viral strains. Introduction of the virus with early induction of tolerance can change into autoimmunity later in life. In addition, a provirus acquired early in life may change into an active virus in later life due to exogenous factors such as ultraviolet light, drugs, and other chemical agents. Autoimmune diseases in man, especially autoimmune hemolytic anemia, are often associated with lymphatic leukemia, lymphosarcoma, and other forms of malignant proliferation of lymphoid tissue. In mice it has been well established that lymphomas and leukemias can be caused by viruses.

If viral infections lead to autoimmunity, then the following mechanisms are possible [60]: (a) Viral disease of the thymus and lymphoid system can result in alterations of the immune system with loss of self recognition and subsequent autoantibody production. (b) Viral infection may evoke transformation of target cells with alteration of host tissue which is recognized as foreign to the host. The resulting sensitized cells and antibodies cross react with normal body constituents.

The alteration of target cell by specific viral infections resulting from a selective and genetic affinity could explain many diseases with an autoimmune pathogenesis. The concept of modification or denaturation of autologous antigens can explain many events in autoimmune diseases.

Talal [57] has presented a theory of interacting genetic, viral, and immunologic factors in the pathogenesis of autoimmunity and malignancy in New Zealand Black mice (animal counterpart of systemic

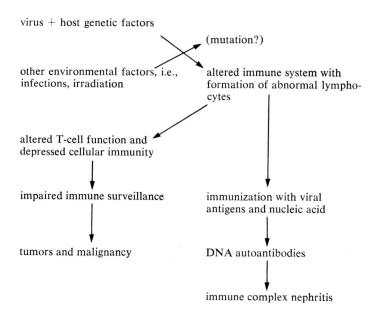

Figure 7-7
Possible immunologic and viral factors in the pathogenesis of systemic lupus erythematosus. (Modified from Talal [57].)

lupus erythematosus in humans). The failure of cellular immune mechanisms to control viral infections, with resulting immunologic and neoplastic transformation of viral action, can explain many interrelationships among immune deficiency disorders, autoimmunity, and lymphoreticular malignancy (Fig. 7-7).

As shown in Fig. 7-7, genetic factors in combination with a virus may initiate alteration of the immune system in the disease of NZB mice or systemic lupus in humans. The altered immune state predisposes to immunization with viral antigens and nucleic acids with production of autoantibodies. An impaired immune system predisposes the host to malignancy. Other environmental factors such as infections, irradiation, and chemical immunosuppression would enhance the development of autoimmunity and malignancy.

Human Cancer and Autoimmunity

In Green's immunologic theory of cancer [25], malignant cells are malignant because they have lost tissue specific antigens and are no longer subject to tissue homeostatic control mechanisms. Autoimmune reactions to damaged or altered tissue may hasten malignant degeneration with adaptive loss of cellular components. However, autoimmune reactions might lead to cancer only when the part of the cell attached is an important specific tissue constituent for effective normal homeostasis.

In support of the immunologic theory of cancer deletion of normal tissue antigen such as A, B, and H, blood antigens have been observed in many human tumors [26]. Deletion of normal tissue antigens has been reported in the following human tumors: carcinoma of skin, thyroid, cervix, colon, stomach, and kidney.

Human cancer and autoimmunity are related in at least two ways [26]: (a) Certain autoimmune disorders are precancerous; and (b) tumors may be accompanied by distant nonmetastatic lesions which may be due to a host immune response to invading tumor.

The relationship between cancer and organ specific autoimmune diseases can be listed as follows:

A. Atrophic gastritis, achlorhydria, and pernicious anemia. In pernicious anemia, humoral antibodies reacting with gastric parietal cells have been demonstrated by fluorescent antibody tests [30]. The risk of stomach cancer is 22 times greater than for the general population of the same age [27].

B. Chronic lymphocytic thyroiditis (including Hashimoto's and chronic focal thyroiditis). The incidence of cancer is 4 times greater than in the general population [35].

C. Ulcerative colitis. Pathogenesis is not yet established, but evidence favors autoimmune disease. Patients demonstrate humoral antibodies in serum which specifically react with extract of colon. Cancer risk in ulcerative colitis is *30 times* the general population of same age and sex [63].

Neuromyopathic Syndromes Associated with Cancer

The host immune response to the invading tumor may initiate tissue injury by immunologic mechanisms such as (a) toxic antigen-antibody complexes or (b) autoantibodies to tumor components cross-reacting with normal tissue components of skin and muscle. Neuromyopathic syndromes often seen with tumors are

DERMATOMYOSITIS.   Connective tissue disorder involving muscles, skin, and blood vessels. Fifteen percent of the patients with dermatomyositis have either a clinically apparent malignancy or are found at autopsy to have a tumor [71]. No predilection for a particular type of tumor has been reported, and tumors at most sites including lymphomas have been reported.

POLYMYOSITIS.   Myopathy, which is similar to dermatomyositis, may occur without skin involvement in cancer [51].

MYASTHENIA GRAVIS.   Fifteen percent of patients with myasthenia gravis have thymomas [11], and the majority of patients have an abnormal thymus gland with germinal centers [7]. Normal individuals do not show germinal centers in the thymus gland. Patients with myasthenic features without true myasthenia gravis have been seen in patients with oat cell carcinoma of the lung [32].

NEUROMYOPATHY.   Incidence of neuromyopathy in cancer [26] varies from 10 to 16% with carcinoma of the lung, ovary, breast, stomach, colon, or prostate—4 to 19%.

MULTIFOCAL LEUKOENCEPHALOPATHY.   The disease shows patchy demyelinization of the white matter of the cerebral hemispheres associated with inclusion bodies in the oligodendroglia. Often seen as a terminal complication of leukemias or generalized Hodgkin's disease, it is now believed to be caused by a virus [56].

Nonneuromyopathic Syndromes
ARTHRITIS.   In arthritis cases clinically indistinguishable from true rheumatoid arthritis, a malignant tumor is often detected. A possible explanation of the pathogenesis of the arthritis may be toxic antigen-antibody complexes.

NEPHROTIC SYNDROMES.   The incidence of malignancy in patients with nephrotic syndromes is approximately 10 times over the expected incidence [33]. The nephrotic syndrome may be due to the immune response of the patient to his neoplasm with deposition of antigen-antibody complexes in the kidney [34].

ACANTHOSIS NIGRICANS.   The lesions consist of confluent areas of hyperpigmentation with velvety raised ridges in the body folds. The pigmented lesion is often associated with a malignant tumor, usually an adenocarcinoma [47].

The association of the various lesions with cancer may result from (a) common genetic factors, (b) immunologic alterations predisposing the host to both cancer and autoimmune lesions which has been discussed in the role of virus in autoimmunity, (c) immunologic injury mechanisms associated with the host immune response to the tumor, or (d) other factors, as response to treatment.

Autoimmunity and Aging

In the last several years, there has been considerable evidence that aging may be related to changes in fundamental immune systems of the host [17, 55, 61]. Walford proposed an immunologic theory of aging which assumes that body cells undergo spontaneous mutations with genetic alterations which lead to the loss of ability of the cells to recognize self

[61]. The ensuing autoimmune reaction would be similar to an experimental graft versus host reaction in transplantation disease. Burnet [8, 10] has pointed out that with advancing age (a) there is a greater frequency of formation of forbidden clones which are capable of attacking a variety of tissues, and (b) the forbidden clones are also less subject to control of the homeostatic mechanisms. There is much experimental evidence to support the immunologic theory of aging [55, 62]. However, actual mutation and genetic diversification does not have to occur for a failure of homeostatic mechanisms for self recognition. The change in homeostasis with ensuing autoimmune reactions will have the same pathogenic effect without requiring genetic alterations.

One group of autoimmune diseases is seen with high frequency in young women, such as systemic lupus erythematosus. The second category of autoimmune diseases is seen with increasing frequency in older individuals, with a higher incidence in males. The age-related autoimmune diseases include various types of periarteritis, senile amyloidosis, cold antibody type of hemolytic anemia, and possibly maturity-onset diabetes [62].

References

1. Allison, A. C., Denman, A. M., and Barnes, R. D.   Cooperating and controlling functions of thymus-derived lymphocytes in relation to autoimmunity. *Lancet* 2:135, 1971.
2. Alpert, E., Isselbacher, K. J., and Schur, P. H.   The pathogenesis of arthritis associated with viral hepatitis. *N. Engl. J. Med.* 285:185, 1971.
3. Ammann, A. J., and Hong, R.   Selective IgA deficiency and autoimmunity. *Clin. Exp. Immunol.* 7:833, 1970.
4. Ammann, A. J., and Hong, R.   Selective IgA deficiency: Presentation of thirty cases and a review of the literature. *Medicine* (Baltimore) 50:233, 1971.
5. Anderson, J. R., Buchanan, W. W., and Goudie, R. B.   *Autoimmunity*. Springfield, Ill.: Thomas, 1967.
6. Burnet, M.   *The Clonal Selection Theory of Acquired Immunity*. London: Cambridge University Press, 1959.
7. Burnet, P. M.   Role of the thymus and related organs in immunity. *Br. Med. J.* 2:807, 1962.
8. Burnet, P. M.   Somatic mutation and chronic disease. *Br. Med. J.* 1:338, 1965.
9. Burnet, M.   *Cellular Immunology*. London: Cambridge University Press, 1969, Books 1 and 2.
10. Burnet, M.   *Autoimmunity and Autoimmune Disease*. Philadelphia: Davis, 1972.
11. Castelman, B.   The pathology of the thymus in myasthenia gravis. *Medicine* (Baltimore) 38:27, 1949.
12. Chiller, J. M., Habicht, G. S., and Weigle, W. O.   Cellular sites of immunologic unresponsiveness. *Proc. Natl. Acad. Sci. U.S.A.* 65:551, 1970.

13. Chiller, J. M., and Weigle, W. O.   Cellular basis of immunological unresponsiveness. In M. G. Hanna, Jr. (ed.), *Contemporary Topics in
Immunobiology*. New York: Plenum Press, 1972, vol. 1, chap. 6.
14. Cinader, B., Dubiski, S., and Wardlaw, A. C.   Distribution, inheritance,
and properties of an antigen MuB_1 and its relation to hemolytic complement. *J. Exp. Med.* 120:897, 1964.
15. Claman, H. N., and Chaperon, E. A.   Immunologic complementation
between thymus and bone marrow cells: A model for the two cell
theory of immunocompetence. *Transplant. Rev.* 1:92, 1969.
16. Cochrane, C. C.   Initiating events in immune complex injury. In
B. Amos (ed.), *Progress in Immunology*. 1st International Congress of
Immunology. New York: Academic, 1971.
17. Comfort, A.   The position of fundamental age studies. *Am. Heart J.*
62:293, 1961.
18. Daniel, P. M., Pratt, O. E., Roitt, I. M., and Torrigiani, G.   The release of thyroglobulin from the thyroid gland into thyroid lymphatics;
the identification of thyroglobulin as the thyroid lymph and in the
blood of monkeys by physical and immunologic methods and its estimation by radioimmunoassay. *Immunology* 12:489, 1967.
19. Dixon, F.   The role of antigen-antibody complexes in disease. *Harvey
Lect.* 58:21, 1963.
20. Dmochowski, L. L.   Review of the clinical implications of the virus-
autoimmune response. *Am. J. Clin. Pathol.* 56:261, 1971.
21. Dutton, R. W., Falkoff, R., Hirst, J. A., Hoffman, M., Kappler, J. W.,
Kettman, J. R., Lesley, J. F., and Vann, D.   Is there any evidence for
a nonantigen specific diffusible chemical mediator from the thymus derived cell in the initiation of the immune response? In B. Amos (ed.),
Progress in Immunology. New York: Academic, 1971.
22. Epstein, W. L.   Granulomatous hypersensitivity. *Prog. Allergy* 11:36,
1967.
23. Fudenberg, H. H.   Are autoimmune diseases immunologic deficiency
states? *Hosp. Pract.* 3:43, 1968.
24. Gocke, D. J., Hsu, K., Morgan, C., Bombardieri, S., Lockshin, M., and
Christian, C. L.   Vasculitis in association with Australia antigen. *J.
Exp. Med.* 134:3305, 1971.
25. Green, H. N.   The immunological theory of cancer: Some implications
in human pathology. *J. Chronic Dis.* 8:123, 1958.
26. Green, H. N., Anthony, H. M., Baldwin, R. W., and Westrop, J. W.   *An
Immunological Approach to Cancer*. London: Butterworth, 1967.
27. Hitchcock, C. R., Maclean, L. D., and Sullivan, W. A.   The secretory
and clinical aspects of achlorhydria and gastric atrophy as precursors
of gastric cancer. *J. Natl. Cancer Inst.* 18:795, 1957.
28. Hotchin, J. E.   The biology of lymphocytic choriomeningitis infection:
Virus-induced autoimmune disease. *Cold Spring Harbor Symp. Quant.
Biol.* 27:479, 1962.
29. Humphrey, J. H., and White, R. G.   *Immunology for Students of
Medicine*. Philadelphia: Davis, 1970, p. 605.
30. Irvine, W. J.   Immunological aspects of pernicious anemia. *N. Engl. J.
Med.* 273:432, 1965.
31. Koffler, D., Sandson, J., and Kunkel, H. G.   Elution studies on tissues

from patients with Goodpasture's syndrome and other forms of sub-acute glomerulonephritis. *J. Clin. Invest.* 47:55A (Abstract), 1968.

32. Lambert, E. H., Rooke, E. D., Easton, L. M., and Hodgson, C. H. Myasthenic syndrome occasionally associated with bronchial neoplasm; neurophysiologic studies. In H. R. Viets (ed.), *Myasthenia Gravis.* Springfield, Ill.: Thomas, 1961, p. 362.

33. Lee, J. C., Yamauchi, H., and Hopper, J., Jr. The association of cancer and the nephrotic syndrome. *Ann. Intern. Med.* 64:41, 1966.

34. Lewis, M. G., Loughridge, L. W., and Phillips, T. M. Immunological studies in nephrotic syndrome associated with extrarenal malignant disease. *Lancet* 2:134, 1971.

35. Lindsay, S., Dailey, M. E., Friedlander, J., Yee, G., and Soley, M. H. Chronic thyroiditis: A clinical and pathological study of 354 patients. *J. Clin. Endocrinol. Metab.* 12:1578, 1952.

36. MacKay, I. R., and Burnet, E. M. *Autoimmune Diseases.* Springfield, Ill.: Thomas, 1963.

37. Mitchison, M. A. Immunocompetent cell populations. In M. Landy and W. Brown (eds.), *Immunological Tolerance.* New York: Academic, 1969, p. 115.

38. Möller, G. Immunocyte triggering cell. *Immunology* 1:573, 1970.

39. Nakamura, R. M., and Weigle, W. O. In vivo behavior of homologous and heterologous thyroglobulin and induction of immunologic unresponsiveness to heterologous thyroglobulin. *J. Immunol.* 98:653, 1967.

40. Nakamura, R. M., and Weigle, W. O. Induction, maintenance and termination of immunologic unresponsiveness to bovine thyroglobulin in rabbits. *J. Immunol.* 99:357, 1967.

41. Nakamura, R. M., and Weigle, W. O. Passive transfer of experimental autoimmune thyroiditis from donor rabbits injected with soluble thyroglobulin without adjuvant. *Int. Arch. Allergy Appl. Immunol.* 32:506, 1967.

42. Nakamura, R. M., Spiegelberg, H. L., Lee, S., and Weigle, W. O. Relationship between molecular size and intra- and extravascular distribution of protein antigens. *J. Immunol.* 100:376, 1968.

43. Nakamura, R. M., and Weigle, W. O. Transfer of experimental autoimmune thyroiditis by serum from thyroidectomized donors. *J. Exp. Med.* 130:263, 1969.

44. Nakamura, R. M., and Weigle, W. O. Suppression of thyroid lesions in rabbits by treatment with cyclophosphamide after induction of thyroiditis. *Clin. Exp. Immunol.* 7:541, 1970.

45. Oldstone, M. B. A., and Dixon, F. J. Pathogenesis of chronic disease associated with persistent lymphocytic choriomeningitis viral infection: I. Relationship of antibody production to disease in neonatally infected mice. *J. Exp. Med.* 129:483, 1969.

46. Oldstone, M. B. A., and Dixon, F. J. Immune complex disease in chronic viral infections. *J. Exp. Med.* 134:325, 1971.

47. Ollendorf, C. H., Helberg, H. W., and Machacek, G. F. The site and histology of the cancer associated with malignant acanthosis nigricans. *Cancer* 15:364, 1962.

48. Orange, R. P., Valentine, M. D., and Austen, K. F. Antigen induced release of reacting substance of anaphylaxis in rats prepared with homologous antibody. *J. Exp. Med.* 127:767, 1968.

49. Pirofsky, B. *Autoimmunization and the Autoimmune Hemolytic Anemia*. Baltimore: Williams & Wilkins, 1969.
50. Roitt, I. M., and Torrigiani, G. Identification and estimation of undegraded thyroglobulin in human sera. *Endocrinology* 81:421, 1967.
51. Rowland, L. P., and Schotland, D. C. Neoplasms and muscle diseases. In R. B. Bain and F. H. Norris (eds.), *The Remote Effects of Cancer on the Nervous System*. New York: Grune & Stratton, 1965, p. 83.
52. Sell, S. Immunopathologic mechanisms: Part I and Part II. *Bull. Rheum. Dis.* 19:546 and 554, 1969.
53. Sell, S. *Immunology, Immunopathology, and Immunity*. Hagerstown, Md.: Harper & Row, 1972.
54. Shulman, S. Thyroid antigens and autoimmunity. In F. J. Dixon and H. G. Kunkel (eds.), *Advances in Immunology*, 14:85, 1971.
55. Siegel, M. M., and Good, R. A. *Tolerance, Autoimmunity and Aging*. Springfield, Ill.: Thomas, 1972.
56. Silverman, L., and Rubinstein, L. J. Electron microscopic observation on a case of progressive multifocal leucoencephalopathy. *Acta Neuropathol.* (Berl.) 15:265, 1965.
57. Talal, N. Immunologic and viral factors in the pathogenesis of systemic lupus erythematosus. *Arthritis Rheum.* 13:887, 1970.
58. Triplett, E. L. On the mechanisms of immunologic self-recognition. *J. Immunol.* 89:505, 1962.
59. Valentine, F. T., and Lawrence, H. S. Cell-mediated immunity. *Adv. Intern. Med.* 17:51, 1971.
60. Van Loghem, J. J. Concepts on the origin of autoimmune diseases—the possible role of viral infection in the etiology of idiopathic autoimmune diseases. In S. E. Bjorkman (ed.), *Concepts of Autoimmunity and Their Application in Hematology. Ser. Haematol.* 9:1, 1965.
61. Walford, R. L.: Autoimmunity and aging. *J. Gerontol.* 17:281, 1962.
62. Walford, R. L. *The Immunological Theory of Aging*. Baltimore: Williams & Wilkins, 1969.
63. Weckesser, E. C., and Chinn, A. B. Carcinoma of the colon complicating chronic ulcerative colitis. *J.A.M.A.* 152:905, 1953.
64. Weigle, W. O. The induction and autoimmunity in rabbits following injection of heterologous or altered homologous thyroglobulin. *J. Exp. Med.* 121:289, 1965.
65. Weigle, W. O. *Natural and Acquired Immunologic Unresponsiveness*. Cleveland: World, 1967.
66. Weigle, W. O., and Nakamura, R. M. The development of autoimmune thyroiditis in rabbits following injection of aqueous preparations of heterologous thyroglobulin. *J. Immunol.* 99:223, 1967.
67. Weigle, W. O., High, G. J., and Nakamura, R. M. The role of mycobacteria and their effect of proteolytic degradation of thyroglobulin on the production of autoimmune thyroiditis. *J. Exp. Med.* 130:243, 1969.
68. Weigle, W. O., Chiller, J. M., and Habicht, G. S. Thymus and bone marrow cells in unresponsiveness. In P. A. Miescher (ed.), *Immunopathology*. 4th International Symposium. New York: Grune & Stratton, 1970.
69. Weigle, W. O. Immunologic unresponsiveness. *Hosp. Practice* 6:121, 1971.

70. Weigle, W. O.   Recent observations and concepts in immunological un-responsiveness and autoimmunity. *Clin. Exp. Immunol.* 9:437, 1971.
71. Williams, R. C., Jr.   Dermatomyositis and malignancy: A review of the literature. *Ann. Intern. Med.* 50:1174, 1959.
72. Yunis, E. J., Fernandes, G., and Stutman, O.   Susceptibility to involution of the thymus-dependent lymphoid system and autoimmunity. *Am. J. Clin. Pathol.* 56:280, 1971.

8

General Approach to the Diagnosis of Autoimmune Disorders

History and Physical Examination

A. Search for possible immune deficiency diseases.
B. Family history of diseases of known immune pathogenesis, i.e., thyroiditis, lupus, etc.
C. Other disease states—increased incidence of autoimmune disease in neoplastic conditions.
D. Physical examination is important in the evaluation of many autoimmune disorders.

Findings in Common Laboratory Tests That May Lead to Suspicion of an Autoimmune Disorder

Some examples are:
A. Hemoglobin may be low, and presence of Coombs' positive test suggests autoimmune hemolytic anemia.
B. Urinalysis with proteinuria and casts—suspect glomerulonephritis with immune pathogenesis.
C. Abnormal serum proteins by chemical or electrophoretic analyses:
   a. Hypogammaglobulinemia—possible immune deficiency diseases.
   b. Hypergammaglobulinemia with elevated γ-globulin levels—possible collagen vascular disease.
D. Abnormal liver profile—suspect "autoallergic" liver disease.
E. Biologic false positive serologic test for syphilis [25].

Observations Which Indicate Involvement of Autoimmune Mechanisms in a Given Disease

MacKay and Burnet [43] have listed the following conditions, which are often seen in diseases with an autoimmune pathogenesis.

225

A. Hypergammaglobulinemia with γ-globulin levels greater than 1.5 gm/100 ml.
B. Presence of amyloid deposits indicated by deposition of denatured γ-globulin.
C. Inflammatory tissue lesions with many lymphocytes and plasma cells.
D. Coexistence of the disease with other lesions consistent with immunologic injury.
E. Improvement of the disease with immunosuppressive therapy such as cortisone, Imuran, and cyclophosphamide.
F. Presence of one or more autoantibodies.

Overlap of Autoimmune Disorders

There is a high frequency of association of many autoimmune diseases in comparison to the expected incidence in a random population [2, 44, 53]. One group involves the organ specific type of autoimmune diseases and is often referred to as the (a) *thyrogastric group,* while the second group concerns the nonorgan specific type of autoimmune disease and is called the (b) *lupus group.* The diseases in each group are related genetically and demonstrate overlap of clinical lesions and type of autoantibodies.

Thyrogastric Group
A. Autoimmune thyroiditis
  a. Hashimoto's disease
  b. Primary myxedema
B. Pernicious anemia with atrophic gastritis
C. Primary Addison's disease
D. Hypoparathyroidism
E. Vitiligo
F. Primary ovarian failure
G. Myasthenia gravis (found also in lupus group)

There is a definite interrelationship between the various endocrine organs and pernicious anemia with atrophic gastritis [2, 38]. The patient with autoimmune thyroiditis has a 10% incidence of pernicious anemia, as compared to 0.2% in the general population. The incidence of anti-parietal cell antibodies in autoimmune thyroiditis patients is 30%, and pernicious anemia patients show a 50% incidence of thyroid antibodies [23, 38].

Lupus Group
(a) Rheumatoid arthritis, (b) dermatomyositis, (c) Sjögren's syndrome, (d) scleroderma, (e) lupoid hepatitis (chronic active hepatitis), (f) myasthenia gravis, (g) autoimmune hemolytic anemia, (h) idio-

pathic thrombocytopenic purpura, (i) idiopathic leukopenia, (j) bullous skin diseases (pemphigus vulgaris, bullous pemphigoid)

Laboratory Diagnosis of Autoimmune Disorders

The serologic diagnosis depends on the demonstration of autoantibodies in patients suspected of an autoimmune disorder. The common methods used in clinical laboratories for demonstrating autoantibodies in sera are [56, 61]: (a) immunofluorescence, (b) enzyme-labeled antibody techniques (peroxidase), (c) antiglobulin reaction (Coombs' test), (d) complement fixation, (e) hemagglutination, (f) latex particle agglutination, (g) immunodiffusion, (h) radioimmunoassay, (i) bioassay.

Immunofluorescence and Enzyme-Labeled Antibody Methods

The immunofluorescence method [13, 52] and the more recently developed peroxidase-labeled antibody method [3, 46, 49] are both very useful in the clinical laboratory to demonstrate (a) autoimmune antibodies in serum, (b) tissue localization of autoantibody, and (c) deposition of antigen-antibody complexes in kidneys and other tissues (Figs. 8-1, 8-2).

The indirect immunofluorescence test in the past has been most widely used in the clinical laboratory to test for serum autoantibodies. However, several investigators have compared the peroxidase and fluorescein-conjugated antisera in an indirect system for antinuclear anti-

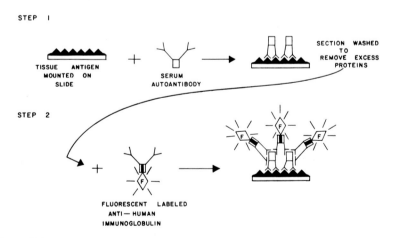

Figure 8-1
Indirect fluorescent-labeled antibody method for the detection of autoimmune antibody.

Table 8.1 Autoantibodies in Various Autoimmune Disorders.

Disorders	Antigen Involved	Common Method of Detection of Antibody
A. Organ Specific Endocrine		
Hashimoto's thyroiditis primary myxedema thyrotoxicosis	Thyroglobulin	a. Indirect Immunofluorescent Test (IFT)—[4] human thyroid tissue fixed in methanol at 56° C for 3 min to fix colloid
		b. Passive hemagglutination [39]
		c. Latex agglutination [1]
	Cytoplasmic microsome	IFT—unfixed human thyroid tissue from patient with thyrotoxicosis is used as substrate [33]. Complement fixation test with thyroid microsomes [15]
Thyrotoxicosis	Thyroid cell surface antigen	Bioassay—mouse thyroid stimulation in vivo [47]
Addison's disease	Adrenal cell cytoplasm	IFT on unfixed human adrenal cortex [10, 12]
Parathyroid	Parathyroid cytoplasmic antigen	IFT human parathyroid gland [11]
B. Alimentary Tract		
Pernicious anemia and atrophic gastritis	Parietal cell microsomes	IFT—human or mouse gastric mucosa substrate [37, 45]
Pernicious anemia	Intrinsic factor	Radioactive vit. B_{12} binding assay [32]
Sjögren's syndrome	Salivary duct cells	IFT—unfixed human salivary gland [7]
Ulcerative colitis	Colon, lipopolysaccharide	IFT—human or rat colon [14]
Coeliac disease	Reticulin	IFT—rat kidney [54]
Active chronic or (lupoid) hepatitis	Smooth muscle	IFT—rat gastric mucosa [59] human cervical tissue
Primary biliary cirrhosis	Mitochondrial	IFT—rat kidney unfixed [21, 22]

C. Nonorgan Specific Diseases

Disease	Antigen	Test
Lupus erythematosus Dermatomyositis Periarteritis nodosa Scleroderma Rheumatoid arthritis Sjögren's disease "Autoallergic" liver diseases	*Nuclear antigens* (a) DNA (b) Nucleoprotein (c) Sm antigen (d) Ribonucleoprotein (e) Nucleolar RNA	IFT—rat kidney substrate [58] Peroxidase enzyme-labeled antibody [6, 27] Hemagglutination [40] Radioactive DNA antigen-binding capacity assay [16] Precipitin test [57]
Rheumatoid arthritis Sjögren's disease Lupus erythematosus Other collagen diseases	Altered γ-globulin	Latex test for rheumatoid factor [51] Rose test, sheep cell agglutination [17]

D. Other

Disease	Antigen	Test
Myasthenia gravis	Skeletal or heart muscle	IFT—rat skeletal muscle and calf thymus [48]
Goodpasture's syndrome	Glomerular and lung basement membrane	Peroxidase-labeled antibody [20] IFT—biopsy of patient's kidney IFT—human kidney substrate with patient's serum [41]
Pemphigus vulgaris	Prickle cell desmosomes	IFT—human skin [8, 9] Peroxidase-labeled antibody [29]
Bullous pemphigoid	Epithelial basement membrane	IFT—human skin [8, 9] Peroxidase-labeled antibody [29]
Dermatitis herpetiformis	Reticulin	IFT—rat kidney [54]
Autoimmune hemolytic anemia	Red cell or closely associated antigen	Coombs' antiglobulin test—direct and indirect tests on patient's cells and serum [50]

bodies, and have found that the sensitivities of both methods are identical. Petts and Roitt [49] have used the peroxidase method for the detection of many tissue antibodies including antithyroid, antinuclear, antimuscle, antimitochondrial, anti-parietal cell, and anti-treponema pallidum antibodies. They have found that the immunofluorescence technique is quicker but that the peroxidase method has certain advantages: (a) A conventional microscope may be used. (b) The test slides are permanent. (c) The preparation can be further studied by other cytochemical methods or with a second antibody labeled with a radioactive or different enzyme marker. (d) Since the enzyme reaction produces an electron dense reaction product, ultrastructural studies can be carried out.

Autoantibodies to Host Tissue
These autoantibodies can be demonstrated by labeled antibody methods in the following diseases: (a) myasthenia gravis—antibody to striated muscle on biopsied skeletal muscle; (b) pemphigus vulgaris—antibody to prickle cell desmosomes on biopsied skin; and (c) bullous pemphigoid—antibody to epithelial basement membrane on skin biopsy from patients.

Immune Complexes
These complexes may be detected in kidney biopsies by labeled antibody techniques. In systemic lupus, antinuclear-nuclear antigen complexes may be seen at the dermal epidermal junction of the skin as well as in kidney biopsies.

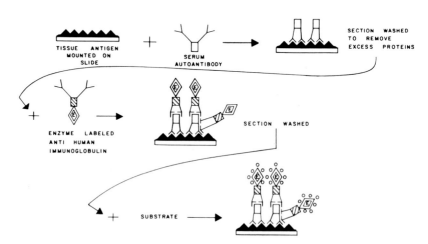

Figure 8-2
Enzyme-labeled antibody method for the detection of autoimmune antibody.

Table 8.2. Antibodies Detected by the Indirect Labeled Antibody Method.

Disease	Antibody to	Substrate*
SLE and related diseases	Nuclear antigens	Rat kidney
Active chronic or lupoid hepatitis	Smooth muscle	Rat stomach or human cervix
Primary biliary cirrhosis	Mitochondria	Unfixed rat kidney
Sjögren's disease	Salivary duct	Unfixed human salivary gland
Ulcerative colitis	Colon	Human or rat colon
Adult celiac disease	Reticulin	Unfixed rat kidney
Myasthenia gravis	Skeletal muscle (myoid)	Rat skeletal muscle; calf thymus
Pemphigus vulgaris	Prickle cell desmosome	Human skin or vagina
Bullous pemphigoid	Epithelial basement membrane	Human skin or vagina
Dermatitis herpetiformis	Reticulin	Unfixed rat kidney
Autoimmune thyroid disease	Thyroglobulin, thyroid cytoplasmic	Fixed human thyroid; unfixed human thyroid from thyrotoxic patient
Pernicious anemia	Parietal cell	Mouse or human stomach
Primary Addison's disease	Adrenal cortical cell	Human adrenal gland
Primary hyperparathyroidism	Parathyroid cell	Human parathyroid gland
Premature gonadal failure	Gonadal cell	Human or rabbit ovary and testes

* Human tissues should be from blood group O individuals so there is no interference with blood group antibodies.

Immunofluorescence Tests for Screening of Patients Suspected of Autoimmune Disorders

Roitt and Doniach [52] have used a composite slide of tissues which include (a) fixed human thyroid tissue, (b) unfixed human thyroid from a thyrotoxic patient, (c) unfixed rat or mouse stomach, and (d) unfixed rat kidney. Five to 6 μ frozen sections are cut and used as substrate material for the indirect immunofluorescence procedure. A polyvalent fluoresceinated antihuman immunoglobulin is used to detect IgG and IgM antibodies. The test will screen for the following:

Substrate	Antibodies to
Fixed human thyroid	Thyroglobulin and soluble proteins of the antinuclear factors (ANF)
Unfixed human thyroid	Cytoplasmic thyroid (complement fixing)
Unfixed rat or mouse stomach	Smooth muscle, parietal cell, mitochondria
Unfixed rat kidney	Mitochondria, nucleus, and reticulin

First a 6 μ frozen section of unfixed thyroid tissue is mounted on a slide and the slide is fixed in absolute methanol at 56° C for 3 min. Then a frozen section is mounted on the same slide from a composite block of unfixed thyroid, stomach, and kidney tissues. Comparison of the various sections is helpful in evaluating fluorescent staining of leukocytes and specific tissue cells.

Coombs' Reaction

The antiglobulin test detects autoantibody to red cells and is helpful in the diagnosis of autoimmune hemolytic anemia, which may be divided into three groups [19, 62]: (a) anemia due to antibody active at warm temperature and includes hemolytic disease caused by α-methyl dopa. IgG antibody active at warm temperature; shows specificity in the Rh system; (b) paroxysmal cold hemoglobinuria. IgG antibody hemolyzes cells after exposure to cold. Patient's red cells show presence of complement only; (c) cold agglutinin syndrome often associated with primary atypical pneumonia. IgM antibody with blood group I specificity. Patient's red cells show presence only of complement.

Complement Fixation Test

This test has been widely used for investigative purposes and has the advantage of specificity when there are several different antibodies and antigens as, e.g., the antinuclear factors in the collagen diseases. Gajdusek [31] and also Roitt and Doniach [52] have utilized a micro-complement fixation test for antibodies to liver and kidney with the use of plastic trays with multiple cups. A commercial test is available for the thyroid complement-fixing antigen from Wellcome.

Hemagglutination Test

The tanned red cell hemagglutination test is used commonly to detect antithyroglobulin and anti-DNA antibodies. The tanned red cell test for antithyroglobulin antibodies is about 1,000 times more sensitive than the precipitin reaction [23]. The procedure developed by Fulthorpe et al. [30] provides a long-lasting stable preparation of formalin-ized coated red cells.

Latex Particle Agglutination
Latex tests are used for the detection of antithyroglobulin antibodies [1] and rheumatoid factor [51]. The latex test for antithyroglobulin antibodies is slightly more sensitive than the precipitin test, and is a convenient screening test. However, because the latex test is not as sensitive as other tests it will not detect the cases of Hashimoto's thyroiditis with a low titer of antithyroglobulin antibodies [23].

The specificity of the latex test for rheumatoid factor can be increased by heat inactivating the test serum 56° C for 30 min [18]. In many cases, sera which are not inactivated will show a false positive test due to interference by C1q component of complement.

Sensitized Sheep Cell Agglutination for Detection of Rheumatoid Factor
The Rose test [17] makes use of sheep cells coated with a subagglutinating dose of rabbit antisheep cell hemolysin. The cells coated with rabbit IgG reacts with rheumatoid factor. The test has greater specificity than the latex test and is still of value since positive reactions rarely occur in conditions other than rheumatoid arthritis, provided that the sheep cells are sensitized with a relatively low dose of rabbit γ-globulin.

Radioimmunoassay for Antibody to Gastric Intrinsic Factor
In this assay [32] the antibody to intrinsic factor interferes with the union of vitamin B_{12} and gastric intrinsic factor. The intrinsic factor is involved in the absorption of vitamin B_{12} from the gastrointestinal tract.

Bioassay for Long-Acting Thyroid Stimulator (LATS) in Hyperthyroidism
LATS is an autoantibody of the IgG class in patients with thyrotoxicosis. The assay [47] depends upon the release of radioiodine from the thyroid gland of thyroxine-treated mice injected with a test sample containing LATS. LATS shows a maximum release of radioiodine from the thyroid gland of the test animal at 8 hours, while the thyroid-stimulating hormone (TSH) shows a rapid effect with a maximum at 2 hours.

Other Laboratory Tests
There are many other tests, such as the LE cell test for systemic lupus, which will be discussed in chapter 9. Nonspecific tests for help in the evaluation, diagnosis, prognosis, and following the course of therapy of various autoimmune diseases include (a) screen complement—total and specific component analysis; (b) serum immunoglobulin evaluation by γ-globulin quantitation by electrophoresis, by immunoelectrophoresis, and by specific immunoglobulin quantitation by radial immunodiffusion and electroimmunodiffusion; and (c) serum cryoglobulins [5].

General Interpretation of Tests for Autoantibodies

The interpretation of a positive test is dependent upon the following characteristics.

Age and Sex

With increasing age, the incidence of a positive test for one or more autoantibodies is increased. At age 60 years, over 50% of the subjects tested demonstrate one or more autoantibodies [60]. If the elderly person appears to be healthy, the level of the autoantibody is usually low. A positive antinuclear test would be significant in a young female since antinuclear antibody is rarely seen in a young person, but low titers of antinuclear antibody are often seen in elderly persons.

In a well-designed study, autoantibodies were detected in 21.6% of 3,492 subjects in a rural Australian town [35]; over 90% of the adult population in the town was included in the study. The prevalence of autoantibody increased with age, and there was a sharp rise in incidence at age 75 to 80 years. Females had an incidence of 27.5% with an increased incidence of antinuclear and gastric parietal cells and thyroid antibodies [35]. The incidence of anti-smooth muscle antibody and rheumatoid factor was similar in females and males; and the number of persons with anti-smooth muscle antibody did not increase with age.

Thus it appears that the following antibodies are age and sex dependent with an increasing incidence in females and older persons: (a) antinuclear antibodies, (b) anti-gastric parietal cell antibody, and (c) antithyroid antibodies. Individuals with autoantibodies may be associated with either the lupus group or the thyrogastric group. The two groups show no definite correlation and may be controlled by independent genetic or other etiologic factors.

The incidence of anti-smooth muscle antibody and rheumatoid factor do not correlate with the age and sex and are non-age-sex dependent. These latter autoantibodies are speculated to be associated with extrinsic factors such as infections [35].

Level of Autoantibodies

In general, the level of antibody is high in patients with autoimmune disorders and low in apparently healthy persons. The level or titer of antibody must be interpreted in relation to the stage and treatment of a particular disorder. Quantitative levels of certain antibodies to DNA are often used to monitor therapy and establish prognosis in the course of the disease.

Specificity of an Autoantibody

The serological diagnosis of a particular autoimmune disease is confirmed by the presence of a specific autoantibody. Also, autoantibodies associated with other closely related autoimmune diseases may be present.

Significance of Various Autoantibodies

Following is a brief comment on some of the autoantibodies. More detailed discussions of the interpretation and significance of antibodies in certain collagen diseases and autoallergic liver diseases are presented in other sections.

Antithyroid Autoantibodies [23, 53]

A. A negative indirect fluorescence test for antithyroglobulin and antithyroid epithelial cell cytoplasmic antibodies rules out Hashimoto's thyroiditis and helps to distinguish it from other diseases such as tumors and goiters. A positive IFT should be followed further by (a) specific tanned red cell agglutination for antithyroglobulin antibodies, and (b) quantitative complement fixation test for the cytoplasmic antibodies before a definite diagnosis of Hashimoto's thyroiditis can be confirmed.

B. A negative IFT practically rules out the diagnosis of myxedema, but a positive IFT is not diagnostic of hypothyroidism. Low titers of antithyroid antibodies are present in nonprogressive focal thyroiditis.

C. A large majority of thyrotoxic patients have low titers of antithyroid antibodies. The test may help in differentiating a mild form of the disease from psychological disorders.

D. 50% of pernicious anemia patients have antithyroid antibodies, often with hypothyroidism.

E. Low titers of antithyroid antibodies are seen in the apparently normal population with a higher incidence in females. The incidence is 20% in middle-age females.

Antigastric Antibody [38]

A. Anti-parietal cell antibodies are seen in 90% of pernicious anemia patients. The test is helpful in differentiating it from other macrocytic anemias.

B. The anti-parietal cell antibody is seen in a large percentage of cases of atrophic gastritis.

C. About one-third of the patients with thyroiditis or Graves' disease have anti-parietal cell antibodies.

D. In normal subjects, anti-parietal cell antibodies are rare under the age of 20 years. There is an increasing incidence with age in females and males, which reflects increasing frequency of atrophic gastritis with age.

Antiadrenal Antibody [10, 12]

One-half of patients with Addison's disease due to primary atrophy show evidence of antibodies. Anti-cortical adrenal cell antibodies are seen in a very small percentage of other autoimmune diseases.

Anti-Striated Muscle Antibody

Anti-myoid cell antibody is seen in less than 50% of cases of myasthenia gravis, and is rarely detected in young women unless the myasthenia gravis is accompanied with a thymoma [61].

Anti-Smooth Muscle Antibody

These antibodies are found in IgG and IgM classes of immunoglobulins, and are seen mainly in the autoallergic liver diseases [22, 42]. The antibodies are probably indicative of acute liver cell damage, since they are seen in acute viral hepatitis [28]. The anti-smooth muscle antibody of acute viral hepatitis is predominantly of the IgM class, and the titers seldom exceed 1:80 [34]. Anti-smooth muscle antibodies are seen in patients with lupoid hepatitis but are absent in patients with systemic lupus erythematosus [59]. More recently, anti-smooth muscle auto-antibodies have been seen in malignant disease and viral infections or infectious mononucleosis [34]. Patients with anti-smooth muscle antibody titers of 1:100 or more usually have a chronic active or aggressive hepatitis.

Anti-Salivary Gland Antibody

In Sjögren's disease, 75% of patients demonstrate antibodies to salivary duct epithelium, although there is a low incidence in cases of rheumatoid arthritis and other collagen diseases [55, 61].

Antimitochondrial Antibody

High titer antimitochondrial antibodies of 1:160 or greater are considered diagnostic of primary biliary cirrhosis [21, 22]. However, low levels of antimitochondrial antibodies are seen in other autoallergic diseases of the liver [23, 39]. Antimitochondrial antibodies similar to those seen in patients with primary biliary cirrhosis, but of low titer and of the IgM type of immunoglobulin, were seen in patients with a chronic false positive reaction for syphilis [25]. Such patients show mitochondrial antibody in the absence of liver disease and may demonstrate antinuclear and other tissue antibodies.

Antireticulin Antibody

An IgG antibody which reacts with connective tissue reticulin in rat and human tissue has been found in certain cases of dermatitis herpetiformis and adult coeliac disease [54]. The pathogenic nature of the antibody remains to be elucidated.

Antinuclear Antibodies

Antinuclear antibodies are found in many of the collagen and other autoimmune diseases. However, a high level of anti-DNA antibodies is quite characteristic of systemic lupus erythematosus. Patients with lupoid hepatitis have usually antinuclear and anti-smooth muscle antibodies, although patients with systemic lupus do not have any anti-smooth muscle antibody [59].

In summary, laboratory tests may be used for aid (a) in the diagnosis of autoimmune disorders, (b) in the evaluation of prognosis of disease, and (c) in the monitoring of therapy of the disease. A wide variety of tests are available, and laboratory confirmation of the clinical diagnosis of an autoimmune disorder depends on the detection and quantitation of the specific autoantibody or antibodies characteristic of the particular disorder.

Combined Immunofluorescence Screening Test for Serum Autoantibodies
(Modified from Roitt and Doniach [52] and Whittingham [61])

SELECTION OF ANTIGEN SUBSTRATES

Thyroid. Fresh thyrotoxic glands are obtained at operation. The tissue should have tall columnar epithelial cells so cytoplasmic fluorescence can be distinguished from nuclear fluorescence. The sections should have many small acini filled with colloid. Sections of tissue 3 × 4 mm are placed in aluminum foil, covered with OCT (optimal cutting temperature compound from Lab-Tek) and snap frozen in liquid nitrogen or isopentane cooled with solid dry ice. The sections may be stored in precooled serum-cap vials for storage in a −70° C freezer.

Stomach. Fresh human gastric mucosa may be taken from the upper end of the gastrectomy specimen. The section is cut so that a longitudinal section of gastric mucosa may be obtained. Tissue from group O blood type human patients is preferable to avoid interference with blood group isoantibodies when screening for autoantibodies.

Rat stomach may be used and will react with human parietal cell and smooth muscle antibodies. However, rat stomach may give false positive reactions for anti-parietal cell antibody, and the preferable substrates are mouse stomach and human stomach tissue [45]. The sections may be snap frozen and stored similar to the thyroid tissue described above.

Recently, it was noted that normal individuals and patients without pernicious anemia contained an antibody which reacted with a distinct antigen of rat gastric parietal cells and renal tubular brush border [36]. The same sera giving a positive reaction with rat tissue did not react with human tissue. Muller and associates [45] have shown that, of 94 human sera which gave a positive indirect fluorescence test with rat gastric parietal cells, 41 or 44% of the sera contained an antibody which was different from the antibody to pernicious anemia autoantigen. Ten of the 94 sera reacted to both parietal antigens. They recommended that mouse gastric mucosa replace rat gastric mucosa for the immunofluorescence tests [45].

Kidney tissue.   Sections of fresh normal human or rat kidney tissue may be obtained, placed in aluminum foil, snap frozen, and stored in the freezer. Rat kidney tissue is useful for the detection of nuclear, mitochondrial, reticulin, and occasionally kidney basement membrane antibodies.

Smooth muscle.   Rat, mouse, or human stomach muscularis sections have been used. Human cervix uteri are also a convenient source of tissue. Since the smooth muscle antigen is not very stable, it is advisable to use fresh tissue if possible.

Adrenal gland.   Fresh post-mortem human glands are desirable. The tissue sections may be collected, snap frozen, and stored similar to thyroid tissue. A positive indirect immunofluorescence test for serum adrenal antibodies will result in a bright fluorescence at the glomerular and reticular zones of the cortex.

Skeletal muscle.   Skeletal muscle may be obtained from fresh human specimens removed during surgery, or rat skeletal muscle may be used. The tissue is frozen and oriented so a longitudinal section is cut for the immunofluorescence test.

Fixation of sections.   Thyroid colloid containing thyroglobulin bleaches out during staining and washing procedures unless the section is fixed. Tissue microsomal antigens such as thyroid and gastric parietal cells are destroyed by fixation. Unfixed tissues are used for the detection of antibodies to microsomal antigens of thyroid and adrenal cortex, antimitochondrial, and anti-smooth muscle antibody. For the immunofluorescence test for autoantibody screening, fixed human thyroid, unfixed human thyroid, unfixed rat or mouse stomach, and unfixed rat kidney are used.

MATERIALS AND REAGENTS

A. Tissues: fixed and unfixed human thyroid, unfixed rat kidney, and unfixed mouse stomach
B. Cryostat
C. Clean glass slides (1.0–1.1 mm in thickness)
D. Coplin jars
E. Absolute methyl alcohol
F. Water bath heated to 56° C
G. Fan (for air drying)
H. Moist chamber
 I. Phosphate-buffered saline solution (pH 7.0–7.2)
J. Cheese-cloth (for drying out sections)
K. Polyvalent fluoresceinated antisera containing anti-human IgG and IgM
L. Slide coverslips. (#1 coverslip 0.17–0.19 mm in thickness)
M. Buffered glycerol
N. Fluorescence microscope with standard filter and light source
O. Immersion oil (nonfluorescent as #188, Harleco immersion oil)

PROCEDURE

1. 6 μ sections of thyroid tissue are cut in the cryostat and mounted on clean glass slides.
2. The slides with thyroid sections are then immersed for 3 min in a Coplin jar containing absolute methyl alcohol heated to 56° C in a heated water bath. The slides are removed and air dried with a fan.
3. 6 μ cryostat sections are cut from a new block of tissue containing human thyroid, rat kidney, and mouse stomach. The sections with 3 pieces of tissue are mounted on the slide containing the fixed thyroid tissue. Sections are mounted so all four pieces of tissue are adjacent to one another in close proximity. The slides are air dried.
4. Test serum samples are diluted 1:10 and reacted in a moist chamber for 30 to 40 min with the above prepared sections containing the four pieces of tissue.
5. The slides are carefully rinsed with phosphate buffered saline solution and washed 2 times for 8 min each in changes of phosphate-buffered saline solution.
6. The excess moisture is removed from the slides with a cheese-cloth without drying out the section. The section is then reacted with a polyvalent fluoresceinated antiserum containing anti-human IgG and IgM for 30–40 min.
7. The slides are carefully rinsed with phosphate buffered saline solution and washed 2 times for 8 min each in changes of phosphate-buffered saline solution.
8. The slides are mounted, coverslipped with buffered glycerol, and examined with a fluorescence microscope.

GENERAL INTERPRETATION

A. The screening test will detect (a) antinuclear antibodies, (b) anti-mitochondrial antibody, (c) anti-parietal cell antibody, (d) anti-reticulin antibody, (e) anti-smooth muscle antibody, (f) antithyroglobulin antibody, (g) anti-thyroid microsomal antibody.
B. Antinuclear antibodies will show a rim, homogeneous, speckled, or nucleolar pattern of the tissue nuclei.
C. Antimitochondrial antibody will usually show a bright granular fluorescence of the entire cytoplasm in distal tubules, gastric parietal cells, and thyroid cells with eosinophilic metaplasia [26].
D. Anti-parietal cell antibody will show cytoplasmic fluorescence of gastric parietal cells and not kidney tubular cells, whereas antimitochondrial antibody will show staining of cells rich in mitochondria.
E. Antireticulin antibody will stain the peritubular fibers, Bowman's capsule, and adventitia of the rat kidney.
F. Anti-smooth muscle antibody will show bright fluorescent staining of smooth muscle tissue in blood vessels and muscularis mucosae.
G. Antithyroglobulin antibody will often demonstrate a floccular bright

staining pattern of the thyroid colloid. The specific anti-thyroid microsomal antibody will stain the cytoplasm of the thyroid epithelium. The apex of thyroid epithelial cells in the unfixed section will show a brighter staining.

H. A positive screening test should be followed by a determination of serum antibody titer. In the interpretation of the screening tests, one should keep in mind that low titers of autoantibodies are very common in the age group beyond 50 years. The presence of the autoantibodies in young persons with symptoms should be investigated with various other ancillary tests.

References

1. Anderson, J. R., Buchanan, W. W., Goudie, R. B., and Gray, K. G. Diagnostic tests for thyroid antibodies: A comparison of the precipitin and latex-fixation (Hyland TA) tests. *J. Clin. Pathol.* 15:462, 1962.
2. Anderson, J. R., Buchanan, W. W., and Goudie, R. B. *Autoimmunity, Clinical and Experimental.* Springfield, Ill.: Thomas, 1967.
3. Avrameas, S., and Bouteille, M. Ultrastructural localization of antibody by antigen labeled with peroxidase. *Exp. Cell Res.* 53:166, 1968.
4. Balfour, B. M., Doniach, D., Roitt, I. M., and Couchman, K. E. Fluorescent antibody studies in human thyroiditis: Autoantibody to an antigen of the thyroid colloid distinct from thyroglobulin. *Br. J. Exp. Pathol.* 42:307, 1961.
5. Barnett, E. V., Bluestone, R., Cracchiolo, A., Goldberg, L. S., Kantor, G. L., and McIntosh, R. M. Cryoglobulin and disease. *Ann. Intern. Med.* 73:95, 1970.
6. Benson, M. D., and Cohen, A. S. Antinuclear antibodies in systemic lupus erythematosus—detection with horseradish peroxidase conjugated antibody. *Ann. Intern. Med.* 73:943, 1970.
7. Bertram, V., and Halberg, P. A specific antibody against the epithelium of the salivary ducts in sera from patients with Sjögren's syndrome. *Acta Allergol.* (Kbh) 14:458, 1964.
8. Beutner, E. H., Gordon, R. E., and Chorzelski, T. P. The immunopathology of pemphigus and bullous pemphigoid. *J. Invest. Dermatol.* 51:64, 1968.
9. Beutner, E. H., Chorzelski, T. P., and Jordon, R. E. *Autosensitization in Pemphigus and Bullous Pemphigoid.* Springfield, Ill.: Thomas, 1970.
10. Blizzard, R. M., and Kyle, M. Studies of adrenal antigens and antibodies on Addison's disease. *J. Clin. Invest.* 42:1653, 1963.
11. Blizzard, R. M., Chee, D., and Davis, W. The incidence of parathyroid and other antibodies in the sera of patients with idiopathic hypoparathyroidism. *Clin. Exp. Immunol.* 1:119, 1966.
12. Blizzard, R. M., Chee, D., and Davis, W. The incidence of adrenal and other antibodies in the sera of patients with idiopathic adrenal insufficiency (Addison's disease). *Clin. Exp. Immunol.* 2:19, 1967.
13. Blundell, G. P. Fluorescent antibody technics. In M. Stefanini (ed.), *Progress in Clinical Pathology.* New York: Grune & Stratton, 1970, vol. 3, chap. 6.

14. Broberger, O., and Perlmann, P.   Autoantibodies in human ulcerative colitis. *J. Exp. Med.* 110:657, 1959.

15. Buchanan, W. W., Koutras, D. A., Crooks, J., Alexander, W. D., Brass, W., Anderson, J. R., Goudie, R. B., and Gray, K. E.   The clinical significance of the complement fixation test in thyrotoxicosis. *J. Endocrinol.* 24:115, 1962.

16. Carr, R. I., Koffler, D., Agnello, V., and Kunkel, H. G.   Studies on DNA antibodies using DNA labeled with actinomycin D (3H) or dimethyl sulfate (3H). *Clin. Exp. Immunol.* 4:527, 1969.

17. Cathcart, E. S.   Rheumatoid factors and serologic technique. In A. S. Cohen (ed.), *Laboratory Diagnostic Procedures in the Rheumatic Diseases*. Boston: Little, Brown, 1967, p. 107.

18. Cheng, C. T., and Persellin, R. H.   Interference by Cl_q in slide latex tests for rheumatoid factor. *Ann. Intern. Med.* 75:683, 1971.

19. Dacie, J. V., and Worlledge, S. M.   Autoimmune hemolytic anemias. In E. B. Brown and C. V. Moore (eds.), *Progress in Hematology*. New York: Grune & Stratton, 1969, vol. 6, p. 81.

20. Davey, F. R., and Busch, G. J.   Immunohistochemistry of glomerulonephritis using horseradish peroxidase and fluorescein labeled antibody—a comparison. *Am. J. Clin. Pathol.* 53:531, 1970.

21. Deodhar, S. D., Yazbek, A., Ochkar, E., and Brown, C. H.   Mitochondrial antibody test—a clue to diagnosis of primary biliary cirrhosis: Report of two interesting cases. *Cleve. Clin. Q.* 36:95, 1969.

22. Doniach, D., Roitt, I. M., Walker, J. G., and Sherlock, S.   Tissue antibodies in primary biliary cirrhosis, active chronic (lupoid) hepatitis, cryptogenic cirrhosis, and other liver diseases and their clinical implications. *Clin. Exp. Immunol.* 1:237, 1966.

23. Doniach, D., and Roitt, I. M.   Thyroid autoallergic disease. In P. C. H. Gill and R. R. A. Coombs (eds.), *Clinical Aspects of Immunology*. Philadelphia: Davis, 1968, 2nd ed., chap. 35.

24. Doniach, D.   The concept of "autoallergic" hepatitis. *Proc. R. Soc. Med.* 63:527, 1970.

25. Doniach, D., Delhanty, J., Lindqvist, H. J., and Catterall, R. D.   Mitochondrial and other tissue autoantibodies in patients with biologic false positive reactions for syphilis. *Clin. Exp. Immunol.* 6:871, 1970.

26. Doniach, D., Lindqvist, H. J., and Berg, P. A.   Nonorgan specific cytoplasmic antibodies detected by immunofluorescence. *Int. Arch. Allergy Appl. Immunol.* 41:501, 1971.

27. Dorling, J., Johnson, G. D., Webb, J. A., and Smith, M. E.   Use of peroxidase conjugated antiglobulin as an alternative to immunofluorescence for the detection of antinuclear factor in serum. *J. Clin. Pathol.* 24:501, 1971.

28. Farrow, L. J., Holborow, E. J., Johnson, G. D., Lamb, S. E., Stewart, J. S., Taylor, P. E., and Zuckerman, A. J.   Autoantibodies and the hepatitis associated antigen in acute infective hepatitis. *Br. Med. J.* 2:693, 1970.

29. Fukuyama, K., Douglas, S. D., Tuffanelli, D. C., and Epstein, W. C.   Immunohistochemical method for localization of antibodies in cutaneous disease. *Am. J. Clin. Pathol.* 54:410, 1970.

30. Fulthorpe, A. J., Roitt, I. M., Doniach, D., and Couchman, K. E.   A

stable sheep cell preparation for detecting thyroglobulin autoantibodies and its clinical applications. *J. Clin. Pathol.* 14:654, 1961.

31. Gajdusek, D. C.   An "autoimmune" reaction against human tissue antigens in certain acute and chronic diseases: I. Serologic investigations. *Arch. Intern. Med.* 101:9, 1958.

32. Gottlieb, C., Lau, K. S., Wasserman, L. R., and Herbert, V.   Rapid charcoal assay for intrinsic factor (IF) gastric juice unsaturated B_{12} binding capacity, antibody to IF and serum unsaturated B_{12} binding capacity. *Blood* 25:875, 1965.

33. Holborow, E. J., Brown, P. C., Roitt, I. M., and Doniach, D.   Cytoplasmic localization of complement fixing autoantigen in human thyroid epithelium. *Br. J. Exp. Pathol.* 40:583, 1959.

34. Holborow, E. J.   Smooth muscle autoantibodies, viral infections and malignant disease. *Proc. R. Soc. Med.* 65:481, 1972.

35. Hooper, B., Whittingham, S., Mathews, J. D., MacKay, I. R., and Curnow, D. H.   Autoimmunity in a rural community. *Clin. Exp. Immunol.* 12:79, 1972.

36. Ireton, H. J. C., Muller, H. K., and McGiven, A. R.   Human antibody against rat gastric parietal cells and kidney brush border. *Clin. Exp. Immunol.* 8:783, 1971.

37. Irvine, W. J.   Gastric antibodies studied by fluorescence microscopy. *Q. J. Exp. Physiol.* 48:427, 1963.

38. Irwin, W. J.   Autoimmune and hypersensitivity phenomenon in alimentary diseases. In S. C. Dyke (ed.), *Recent Advances in Clinical Pathology*. Boston: Little, Brown, 1968, series V, chap. 29.

39. Klatskin, G., and Kantor, F. S.   Mitochondrial antibody in primary biliary cirrhosis and other diseases. *Ann. Intern. Med.* 77:533, 1972.

40. Koffler, D., Carr, R., Agnello, V., Thoburn, R., and Kunkel, H. G.   Antibodies to polynucleotides in human sera: Antigenic specificity and relation to disease. *J. Exp. Med.* 134:294, 1971.

41. Lerner, R. A., Glassock, R. J., and Dixon, F. J.   The role of antiglomerular basement membrane antibody in the pathogenesis of human glomerulonephritis. *J. Exp. Med.* 126:989, 1967.

42. Ludwig, R. N., Deodhar, S. D., and Brown, C. H.   Autoimmune tests in chronic active disease of the liver. *Cleve. Clin. Q.* 38:105, 1971.

43. MacKay, I. R., and Burnet, E. M.   *Autoimmune Diseases*. Springfield, Ill.: Thomas, 1963.

44. MacKay, I. R.   Cirrhosis and other diseases of the liver. In M. Samter (ed.), *Immunological Diseases*. Boston: Little, Brown, 1970, 2nd ed., chap. 81.

45. Muller, H. K., McGwen, A. R., and Nairn, R. C.   Immunofluorescent staining of rat gastric parietal cell by human antibody unrelated to pernicious anemia. *J. Clin. Pathol.* 24:13, 1971.

46. Nakane, P. K., and Pierce, G. B.   Enzyme labeled antibodies for the light and electron microscope localization of tissue antigens. *J. Cell Biol.* 33:307, 1967.

47. Ochi, Y., and DeGroot, L. J.   Long-acting thyroid stimulator of Graves' disease. *N. Engl. J. Med.* 278:718, 1968.

48. Osserman, K. E., and Weiner, L. B.   Studies in myasthenia gravis: Immunofluorescent tagging of muscle striation with antibody from serum of 256 myasthenia patients. *Ann. N.Y. Acad. Sci.* 124(II):730, 1965.

49. Petts, V., and Roitt, I. M.   Peroxidase conjugates for demonstration of tissue antibodies: Evaluation of the technique. *Clin. Exp. Immunol.* 9:407, 1971.
50. Pirofsky, B.   *Autoimmunization and the Autoimmune Hemolytic Anemias.* Baltimore: Williams & Wilkins, 1969.
51. Rheins, M. S., McCoy, F. W., Burell, R. G., and Beuhler, E. V.   A modification of the latex fixation test for the study of rheumatoid arthritis. *J. Lab. Clin. Med.* 50:113, 1957.
52. Roitt, I. M., and Doniach, D.   *Manual of Autoimmune Serology.* Geneva: World Health Organization, 1969.
53. Roitt, I. M.   *Essential Immunology.* Oxford: Blackwell, 1971, p. 186.
54. Seah, P. P., Fry, L., Hoffbrand, A. V., and Holborow, E. J.   Tissue antibodies in dermatitis herpetiformis and adult coeliac disease. *Lancet* 1:834, 1971.
55. Smith, L. H., Martin, D. W., Schrier, R. W., et al.   Clinical spectrum of Sjögren's syndrome—medical staff conference, University of California, San Francisco. *Calif. Med.* 117:63, 1972.
56. Steffen, C.   Antibodies to tissues. In M. Stefanini (ed.), *Progress in Clinical Pathology.* New York: Grune & Stratton, 1970, vol. 3, chap. 7.
57. Tan, E. M., Schur, P. H., Carr, R. I., and Kunkel, H. G.   Desoxyribonucleic acid (DNA) and antibodies to DNA in the serum of patients with systemic lupus erythematosus. *J. Clin. Invest.* 45:1732, 1966.
58. Tan, E. M.   Relationship of nuclear staining patterns with precipitating antibodies in systemic lupus erythematosus. *J. Clin. Lab. Med.* 70:800, 1967.
59. Whittingham, S., Irwin, J., MacKay, I. R., and Smalley, M.   Smooth muscle autoantibody in "autoimmune hepatitis." *Gastroenterology* 51:499, 1966.
60. Whittingham, S., Irwin, J., MacKay, I. R., Marsh, S., and Cowling, D. C.   Autoantibodies in healthy subjects. *Aust. Ann. Med.* 18:130, 1969.
61. Whittingham, S.   Serological methods in autoimmune disease in man. In J. B. G. Kwapinski (ed.), *Research in Immunochemistry and Immunobiology.* Baltimore: University Park Press, 1972, vol. 1, p. 121.
62. Worlledge, S.   Autoimmunity and blood diseases. *Practitioner* 199:171, 1967.

II

Assessment of Specific Autoimmune Disorders

9

Laboratory Tests for the Evaluation of Systemic Lupus Erythematosus and Related Collagen Disorders

S ystemic lupus erythematosus (SLE) is a clinically complex disorder characterized by serum antinuclear factors and autoantibodies directed at other non-organ specific cellular antigens. It is now believed that these are signs of a fundamental disturbance of the immune system that leads to the appearance of the characteristic disseminated lesions.

Pathogenesis of Systemic Lupus Erythematosus

In SLE there is production of antibodies to many cellular constituents and native DNA. Antibody production to native DNA has not been induced experimentally, although certain strains of experimental animals such as mice [23] and dogs [45] demonstrate a spontaneous lupus-like syndrome similar to the human disease. The New Zealand Black (NZB) strain of mice has a high incidence of autoimmune antihemolytic and anti-DNA antibodies, and recently the mice were discovered to have a natural thymocytoxic autoantibody [62, 63]. When NZB mice are mated with the New Zealand white strain, the female hybrid mice have a very high prevalence of a lupus-like disease [23]. The thymocytoxic autoantibody may play a role in the disturbed tolerance noted in the disease. It is noteworthy that lymphocytotoxic antibodies were found in the serum of patients with systemic lupus erythematosus and rheumatoid arthritis [76].

The disease may be diagnosed [29] when there is (a) multisystem involvement, often with glomerulonephritis; (b) nondestructive polyarthritis; and (c) presence of LE cell or antinuclear antibodies. Antibodies to a wide variety of nuclear antigens are seen. Characteristic of lupus erythematosus are anti-native DNA antibodies. The patient often shows the presence of anti-DNA antibodies, which can be detected by various tests. During an acute exacerbation of the disease, such as after exposure to sunlight, DNA may appear in the circulation [69]. Excess

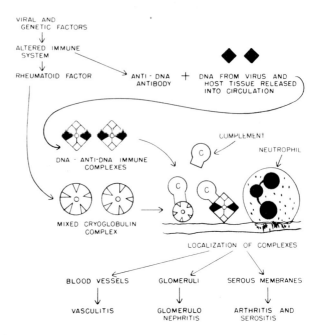

Figure 9-1
Pathogenesis of systemic lupus erythematosus.

tissue destruction with release of DNA into the circulation will form DNA–anti-DNA immune complexes, and with an excess of DNA, there will be evidence of free DNA. With the appearance of DNA in the circulation, there is fever and proteinuria (Fig. 9-2). Treatment with prednisone will result in the disappearance of free DNA or DNA–anti-DNA immune complexes. The DNA antigen-antibody complexes are pathogenic and responsible for the nephritis, vasculitis, and serositis which are the hallmarks of an immune complex disease [11, 69] (Fig. 9-1).

Cryoglobulins and Systemic Lupus Erythematosus

Cryoglobulins have been observed in a significant number of patients with systematic lupus erythematosus [65]. Such cryoglobulins possess biologic properties similar to circulating DNA–anti-DNA immune complexes in lupus nephritis [2, 65].

In systemic lupus erythematosus, high molecular weight complexes (greater than 19S), independent of the DNA–anti-DNA system, may play a role in lupus nephritis [1, 2]. Rheumatoid factor has been detected in the cryoprecipitates from patients with SLE, and in addition, fluorescent localization studies with labeled aggregated γ-globulin demonstrated rheumatoid factor in the glomeruli of SLE patients. Complement

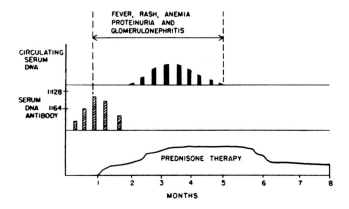

CORRELATION OF CIRCULATING DNA ANTIBODY AND FREE
SERUM DNA WITH THE CLINICAL COURSE IN A CASE OF
SYSTEMIC LUPUS ERYTHEMATOSUS

Figure 9-2
Clinical course of systemic lupus erythematosus.

and rheumatoid factor interact and become a part of the cryoglobulin complex which contributes to the renal injury of SLE patients [43].

Lupus Erythematosus-Like Syndrome with a Hereditary Defect in Complement

Recently there have been two siblings with illnesses suggesting a lupus-like connective tissue syndrome with fever, skin lesions, vasculitis, arthralgia, and glomerular lesions [49]. The patients did not have evidence of antinuclear antibodies. The first component of complement was abnormally low. The other components which are usually depressed in active cases of lupus were normal.

Familial hereditary deficiency of second component of complement has been described [56]. Agnello and co-workers [3] have shown that a patient homozygous for the C2 complement deficiency trait developed a lupus-like syndrome with widespread recurrent skin rashes. The laboratory tests were positive for LE cells and anti-DNA antibodies. The association of hereditary C2 deficiency and SLE may not be due just to coincidence.

Mixed Connective Tissue Disease and Its Relation to Systemic Lupus Erythematosus

Sharp and associates [61] have recently described a syndrome which had features similar to systemic lupus erythematosus, scleroderma, and polymyositis. The 25 patients described had the following features, which seem to distinguish the mixed connective tissue disease from the usual case of systemic lupus erythematosus:

A. High titers of antibody to extractable nuclear antigen (ENA) [34] with a definite specificity. The ENA consists of protein and ribonucleic acid (RNA) [61]. In mixed connective tissue diseases the antibody to ENA does not react with ENA which has been treated with ribonuclease. Antibodies to ENA occur in 50% of systemic lupus patients, but the reaction is not affected by ribonuclease treatment of the ENA antigen.

B. The Sm antigen [68] is found in the ENA fraction and is a carbohydrate containing protein. No detectable Sm antibody was noted in mixed connective tissue disease [61].

C. Antibody to native desoxyribonucleic acid (DNA) was infrequent or of low titer.

D. The disease has a favorable prognosis and usually has an excellent response to corticosteroid therapy.

Nuclear Antigens and Antibodies

In the various collagen diseases, antibodies to many different nuclear antigens are seen. The nuclear antigens can be listed as follows:

A. Native DNA or double-stranded DNA [69]

B. Heat-denatured DNA [69] or ultraviolet-denatured DNA [72]

C. Nucleoproteins [70]

D. Saline extractable antigens. One of the antigens is a carbohydrate containing protein which has been identified as Sm antigen [68]. Also in this fraction, ribonucleoproteins have been identified [46, 61]. Extractable nuclear antigen (ENA), first described by Holman [6], is now believed to contain both the Sm and ribonucleoprotein antigens [61].

E. Nucleolar (RNA) antigen. Antibody to nucleolar RNA may be frequently seen in progressive systemic sclerosis [54].

F. Double-stranded RNA [58, 59]

G. Polyribonucleotides [57]

Antibodies to native DNA are found in systemic lupus erythematosus, and such native anti-DNA antibodies cannot be experimentally induced by the immunization of healthy animals. The Sm antigen is difficult to obtain in the purified state, and antibodies to the Sm antigen may be specific for systemic lupus erythematosus and found in approximately 30 to 50% of the cases [61]. A satisfactory test for the antibody to the Sm antigen is not widely available in the clinical laboratory at the present time.

Antinuclear antibodies have been identified in the IgG and IgM fractions. Antibodies of different immunoglobulin classes can be detected with fluorescein-conjugated antisera to the corresponding heavy chains, and antibodies to IgG, IgA, and IgM may be present in any combination [9]. In addition, various subclasses of IgG have also been found to be present in SLE [31, 39]. The detection of antinuclear antibodies in all three immunoglobulin classes rules against the likelihood that these autoantibodies are produced by a single abnormal clone of cells.

Cellular Immunity in SLE and Reactions to Nuclear Antigens

Many of the patients with SLE were noted to have lymphocytotoxic antibodies [76], and one wonders about the cell-mediated immune mechanisms in these patients. Recently, Bitter and co-workers [18] studied 10 patients with early active SLE, who were not on treatment and who were found to be anergic to a battery of skin test antigens. Further, these 10 untreated patients showed no significant stimulation of their lymphocytes in culture with phytohemagglutinin.

On the other hand, a recent study has demonstrated that the cellular immune system in SLE patients is not impaired [32]. Twenty-four patients with SLE were skin tested with a variety of antigens as PPD, histoplasmin, Candida, and Trichophyton, and in addition an in vitro lymphocyte transformation test with phytohemagglutinin was conducted. Although most of the patients in this study had SLE for an extended period of time, marked anergic skin tests to a battery of antigens were not observed in 2 patients who had active SLE of less than 6 weeks' duration [32].

There have been variable reports of delayed type skin reactivity to nuclear antigens in systemic lupus erythematosus [19, 51]. In one study, no difference in skin reactivity to calf thymus DNA was observed between the SLE group and the controls [19]. However, in a more recent study, the same 24 SLE patients discussed above were tested with a variety of nuclear antigens, e.g., rabbit thymus DNA, calf thymus DNA, and rabbit thymus soluble nucleohistone. Of the SLE patients, 83% were positive to at least one of the nuclear antigens, and 46% were positive with the lymphocyte transformation test [32]. Compared to a control group, the SLE patients showed a significantly greater reactivity to the cellular immune tests with the nuclear antigens. A positive lymphocyte transformation test to rabbit native DNA correlated with the presence of active renal disease in the patients with SLE.

Laboratory Tests for Antinuclear Antibodies

In a laboratory test for the diagnosis of systemic lupus erythematosus, one would prefer a very sensitive test which can detect the presence or absence of antinuclear antibodies in patients' sera and still have a low incidence of false positive tests in an "apparently normal" population.

The absence of antinuclear antibodies, for all practical purposes, would rule out the possibility of systemic lupus erythematosus, if the patient had not been treated with corticosteroids or immunosuppressive drugs.

The various diagnostic tests for antinuclear antibodies available in the clinical laboratory may be numerated as follows: (a) the LE cell test [35]; (b) antiglobulin consumption test [48]; (c) complement fixation tests [5, 67]; (d) precipitin tests [46, 69]; (e) agglutination tests [28, 37, 41, 42, 44]; (f) radioimmunoassay for DNA and DNA antibody [24, 52, 78]; (g) indirect immunofluorescence test [15, 71]; and (h) peroxidase enzyme-conjugated antibody technique [17, 27].

The LE Cell Test [35]

The LE cell test is quite insensitive and positive in only 50–80% of the cases. The LE cell reaction occurs in three phases [16].

1. There is a reaction of the LE cell humoral factor with extracted nuclear material.
2. The humoral factor has been identified as a 7S complement-fixing antibody and reacts with nucleoproteins. After combining with extracted nuclei, there is a modification of the nuclear material with the formation of hematoxylin bodies.
3. The last phase consists of phagocytosis of the hematoxylin body by living polymorphs. In the performance of the LE cell test there should be traumatization of the cellular material with extrusion of the nuclei. The nuclear material then reacts with the antibody, causing

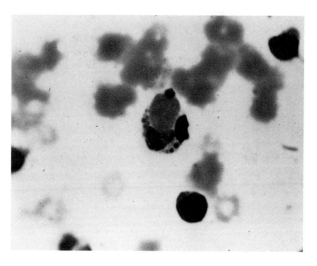

Figure 9-3
Positive lupus erythematosus cell. Note homogeneous body within polymorphonuclear leukocyte. (Wright's stain; 1,000× before 30% reduction.)

formation of the hematoxylin body. Phagocytosis of the hematoxylin body by polymorphs occurs in the presence of complement. The test is dependent upon many variables and does not have the desirable sensitivity. It is not recommended as a screening test. (Fig. 9-3).

Antiglobulin Consumption Test [48]
The antiglobulin consumption test is a cumbersome test in which nuclear stroma is first reacted with the patient serum. The antinuclear antibodies in the serum adhere to the nuclear stroma. After repeated washings, the antinuclear antibodies are eluted from the nuclear stroma and quantitated by inhibition of the Coombs' test.

Complement Fixation Tests [5, 67]
The complement fixation test is a sensitive test and is useful in that specific nuclear antigens may be utilized. However, these tests are unwieldy for the clinical laboratory, and the patient's serum often contains anticomplementary substances.

Precipitin Tests [46, 69]
The precipitin test is a secondary manifestation of antigen-antibody reaction and is relatively insensitive. However, when large agar plates are used, DNA may be detected in the very low concentrations of 1 to 5 μg/ml [69]. DNA has been found in a patient's serum just prior to the detection of anti-DNA antibody in cases of systemic lupus with exacerbation of the disease syndrome [69]. Often in lupus patients one can detect antibodies to native DNA, single stranded, or to heat-denatured DNA [42] (Fig. 9-4).

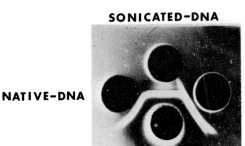

SONICATED-DNA

NATIVE-DNA

HEAT DENATURED-DNA

SLE SERUM

Figure 9-4
Agar gel precipitin reaction of anti-DNA antibodies in a case of systemic lupus erythematosus. Note that native DNA and sonicated DNA show line of identity. A cross-reactive spur is seen when the SLE serum is reacted with sonicated DNA and heat-denatured DNA (single-stranded DNA).

A precipitin test can be performed to detect serum-precipitating antibodies to a soluble ribonucleoprotein antigen [46]. The presence of antibodies to such ribonucleoproteins correlates with a low incidence of nephritis in patients with systemic lupus erythematosus [53].

Agglutination Tests [28, 37, 41, 42, 44]
Several different agglutination tests for the detection of antinuclear antibodies have been published and include passive hemagglutination of DNA coated red cells, and agglutination of coated latex particles and coated bentonite particles. A latex agglutination test for anti-DNA-histone is marketed commercially and has proved fairly specific in routine use, but has the great disadvantage of poor sensitivity [28]. ·A modified assay by antibodies to DNA utilizing formalinized and tanned red blood cells has been developed by Lawlis [44] and by Koffler et al. [41, 42]. The hemagglutination technique was found to be a useful method for detecting antibodies to photo-oxidized DNA, UV-irradiated DNA, and single-stranded DNA, as well as native DNA [42]. Positive hemagglutinating DNA antibodies have been demonstrated in patients who show no detectable precipitating antibodies by the agar double-diffusion test [42]. Sharp and co-workers have used the hemagglutination technique for the detection of antibodies to DNA and ENA [60, 61].

It is extremely useful in most clinical laboratories to detect antibodies to DNA with the red cell hemagglutination method. A microhemagglutination test has been developed [37] and will be described later. The microtiter method has been used to test sera of patients for the presence

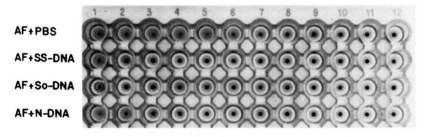

AF+PBS

AF+SS-DNA

AF+So-DNA

AF+N-DNA

Figure 9-5
Hemagglutination test for anti-DNA antibodies. Hemagglutination patterns are shown when the serum of a patient with SLE (AF) is reacted with sonicated DNA coated human red cells under different conditions. First row (AF + PBS) shows positive hemagglutination to dilution of 1/64. In the next three rows, the test was performed in the presence of added single-strand DNA (SSDNA), sonicated DNA (SoDNA), and native DNA (NDNA) and shows inhibition of agglutination, demonstrating that specificity of AF serum is against single-strand, sonicated, and native DNA.

of DNA antibodies and also for the presence of circulating DNA. A specific test for anti-DNA antibodies is most useful for monitoring the course of therapy (Fig. 9-5).

Radioimmunoassay for DNA and Anti-DNA Antibody [24, 52, 78]
Binding of radio-labeled DNA antigen in which DNA is labeled by incorporation with tritiated actinomycin D or tritiated dimethylsulfate is the most sensitive test available today for the detection of free DNA or anti-DNA antibody [24]. The ammonium sulfate technique of Farr [30] can be used to measure antigen-binding capacity, if the antigen, such as DNA, is soluble in 50% saturated ammonium sulfate, since the antigen bound to antibody may be separated from the unbound free antigen. Antibodies to DNA contained in the serum will bind with DNA to form DNA–anti-DNA complexes which are insoluble in 50% ammonium sulfate, while free DNA is soluble and found in the supernate. Also by this technique, one can demonstrate the presence of free DNA in the serum. The concentrations of DNA or DNA antibody may be determined by the ratio of binding to radio-labeled DNA in comparison with a standard curve. The ammonium sulfate method has the advantage of detecting a wider spectrum of antibodies. Certain populations of antibodies do not fix complement and have low precipitating and agglutinating ability. The main limitation of the test is the requirement for radioactive DNA (Fig. 9-6).

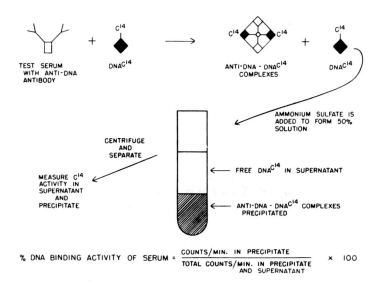

Figure 9-6
Determination of serum DNA binding activity with DNA–C14

The radio-labeled method for the detection of DNA and anti-DNA antibodies was first reported by Wold et al. [78]; labeled DNA was extracted from the growth of microorganisms in a medium containing radioactive nucleic acid precursors. Subsequently, Pincus and associates [52] have used C^{14}-labeled DNA obtained from cultured human tumor cells to detect antibodies to DNA. Their work revealed DNA-binding capacity in 66% of SLE serum shown to be negative by other tests. Carr and associates [24] have used calf thymus DNA labeled in vitro with actinomycin (H^3) or dimethyl (H^3) sulfate. The labeling procedure is not difficult and does not result in the alteration of the precipitability of the DNA. The sensitivity of the ammonium sulfate precipitation technique for the detection of DNA antibodies was shown by the fact that certain sera at 1:10,000 to 1:25,000 dilution showed a significant reaction to actinomycin-labeled DNA. In contrast, precipitins were not demonstrable with sera diluted 1:100, and hemagglutination with the same sera gave titers of less than 1:512. The maximum titer by complement fixation test was 1:1,000, and several sera demonstrating DNA antibodies by the ammonium sulfate method showed no complement fixation.

Indirect Immunofluorescence Test [15, 71]
The indirect immunofluorescence test is the most practical in the clinical laboratory today. The patient's serum is reacted with a section of substrate containing nuclei, and after washing the section is reacted with fluoresceinated antihuman globulin. The test allows the two significant characteristics of the antisera (specificity and sensitivity) to be linked with precise microscopic examination for the localization of antigens in tissue sections and smears. The fluorescence test is very sensitive and it can be developed to the point where a negative test may, for all practical purposes, rule out the diagnosis of systemic lupus erythematosus if the patient is not treated with corticosteroids or immunosuppressive drugs. By the pattern of fluorescence and titer one can derive some idea as to the type of antinuclear antibody. When the serum is tested in various dilutions, the antibody with the strongest titer will show a characteristic fluorescence pattern. A membranous ring or homogeneous pattern may be seen with antibodies to DNA or nucleoproteins. The speckled pattern quite often is seen with antibodies to saline extractable antigens, which include ribonucleoproteins and Sm antigens. A nucleolar pattern is seen with antibodies to nucleolar RNA; this antibody is most easily detected by the indirect immunofluorescence test today (Fig. 9-7).

Peroxidase Enzyme-Conjugated Antibody Technique [17, 27]
This technique may be used to test for the presence of antinuclear antibody. Antibody to human IgG is conjugated to horseradish peroxidase and used to demonstrate adherence of antinuclear antibodies to substrate nuclei. Localization of the enzyme is shown by reactions with

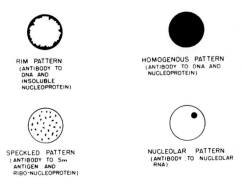

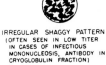

Figure 9-7
Fluorescent staining patterns seen in the indirect antinuclear antibody test.

PATTERNS MAY INDICATE TYPE OF ANTIBODY PRESENT BUT IS NOT DIAGNOSTIC. ALSO, THE FLUORESCENT PATTERN MAY CHANGE UPON SERIAL DILUTION OF TEST SERUM.

3,3'-diaminobenzidine, which gives an insoluble main reaction product. Patterns of nuclear staining are observed with this technique and correlate with the patterns seen by the fluorescence method (Fig. 9-8a, b, c). Comparison of the titers of antinuclear antibody showed the peroxidase method to be as sensitive as the fluorescence technique [17, 27]. A conventional microscope may be used, and no special equipment is necessary for the peroxidase enzyme method.

The disadvantages of the test are that the reagents are difficult to standardize and also that a wide variety of peroxidase-labeled antibodies to the specific immunoglobulins and complement components are not readily available.

Indirect Fluorescent Antinuclear Antibody Test (ANA)

In the detection of antinuclear antibodies, the most widely used fluorescence method is the indirect technique. The tissue is exposed to the patient's serum in a moist chamber to prevent evaporation for at least 30 minutes to allow attachment of the antinuclear antibody. The unattached serum proteins are then removed by washing with neutral buffered saline solution. After removal of excess washing fluid, the tissue is treated with fluorescein isothiocyanate-conjugated anti-human immunoglobulin serum. The excess conjugate is removed by washing and the tissue is mounted in buffered glycerol. The specimens are then examined with the fluorescence microscope.

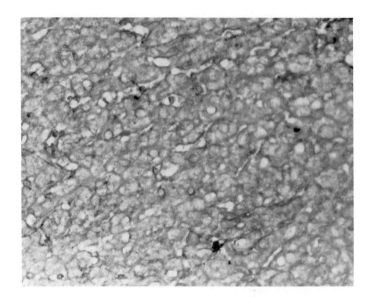

a

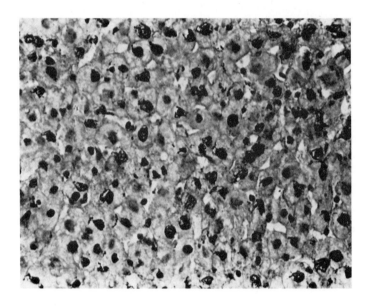

b

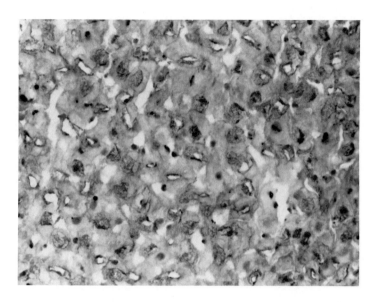

c

Figure 9-8
Peroxidase-labeled antibody test for the detection of anti-DNA antibody.
(a) Fixed rat liver reacted with normal serum. No staining of nuclei is
seen. (b) Fixed rat liver reacted with SLE serum and shows dense positive
staining of liver cell nuclei. (c) Fixed rat liver reacted with serum from
patient with mixed connective tissue disorder. Note speckled staining pattern.
Frozen rat liver sections were first fixed in acetone and then reacted with
test serum samples. After being washed, the sections were reacted with peroxidase-labeled goat anti-human IgG antiserum. The sections were washed and
peroxidase-labeled antibody was localized by reaction with specific substrate. (400× before 20% reduction.)

SUBSTRATES IN THE ANA TESTS.   There is much confusion about the indirect fluorescent nuclear antibody test since there are numerous substrates being utilized. The common substrates used today are:

Chicken erythrocytes.   Nucleated chicken red cells have certain disadvantages in that they lack sensitivity [77]. In addition, the hemoglobin may have a quenching effect and interfere with fluorescence. Also, certain sera from patients with collagen disease give a speckled fluorescent nuclear pattern and react with mammalian nuclei only [13]. More recently, a technique using formalinized chicken red cell nuclei [75] appears to show some promise as a possible antigen for a standardized test. We have evaluated the feasibility of formalinized chicken red cell nuclei and found that the chick nuclei are poor for demonstration of the speckled pattern [25], which is produced by antibodies to saline extractable antigen or soluble ribonucleoproteins. This is understandable since mammalian and nonmammalian proteins usually do not cross react.

Human leukocytes.   Leukocytes are a convenient source of nuclear antigen and have been used for the immunofluorescence test for the detection of antinuclear antibodies [8, 36]. However, the test is very sensitive, and many low-titered false positive fluorescence reactions are seen which are not specific for antinuclear antibodies. The test may have some interference with blood group and antileukocyte antibodies. Many patients with lupus erythematosus have many other anti-red cell, platelet, and tissue antibodies in addition to antinuclear antibodies. The difficulties in the interpretation of fluorescence patterns occur in the serum samples with low titers of antinuclear antibodies. Also Bruchhausen and co-workers [22] have shown that nonspecific nuclear staining in the fluorescent antibody methods may be due to minute amounts of labeled basic protein present in the labeled sera. The attraction of the basic proteins is caused by electrostatic forces.

Human skin tissue.   This is a convenient and useful substrate if hemorrhoidal tissue is used [21]. However, some interference may occur with blood and antitissue antibodies depending on the blood type and tissue type of the donor. The interfering antibodies will definitely increase the background fluorescence, and the detection of low titers of antinuclear antibodies is difficult.

Tissue culture cells.   Human tissue has been used [50] and satisfactory results may be obtained, but questions raised in the use of human skin also apply here.

Rat or mouse kidney and liver tissue.   Rat or mouse tissue is recommended since interference of the test with blood group antibodies as well as with certain antitissue antibodies is minimized. The test can be made sensitive enough, and if carefully performed with a conjugated antiserum which has a very low background with negative control tissue, satisfactory results can be obtained. One can, for practical purposes, rule out the diagnosis of untreated systemic lupus erythematosus if a negative antinuclear fluorescence test is observed.

RELATIONSHIPS OF FLUORESCENT NUCLEAR STAINING PATTERNS TO ANTINUCLEAR ANTIBODIES. Different patterns of nuclear staining which have been observed include homogeneous, shaggy or peripheral, speckled, and nucleolar [71]. Nuclear, rim, and intranuclear fibrillar staining were shown to be produced by antibody to native DNA and antibody to soluble nucleoprotein. Speckled nuclear staining is produced by antibodies to saline solution soluble nuclear proteins, e.g., Sm antigen [68] and ribonucleoprotein [46, 53, 61]. Homogeneous nuclear staining is produced by an antibody reacting with nucleoprotein. The nucleolar pattern is produced by antibodies to a constituent of the nucleoli, and the antigen probably contains RNA and associated protein. It was also shown that many sera with one pattern of nuclear staining would change to other patterns on serial dilution, due to the presence of different types of antinuclear antibody and the effect of some antibodies interferes with the reactivity of others. Nuclear staining patterns can be interpreted in terms of specific antinuclear antibodies with the understanding that some patterns may be produced by more than one antibody, and that some antibodies may interfere with the staining of others (Fig. 9-9).

Patients with mixed connective tissue disease may have a high titer of speckled pattern fluorescent antinuclear antibody [61]. No detectable Sm antibody was found.

INTERPRETATION OF FLUORESCENCE ANTINUCLEAR ANTIBODY TEST. Sera are screened at 1:4 and 1:16 dilution. The incidence of positive fluorescence at a 1:4 dilution is 2% in an apparently normal population [74]. If the serum shows a positive result at the 1:16 titer, then it is further tested at 1:64 and 1:256 dilutions.

In the fluorescence test, one should be careful that the substrate is fixed in acetone, since nonfixation of the substrate may result in the elution of some of the nuclear constituents. Nonfixation of the substrate will tend to give rise to a "comet" pattern of nuclear staining with the indirect fluorescent antibody test [38]. The nuclei are streaked in the shape of a comet (Fig. 9-10). The comet staining was observed when (a) tissues were unfixed and pretreated with ANA-negative serum or even with neutral isotonic saline solution, and (b) when the serum had a low titer of ANA [38]. A strongly positive serum with high levels of ANA prevents the nuclear antigen from diffusing, and no comet pattern was noted. The weakly reactive ANA sera may allow diffusion of nuclear material.

A significant result of nonfixation of the substrate may be a negative fluorescent test with a positive LE cell phenomenon. We have observed two lupus erythematosus cases, referred by other laboratories, in which the initial tests showed positive LE cell tests and negative indirect fluorescent antibody tests. Both cases showed a positive speckled pattern with fixed rat kidney substrate. One case showed a lower fluorescent test

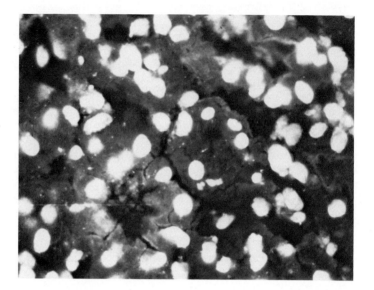

a

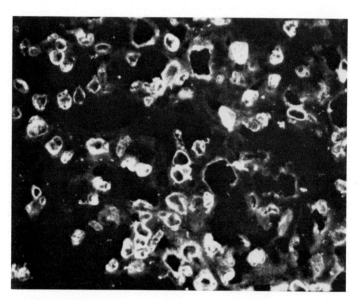

b

Figure 9-9
Fluorescent staining patterns seen in antinuclear antibody tests. Substrate used was acetone-fixed rat kidney which was first reacted with various sera. After being washed, the sections were then reacted with fluorescein isothio-

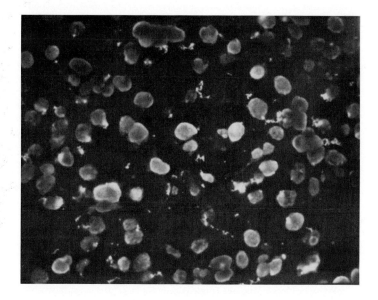

c

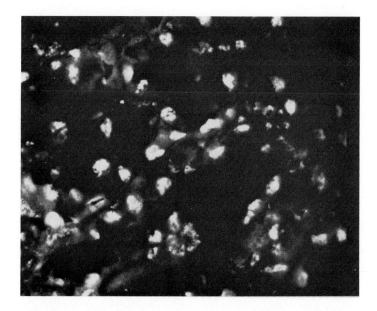

d

cyanate-labeled rabbit anti-human IgG. (a) homogeneous pattern (400×);
(b) rim pattern (400×); (c) rim and homogeneous pattern (40×); (d)
coarsely granular speckled pattern (400×).

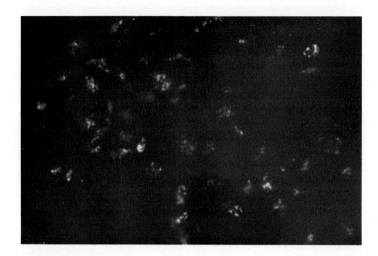

e

Figure 9-9 (*Continued*)
(e) irregular speckled pattern (400×)—all before 20% reduction. The rim and homogeneous pattern is noted with antibodies to DNA and nucleoproteins. The speckled pattern is seen with antibodies to the Sm antigen and ribonucleoprotein.

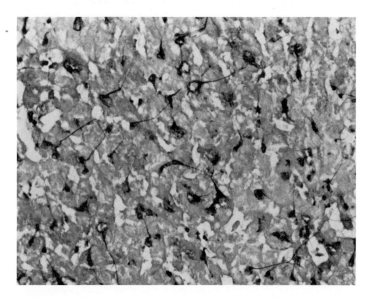

Figure 9-10
Comet pattern seen in antinuclear antibody tests. Unfixed section of rat liver
was reacted with serum from patient with SLE. Nuclear antibodies were
localized by peroxidase-labeled goat anti-human IgG. Note nuclear comet
streaks. This pattern may be seen when substrate sections are not fixed and
when there is diffusion of soluble nuclear antigens. (400× before 20%
reduction.)

titer with unfixed rat kidney, and the second case was negative when
tested with chicken red cell nuclei [25].

A fluorescence titer of at least 1:16 or greater is usually present before
there is evidence of a positive LE cell test [10]. The various patterns of
fluorescence by utilization of the rat and mouse kidney are homogeneous,
rim, and fibrillar, combined rim and homogeneous, shaggy, and speckled.
Also, there is a nucleolar pattern as seen quite often in lupus and systemic scleroderma. In infectious mononucleosis, there is often a low
titer, irregular, shaggy type of pattern (Fig. 9-11). The antinuclear
antibodies were of the IgG and IgM class and appeared in the cryoprecipitates when sera were stored at 4° C [40]. The antinuclear antibodies in infectious mononucleosis did not cause the LE cell phenomenon [40].

In the collagen diseases, the incidence of various antinuclear antibodies in systemic lupus is 99% or greater; in Sjögren's syndrome, 68%;
in scleroderma, 40%; in adult rheumatoid arthritis, 15–25%; in juvenile
rheumatoid arthritis, 22% [14]. Approximately 50% of the cases of discoid lupus have been reported to react positively in immunofluorescence
tests [64]. A low incidence of antinuclear antibodies can be observed in

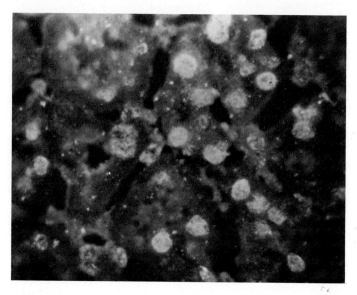

Figure 9-11
Positive antinuclear antibody test in infectious mononucleosis. The rat kidney section shows a positive indirect fluorescent antinuclear antibody test with irregular moth-eaten type of nuclear fluorescence. The serum from a patient showed a titer of 1:8 of antinuclear antibody. The antinuclear antibodies in infectious mononucleosis are usually of low titer and may occur in the cryoprotein fraction.

many other diseases, e.g., Addison's disease, pernicious anemia, Felty's syndrome, Sjögren's syndrome, chronic active hepatitis, and viral hepatitis.

Anticonvulsants such as the hydantoins, trimethadione, and primidone have a potential to induce the development of antinuclear antibodies [7]. Most of the anticonvulsant drugs elicit antibodies primarily directed to a soluble nucleoprotein. The soluble nucleoprotein antigen used in the studies was initially characterized by Tan [70]. Patients on hydantoin therapy have been observed to develop anti-DNA antibodies [7]. However, patients on anticonvulsant therapy who develop significant levels of anti-DNA antibodies should be suspected of having an underlying SLE.

The serum antinuclear antibody titers by the fluorescence test in drug-induced cases are usually lower than those in the collagen diseases. Furthermore, withdrawal of the drug may be associated with a disappearance of the nuclear antibody. If the level of antinuclear antibody titer rises after withdrawal of the drug, or if there is a significant level of anti-DNA, then the possibility of an SLE triggered by a drug should be considered.

In general, the higher the titer of antinuclear antibodies, the more likely is the diagnosis of systemic lupus erythematosus. In systemic lupus erythematosus, the reciprocal titers are often high, usually 64 to 256, whereas in other diseases such as rheumatoid arthritis, Addison's disease, and pernicious anemia, the antibody titers are often 64 or less [14].

Organ specific autoantibodies as seen in Hashimoto's thyroiditis, pernicious anemia, and idiopathic Addison's disease are rarely found in systemic lupus erythematosus (SLE). Also in SLE the titer to antinuclear antibodies is usually quite high, and antibodies to collagen, heart or blood vessel homogenates, leukocytes, and platelets may be found. In Felty's syndrome, antibodies to leukocytes are seen. In Sjögren's syndrome, antibodies to collagen and epithelial cells of the parotid glands are seen. In scleroderma, antibodies to collagen, nuclei, and blood vessel nucleoli are frequently seen [66] (Fig. 9-12).

The demonstration of serum antinucleolar antibodies can be of help to differentiate systemic sclerosis from other rheumatic diseases. The highest titer of antinucleolar antibodies is seen in cases of systemic sclerosis. In patients with rheumatic syndrome, Ritchie has reported [54] in 2,449 cases an overall incidence of 203 positive antinucleolar antibody tests (8.3%). Thirteen (54%) of 24 with systemic sclerosis had antinucleolar antibodies, whereas 26% with SLE and only 9% with rheumatoid arthritis had such antibodies.

Tests to Follow Therapy in Systemic Lupus Erythematosus

Tests useful in following the course of therapy of lupus erythematosus may be different from those used for initial diagnostic purposes. In the initial screening tests for diagnosis, one would prefer a very sensitive test for all types of antinuclear antibodies, such as the indirect fluorescence test or the peroxidase enzyme method, whereas in lupus erythematosus, the important pathogenic antibody is the anti-DNA antibody. When DNA is released from tissues into the circulation and combines with anti-DNA antibody, immune complexes are formed with the development of the clinical symptoms of fever, rash, and proteinuria.

During the acute phase with circulating DNA–anti-DNA complexes, there may be an excess of DNA in the circulation with an absence of anti-DNA antibody. Serum-circulating DNA may be detected by the agar gel double-diffusion method upon reaction with a known serum sample from a known SLE patient who has precipitating antibody to native DNA. The DNA in the serum can be detected by the inhibition of hemagglutination of DNA-coated red cells when reacted with a known serum sample containing anti-DNA antibodies.

Almost all cases of active LE nephritis will sooner or later demonstrate antibodies to double-stranded DNA as well as antibody to denatured DNA. Antibodies to DNA may be detected by the agar gel double-diffusion, hemagglutination, complement fixation, or radioimmunoassay test for anti-DNA antibody. When patients with lupus erythe-

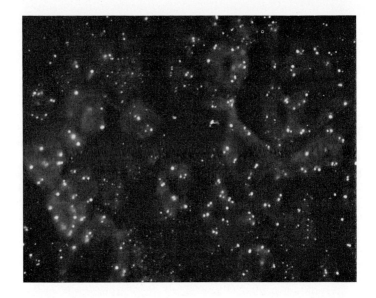

a

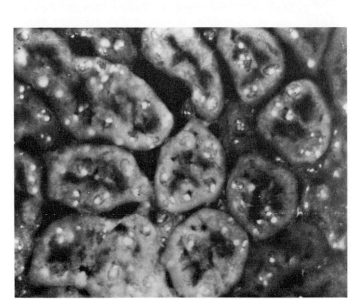

b

Figure 9-12
Positive indirect fluorescence test for antinucleolar antibodies. (a) Fixed rat kidney substrate reacted with serum from patients with nonspecific collagen disease. Section was washed and overlayed with fluorescein isothiocyanate-labeled anti-human IgG. (100×.) (b) Fixed rat kidney substrate reacted with serum from patient with systemic scleroderma. The section was processed similar to Figure 12a. (400×.)

matosus respond to treatment with prednisone and immunosuppressive agents, the anti-DNA antibody level will decrease and eventually disappear. Thus, the specific test for antibodies to native DNA is more useful than the fluorescent antibody test for monitoring the clinical course of systemic lupus erythematosus.

After treatment of SLE with corticosteroids, antinuclear antibodies other than anti-DNA antibody may still be present and be detected by the immunofluorescence test. Therefore, antinuclear antibody titers determined by the indirect immunofluorescence test may not be as useful as specific tests for DNA antibody to monitor therapy. More recently, Sharp and co-workers [60] have reported that individuals with SLE and renal disease which will respond to treatment show antibodies to DNA, and 86% of patients have antibodies to ENA (extractable nuclear antigen, which contains protein and ribonucleoprotein). In cases with renal disease and SLE which fail to respond to therapy, antibodies to DNA are persistent and the incidence of antibodies to the extractable nuclear antigen is only 8% [60]. Apparently, patients with systemic lupus tend to have a favorable prognosis when they have high titers of antibodies to the soluble ribonucleoproteins [53].

The immune complexes of DNA–anti-DNA may be detected by the C1q precipitin reaction described in Chapter 6. Other tests which are helpful in the diagnosis and monitoring of the course of the disease in SLE are tests for rheumatoid factor, cryoglobulins, and serum complement.

Summary of Recommended Laboratory Tests for Lupus Erythematosus and Other Related Collagen Diseases

Diagnostic Tests

SCREENING TESTS. Fluorescent antinuclear antibody ANA test or peroxidase enzyme-labeled antibody test for ANA. A negative test in the absence of corticosteroid, steroid, or immunosuppressive therapy rules out the diagnosis of systemic lupus erythematosus.

Sera are initially screened at a 1:4 dilution. Positive fluorescent ANA tests are titered at doubling dilutions 1:16, 1:64, and 1:256, and staining patterns are noted. (a) A titer of less than 1:16 has not been found to demonstrate a positive LE cell test. (b) High titers, such as 1:256 with rim and fibrillar or homogeneous patterns, are consistent with the diagnosis of systemic lupus erythematosus. (c) Low fluorescent ANA titers are seen in many diseases. (d) A high titered fluorescent ANA with a speckled pattern would make one suspicious of the diagnosis of a mixed connective disorder.

The presence of anti-native DNA antibodies is characteristic of systemic lupus erythematosus, and sera positive for ANA should be tested for the presence of anti-DNA antibodies. Three types of antigenic sites on the DNA molecule are probably present: (a) determinant unique to native DNA, (b) determinants crossreactive to native and single-stranded DNA, and (c) sites which are specific for single-stranded DNA only. Sera with anti-DNA antibodies may have antibodies reactive with all three determinants on the DNA molecule [26].

Patients with procainamide-induced lupus may have antibody to denatured DNA and nucleoprotein but little or no anti-native DNA antibody [20]. In patients with hydralazine drug-induced lupus erythematosus, circulating antibodies to native DNA may be seen [33]. Also such patients with active hydralazine lupus show circulating antibodies and in vitro lymphocyte transformation to hydralazine [33].

Sera positive for ANA may be tested for antibodies to ENA. This test is helpful in differentiating systemic lupus erythematosus from the mixed connective tissue syndrome. The antigen is not commercially available at the present time. The tests are helpful (a) to differentiate SLE from mixed connective tissue disorders; and (b) to monitor therapy. It is also of prognostic value.

OTHER HELPFUL LABORATORY TESTS

Serum cryoglobulins.   SLE is associated with a high incidence of cryoglobulins [64], although cryoglobulins are also seen in many other diseases.

Serum rheumatoid factor.   Rheumatoid factor in the serum of SLE is frequently observed. Conversely, antinuclear antibodies are a common finding in patients with rheumatoid arthritis and play a role in articular inflammation [78].

Tests for serum immune complexes and immune complex glomerulonephritis.   The typical case will show fluorescent localization of IgG, IgM, and C3 in an irregular pattern along the basement membrane. Also, in a significant number of cases the nuclei of kidney cells will demonstrate localization of IgG and IgM immunoglobulins [47].

Properdin was demonstrated by indirect immunofluorescence in the glomeruli of patients with lupus nephritis [55]. Data suggest that the properdin system participates in complement activation in the disease. Thus, it appears that both the conventional complement activation and the alternate pathway of complement activation play a role in the pathogenesis of glomerular lesions in systemic lupus.

Other autoimmune antibodies.   Antibodies to thyroid, parietal cell, mitochondria, smooth muscle, etc. may be present.

Hepatitis-associated antigen (HAA).   In one study, HAA was found in 41% of 116 patients with SLE [6]. There was no correlation between the presence of HAA and disease activity. HAA antigenemia is probably a complication rather than an etiologic factor in the immune disorder seen in SLE.

Tests to Monitor Therapy of Systemic Lupus Erythematosus
A. Circulating DNA and anti-DNA antibody
B. Serum cryoglobulins

C. Serum rheumatoid factors
D. Serum immune complexes and immune complex glomerulonephritis
E. Serum complement levels

Indirect Fluorescent Antinuclear Antibody Test Using
Sections of Mouse or Rat Kidneys
(Modified from Tan [71])

MATERIALS AND REAGENTS
A. Tissues: fresh rat or mouse kidney—3 mm cross sections
B. Stopper test tube and −70° C frost-free freezer (if desired for storing cross sections)
C. Dry ice and acetone or liquid nitrogen (for snap freezing)
D. OCT (optimal cutting temperature compound [Lab-Tek])
E. Flat-bottomed container (for snap freezing; made from aluminum wrapping sheets)
F. Cryostat
G. Water
H. Glass slides
 I. Acetone
 J. Fan (for air drying)
K. Serum
L. Buffered saline solution (pH 7.2 phosphate 0.01 M)
M. Moist chamber
N. Fluorescein-conjugated antiserum to human IgG immunoglobulin
O. Conjugated polyvalent antiserum to IgG, IgA, and IgM
P. Buffered glycerol (for mounting slides)
Q. Fluorescence microscope

PROCEDURE
1. Three mm cross sections of fresh rat or mouse kidney are snap frozen in dry ice and acetone or liquid nitrogen. They may be first embedded in OCT in a small square boat made from aluminum wrapping sheets. The flat surface of the kidney section is placed on the bottom of the boat, covered with OCT, and then snap frozen. The frozen tissue may be stored for a few months in a stoppered test tube or bottle in a nonfrost free freezer at −20° C for short periods or −70° C for periods of longer than a month.
2. The block is mounted on a cryostat block with a small amount of water; care should be taken so the kidney section does not thaw. 5 μ sections of kidney are cut and mounted on glass slides. Several sections may be cut and stored in a used slide box in the refrigerator and can be used for a few days. Freshly cut sections give sharper staining patterns and better results.
3. The sections are fixed in acetone for 10 min at room temperature and air dried just prior to use. Fixation of the section just prior to use appears to give more satisfactory results. Acetone treatment "fixes" the saline-soluble nuclear component, such as ribonucleoprotein and

Sm antigen, and prevents their leaching from cell nuclei during subsequent washings, but does not alter their reactivity. Acetone-fixed sections have the further advantage in that they can be thoroughly washed to get rid of nonspecific staining.

4. After acetone fixation, the kidney section is reacted with serum for 30 min at room temperature, and excess serum is removed with a rinse followed by 2 separate 5-min washings in buffered saline solution. The reaction is carried out in a moist chamber so that evaporation is minimal.

5. Fluorescein-conjugated antiserum to human IgG immunoglobulin is then applied to the section for 30 min at room temperature. The sections are then given two 8-min washings in buffered saline solution. A conjugated polyvalent antiserum to IgG, IgA, and IgM is the preferred reagent. Care should be taken that evaporation and drying of the fluorescent material do not occur.

6. The section is mounted in saline solution and buffered glycerol and examined with a fluorescence microscope.

Serum samples are screened at both 1:4 and 1:16 dilutions. Positive samples are serially diluted and the test is repeated. Serial dilutions of serum samples may produce different patterns of staining. A change in pattern most frequently observed is with rim and fibrillar staining changing to homogeneous or speckled stainings at higher dilutions of serum.

Indirect Antinuclear Antibody Test with Peroxidase-
Labeled Anti-Human IgG
(Modified from Dorling et al. [27])

MATERIALS AND REAGENTS

A. Rat kidney sections
   a. A rat kidney section is quick frozen in a cryostat
   b. Sections of rat kidney are cut at 6 μ and placed on slides. Slides with sections may be stored for 3 to 4 weeks at $-20°$ C and indefinitely at $-70°$ C
B. Acetone
C. Moist chamber
D. Peroxidase-labeled anti-human IgG (Bioware)
E. Phosphate-buffered saline solution (pH 7.2)
F. Agitator
G. Peroxidase substrate solution (freshly prepared; H_2O_2 is added just before use)
   a. 0.05 M Tris/HCl buffer (pH 7.6)—50 ml
   b. Hydrogen peroxide (3%)—0.15 ml
   c. 3,3'-diaminobenzidine tetrahydrochloride (Sigma)—25 mg
   d. Sucrose 4.28 gm to make 0.25 M solution
H. Distilled water
 I. Dehydrating alcohol (reagent alcohol, 95%, 100%)

J. Xylene
K. Permount

PROCEDURE

1. Fix slide in acetone for 10 min at room temperature just prior to use.
2. Incubate 1 drop of patient's serum on rat kidney section for 30 min in a moist chamber at room temperature.
3. Remove serum from slide with a rinse in buffered saline solution and follow with two separate washes of 5 min each.
4. Incubate 1 drop of peroxidase-labeled anti-human IgG on tissue for 30 min in a moist chamber at room temperature.
5. Wash anti-human IgG from slides with a few drops of buffered saline solution.
6. Wash in buffered saline solution with agitation for 8 min, change solution, and repeat wash.
7. Flood slides with peroxidase substrate solution and incubate for 30 min in a moist chamber at room temperature.
8. Wash with distilled water.
9. Dehydrate in 95% alcohol, then place in absolute or 100% alcohol.
10. Clear in two changes in xylene and mount with permount.
11. A positive reaction is indicated by a brown to black staining of nucleus or nucleoli.

Microhemagglutination Test for the Simultaneous Detection of Antibodies to Native and Denatured DNA, and for the Determination of Circulating DNA (Inami, Nakamura, and Tan [37])

REAGENTS

A. Sodium hydroxide solution, approximately 2N. Dissolve approximately 8 gm sodium hydroxide in 100 ml distilled water.
B. Hydrochloric acid solution, approximately 2N. Dilute with distilled water, 17 ml concentrated HCl (12N) to 100 ml.
C. Saline stock solution (0.9% NaCl). Dissolve 9 gm sodium chloride in a sufficient quantity of distilled water to make one liter.
D. Phosphate buffer solutions (0.15 M phosphate)
   a. KH_2PO_4: Dissolve 20.41 gm KH_2PO_4 in distilled water to make one liter of solution.
   b. K_2HPO_4: Dissolve 26.13 gm K_2HPO_4 in distilled water to make one liter of solution.
   c. K_2HPO_4–KH_2PO_4: Mix 3 volumes of K_2HPO_4 solution and one volume of KH_2PO_4 solution.
E. Phosphate-buffered saline working solutions
   a. Phosphate (0.075 M)–NaCl (0.45%): Mix equal volumes of K_2HPO_4–KH_2PO_4 solution and saline stock solution. Adjust pH to 7.3 with 2N NaOH or HCl. This solution will be designated as PBS(I).

  b. Phosphate (0.01 M)–NaCl (0.84%): Dilute 66.7 ml K_2HPO_4–KH_2PO_4 solution to one liter with 0.9% saline stock solution. Adjust pH to 7.3 with NaOH or HCl. This buffer solution will be referred to as PBS(II).

  c. Phosphate (0.01 M)–NaCl (0.6%): Mix 66.7 ml K_2HPO_4–KH_2PO_4 solution with 667 ml 0.9% saline and add distilled water to make one liter. Adjust pH to 7.3. This will be called PBS(III).

F. Tannic acid solution

  a. Tannic acid stock solution: Prepare 25 ml 10 mg/ml tannic acid stock solution by dissolving 250 mg tannic acid in 25 ml water.

  b. Tannic acid working solution: 0.5 ml stock solution is diluted to 100 ml with PBS(II).

G. McIlvaine buffer solution: Mix equal volumes of 0.1 M citric acid (19.21 gm anhydrous or 21.01 gm monohydrate to one liter with distilled water) and 0.2 M Na_2HPO_4 (28.41 gm anhydrous to one liter with water) and adjust pH to 4.9 with NaOH or H_3PO_4.

H. Stock formalin solution (37% formaldehyde, J. T. Baker analyzed reagent).

I. Sodium azide solution: Prepare 100 ml 100 mg/ml NaN_3 solution.

J. Calf thymus DNA (Worthington)

  a. Native DNA stock solution (NDNA): Dissolve 100 mg calf thymus DNA in sufficient PBS(II) to make 100 ml solution. Agitate overnight at 4° C to complete dissolution. Also prepare 100 ml 1 mg NDNA/ml in McIlvaine buffer.

  b. Sonicated DNA (SoDNA): Sonically disrupt NDNA dissolved in McIlvaine buffer for 2 min using a power sonifier (Branson Sonic Power Sonifier, Model 9110). Cool the solution in ice bath to avoid excessive heating during sonication.

  c. Single-stranded DNA (SSDNA): Dilute native DNA solution with PBS(III) to give 0.200 mg DNA/ml. Heat this solution in a boiling water bath for 10 min and then immediately cool in an ice bath. Prepare daily.

K. Bovine albumin, 30% (Hyland Laboratories).

FORMALIZATION OF HUMAN TYPE O RH NEGATIVE ERYTHROCYTES

1. Pack fresh human type O Rh negative cells at 900 g (2,000 rpm with 19.8 cm radius) for 5 min and wash 4 times, each time with 7–10 volumes of PBS(I). Use this buffer for subsequent steps of this section.

2. Resuspend the cells to a concentration of 10% in PBS(I).

3. Mix equal volumes 10% cell suspension and diluted formalin (3.7% formalin in PBS) and incubate at room temperature for 4–6 hours, with occasional stirring. Then incubate at 37° C for 15–18 hours.

4. Pack and wash formalinized cells four times, each time with 10 volumes of PBS(I).

5. Make a 10% cell suspension in PBS(I) with 0.1% NaN$_3$, divide into 10 ml aliquots and store at 4° C.

PREPARATION OF DNA-COATED CELLS
1. Pack 10 ml 10% suspension of formalinized human red blood cells.
2. Wash one time with PBS(II).
3. Resuspend the 1 ml packed cells in 50 ml tannic acid working solution.
4. Incubate the cell suspension at 37° C for 45 min with frequent shaking.
5. Wash four times, each time with 20 volumes of PBS(II).
6. Wash cells once with 20 ml McIlvaine buffer.
7. Pack and decant supernate; to the packed cells add approximately 15 ml McIlvaine buffer, 1.25 mg DNA (1.25 ml 1 mg/ml DNA solution) and then bring to a total volume of 25 ml with McIlvaine buffer. DNA concentration corresponds to 50 μg per ml cell suspension.
8. Incubate at 37° C for one hour with frequent shaking.
9. Pack and wash four times, each time with 20 volumes PBS(II), and resuspend in this buffer with 0.07% bovine albumin to a final cell concentration of 1.3%.

MATERIALS FOR HEMAGGLUTINATION TEST
A. Pipette droppers: 0.025 ml calibration (Cooke Engineering).
B. Microdiluters: 0.025 ml calibration (Cooke Engineering).
C. Disposable V-shaped plates (Linbro of the Pacific).
D. Diluent: PBS(III), with 0.2% bovine albumin.
E. Sera for titration (inactivated at 56° C for 30 min).
F. Coated, tanned, formalinized cells (1.3% suspension).
G. Antigens: Native, sonicated, and single-stranded DNA in PBS(II), each at a concentration of 0.200 mg DNA/ml.

PROCEDURE OF HEMAGGLUTINATION TEST
1. With pipette dropper add 0.025 ml diluent to each well of the V plate.
2. Immerse tip of each diluter into saline solution prior to dilution and check calibration on "Go/NoGo" delivery tester. Blot off excess solution on outer surface of the prongs.
3. Dip the tip of the diluter into serum so that no bubbles are caught in the prongs. Place diluter into the first well.
4. Twirl diluters about 10 times in each well. Then proceed to the next well and repeat until serial dilutions are complete.
5. With a pipette dropper add one drop (0.025 ml) of coated cell preparation to each well.
6. Tap plate several times but avoid splashing liquid from the wells. Examine and remove bubbles on the bottoms of the wells. Cover plate with sealers.

7. Allow cells to settle 1–4 hours, then observe the hemagglutination reaction in each well. A smooth mat at the bottom of the wells is recorded as positive (+), and a clearly defined button of cells centered at the bottom of the wells is designated negative (−); intermediate reactions are called (±). The last well giving a positive reaction (highest dilution) is taken as the endpoint.

HEMAGGLUTINATION INHIBITION PROCEDURE
(provides a measure of antibody specificity)
1. With a pipette dropper add 0.025 ml diluent to all but the first well of each row.
2. Add one drop (0.025 ml) DNA inhibitor at a concentration of 0.200 mg DNA/ml in PBS(III) to the first well. Then, using a microdiluter, place in the same well 0.025 ml test serum and carry out the serial double dilution steps as described above.
3. Incubate the inhibitor-serum dilutions for 20 min at room temperature.
4. Add one drop of coated cells to each well.
5. Specificity is indicated by a drop in hemagglutination titer.

QUANTITATIVE INHIBITION PROCEDURE
1. With a pipette dropper dispense 0.025 ml diluent to each well.
2. Check calibration of the diluter.
3. Using the diluter pick up and transfer 0.025 ml DNA solution at a concentration of 0.200 mg/ml to the first well.
4. Perform serial dilutions as already outlined.
5. To each well add 0.025 ml antiserum (preferably that which contains both anti-native DNA and anti-denatured DNA) whose concentration corresponds to approximately 2 times the endpoint titer. Dilution is made with PBS(II).
6. Incubate the plate for 20 min at room temperature.
7. Add 0.025 ml coated cell preparation to each well.
8. Sensitivity is given by the last well exhibiting no hemagglutination.

DETERMINATION OF CIRCULATING DNA
1. Dispense with a pipette dropper 0.025 ml diluent to each well.
2. Check calibration of a diluter.
3. Using this diluter transfer 0.025 ml test serum to the first well.
4. Carry out serial double dilution as described earlier.
5. To each well add 0.025 ml (one drop from a pipette dropper) of DNA antiserum, preferably known to contain both anti-native DNA and anti-denatured DNA. Dilute the antiserum with PBS(II) to a concentration approximately twice the hemagglutination endpoint titer.
6. Incubate the plate for 20 min at room temperature.
7. Add 0.025 ml DNA-coated cells to each well.

8. Tap plate gently so as to achieve thorough mixing of the solutions.
9. Record the last well exhibiting no hemagglutination. This datum, in conjunction with those data obtained by quantitative inhibition experiments, permits the determination of the amount of circulating DNA in the test serum.

CLEANING DROPPERS AND DILUTERS
1. Rinse droppers several times with distilled water.
2. Rinse diluters in distilled water, flame them to incandescence (cherry red), and plunge into distilled water.
3. Place in holders.

COMMENT.   The microhemagglutination test in our laboratory has been very sensitive and reproducible. The test has the sensitivity of detecting antibody levels capable of reacting with less than 1 μgr DNA/ml. A significant titer is 1:4 or greater. A good procedure is to recheck positive tests for anti-DNA with the addition of DNA to the serum containing antibodies which should result in an inhibition of the agglutination pattern (Fig. 9-13).

Macrohemagglutination Test for Anti-DNA Antibodies
(Method of Koffler et al. [41, 42])

PREPARATION OF FORMALINIZED HUMAN RED CELLS
1. Pack and wash human 0+ or 0− cells in Alsever's solution 4 times with 0.9% saline solution.
2. Resuspend the cells to a concentration of 8% in buffered saline solution (pH 7.2, phosphate 0.01 M).
3. Dilute stock formalin (37%) to 3.7% with buffered saline solution.
4. Mix equal volumes of cells from step 2 and diluted formalin (step 3), and incubate at 37° C for 18–24 hours.
5. Pack the formalinized cells and wash 4 times with 10 volumes distilled water.
6. Resuspend the washed formalinized cells and follow procedure below for tanning and coating with DNA.

PREPARATION OF DNA-COATED RED CELLS
1. Pack 10 ml 10% suspension of formalinized erythrocytes (human, 0+ or 0−) in a Serofuge (Clay Adams).
2. Wash 4 times with buffered saline solution (pH 7.2, phosphate 0.02 M, saline 0.15 M).
3. Resuspend 1 ml packed cells in 50 ml 1:20,000 solution of tannic acid in buffered saline solution.
4. Incubate at 37° C for 30 min with frequent shaking.
5. Wash 4 times as above with buffered saline solution.
6. Resuspend 1 ml packed cells in 25 ml buffered saline solution.

Ab+PBS

JP+PBS

So-DNA+PBS+Ab

IH+PBS+Ab

JC+PBS+Ab

RS+PBS+Ab

CB+PBS+Ab

MB+PBS+Ab

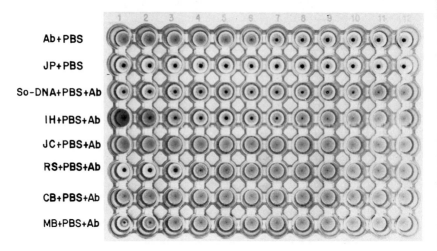

Figure 9-13
Microhemagglutination test for the detection of anti-DNA antibody and inhibition test for the determination of free circulating DNA in serum. Hemagglutination patterns for reference antiserum (Ab), negative sera (JP, CB, MB), control DNA (SoDNA), and positive SLE sera (IH, JC, RS) against red cells coated with sonicated DNA. Row 1 (Ab + PBS) shows positive hemagglutination to dilution of 1/64. Negative hemagglutination in row 2 indicates absence of anti-DNA antibodies. In the next 6 rows, the quantitative inhibition test was performed, using reference antiserum diluted 1:32. In row 3, 200 μg/ml SoDNA was serially diluted, and a HA inhibition of 10 wells was achieved. Rows 4 and 6 illustrate, respectively, the presence of 40 and 1.6 μg/ml of circulating DNA. In row 5, no inhibition is observed because the serum contains antibodies to DNA. Row 8 exemplifies that nonspecific inhibition of one well may be observed in some normal sera; in others, as demonstrated by the pattern in row 7, no inhibition is observed.

7. Pack 1 ml 4% suspension from step 6 and wash 1 time with McIlvaine's buffer (pH 4.9, mixture of 0.1 M citric acid and 0.2 M disodium phosphate)
8. Resuspend in 1 ml McIlvaine's buffer.
9. Dilute native DNA to 50 μg/ml in McIlvaine's buffer.
10. Add an equal volume of DNA solution from step 9 to 4% cell suspension from step 8.
11. Incubate at 37° C for one hour with *constant agitation*.
12. Pack cells and wash 4 times with buffered saline solution, containing 1% normal rabbit serum.
13. Resuspend in solution to a final cell concentration of 3%.

For the preparation of cells coated with denatured DNA, use *pH 4.7* McIlvaine's buffer in place of the *pH 4.9* buffer, and add denatured DNA diluted to 10 μg/ml. Thermal denaturation may be carried out by heating solutions of 0.5 mg/ml for 10 min in a boiling water bath and immediately cooling in an ice bath [69].

PERFORMANCE OF HEMAGGLUTINATION TEST
1. Absorb sera with formalinized tanned 0+ or 0− erythrocytes 4 times.*
2. Inactivate absorbed sera at 56° C for 30 min.
3. Set up the rack for serial dilutions with an appropriate number of tubes.
4. With an automatic syringe add 0.3 ml phosphate-buffered saline solution (pH 7.2) containing 1% NRS to the first tube, and 0.2 ml to the others.
5. Add 0.1 ml undiluted serum from step 2 to the first tube.
6. Transfer 0.2 ml serially (with Biopette [Schwartz Bioresearch]).
7. Add 0.05 ml of the 3% suspension of DNA or HDNA-coated cells to all tubes (added with microtiter 0.05 ml dropper).
8. Shake vigorously and allow to stand at room temperature overnight.
9. Read and record results as number of tubes in which at least 2+ hemagglutination occurs.

For inhibition studies, add inhibitor to sera from step 2. Incubate at 37° C for one hour, centrifuge to clear, and add supernatant as in step 5. In calculating the titer, make the appropriate correction necessary because of the dilution of the serum by the addition of the inhibitor.

Agar Double-Diffusion Precipitin Test for Detection of DNA Antibodies [69]

MATERIALS
A. Heating equipment
B. Filter paper
C. Petri dish
D. Calf thymus DNA (Worthington)
E. Standard anti-DNA antiserum

REAGENTS
1. Agarose (Seakem)
2. Buffered saline solution (pH 7.0, 7.2; phosphate 0.01 M).
3. Sodium azide (Sigma)

PROCEDURE
1. A 0.4% agarose in phosphate-buffered saline solution (pH 7.2) with 0.1% sodium azide is heated to dissolve the agarose.
2. The hot solution is passed through a filter paper to obtain clarity.

* Sera may be screened for anti-DNA antibodies without absorption with formalinized tanned red cells. A significant number of positive lupus sera may contain antitissue antibodies and react with uncoated red cells. 0− red cells are preferable, but 0+ cells may be used.

3. 25 ml clarified agarose solution is poured into a petri dish (100 × 15 mm). After cooling of the gel, 8 mm diameter wells are made in the agar and placed 4 mm apart.
4. Calf thymus DNA (Worthington) is dissolved in phosphate-buffered saline solution (pH 7.0) at a concentration of 1 mg/ml as the stock solution. Denatured DNA is produced by heating solutions containing 0.5 mg per ml of native DNA for 10 min in a boiling water bath and immediately cooling in an ice bath.
5. For precipitin reactions native DNA or denatured DNA is used at a concentration of 0.5 mg/ml.
6. Reactions are allowed to proceed for 48 to 72 hours. With the use of a standard anti-DNA antiserum, the presence of DNA in an unknown serum may be detected.

Preparation of Extractable Nuclear Antigen (ENA)
Procedure Similar to Method Described by Holman [34]

MATERIALS AND REAGENTS
A. Calf thymus glands obtained immediately after slaughter, transported to the laboratory in ice
B. Cold (4° C) 0.25 M sucrose solution containing 0.003 M $CaCl_2$
C. Waring blender
D. Refrigeration equipment (to 4° C)
E. Cheesecloth
F. Refrigerated centrifuges (International, Sorvell)
G. Cold buffered saline solution (pH 7.0, phosphate 0.01 M, saline, 0.15 M)
H. Agitator
I. Sodium acetate
J. Cold absolute ethanol
K. 0.15 M NaCl

PROCEDURE
1. Transport to the laboratory packed in ice calf thymus glands obtained immediately after slaughter of the animal.
2. Trim fat and connective tissue from cold thymus. Mince into bite size pieces.
3. Rinse them in cold (4° C) 0.25 M sucrose solution containing 0.003 M $CaCl_2$ to remove blood.
4. Homogenize in a Waring blender at low speed for 4 min, 50 gm thymus with 450 ml cold sucrose solution. Keep temperature of homogenate as close to 4° C as practical.
5. Filter the homogenate through two layers of cheesecloth. Repeat.
6. Centrifuge the filtrate at 600 g (International refrigerated centrifuge, 1,500 rpm with 24.4 cm radius) 10 min and collect the sedimented nuclei.

7. Add 2 volumes cold buffered saline solution to one volume of sedimented nuclei.
8. Disrupt nuclei in Waring blender at high speed for 4 min. Keep the temperature of the homogenate as close to 4° C as practical.
9. Extract the nucleoprotein by agitating at least 30 min at 4° C.
10. Centrifuge at 27,000 g (Sorvall refrigerator centrifuge. 15,000 rpm using SS34 rotor) 30 min at 4° C.
11. Collect the slightly pink supernatant.
12. Add 10 mg sodium acetate to each milliliter of supernatant. Stir to effect complete dissolution of sodium acetate.
13. Add 6 volumes of cold absolute ethanol. A flocculant precipitate is produced.
14. Centrifuge at 1,100 g (International refrigerated centrifuge, 2,000 rpm with 24.4 cm radius) 10 min. A white precipitate is formed. Remove supernatant.
15. Dissolve the white precipitate in 0.15 M NaCl. (Use approximately 20 ml saline solution for each 50 g thymus processed.) The major portion of the precipitate will dissolve. Centrifuge at 1,100 g 10 min and collect supernate.
16. The opalescent solution is lyophilized or stored at −60° C.

MODIFIED METHOD OF PREPARATION OF EXTRACTABLE
NUCLEAR ANTIGENS

1. Take 500 ml slightly pink supernatant from step 11 in preceding Procedure and make it 35% w/v in $(NH_4)_2SO_4$.
2. Centrifuge and save the supernate. Discard the precipitate.
3. Make supernate 60% in $(NH_4)_2SO_4$.
4. Centrifuge at 1,100 g 10 min (International refrigerated centrifuge, 2,000 rpm with a 24.4 cm radius) at 4° C.
5. Discard the supernatant and dissolve the pink precipitate in 50 ml 0.15 M saline solution.
6. Repeat steps 4–6.
7. Dialyze the ENA in saline against 20 volumes buffered saline solution (phosphate 0.01 M, salt 0.15 M). This step is used to remove $(NH_4)_2SO_4$.
8. The resulting pink solution is lyophilized or stored at −60° C.

Tanned Red Cell Hemagglutination Test for ENA Antibody
(Method of Sharp et al. [60])

REAGENTS
A. Buffer solution: Veronal saline buffer (VSB), stock solution ×5
     85.0 gm NaCl
     5.75 gm 5,5 diethyl barbituric acid (barbital)
     3.75 gm sodium 5,5 diethyl barbiturate (barbital sodium)
   1. Dissolve NaCl and barbital sodium in 600 ml distilled water.

2. Dissolve the acid in 500 ml hot distilled water and add to the solution prepared in step 1.
3. Cool and make up to 2 liters with distilled water.
4. After dilution add: 0.0332 gm $CaCl_2$
$$0.2034 \text{ gm Mg } Cl_2 \cdot 6H_2O$$
$$pH = 7.3\text{--}7.4$$
To use, dilute 1:5 with HOH. Must be made up fresh.
B. Tannic Acid
1. 50 mg tannic acid | 10 ml distilled water. Add acid to the water and allow it to settle into solution. Do NOT agitate. 1:200 dilution.
2. Dilute 1:200 solution of tannic acid 1:10 with VSB to a final dilution of 1:2,000.
3. Make a second dilution of tannic acid by diluting 4 ml of the 1:2,000 tannic acid solution with 46 ml VSB so that final dilution is 1:25,000.
C. Sheep RBC (sheep red cells approximately 7–14 days old)
1. Spin off Alsever's solution.
2. Wash cells 2 times in VSB.
3. Make 4% suspension—2 ml packed cells and 48 ml VSB.
D. Normal rabbit serum (NRS) (absorbed with sheep red blood cells)

During the entire process reagents and cells must be handled gently. All centrifugation at 10° C, 1,200–1,400 rpm for 12–15 min.

MATERIALS
A. Incubator
B. Agitator
C. Plastic tubes—2
D. Centrifuge
E. Pasteur pipette
F. Centrifuge tubes—2
G. Coleman Junior spectrophotometer model 620
H. Refrigeration to 4° C

PROCEDURE
Preparation of tanned red cells
1. Gently pour a 4% suspension of red cells into an equal volume of tannic acid solution 1:25,000.
2. Incubate 30 min at room temperature. Mix gently by swirling at intervals.
3. Pour into two plastic tubes. Spin off the solution.
4. Wash with VSB—add VSB in *small* amounts and separate clumped cells gently with a Pasteur pipette.
5. For the second wash, resuspend cells—same precaution as above. Combine in one tube 20 ml total.

6. Pour into two centrifuge tubes. Spin ½ control cells, ½ to be sensitized.

Sensitization of tanned red cells
1. To packed tanned cells, add 2× volume VSB.
2. 5 mg ENA is used to coat 1 ml 33% suspension of tanned sheep red blood cells.
3. Incubate exactly 30 min at room temperature.
4. Add a small amount of NRS 1:150 in VSB to stop the reaction.
5. Spin and wash 2 times with NRS 1:150 in VSB.
   (Wash volume approximately 15 to 20× volume of packed RBC.)

STANDARDIZATION OF FINAL RED CELL SUSPENSION
WITH THE USE OF A COLEMAN JUNIOR SPECTROPHOTOMETER
MODEL 620
1. At 650 nm, zero machine with 1:150 NRS.
2. Add an equal volume of red cell suspension.
3. Mix.
4. Dilute the red cell suspension to 39% transmission.

TEST PROCEDURE
1. Inactivate all sera to be tested and NRS at 56° C for 30 min and absorb with one-half volume packed sheep RBC at 37° C for 30 min 2 times.
2. Initial serum dilution 1:10, 0.1 ml serum diluted with 1:150 NRS and further dilutions are made in 1:150 NRS.
3. Control test 0.25 ml serum dilution + 0.25 ml nonsensitized red cell suspension.
4. Test 0.25 ml serum dilution + 0.25 ml sensitized red blood cells.
5. Mix and let stand in cold at 4° C overnight. Titers were expressed as the highest dilution of antiserum which gives a 1 to 2+ agglutination of cells on the bottom of the tube. Parallel controls at each dilution with nonsensitized tanned red cells and serum.

COMMENT.   A positive titer was considered to be 1:10 or greater. There is a tendency for nonspecific agglutination at a very low titer.

The ENA hemagglutination test may not be feasible to perform as an occasional test in the clinical laboratory. The parameters have not been established to perform microhemagglutination with formalinized human cells in order to avoid absorption of the serum samples for antibodies to the heterologous sheep red cells. So far today, for the demonstration of antibodies to ENA, the procedure of Sharp et al. [60] with use of sheep cells has been the most reproducible.

Current work is in progress to develop specific tests for the Sm antigen, which is a saline extractable carbohydrate-containing protein in nuclei. A specific test for antibodies to Sm antigen will help in the diagnosis of systemic lupus erythematosus. Patients with mixed connective tissue disease having a high titer of ENA antibodies most likely have antibodies to ribonucleoproteins and would not have antibodies to Sm antigen [61].

References

1. Agnello, V., Winchester, R. J., and Kunkel, H. G.   Precipitin reactions of the Cl_q component of complement with aggregated γ-globulin and immune complex in gel diffusion. *Immunology* 19:909, 1970.
2. Agnello, V., Koffler, D., Eisenberg, J. A., Winchester, R. J., and Kunkel, H. G. Cl_q precipitins in the sera of patients with systemic lupus erythematosus and other hypocomplementemic states: Characterization of high and low molecular weight types. *J. Exp. Med.* 134:228s, 1971.
3. Agnello, V., de Bracco, M. M. E., and Kunkel, H. G.   Hereditary C2 deficiency with some manifestations of systemic lupus erythematosus. *J. Immunol.* 108:837, 1972.
4. Alarcón-Segovia, D.   Drug-induced lupus syndromes. *Mayo Clin. Proc.* 44:664, 1969.
5. Alarcón-Segovia, D., Fishbein, E., Alcacá, H., Olguin-Palacios, E., and Estrada-Parra, S.   The range and specificity of antinuclear antibodies in systemic lupus erythematosus. *Clin. Exp. Immunol.* 6:557, 1970.
6. Alarcón-Segovia, D., Fishbein, E., and Diaz-Jouanen, E.   Presence of hepatitis associated antigen in systemic lupus erythematosus. *Clin. Exp. Immunol.* 12:9, 1972.
7. Alarcón-Segovia, D., Fishbein, E., Reyes, P. A., Diés, H., and Shwadsky, S.   Antinuclear antibodies in patients on anticonvulsant therapy. *Clin. Exp. Immunol.* 12:39, 1972.
8. Alexander, W. R. M., Bremner, J. M., and Duthie, J. J. R.   Incidence of the antinuclear factor in human sera. *Ann. Rheum. Dis.* 19:338, 1960.
9. Barnett, E. V., Condemi, J. J., Leddy, J. P., and Vaughan, J. H.   Gamma 2, gamma 1A, and gamma 1M antinuclear factors in human sera. *J. Clin. Invest.* 43:1104, 1964.
10. Barnett, E. V.   Diagnostic aspects of lupus erythematosus cells and antinuclear factors in disease states. *Mayo Clin. Proc.* 44:645, 1969.
11. Barnett, E. V., Kantor, G., Bickel, Y. B., Foresen, R., and Gonick, H. C.   Systemic lupus erythematosus. *Calif. Med.* 11:467, 1969.
12. Barnett, E. V., Bluestone, R., Cracchiolo, A., Goldberg, L. S., Kantor, G. L., and McIntosh, R. M.   Cryoglobulinemia and disease. *Ann. Intern. Med.* 73:95, 1970.
13. Beck, J. S.   Variations in the morphological patterns of "autoimmune" nuclear fluorescence. *Lancet* 1:1203, 1961.
14. Beck, J. S.   Autoantibodies to cell nuclei. *Scott. Med. J.* 8:373, 1963.
15. Beck, J. S.   Antinuclear antibodies: Methods of detection and significance. *Mayo Clin. Proc.* 44:600, 1969.
16. Beerman, H.   The L.E. cell and phenomenon in lupus erythematosus. *Am. J. Med. Sci.* 222:473, 1951.
17. Benson, M. D., and Cohen, A. S.   Antinuclear antibodies in systemic lupus erythematosus. *Ann. Intern. Med.* 73:943, 1970.

18. Bitter, T., Bitter, F., Silberschmidt, R., and Dubois, E. L. In vivo and in vitro study of cell mediated immunity (CMI) during onset of systemic lupus erythematosus (SLE). *Arthritis Rheum.* 14:152, 1971 (Abstract).

19. Block, S. R., Gibbs, C. B., Stevens, M. B., and Shulman, L. E. Delayed hypersensitivity in systemic lupus erythematosus. *Ann. Rheum. Dis.* 27:311, 1968.

20. Blomgren, S. E., Condemi, J. J., and Vaughan, J. H. Procainamide-induced lupus erythematosus. *Am. J. Med.* 52:338, 1972.

21. Blundell, G. P. Fluorescent antibody methods. In M. Stefanini (ed.), *Progress in Clinical Pathology.* New York: Grune & Stratton, 1970, vol. 3, p. 211.

22. Bruchhausen, D., Hofermann, R., and Mayersbach, H. V. Studies on nuclear staining by the fluorescent antibody method: I. Nonimmunological factors leading to nuclear fluorescence. *Immunology* 19:1, 1970.

23. Burnet, M. Implications for autoimmune disease in man, studies on NZB mice and their hybrids. II. Renal and thymic disease. *R. Inst. Public Health Hyg. J.* 29:95, 1966.

24. Carr, R. I., Koffler, D., Agnello, V., and Kunkel, H. G. Studies on DNA antibodies using DNA labeled with actinomycin-D (3H) or dimethyl (3H) sulfate. *Clin. Exp. Immunol.* 4:527, 1969.

25. Cleymaet, J. E., and Nakamura, R. M. Indirect immunofluorescent antinuclear tests: Comparison of sensitivity and specificity of different substrates. *Am. J. Clin. Pathol.* 58:388, 1972.

26. Cohen, S. A., Hughes, G. R. V., Noel, G. L., and Christian, C. L. Character of anti-DNA antibodies in systemic lupus erythematosus. *Clin. Exp. Immunol.* 8:551, 1971.

27. Dorling, J., Johnson, G. D., Webb, J. A., and Smith, M. E. Use of peroxidase conjugated antiglobulin as an alternative to immunofluorescence for the detection of antinuclear factor in serum. *J. Clin. Pathol.* 24:501, 1971.

28. Dubois, E. L., Drexler, E., and Arterberry, J. D. A latex nucleoprotein test for diagnosis of systemic lupus erythematosus: A comparative evaluation. *J.A.M.A.* 177:141, 1961.

29. Dubois, E. L. *Lupus Erythematosus.* New York: Blakiston Div., McGraw-Hill, 1966.

30. Farr, R. S. A quantitative immunochemical measure of primary interaction between I*BSA and antibody. *J. Infect. Dis.* 103:239, 1958.

31. Friou, G. J., Tojo, T., and Spiegelberg, H. C. IgG subclasses of human antinuclear antibodies. *Fed. Proc.* 28:695, 1969.

32. Goldman, J. A., Litwin, A., Adams, L. E., Krueger, R. C., and Hess, E. V. Cellular immunity to nuclear antigens in systemic lupus erythematosus. *J. Clin. Invest.* 51:2669, 1972.

33. Hahn, B. H., Sharp, G. C., Irvin, W. S., Kantor, O. S., Gardner, C. A., Bagby, M. K., Perry, H. M., and Osterland, C. K. Immune responses to hydralazine and nuclear antigens in hydralazine-induced lupus erythematosus. *Ann. Intern. Med.* 76:365, 1972.

34. Hargraves, M. M., Richmond, H., and Morton, R. Presentation of two bone marrow elements: The "tart" cell and the "L.E." cell. *Proc. Staff Meet. Mayo Clin.* 23:25, 1948.

35. Hijmans, W., Schuit, H. R. E., Mandema, E., Nienhuis, R. L. F., Feltkamp, T. E. W., Holborow, E. J., and Johnson, G. D. Comparative
study for the detection of antinuclear factors with the fluorescent antibody technique. *Ann. Rheum. Dis.* 23:73, 1964.
36. Holman, H. R. Partial purification and characterization of an extractable nuclear antigen which reacts with SLE sera. *Ann. N.Y. Acad. Sci.*
124:800, 1965.
37. Inami, Y. H., Nakamura, R. M., and Tan, E. M. Microhemagglutination test for the simultaneous detection of antibodies to native and
denatured DNA and for the determination of circulating serum DNA.
J. Immunol. Methods 3:287, 1973.
38. Johnson, G. D., Smith, M. E., and Holborow, E. J. The comet pattern
of nuclear immunofluorescence. *Clin. Exp. Immunol.* 10:463, 1972.
39. Kacaki, J. N., Callerame, M. L., Blomgren, S. G., and Vaughan, J. H.
Immunoglobulin G subclasses and antinuclear antibodies and renal deposits. *Arthritis Rheum.* 14:276, 1971.
40. Kaplan, M. E., and Tan, E. M. Antinuclear antibodies in infectious
mononucleosis. *Lancet* 1:561, 1966.
41. Koffler, D., Carr, F. I., Agnello, V., and Kunkel, H. G. Assay of
antibodies to DNA by hemagglutination and their procedures. *Fed.
Proc.* 28:486, 1969.
42. Koffler, D., Carr, R., Agnello, V., Thoburn, R., and Kunkel, H. G.
Antibodies to polynucleotide in human sera: Antigenic specificity and
relation to disease. *J. Exp. Med.* 134:294, 1971.
43. Koffler, D., Agnello, V., Thoburn, R., and Kunkel, H. G. Systemic
lupus erythematosus: Prototype of immune complex nephritis in man.
J. Exp. Med. 134:169s, 1971.
44. Lawlis, J. F. Serological detection of deoxyribonucleic acid (DNA)
adsorbed to formalinized erythrocytes. *Proc. Soc. Exp. Biol. Med.*
98:300, 1958.
45. Lewis, R. M., and Schwartz, R. S. Canine systemic lupus erythematosus. Genetic analysis of an established breeding colony. *J. Exp. Med.*
134:417, 1971.
46. Mattioli, M., and Reichlin, M. Characterization of a soluble nuclear
ribonucleoprotein antigen reactive with SLE sera. *J. Immunol.* 107:
1281, 1971.
47. McCoy, R. C. Nuclear localization of immunoglobulins in renal
biopsies of patients with lupus nephritis. *Am. J. Pathol.* 68:469, 1972.
48. Miescher, P. Mise en evidence du facteur L.E. par la reaction de con-
sommation d'anti-globuline. *Vox Sang.* 5:116, 1955.
49. Moncada, B., Day, N. K. B., Good, R. A., and Windhorst, D. B. Lupus
erythematosus-like syndrome with a familial defect of complement.
N. Engl. J. Med. 286:689, 1972.
50. Muna, N. M., Verner, J. L., and Hammond, D. F. Fluorescent antibody technique as a routine procedure in the diagnosis of lupus erythematosus using stored tissue culture cells. *Am. J. Clin. Pathol.* 45:117,
1966.
51. Patrucco, A., Rothfield, N. F., and Hirschorn, K. The response of
cultured lymphocytes from patients with systemic lupus erythematosus
to DNA. *Arthritis Rheum.* 10:32, 1967.

52. Pincus, T., Schur, P. H., Rose, J. A., Decker, J. L., and Talal, N. Measurement of serum DNA-binding activity in systemic lupus erythematosus. *N. Engl. J. Med.* 281:701, 1969.
53. Reichlin, M., and Mattioli, M. Correlation of a precipitin reaction to a RNA protein antigen and low prevalence of nephritis in patients with systemic lupus erythematosus. *N. Engl. J. Med.* 286:408, 1972.
54. Ritchie, R. F. Antinucleolar antibodies. *N. Engl. J. Med.* 282:1174, 1970.
55. Rothfield, N., Ross, H. A., Minta, J. O., and Lepow, I. H. Glomerular and dermal deposition of properdin in systemic lupus erythematosus. *N. Engl. J. Med.* 287:681, 1972.
56. Ruddy, S., Klemperer, M. R., Rosen, F. S., Austen, K. F., and Kumate, J. Hereditary deficiency of the second component of complement (C2) in man: Correlation of C2 haemolytic activity with immunochemical measurements of C2 protein. *Immunology* 18:943, 1970.
57. Schur, P., Moroz, L. A., and Kunkel, H. G. Precipitating antibodies to ribosomes in the serum of patients with systemic lupus erythematosus. *Immunochemistry* 4:445, 1967.
58. Schur, P. H., and Monroe, W. Antibodies to ribonucleic acid in systemic lupus erythematosus. *Proc. Natl. Acad. Sci. U.S.A.* 63:1108, 1969.
59. Schur, P. H., Stoller, B. D., Steinberg, A. D., and Talal, N. Incidence of antibodies to double stranded RNA in systemic lupus erythematosus and related diseases. *Arthritis Rheum.* 14:342, 1971.
60. Sharp, G. C., Irvin, W. S., LaRoque, R. L., Velez, C., Daly, V., Kaiser, A. D., and Holman, H. R. Association of autoantibodies to different nuclear antigens with clinical patterns of rheumatic disease and responsiveness to therapy. *J. Clin. Invest.* 50:350, 1971.
61. Sharp, G. C., Irvin, W. S., Tan, E. M., Gould, R. G., and Holman, H. R. Mixed connective tissue disease: An apparently distinct rheumatic disease syndrome associated with a specific antibody to an extractable nuclear antigen (ENA). *Am. J. Med.* 52:148, 1972.
62. Shirai, T., and Mellors, R. C. Natural thymocytotoxic autoantibody and reactive antigen in New Zealand black and other mice. *Proc. Natl. Acad. Sci. U.S.A.* 68:1412, 1971.
63. Shirai, T., and Mellors, R. C. Natural cytotoxic autoantibody against thymocytes in NZB mice. *Clin. Exp. Immunol.* 12:133, 1972.
64. Shrank, A. B., and Doniach, D. Discoid lupus erythematosus; correlation of clinical features with serum autoantibody pattern. *Arch. Dermatol.* 87:677, 1963.
65. Stastny, P., and Ziff, M. Cold-insoluble complexes in complement levels in systemic lupus erythematosus. *N. Engl. J. Med.* 280:1376, 1969.
66. Steffen, C. Antibodies to tissues. In M. Stefanini (ed.), *Progress in Clinical Pathology.* New York: Grune & Stratton, 1970, vol. 3, p. 226.
67. Stollar, D., Levine, L., and Marmur, J. Antibodies to denatured desoxyribonucleic acid in lupus erythematosus serum: II. Characterization of antibodies in several sera. *Biochim. Biophys. Acta* 61:7, 1962.
68. Tan, E. M., and Kunkel, H. G. Characteristics of a soluble nuclear antigen precipitating with sera of patients with systemic lupus erythematosus. *J. Immunol.* 96:464, 1966.

69. Tan, E. M., Schur, P. H., Can, R. I., and Kunkel, H. G.   Deoxyribo-
    nucleic acid (DNA) and antibodies to DNA in the serum of patients
    with systemic lupus erythematosus. *J. Clin. Invest.* 45:1732, 1966.
70. Tan, E. M.   An immunologic precipitin system between soluble nucleo-
    protein and serum antibody in systemic lupus erythematosus. *J. Clin.
    Invest.* 46:735, 1967.
71. Tan, E. M.   Relationship of nuclear staining patterns with precipitating
    antibodies in systemic lupus erythematosus. *J. Clin. Lab. Med.* 70:800,
    1967.
72. Tan, E. M.   Antibodies to deoxyribonucleic acid irradiated with ultra-
    violet light: Detection by precipitin and immunofluorescence. *Science*
    161:1353, 1968.
73. Tan, E. M.   The influence of hydralazine on nuclear antigen-antibody
    reactions. *Arthritis Rheum.* 11:515, 1968.
74. Tan, E. M.   Scripps Clinic and Research Foundation. Personal com-
    munication, 1972.
75. TenVeen, J. H., and Feltkamp, T. E. W.   Formalinized chicken red
    cell nuclei as a simple antigen for standardized antinuclear factor de-
    termination. *Clin. Exp. Immunol.* 5:673, 1969.
76. Terasaki, P. I., Mottironi, V. D., and Barnett, E. V.   Cytotoxins in
    disease—autocytotoxins in lupus. *N. Engl. J. Med.* 283:724, 1970.
77. Widelock, D., Gilbert, C., Siegel, M., and Lee, S.   Fluorescent anti-
    body procedure for lupus erythematosus: Comparative use of nucleated
    erythrocytes and calf thymus cells. *Am. J. Public Health* 51:829, 1961.
78. Wold, R. T., Young, F. E., Tan, E. M., and Farr, R. S.   Desoxyribo-
    nucleic acid antibody: A method to detect its primary interaction with
    desoxyribonucleic acid. *Science* 161:806, 1968.
79. Zvaifler, N. J., and Martinez, M. M.   Antinuclear factors and chronic
    articular inflammation. *Clin. Exp. Immunol.* 8:271, 1971.

10

Immunologic Tests in the Diagnosis of Autoallergic Liver Disorders

Introduction and Classification of Autoallergic Liver Diseases

In liver diseases, the concept of a primary autoallergic disorder is a speculative one. Experimentally, immunization of animals with liver extracts has not given rise to a convincing form of hepatitis or progressive cirrhosis, and definite liver specific antibodies have not been demonstrated [29]. Experimental liver tissue damage has been induced by non-liver specific antigen-antibody complexes [28], which can exert a local cytotoxic effect by binding complement.

However, there is increasing evidence that there are various forms of human liver disease which are characterized by underlying processes closely associated with autoimmune phenomenon and can be accepted as autoallergic disorders [17]. The three chronic liver syndromes are (a) primary biliary cirrhosis; (b) active chronic hepatitis ("lupoid" hepatitis or juvenile cirrhosis); and (c) cryptogenic cirrhosis.

Primary biliary cirrhosis is a progressive disease seen most commonly in women in the second half of their reproductive period. There is progressive evidence of jaundice with relative well being, and late development of cirrhosis. The characteristic liver lesion is nonsuppurative necrosis of bile ducts which may progress to an advanced cirrhosis histologically indistinguishable from other forms of cirrhosis (Fig. 10-1). This disorder has characteristic immunologic features particularly in the early stages [5, 6, 7, 20]. A relatively high titer of nonspecific antimitochondrial antibodies is seen. In addition, often other antibodies noted are antinuclear, rheumatoid factor, and anti-liver duct antibodies. A specific etiology in primary biliary cirrhosis has not been established, and some cases seem to follow viral hepatitis or obstructive biliary tract disease.

Active chronic hepatitis is a disease of unknown etiology, predominantly in young women, which has a progressive course characterized by

289

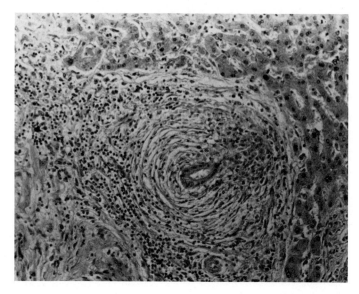

Figure 10-1
Microscopic section of liver lesion in primary biliary cirrhosis. There is a
nonsuppurative inflammatory necrosis of the bile duct epithelium with surrounding mononuclear inflammatory cells. (H&E stain; 100× before 20%
reduction.)

laboratory, clinical, and histologic features of both acute and chronic
hepatitis [22]. Depending upon the stage, signs of cirrhosis may be
present, but the characteristic lesion is the so-called "piecemeal" necrosis.
This is characterized by infiltration of the portal tracts by lymphoid cells,
plasma cells, histiocytes, and fibroblasts as well as proliferation of bile
ductules. The limiting plate of liver parenchymal cells is disrupted, and
the inflammatory cells are in close approximation to the liver cells with
individual cell necrosis (Fig. 10-2).

Active chronic hepatitis is usually associated with a variety of systemic and serologic reactions. If associated with a positive LE cell test,
the disease is often called *lupoid hepatitis*. The etiologic role of hepatitis
virus or viruses in the initiation of certain diseases in active chronic
hepatitis is under active investigation. The finding of Australia antigen in
some cases of active chronic hepatitis suggests that a chronic viral infection is present [17].

Cryptogenic cirrhosis undoubtedly represents a heterologous group
of liver diseases resulting from a number of unrelated injuries [7].
There is no history of acute liver damage in these cases (Fig. 10-3).

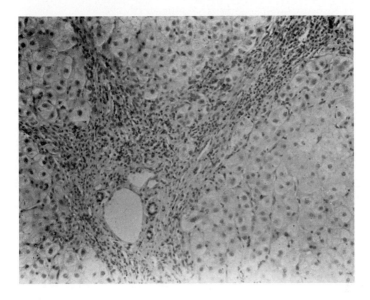

Figure 10-2
Microscopic section of liver lesion in chronic active hepatitis. There is evidence of necrosis and fibrosis in the periphery of the liver lobule adjacent to the portal areas. The limiting plate of liver parenchymal cells is disrupted, and the inflammatory cells are in close approximation to the liver cells with individual cell necrosis. (H&E section; 40× before 20% reduction.)

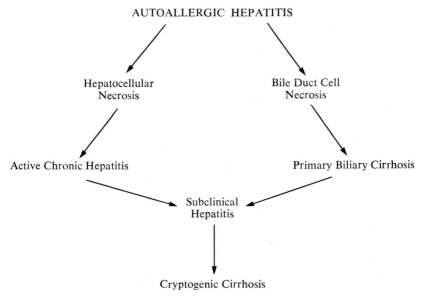

Figure 10-3
Autoallergic hepatitis. (Modified from Doniach and Walker [6].)

Common Immunologic Tests and Autoantibodies in Liver Diseases

Various serologic techniques have been used in the study of liver diseases [36]. Among the methods have been complement fixation, colloidin-particle reaction, passive hemagglutination, antiglobulin consumption test, and immunofluorescence. Antigens for the tests have varied from water, saline, and phenol-water extracts of liver to homogenates of liver, sections of liver and other tissues, and subcellular fractions of liver and other organs. Various different types of antibody are found in patients with liver disease.

Serologic techniques have proved of diagnostic value in the differentiation of primary biliary cirrhosis and long-lasting extrahepatic biliary occlusion and in the diagnosis of chronic active hepatitis. Of the several tests available, the immunofluorescence tests are easily performed in most clinical laboratories and will be discussed in further detail.

The following types of autoantibodies have been reported in the autoallergic liver diseases [36]: (a) antinuclear antibodies, (b) antimitochondrial antibody, (c) anti-smooth muscle antibody, (d) antiglomerular antibody, and (e) anti-bile duct antibody.

Antinuclear Antibodies

Antinuclear antibodies are detected in 75% of patients with chronic active hepatitis, 46% of patients with primary biliary cirrhosis, and 38% of those with cryptogenic cirrhosis. Positive LE cell tests are found in a high incidence of chronic active hepatitis, and often the disease is classified as lupoid hepatitis. Antinuclear antibodies are found in primary biliary cirrhosis patients in a higher percentage than in controls [5]. Antinuclear antibodies showing fluorescent patterns of diffuse, speckled nucleolar types are all seen in the autoallergic liver disorders.

Antimitochondrial Antibody

This antibody is non-organ and non-species specific, and is directed against a lipoprotein constituent of mitochondrial inner membrane. It occurs in 94% of patients with primary biliary cirrhosis and in 3% of the *acute* cases of extrahepatic biliary tract obstruction [5, 7]. Positive antimitochondrial antibody tests were observed in chronic cases of extrahepatic biliary obstruction during the third month of obstruction [21]. The antibody is found in all the immunoglobulin fractions [29] and is complement fixing [2]. The antigen is found on the inner membrane of the mitochondria and contains a lipid substance. The mitochondrial antigen is destroyed by fixation with lipid solvents (ethanol, butanol, acetone) and protein fixatives. The antibodies are adsorbed by purified preparations of mitochondria, and there seems to be a high correlation between antigen content and the enzyme succinic dehydrogenase [1] (Fig. 10-4).

In primary biliary cirrhosis, the level of antimitochondrial antibodies in the serum varies from a trace to very high titers. In patients followed for several years, the level of antimitochondrial antibodies has no relation to the severity or duration of the disease. The antibody level did not necessarily decrease after treatment with corticoids and immunosuppressive agents [7]. The exact role of the antimitochondrial antibodies in the pathogenesis of primary biliary cirrhosis is unknown.

Anti-Smooth Muscle Antibody
The antibody is non-organ specific and non-species specific. The anti-smooth muscle antibodies are not complement fixing, and are of the IgG and IgM type. Although anti-smooth muscle antibodies are found in all three chronic liver disorders, they are found mainly in active chronic hepatitis. The role of the antibody in the pathogenesis of chronic liver disease is unknown. They are seen in less than 2% of normal subjects [41, 42]. The anti-smooth muscle antibody is helpful in differentiating

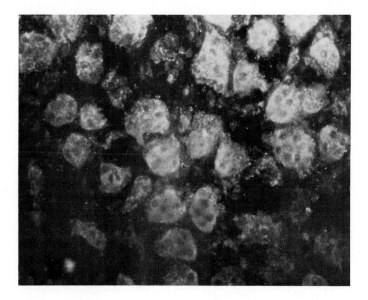

Figure 10-4
Positive indirect fluorescence test for antimitochondrial antibody. Substrate tissue is unfixed rat kidney. The section was first reacted with serum containing antimitochondrial antibody and then reacted with fluorescein isothiocyanate-labeled goat anti-human immunoglobulin. Note the bright granular fluorescence of cytoplasm of the kidney tubular cells. (Approximately 150× before 20% reduction.)

active chronic hepatitis from systemic lupus erythematosus, as anti-smooth muscle antibodies are not usually seen in systemic lupus, whereas the positive LE cell phenomenon is often observed in active chronic hepatitis.

Anti-smooth muscle antibodies of the IgM or IgG type were found in acute viral hepatitis [14]. The antibody was found independently of Australia antigen, and is probably more directly related to liver cell damage than to the presence of Australia antigen. The anti-smooth muscle antibody found in human hepatitis is reactive with a component resembling smooth muscle actomyosin present in liver cells as well as in other cells [15]. It is possible that viral infection of liver cells reveals or alters liver cell components which become autoantigenic [15]. Anti-smooth muscle antibodies are also found in infectious mononucleosis and other viral diseases, as well as in patients with proved malignancy [18] (Fig. 10-5).

Liver cells and other cells probably contain antigen in the cell membrane related to smooth muscle actomyosin [15, 18]. The smooth muscle-like antigen is not accessible to the surface of normal liver cells; however, the antigen can be exposed by treatment of monolayers of liver cells with isopentane at the temperature of liquid nitrogen [15]. The exposed antigen is then readily reactive with anti-smooth muscle antibody.

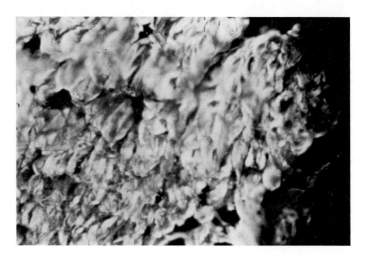

Figure 10-5
Positive indirect fluorescence test for anti-smooth muscle antibody. The substrate consists of unfixed rat stomach. The section was first reacted with serum containing anti-smooth muscle antibody. After washing, the section was reacted with fluorescein isothiocyanate-labeled goat anti-human immunoglobulin. The smooth muscle fibers of the stomach wall show a bright fluorescence. (100× before 20% reduction.)

Antiglomerular Antibody

Sera containing anti-smooth muscle antibodies have been noted to stain renal glomeruli [42] and liver cells themselves in a polygonal pattern [18]. When the serum-containing anti-smooth muscle antibody was adsorbed with extracts containing human smooth muscle actomyosin, the three patterns of staining of smooth muscle, kidney glomerular, and polygonal liver tissue were abolished [18]. The other autoantibodies present in the serum, such as antinuclear antibodies, were not affected by absorption with smooth muscle tissue (Fig. 10-6).

Serum from 61% of the cases of chronic active hepatitis with positive LE cell tests reacted with cells of the renal glomeruli of man and rat by the indirect immunofluorescence test [42]. In these cases, microscopic evidence of membranous glomerular lesions has been observed. The antiglomerular antibody is most likely directed toward the basement membrane of the kidney. However, many cases of lupoid hepatitis with antiglomerular antibody do not develop nephritis, while nephritis is a frequent complication of systemic lupus erythematosus. Further, in

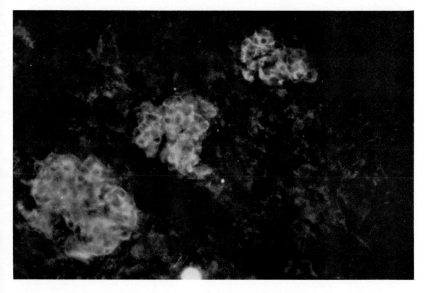

Figure 10-6
Positive indirect fluorescence test for antiglomerular antibody in a case of chronic active hepatitis with anti-smooth muscle antibody. The substrate is unfixed rat kidney, first reacted with test serum. The section is washed and then reacted with fluorescein isothiocyanate-labeled goat anti-human immunoglobulin. The sections show a linear pattern of fluorescence of glomerular membrane (100× before 5% reduction). The antiglomerular antibody seen in liver disease cross reacts with smooth muscle tissue and is not associated with glomerulonephritis.

systemic lupus erythematosus, there is an absence of antiglomerular antibody. In systemic lupus erythematosus, there is deposition of anti-gen-antibody complexes (often DNA–anti-DNA) in the glomeruli. The antiglomerular antibody in lupoid hepatitis may play a protective role, but the exact role remains to be elucidated.

Anti-Bile Duct Antibody

Antibodies to epithelial cells of bile ductules and/or mitochondria can be seen with immunofluorescence tests in 71 to 90% of cases with primary biliary cirrhosis, but in practically no cases with extrahepatic obstruction. Alcoholic cirrhosis and postnecrotic cirrhosis have been reported to demonstrate antibodies reactive with duct tissue of liver by immunofluorescence in about one-fourth of the cases [25].

Antibodies to bile canaliculi were observed in 16 of 24 patients with active chronic liver disease, but were rarely observed in other hepatic diseases [13]. Active chronic liver disease was defined as a disease lasting for more than 6 months with the histologic appearance of chronic aggressive hepatitis, chronic persistent hepatitis, and cirrhosis [13]. The anti-bile duct canalicular antibody was demonstrated in serum samples by an indirect immunofluorescence technique with use of frozen bovine liver sections and found to be predominantly in IgG immunoglobulin [13, 24]. In one half of the cases, the antibody reacted with normal human liver as well as bovine liver tissue. The bile canalicular antibody was often observed with anti-nuclear antibodies but infrequently seen in the presence of mitochondrial antibody [13].

Serum Immunoglobulins and Autoallergic Liver Diseases

In most chronic parenchymal liver diseases, there is elevation of all three major immunoglobulins [16]. IgG is most prominently elevated in chronic active hepatitis. Serum IgA elevations were observed in primary biliary cirrhosis, cryptogenic cirrhosis, and chronic active hepatitis [22]. Serum IgM level may reach as high as our 1,000 mg per 100 ml in primary biliary cirrhosis [22]. Significant elevations of IgM were also seen in patients with cryptogenic cirrhosis.

Cell-Mediated Immunity in Active Chronic Hepatitis and Primary Biliary Cirrhosis

No primary role has been demonstrated for circulating antibodies in the production of lesions observed in liver disease. However, cell-mediated immunity may play a significant role in autoallergic liver disease [11].

Smith and co-workers [34] measured delayed sensitivity responses to liver antigens in vitro in cases of active chronic hepatitis and primary biliary cirrhosis. The method employed for the study was the leukocyte migration test described by Søbørg [35]. In the modified technique employed by Smith et al. [34],

1. High molecular weight dextran was used to sediment red cells and separate leukocytes from the peripheral blood of patients.
2. The leukocytes were washed in Hank's balanced salt solution and packed into capillary tubes and incubated in tissue culture medium for 20 hours.
3. The cells migrate to form circular areas on the coverslip.
4. The migration index is calculated by dividing the mean area of migration in the antigen container. A figure of less than 1.0 is indicative of inhibition of migration.

In the studies of Smith et al. [34], the liver antigen was prepared as follows:

1. Fresh human fetal liver obtained at autopsy was pooled.
2. The liver is homogenized in an equal volume of Hank's balanced salt solution and centrifuged at 1,500 g for 20 min.
3. The supernatant is used as antigen in concentrations of 40–400 μg of protein per ml of tissue culture medium.

Inhibition of migration of leukocytes to fetal liver antigens was noted in a significant number of patients with active chronic hepatitis and primary biliary cirrhosis [34]. Negative results were seen in cases of inactive cirrhosis and of extrahepatic biliary obstruction, and in controls. Only one of 16 cases of acute viral hepatitis demonstrated inhibition of migration.

The above studies demonstrate that there are delayed sensitivity responses to fetal liver antigens in cases of active chronic hepatitis and primary biliary cirrhosis. Further cell-mediated sensitivity studies are needed with purified liver antigens to increase the sensitivity and specificity of the response.

Immunofluorescence Test for Antimitochondrial Antibody

PROCEDURE.   Many different sources of tissues may be used for substrate, since the antibody is non-organ and non-species specific. The rat or mouse kidney substrate used for the antinuclear antibody test has worked very well for the detection of antimitochrondrial antibodies. Fresh *unfixed* sections of rat kidney were used. Tests are performed on both a 1:1 and 1:10 dilution of serum. Also anti-C3 complement conjugate may be used, since the antibody usually fixes complement. In the latter test, fresh human serum is added to the test serum for a source of complement.

1. 3 mm cross sections of fresh rat kidney are snap frozen in dry ice or acetone as outlined in the procedure for detection of antinuclear antibodies.

2. 5 μ sections of fresh rat kidney are cut with the use of a cryostat.
3. The sections are used fresh and *unfixed* and reacted with serum for 30 min at room temperature. Excess serum is first removed by a rinse and then followed by 2 separate 5-min washings in buffered saline solution (pH 7.0, phosphate 0.01 M).
4. Fluorescein-conjugated antiserum to human immunoglobulins is then applied to the section for 30 min at room temperature. The sections are first rinsed and then washed twice in buffered saline solution for 8 min each. Polyvalent fluorescein-labeled antiserum to human IgG, IgM, and IgA may be used, or separate tests may be performed with anti-IgM and anti-IgG labeled antisera, respectively.
5. The sections are mounted in buffered glycerol and examined with a fluorescence microscope equipped with standard filters.

INTERPRETATION OF TEST.   M fluorescence pattern is the abbreviation used for the fluorescence pattern observed in the detection of antimitochondrial antibodies characteristically seen in cases of primary biliary cirrhosis and in some cases of active chronic hepatitis and cryptogenic cirrhosis [9, 10, 22]. Positive tests with M fluorescence show a bright and densely granular fluorescence, maximal over the entire cytoplasm in distal renal tubular cells [9]. Antimitochondrial antibodies are found in 90% or more of patients with primary biliary cirrhosis, often in very high titer cases, and in 25 to 30% of patients with active chronic hepatitis and cryptogenic cirrhosis. The level of antimitochondrial antibodies in the serum in primary biliary cirrhosis may vary from trace amounts to titers of 1:6,000 in the fluorescence test [7]. Ten percent have low titers of less than 1:16 with a negative complement fixation test [7, 8]. The antibody has not been recovered from the bile, and antibody levels have usually remained constant on repeated testing. The level of antibody did not correlate with the severity or duration of the disease. A small percentage of patients with primary biliary cirrhosis had negative tests for antimitochondrial antibodies, and their clinical and histologic features could be distinguished from those of patients with high levels of antibodies.

Antimitochondrial antibodies are usually absent in jaundice patients with acute extrahepatic obstruction, drug sensitivity, and viral hepatitis, and thus the test is helpful in the differentiation of surgical and nonsurgical cases of obstructive jaundice. Cases of chronic extrahepatic obstruction of two and one-half months' duration may show a positive test for antimitochondrial antibodies [21]. In patients developing jaundice due to chlorpromazine or halothane sensitivity, a low titer of (less than 1:20) antimitochondrial antibody may be seen which disappears upon recovery [31]. The antibody is usually absent in alcoholic cirrhosis. Antimitochondrial antibodies are not found in normal people, and an incidence of 1% has been reported in a mixed hospital population. Most of the positive reactors have some sort of collagen or other autoimmune disease [7]. Ludwig and co-workers [22] feel that the antimitochondrial antibody test is useful diagnostically, the antibody being present in 8 patients with proved primary biliary cirrhosis in a titer of 1:160, yet absent in 17 patients with proved bile duct obstruction.

Cardiolipin Fluorescent Antibody (CLF) and Its Relation to Mitochondrial M Antigen

The classic Wasserman antibodies which react with cardiolipin do not usually demonstrate a positive mitochondrial fluorescence test when applied to tissue sections. However, certain untreated cases of active secondary syphilis may produce a positive mitochondrial staining pattern resembling primary biliary cirrhosis sera which can be completely abolished with purified cardiolipin or VDRL antigen [10]. The M fluorescence patterns of primary biliary cirrhosis generally give negative reactions in serologic tests for syphilis and are unaffected by cardiolipin absorption [10]. Cardiolipin, which is a phospholipid present in the inner mitochondrial membrane, is very close to the separate but distinct M antigen. There are qualitative differences in the staining patterns of M and CLF antibodies in the indirect fluorescence test. The cardiolipin fluorescent (CLF) antibodies of active secondary syphilis show diffuse cytoplasmic staining with indefinite edges on most tissues, whereas the M antibodies of primary biliary cirrhosis show a dense granularity [10].

Mitochondrial Antibodies and Chronic Biologic False Positive Reactions in Syphilis

Mitochondrial antibodies of low titer (M fluorescence) similar to those seen in primary biliary cirrhosis and predominantly of IgM class were found in 51% of 41 patients with chronic false positive reactions for syphilis in the absence of detectable liver disease [9]. The presence of M fluorescence in the biological false positive test for syphilis is correlated with systemic disease. This test, along with those for antinuclear and other autoantibodies, may be helpful in the diagnosis of unusual connective tissue and so-called autoimmune disorders. These cases are complex since only one-half of patients with low VDRL titers with a collagen disorder had a mitochondrial fluorescence which was not abolished by adsorption of the individual serum with VDRL antigen [10].

Immunofluorescence Test for Anti-Smooth Muscle Antibody

MATERIALS AND REAGENTS

A. Tissues: Fresh rat stomach or human uterine cervical from blood group O, snap frozen
B. Cryostat
C. Glass slides
D. Test serum
E. Moist chamber

F. Buffered saline solution (pH 7.0, phosphate 0.01 M)
G. Fluorescein-conjugated antiserum to human IgG and IgM
H. Buffered glycerol (for slide mounts)
 I. Fluorescence microscope

Antibodies, which are not usually complement fixing, may be either
IgM or IgG. The nature of the antigen is unknown. The staining is
abolished by pretreatment of the secretion with acid citrate (pH 3.2)
buffer and formalin but not by some lipid solvents or acetone [29].
Serum is tested at a 1:2 and 1:10 dilution with use of an indirect immunofluorescence method.

PROCEDURE
1. Fresh tissue is obtained from rat stomach or human uterine cervical
    tissue from patients of blood group O, and snap frozen. It is ad-
    visable to use fresh tissue since the smooth muscle antigen is unstable.
2. 5 μ sections of fresh rat stomach or human cervical tissue are cut
    with the use of a cryostat.
3. The sections are mounted on a clean glass slide and used *unfixed*.
    The test serum is overlayed onto the section and incubated at room
    temperature for 30 min in a moist chamber.
4. The excess serum is removed by a rinse and then followed by two
    separate 5-min washings in buffered saline solution.
5. Fluorescein-conjugated antiserum to human IgG and IgM is applied
    to different sections for 30 min at room temperature in a moist
    chamber.
6. The sections are first rinsed and then washed in two 8-min washings
    twice in phosphate buffered saline solution.
7. The sections are mounted in buffered glycerol and examined with a
    fluorescence microscope.

Specificity of smooth muscle antibody may be checked by (a) use of
different types of muscle antigens; (b) use of normal control serum; or
(c) absorption of test serum by homogenates of human uterus, liver
(which contains very little smooth muscle), and human AB cells.

INTERPRETATION OF TEST. A positive test shows diffuse staining of
the muscle layers of the vessels, muscularis mucosae, and muscle coat
in both unfixed and acetone-fixed slides.
      Sera which give a bright staining pattern for anti-smooth muscle
antibody at titers of up to 1:100 or more are usually from patients with
chronic active hepatitis whose liver biopsies show characteristic portal
tract mononuclear inflammatory cell infiltration with destruction of
adjacent liver cells and accompanying fibrosis [18].
      Anti-smooth muscle antibodies in chronic liver disorders associated
with autoimmune phenomenon or active chronic hepatitis (lupoid) and
primary biliary cirrhosis are usually non-complement fixing. They are

seen in less than 2% of normal subjects. A uniform fluorescence of all smooth muscle fibers, including vascular and uterine muscle, is seen and is quite distinct from that found in myasthenia gravis. The anti-smooth muscle antibody was demonstrated in the serum of 28 of 34 cases (82%) of active chronic hepatitis with positive LE cell phenomenon (lupoid hepatitis) and in 9 of 19 or 48% of active chronic hepatitis [41, 42]. In 42 cases of systemic lupus erythematosus with positive tests for antinuclear factor, none were positive for anti-smooth muscle antibody [41]. The anti-smooth muscle antibody tended to accompany the antinuclear factor in chronic active hepatitis. A positive anti-smooth antibody test may be seen in a wide variety of conditions besides a primary liver disease, as discussed below.

Anti-Smooth Muscle Antibody and Viral Infections
Anti-smooth muscle antibodies of the IgM and IgG types were found in acute viral hepatitis [14]. The anti-smooth muscle antibody of acute viral hepatitis is usually predominantly of IgM class and the titers seldom exceed 1:80 [18]. In 39 unselected patients with acute infectious hepatitis, the anti-smooth muscle antibody was found in 87% and hepatitis-associated antigen was noted in 33% [14]. Anti-smooth muscle antibody was found independently of Australia antigen (hepatitis-associated antigen), and is probably more directly related to liver cell damage than to the presence of Australia antigen. Anti-smooth muscle antibodies may appear independently from either antinuclear factor or antimitochondrial antibody. However, the anti-smooth muscle antibody and antinuclear antibody titers used together may be helpful in selecting patients with chronic active (lupoid) hepatitis for immunosuppressive therapy [22].

Positive tests for anti-smooth muscle antibody have been seen in infectious mononucleosis [18]. Of those sera positive for heterophile antibody, 80% were positive for anti-smooth muscle antibody at titers from 1:20 to 1:320, often for both IgG and IgM [18]. Nine percent of infectious mononucleosis cases showed anti-smooth muscle antibody at a titer of 1:10.

ANTI-SMOOTH MUSCLE ANTIBODY AND TUMORS. Anti-smooth muscle antibody appears to be present in a majority of patients with malignant tumors [40]. In 80 patients with diagnosed malignant tumors, anti-smooth muscle antibody titers of 1:10 or more were noted in 67% of 80 patients and 20% of 46 normal control subjects [40]. The incidence ranged from 60% in malignant melanoma to 83% in carcinoma of the ovary. Both IgG and IgM types of anti-smooth muscle antibody were detected.

ANTI-SMOOTH MUSCLE ANTIBODY AND INTRINSIC ASTHMA. Serum IgG and IgM anti-smooth muscle antibodies have been reported in 21%

of patients with intrinsic asthma, contrasting with an incidence of 2.9% and 3.7% in extrinsic asthma and chronic bronchitis, respectively. The antibody is neither species nor organ specific and does not cross react with cardiac or skeletal muscle [39]. The titers were usually low and ranged from 1:10 to 1:20. In vitro complement fixation of the antibody was demonstrated in sera obtained from several patients. The pattern of fluorescence is distinct from that commonly seen in patients with liver disease. The fluorescence pattern has a "streaky" appearance surrounding the surface of individual smooth muscle fibers.

Relationship of Australia and Milan Antigens to Autoantibodies in Chronic Hepatitis

Australia Antigen

In a study of 110 patients with chronic hepatitis, no definite relationship between Australia antigen and anti-smooth muscle and antimitochondrial antibodies was seen [38]. Thirty-three patients with chronic hepatitis who demonstrated both antimitochondrial and anti-smooth muscle antibody had Australia antigen when tested by a modified micro-Ouchterlony immunodiffusion technique [38]. Twenty-two of 78 (28%) patients with chronic hepatitis who were positive for Australia antigen had no evidence of autoantibodies.

Milan Antigen

The Milan antigen is a new antigen detected by gel diffusion, with an antiserum obtained from a multiply transfused patient [3]. The antiserum to Milan antigen produces a precipitin line by gel diffusion when it reacts with sera from patients with both long and short incubation hepatitis [3, 4]. The Milan antiserum contains at least two antibodies, one related to SH or long incubation hepatitis, and another related to short incubation hepatitis. The Milan antigen has been referred to as epidemic hepatitis-associated antigen (EHAA) [4].

The Milan antigen is labile at $-20°$ C and does not survive storage at $-20°$ C for a long period [3]. The sedimentation coefficient of the Milan particle was from 11 to 14S, and the antigen appears to differ from HAA in its molecular properties [4]. The Milan antigen has a high lipid content and may represent an abnormal lipoprotein rather than a virus-related component [11, 37].

Doniach and co-workers [12] have noted that the Milan antigen has been detected in 38% of 94 primary biliary cirrhosis cases irrespective of the degree of obstructive jaundice or the presence of lipoprotein X [32, 33] in the serum. There is no definite correlation of the Milan antigen with the various autoimmune antibodies in liver disease. Patients with high titers of antinuclear and anti-smooth muscle antibodies often were negative for virus associated antigens [11].

Approach to the Use of Laboratory Tests for the Diagnosis and Therapy of Autoallergic Liver Diseases

In suspected cases of *autoallergic liver diseases,* the following tests are helpful in addition to the various biochemical liver function tests: (a) antimitochondrial antibody, (b) anti-smooth muscle antibody, (c) antinuclear antibody, (d) Australia antigen, (e) heterophile antibody test for infectious mononucleosis, and (f) protein electrophoresis (immunoelectrophoresis) serum immunoglobulin quantitation.

A. In cases of primary biliary cirrhosis, a titer of 1:160 or greater of antimitochondrial antibody is practically diagnostic [19]. Ten percent of cases of primary biliary cirrhosis may have titers less than 1:16 of antimitochondrial antibody [7, 8]. Antimitochondrial antibody provides reliable confirmatory evidence of primary biliary cirrhosis when the biopsy findings are consistent [20].

   Antimitochondrial antibodies are usually absent in jaundiced patients with acute extrahepatic obstruction, drug sensitivity, and viral hepatitis. The test is helpful in the differentiation of surgical and nonsurgical jaundice. However, in chronic cases of extrahepatic obstruction, the antimitochondrial antibody test may be positive [21].

B. Anti-smooth muscle antibodies are observed not only in the various autoallergic liver diseases but in other diseases such as viral hepatitis, infectious mononucleosis, malignancy, and intrinsic bronchial asthma.

   In cases of chronic active hepatitis, an anti-smooth muscle antibody titer of 1:100 or more indicates an active and progressive lesion in the liver [18]. The test for anti-smooth muscle antibody is helpful in differentiating chronic active lupoid hepatitis from systemic lupus erythematosus. Cases of systemic lupus erythematosus are usually negative for anti-smooth muscle antibodies.

C. The antinuclear antibody test may be used as a screening test for autoimmune factors in liver disease since antinuclear antibodies are present in a wide variety of diseases including the autoallergic liver diseases. The antinuclear antibody titer is helpful since patients with chronic active hepatitis with titers of 1:20 or greater are likely subjects for immunosuppressive treatment [22].

D. The Australia antigen test aids in the diagnosis of varying states of serum hepatitis infection.

E. Heterophile antibody tests for infectious mononucleosis are helpful since infectious mononucleosis patients may demonstrate anti-smooth muscle antibody titers from 1:10 to 1:320 [18].

F. Serum protein electrophoresis and immunoelectrophoresis are helpful in the assessment of serum protein abnormalities. Quantitations of immunoglobulins are helpful. Various types of autoallergic liver diseases demonstrate IgA elevation; IgM elevations are suggestive of primary biliary cirrhosis; and moderate increases in IgG concentrations are most often seen in chronic active (lupoid) hepatitis [22]. In most chronic parenchymal liver diseases, elevation of all three immunoglobulins of IgG, IgM, and IgA type is present.

Liver biopsy studies are important and cannot be overemphasized. Other studies such as immunofluorescence and electron microscopy for the detection of Australia antigen or hepatitis-associated antigen and immune complexes in tissue are helpful [19, 25].

Laboratory Tests in the Therapy of Autoallergic Liver Disease
Patients with chronic active hepatitis with positive anti-smooth muscle antibody of 1:100 or greater and an antinuclear antibody titer of 1:20 or greater in the active phase of the disease should be seriously considered for immunosuppressive treatment. Therapy should be started early in the course of the illness before progressive irreversible cirrhosis has developed [22]. Patients with primary biliary cirrhosis have not responded to immunosuppressive treatment as well as patients with chronic active hepatitis [22].

Summary and Possible Pathogenesis of Autoallergic Liver Diseases

Immunologic tests have diagnostic value in the differentiation between primary biliary cirrhosis and long-lasting extrahepatic biliary cirrhosis, and in the diagnosis of active chronic hepatitis (lupoid hepatitis). Antibodies to mitochondria can be demonstrated with immunofluorescence tests in 71 to 90% of cases with primary biliary cirrhosis, but they are rare in cases of acute extrahepatic biliary obstruction. The incidence of antimitochondrial antibodies in active chronic hepatitis varies from 28 to 30%, whereas positive results are found in 8% of cases of acute or chronic hepatitis of other origin. Antimitochondrial antibodies of low titer may be seen in patients with chronic false positive reactions for syphilis in the absence of detectable liver disease. The antinuclear antibody test is a useful screening test for autoimmune factors in liver disease since a high incidence of antinuclear antibodies is seen in the autoallergic liver disorders.

The anti-smooth muscle antibody was demonstrated in 82% of cases of active chronic hepatitis with a positive LE cell phenomenon, and in 48% of active chronic hepatitis. The anti-smooth muscle antibody tended to accompany the antinuclear factor in active chronic hepatitis. Surprisingly, the anti-smooth muscle antibody is absent in cases of systemic lupus erythematosus with significant levels of antinuclear antibody.

The anti-smooth muscle antibody has been noted in cases of acute viral hepatitis and appears to correlate with liver cell damage. It is extremely puzzling that anti-smooth muscle antibody is also seen in a wide variety of other diseases.

The role of the various circulating antibodies in the pathogenesis of the autoallergic liver disease is unknown. There is no definite correlation between the level of the various antibodies and the severity or duration of the liver disease process. Similarly, no definite relationship between the autoantibodies and Australia antigen in chronic liver disease is seen. Evidence is accumulating that cellular sensitivity to liver antigens may play a role in the pathogenesis of the autoallergic liver diseases. There is much speculation that viruses or drugs cause alteration of liver tissue. The resulting inflammation and immune response evoke release of sequestered antigens of mitochondrial and liver cell membranes which give rise to non-organ specific autoantibodies reactive with mitochondrial membranes and smooth muscle actomyosin [8, 11, 18].

Oxyphenisatin, which is a common laxative, may be the etiologic factor in certain cases of chronic active hepatitis [30]. Improvement of the liver disease was seen when patients discontinued use of oxyphenisatin.

References

1. Berg, P. A., Doniach, D., and Roitt, I. M.   Mitochondrial antibodies in primary biliary cirrhosis: I. Localization of the antigen to mitochondrial membranes. *J. Exp. Med.* 126:277, 1967.
2. Berg, P. A., Roitt, I. M., Doniach, D., and Cooper, H. M.   Mitochondrial antibodies in primary biliary cirrhosis: IV. Significance of membrane structure for the complement fixing antigen. *Immunology* 17:281, 1969.
3. Del Prete, S., Constantino, D., Doglia, M., Grazuna, A., Ajdukiewicz, A., Dudley, F. J., Fox, R. A., and Sherlock, S.   Detection of a new serum antigen in three epidemics of short incubation hepatitis. *Lancet* 2:579, 1970.
4. Del Prete, S., Constantino, D., Doglia, M., Fabiani, M. P., Borin, R., and Jacini, A.   Epidemic hepatitis associated antigen (Milan antigen) study on normal population and sporadic acute viral hepatitis. *Am. J. Dis. Child.* 123:326, 1972.
5. Doniach, D., Roitt, I. M., Walker, J. G., and Sherlock, S.   Tissue antibodies in primary biliary cirrhosis, active chronic (lupoid) hepatitis, cryptogenic cirrhosis and other liver diseases and their clinical implications. *Clin. Exp. Immunol.* 1:237, 1966.
6. Doniach, D., and Walker, J. G.   A unified concept of autoimmune hepatitis. *Lancet* 1:813, 1969.
7. Doniach, D., Walker, J. G., Roitt, I. M., and Berg, P. A.   "Autoallergic" hepatitis. *N. Engl. J. Med.* 282:86, 1970.
8. Doniach, D.   The concept of an autoallergic hepatitis. *Proc. R. Soc. Med.* 63:21, 1970.

9. Doniach, D., Delhanty, J., Lindqvist, H. J., and Catterall, R. D. Mitochondrial and other tissue antibodies in patients with biological false positive reactions for syphilis. *Clin. Exp. Immunol.* 6:871, 1971.
10. Doniach, D., Lindqvist, H. L., and Berg, P. A. Nonorgan specific cytoplasmic antibodies detected by immunofluorescence. *Int. Arch. Allergy Appl. Immunol.* 41:501, 1971.
11. Doniach, D. Autoimmune aspects of liver disease. *Br. Med. Bull.* 28:145, 1972.
12. Doniach, D., Del Prete, S., Dane, D. S., and Walsh, J. H. Viral hepatitis related antigens in autoimmune hepatic disorders. *Can. Med. Assoc. J.* 106:513, 1972.
13. Diederichsen,, H., Linde, N. C., Møller-Nielsen, P. Antibodies to bile canaliculi in patients with chronic active liver disease. In M. Smith and R. Williams (eds.), *Immunology of the Liver*. Philadelphia: Davis, 1971, p. 82.
14. Farrow, L. J., Holborow, E. J., Johnson, G. D., Lamb, S. E., Stewart, J. S., Taylor, P. E., and Zuckerman, A. J. Autoantibodies and the hepatitis associated antigen in acute infective hepatitis. *Br. Med. J.* 2:693, 1970.
15. Farrow, L. J., Holborow, E. J., and Brighton, W. D. Reaction of smooth muscle antibody with liver cells. *Nature [New Biol.]* 232:186, 1971.
16. Feizi, T. Immunoglobulins in chronic liver disease. *Gut* 9:193, 1968.
17. Gitnick, G. L., Gleich, G. J., Schoenfield, L. J., Baggenstoss, A. H., Sutnick, A. L., Blumberg, B. S., London, W. E., and Summerskill, W. H. J. Australia antigen in chronic active liver disease with cirrhosis. *Lancet* 2:285, 1969.
18. Holborow, E. J. Smooth muscle autoantibodies, viral infections and malignant disease. *Proc. R. Soc. Med.* 65:481, 1972.
19. Huang, S. M., Millman, I., O'Connell, A., Aronoff, A., Gault, H., and Blumberg, B. S. Virus-like particles in Australia antigen associated hepatitis: An immunoelectron microscopic study of human liver. *Am. J. Pathol.* 67:453, 1972.
20. Klatskin, G., and Kantor, F. S. Mitochondrial antibody in primary biliary cirrhosis and other diseases. *Ann. Intern. Med.* 77:533, 1972.
21. Lam, K. C., Mistilis, S. P., and Perrott, M. Positive tissue antibody tests in patients with prolonged extrahepatic biliary obstruction. *N. Engl. J. Med.* 286:1400, 1972.
22. Ludwig, R. N., Deodhar, S. D., and Brown, C. H. Autoimmune tests in chronic active disease of the liver. *Cleve. Clin. Q.* 38:105, 1971.
23. Mistilis, S. P., and Blackburn, C. R. B. Active chronic hepatitis. *Am. J. Med.* 48:434, 1970.
24. Møller-Nielsen, P., Diederichsen, H., and Linde, N. C. Immunofluorescent and enzymatic staining of bile canaliculi in the same sections of the liver. *Am. J. Clin. Pathol.* 58:123, 1972.
25. Nowoslawski, A., Krawczynski, K., Brzosko, W. J., and Madalinski, K. Tissue localization of Australia antigen immune complexes in acute and chronic hepatitis and liver cirrhosis. *Am. J. Pathol.* 68:31, 1972.
26. Paronetto, F., Schaffner, F., Mutter, R. D., Kniffen, J. C., and Popper, H. Circulating antibodies to bile ductular cells in various liver diseases. *J.A.M.A.* 187:503, 1964.

27. Paronetto, F., Schaffner, F., and Popper, H.   Immunochemical and serological observations in primary biliary cirrhosis. *N. Engl. J. Med.* 271:1123, 1964.
28. Paronetto, F., and Popper, H.   Chronic liver injury induced by immunologic reactions; cirrhosis following immunization with heterologous sera. *Am. J. Pathol.* 49:1087, 1966.
29. Paronetto, F.   Immunologic aspects of liver disease. In H. Popper (ed.), *Progress in Liver Disease.* New York: Grune & Stratton, 1970, vol. 3, p. 299.
30. Reynolds, T. B., Peters, R. L., and Yamada, S.   Chronic active and lupoid hepatitis caused by a laxative oxyphenisatin. *N. Engl. J. Med.* 285:813, 1971.
31. Rodriguez, M., Paronetto, F., Schaffner, F., and Popper, H.   Antimitochondrial antibodies in jaundice following drug administration. *J.A.M.A.* 208:148, 1969.
32. Seidel, D., Alaupovic, P., and Furman, R. H.   A lipoprotein characterizing obstructive jaundice: I. Method for quantitative reparation and identification of lipoproteins in jaundiced patients. *J. Clin. Invest.* 48:1211, 1969.
33. Seidel, D., Schmitt, E. A., and Alaupovic, P.   An abnormal low density lipoprotein in obstructive jaundice: II. Its significance in the differential diagnosis of jaundice. *Ger. Med. Mon.* 15:671, 1970.
34. Smith, M. G. M., Eddleston, A. L. W. F., and Williams, R.   Leukocyte migration in active chronic hepatitis and primary biliary cirrhosis. In M. Smith and R. Williams (eds.), *Immunology of the Liver.* Philadelphia: Davis, 1971, p. 155.
35. Sobørg, M.   The leucocyte migration technique for in vitro detection of cellular hypersensitivity. In B. R. Bloom and P. R. Globe (eds.), *In Vitro Methods in Cell Mediated Immunity.* New York: Academic, 1971, p. 289.
36. Steffen, C.   Antibodies to tissues. In M. Stefanini (ed.), *Progress in Clinical Pathology.* New York: Grune & Stratton, 1970, vol. 3, p. 226.
37. Taylor, P. E., Almeida, J. D., Zuckerman, A. J., and Leach, J. M.   Relationship of Milan antigen to abnormal serum lipoprotein. *Am. J. Dis. Child.* 123:329, 1972.
38. Vischer, T. L.   Australia antigen and autoantibodies in chronic hepatitis. *Br. Med. J.* 2:695, 1970.
39. Warwick, M. T., and Haslam, P.   Smooth muscle antibody in bronchial asthma. *Clin. Exp. Immunol.* 7:31, 1970.
40. Whitehouse, J. M., and Holborow, E. J.   Smooth muscle antibody in malignant disease. *Br. Med. J.* 4:511, 1971.
41. Whittingham, S., Irwin, J., MacKay, I. R., and Smalley, M.   Smooth muscle autoantibody in "autoimmune hepatitis." *Gastroenterology* 51:499, 1966.
42. Whittingham, S., MacKay, I. R., and Irwin, J.   Autoimmune hepatitis —immunofluorescence reactions with cytoplasm of smooth muscle and renal glomerular cells. *Lancet* 1:1333, 1966.

11

Autoimmune Disorders of the Thyroid Gland

Introduction

Autoimmune thyroiditis is characterized by the production of organ specific autoantibodies. The exact etiology of thyroiditis in humans is unknown, although some of the factors which may have been considered are (a) viral [17]; (b) genetic [16, 22]; (c) basement membrane alteration [36, 37]; and (d) thyroid hyperplasia [38]. The increased incidence in females in certain families is well documented [13, 16, 22]. There is also a tendency for overlap of one or more autoimmune disorders, with the existence of several autoantibodies, to occur in the same individual. This condition is especially prevalent in the various organ specific autoimmune diseases such as thyroiditis [13].

Recent Concepts in the Pathogenesis of Experimental and Human Thyroiditis
The demonstration of an antibody or sensitization to an autoantigen does not necessarily indicate that the disturbance in the immune mechanism is responsible for the lesions. Witebsky and co-workers [24, 44] proposed some years ago several postulates to prove that immune mechanisms were responsible for the injury in a particular disease. The postulates can be stated as follows:
A. An immune response at some stage of the disease (humoral antibodies or cellular sensitivity to autoantigen)
B. Recognition of a self component as being antigenic
C. Production of antibodies against the same antigen in experimental animals
D. Appearance of tissue lesions similar to human disease in sensitized animals
E. Diseases of experimental animals capable of reproduction in a normal recipient by transfer of antibody in serum or in immunologically competent cells

During the past several years, investigators have shown that experimental thyroiditis can be manipulated to fulfill all of the above postulates.

There is very little question that various animals and humans are normally unresponsive to their own thyroglobulin [10, 25, 29]. In the development of experimental or autoimmune thyroiditis there is probably alteration of the host thyroglobulin and thyroid antigen by genetic and/or other factors. Experimental thyroiditis has been transferred from various experimental animals to normal recipients by cell and serum [35]. Cell transfer was performed in experimental rabbits under experimental conditions in which the soluble altered thyroglobulin was used as an antigen. It was rapidly catabolized and cell transfer was accomplished at the time in the absence of activated antigenic material [26]. Serum and antibody transfer was accomplished from thyroidectomized donors, and antibody which was recovered from donor animals caused small lesions in 50% of the recipient animals [27].

Cellular and Humoral Mechanisms in Thyroiditis
Weigle, Chiller, and co-workers [7, 8, 39, 40] have shown that unresponsiveness and recognition sites for antibody production occur at the level of both the thymus-derived and the bone marrow cells. Further, the kinetics and the dose response for the induction and the maintenance of the unresponsive state to a specific antigen of the thymus-derived and of the bone marrow cells are different [39]. The antibody response to a particular antigen as thyroglobulin requires the interaction of both the thymus-derived and bone marrow cells [39, 40].

Thyroglobulin is found in the peripheral circulation in extremely small concentrations [29]. The concentrations are probably just sufficient to maintain unresponsiveness with tolerance of the thymus-derived cells (T-cells) but not to the B-cells, or antibody-producing cells found in the bone marrow. The host would appear completely normal since unresponsiveness at the T-cell level is sufficient to keep the host tolerant and inhibit any immune response with antibody production [39, 40].

When chemically or enzymatically altered homologous thyroglobulin is injected for induction of experimental thyroiditis in rabbits, a separate population of T-cells can react with the unrelated determinants of the altered thyroglobulin and permit the B-cells in bone marrow to produce autoantibody to thyroglobulin. Thus, B-cells in bone marrow at the cellular level may not have been tolerant since birth, or the level of antigen concentration in circulation may not be sufficient to maintain unresponsiveness in the B-cells. This is consistent with the observations of Nakamura and Weigle [27], who have shown that the circulating antibody is probably the major effector of experimental thyroiditis in rabbits.

In human autoimmune thyroiditis, alteration in thyroid tissue may occur by viral transformation or genetic mutation, thus allowing the thymus cells to react with the altered portions of the self antigens. The T-cells in turn will react with the already immunocompetent bone marrow cells with production of autoimmune antibodies, resulting in injury.

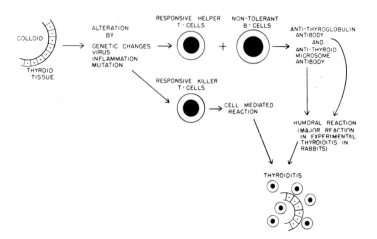

Figure 11-1
Proposed pathogenesis of thyroiditis.

The above hypothesis may explain the pathogenesis of other organ specific autoimmune diseases, such as atrophic gastritis, allergic aspermatogenesis, and allergic encephalitis, in which there are extremely low concentrations of self antigen in circulation (Fig. 11–1).

Thyroid Autoimmune Disorders in Humans

Classification
A. Diffuse Goitrous Lymphocytic Thyroiditis
   a. Struma lymphomatosa (Hashimoto's thyroiditis): (1) fibrous variant and (2) hypercellular variants
   b. Juvenile lymphocytic thyroiditis
B. Diffuse Nongoitrous Thyroiditis
   a. Severe atrophic (myxedema)
   b. Asymptomatic mild
C. Multifocal Lymphocytic Thyroiditis
   a. Associated with primary thyrotoxicosis
   b. Adenomatous goiters
   c. Carcinoma

The presence of autoantibodies to normal thyroid antigens is the hallmark of thyroiditis. The production of autoantibodies is partially related to the extent of lymphocytic inflammatory change within the gland. In the severe forms of autoimmune thyroiditis, the glandular architecture is effaced, may show large collections of lymphoid follicles with destruction of thyroid tissue (Fig. 11–2). The lymphoid follicles may show

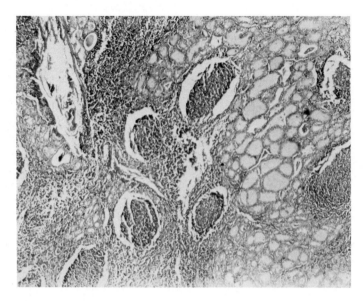

Figure 11-2
Diffuse lymphocytic thyroiditis. H & E microscopic section of human thyroiditis has many lymphoid follicles. (40× before 20% reduction.)

active germinal centers, and thyroid follicular cells show enlarged eosinophilic cells (Fig. 11–3). The gland may be enlarged to several times normal size. The disease may progress to form a fibrous variant with eventual myxedema and atrophy.

There are several other milder forms of lymphocytic goiter which do not fit into the clinical picture of Hashimoto's disease and which may not lead to myxedema. There are numerous focal types of thyroiditis which may lead to antibody formation to the same thyroid antigens [12, 13].

Population Studies and Genetic Aspects
Thyroid antibodies of low titer are frequently present in apparently normal individuals, a finding which corresponds to an incidence of focal lymphocytic infiltration of the thyroid glands examined at necropsy. The tanned red cell test for antithyroglobulin antibody is seldom positive in children, and the incidence of the positive test rises in both sexes, in females up to the age of 70 [13, 42]. A number of studies with thyroid autoimmune disease suggests that there is an increase in incidence of the organ specific type of autoimmune antibodies within families [31, 43].

Overlap of Thyroid Autoimmunity with Other Diseases
The most conspicuous relationship is with autoimmune atrophic gastritis and pernicious anemia, since 30% of patients with thyroiditis have anti-

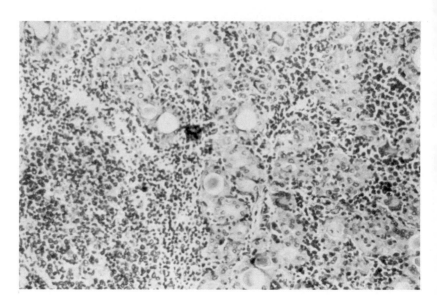

Figure 11-3
Section of thyroid gland from patient with Hashimoto's thyroiditis. Note eosinophilic acinar cells and a portion of a lymphoid follicle seen along one edge of the section. (H&E stain, 100×.)

gastric parietal antibodies, and conversely 50% of patients with pernicious anemia have antithyroid antibodies [30, 31, 43]. There is, in addition, an overlap of thyroid antibodies with autoimmune adrenalitis, myasthenia gravis, and other connective tissue diseases. The existence of autoimmunity to several organs favors the view that these diseases are related to a disorder of the immune system.

When Does One Suspect an Autoimmune Thyroid Disorder?
A. Family history of thyroid or autoimmune disease
B. Abnormal thyroid gland by physical examination which shows a nodular goiter or an enlarged diffuse goiter or atrophic gland
C. Abnormal thyroid function test which leads one to suspect hypothyroidism or hyperthyroidism
D. Concomitant findings which indicate presence of other autoimmune disorders such as pernicious anemia, glomerulonephritis, immune complex vasculitis, or cryoglobulinemia

Thyroid Antigen-Antibody Systems

The three distinct organ specific antigen-antibody systems were identified in human thyroiditis. The antigens are thyroglobulin, microsomal antigen, and the second antigen of the acinar colloid. In patients with mild nonprogressive thyroiditis, antibodies to all three antigens are found, while in severe Hashimoto's disease the titers of these three antibodies are usually much higher. In focal thyroiditis only one or more of the antibodies may be detected in very low levels.

Thyroglobulin

Thyroglobulin has a molecular weight of approximately 660,000 and is the main storage protein in the colloid of the gland. In the immuno-fluorescence test with use of fixed thyroid substrate, serum antithyro-globulin antibodies will give a lobular, floccular type of fluorescent pattern of the colloid material (Fig. 11-4a). The tanned red cell ag-glutination (TRC) test is a very sensitive test for thyroglobulin. The antithyroglobulin antibody is the most common test in thyroid disease and the tanned red cell test may be the only positive test in long standing primary myxedema.

Microsomal Antigen

The antigen, present in low concentrations in normal thyroid tissue, is found in much higher concentrations in thyrotoxic glands. The location of the antigen is in the lipoprotein membranes of the epithelial micro-somes. The antibody to this antigen has been found in human and ex-perimental monkey thyroiditis [35]. A sensitive test for the detection of the microsomal antibody is the indirect fluorescence test on unfixed thyroid sections in which a positive serum will give a bright specific apical staining of the cytoplasm of the thyroid epithelial cells (Fig. 11-4b). The complement fixation test is convenient and useful for detection of these antibodies, and is rarely positive except in cases of active thyroid-itis. In the performance of the immunofluorescence test for the micro-somal antibodies of the thyroid gland it is important to establish the organ specificity of the cytoplasmic antibody with the use of the kidney section, since there are other antibodies which react with cytoplasmic tissue, such as antimitochondrial antibody [14].

The Second Antigen of the Acinar Colloid

Few patients with Hashimoto's thyroiditis may show elevated γ-globu-lin without serum complement fixing or antithyroglobulin antibody. By the indirect fluorescence technique the fixed thyroid tissue may show uniform bright specific staining, in contrast to a floccular pattern ob-tained with sera containing antithyroglobulin antibody [13]. The sec-ond antigen was found to be distinct from thyroglobulin and is fre-quently demonstrable in thyroid tissue. The antibodies to the second colloid antigen have no real diagnostic usefulness since they are found in 10% of normal people and in other forms of autoimmune thyroiditis [13].

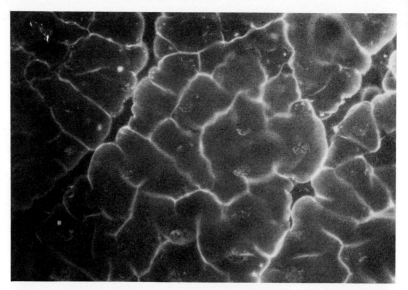

a

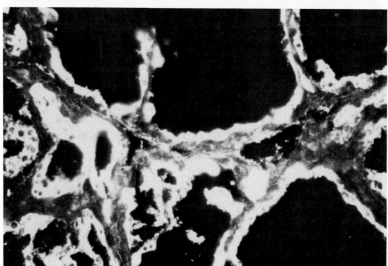

b

Figure 11-4
Positive indirect fluorescent antibody test for antithyroid antibodies.
(a) Positive indirect fluorescent test for antithyroglobulin antibody. The substrate is methyl alcohol fixed human thyroid tissue from a blood group O patient. The section is first reacted with test serum. After washing, the section is treated with fluorescein isothiocyanate labeled rabbit anti-human IgG. Note the irregular floccular fluorescence of colloid within the thyroid follicles. (×100 before 15% reduction.)
(b) Positive indirect fluorescent test for antithyroid epithelial microsome antibody. Substrate is unfixed thyroid tissue from thyrotoxic patient. (×100 before 15% reduction.)

314

Table 11.1. Thyroid Antigens and Common Tests for Detection of Specific Antibody in the Clinical Laboratory. (Modified from Doniach and Roitt [13].)

Thyroid Antigen	Characteristics of Antigen	Tests
Microsomal antigen	Lipoprotein membrane of microsomes in thyroid epithelial cells	a. Immunofluorescence test on unfixed human thyrotoxic gland substrate b. Complement fixation test
Thyroglobulin	660,000, M.W. Main storage protein in colloid of thyroid gland	a. Immunofluorescence test on fixed thyroid tissue b. Tanned red cell agglutination c. Latex test
Second colloid	Less than 1% of colloid protein	a. Immunofluorescence test on fixed thyroid tissue

Useful Laboratory Tests for the Evaluation of Autoimmune Disorders of the Thyroid Gland (see Chapter 8)

The recommended sensitive test in screening for thyroid and other autoimmune antibodies is the *indirect immunofluorescence test* on a composite section of antibodies consisting of fixed thyroid tissues, unfixed thyroid tissue, and stomach and kidney tissue [14, 30, 43].

The *precipitin test by the double diffusion technique* for antithyroglobulin antibody is quite insensitive and not useful for routine screening. However, a positive precipitin test for antithyroglobulin antibody is practically diagnostic for Hashimoto's thyroiditis [13].

The *latex agglutination test* for thyroglobulin-coated particles is slightly more sensitive than the precipitin test; however, like the precipitin test, it is not satisfactory for screening, since it will miss many cases of thyroiditis with low antithyroglobulin antibody [2]. This test can be performed as recommended by its commercial manufacturer (Hyland) by using a 1:20 dilution of the patient's serum, since there may be some false positive reactions. The false positive reactions may be due to the presence of rheumatoid factor, which reacts with traces of macroglobulins present in the thyroglobulin antigen coating the particles [2].

When a positive immunofluorescence screening test is obtained, there should be a further follow-up for the level of antithyroglobulin antibodies by the *tanned red cell agglutination (TRC) test* and a *test for complement-fixing antibody* to thyroid microsomal antigen. A test kit for the tanned red cell agglutination test for antithyroglobulin antibody is commercially available from Wellcome. This test, developed by Fulthorpe et al. [18], is approximately 1,000 times as sensitive as the precipitin reaction (Fig. 11-5). The complement fixation test for thyroid microsome should be performed in conjunction with the tanned red cell test (TRC), since certain cases of Hashimoto's disease may show significant levels only of the complement-fixing antibody. It is easily performed with reagents which may be obtained from Wellcome, and with a microtiter set (Cooke Engineering). It is likely that, with severe inflammation of the thyroid gland, large amounts of thyroglobulin may be released into the circulation and neutralize circulating antithyroglobulin antibodies. Thus, the level of antithyroglobulin antibodies may not necessarily correlate with the extent and severity of the inflammatory lesions within the gland.

Other supplemental tests which are helpful are (a) test for rheumatoid factor, (b) anti-parietal cell antibody test, and (c) bioassay for long-acting thyroid stimulator (LATS) and thyrotoxicosis [22, 28]. Another useful procedure is the biopsy of thyroid tissue for *direct tissue immunofluorescence studies* [12]. The possible fixation of IgG, IgM, IgE, and complement in the thyroid tissue may be examined [12, 41]. The *determination of quantitative serum immunoglobulins* may be helpful in differentiating certain cases of thyroiditis from thyroid carcinoma, since generally the immunoglobulins are elevated in progressive thyroiditis, whereas they are rarely elevated in carcinoma [13, 21]. The various *thyroid function tests,* such as radioiodine uptake, triiodothyronine up-

THYROGLOBULIN TITRATION

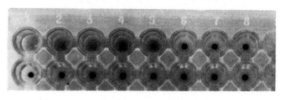

TEST SERUM

NEGATIVE SERUM

Figure 11-5
Microhemagglutination Test for Antithyroglobulin Antibodies
    Hemagglutination patterns for test and negative sera against unsensitized and thyroglobulin sensitized sheep red blood cells (SRBC). In the first row, there is hemagglutination of sensitized red cells with a serum dilution of 1/25,000. The 8th well shows no agglutination of ⅕ diluted serum against unsensitized SRBC. In the second row, there is agglutination for negative serum under similar conditions.

take, and total volume of thyroxine, are helpful in the evaluation of the patient.

When Should the Various Thyroid Antibody Tests Be Performed?
The antibody tests are helpful in the study of goiters and for the differential diagnosis of Hashimoto type thyroiditis from the following lesions: (a) nontoxic nodular goiter, (b) thyroid tumors, (c) viral thyroiditis (DeQuervain), and (d) Reidel's disease. They are useful also for the detection of significant thyroiditis in patients with thyrotoxicosis and in the differentiation of mild thyrotoxicosis from anxiety states.

Antithyroid antibody tests should be performed in the evaluation of unilateral ocular proptosis, for the presence of antithyroid antibodies would indicate an endocrine abnormality instead of a space-occupying mass or tumor. They are helpful also in (a) the diagnosis of myxedema, since the absence of antithyroid antibodies rules against the diagnosis of primary myxedema [30], and (b) in familial studies for thyroid disease and (c) the evaluation of other autoimmune diseases.

Interpretation of Laboratory Tests for Thyroid Antibodies

Interpretation of the Indirect Immunofluorescence Screening Test for Thyroglobulin and Antithyroid Microsomal Antibodies
A. A negative test for antibodies in the thyroglobulin and cytoplasmic microsomes rules out Hashimoto's thyroiditis and is of value in distinguishing this disease from thyroid cancer and nontoxic goiters of other types.
B. A positive fluorescence test is not sufficient for the diagnosis of Hashimoto's disease, since antibodies are present in many thyroid diseases such as thyrotoxicosis. The incidence of antithyroid antibodies of low titers in this test are found in apparently normal people and reflect in the general population a known frequency of focal lymphocytic thyroiditis which is asymptomatic [13].
C. A negative fluorescence test virtually excludes the diagnosis of primary myxedema, although in some long-standing cases only the tanned red cell test is positive at a low titer in primary myxedema. A positive test is insufficient to make a diagnosis of hypothyroidism.
D. Positive tests are seen in cases of thyrotoxicosis, pernicious anemia, and other autoimmune disorders. The thyroid's specific autoantibodies are found in thyroid diseases other than Hashimoto's disease; they are also present in the serum of patients with systemic lupus erythematosus, rheumatoid arthritis, and pernicious anemia. For example, 30% of patients with thyroiditis have anti-gastric parietal cell antibodies, and 50% of patients with pernicious anemia have antithyroid antibodies [13].

After observing a positive indirect fluorescence test for antithyroid antibodies, two tests which are recommended for further studies are the tanned red cell test for hemagglutinating antibodies to thyroglobulin, and the complement fixation test for thyroid microsomes. The hemagglutinating antibodies appear to be IgG and are found in practically all cases of Hashimoto's disease. The titers in the apparently normal population rarely exceed 1 to 10. The incidence of antithyroglobulin antibodies is greater in females and increases with the age of the population. Many patients with Hashimoto's disease have extremely high titers of hemagglutinating antibodies which may be from 1,000 to 5,000 or greater. In general, the frequency of detection of thyroglobulin in antibodies can be correlated with the extent of focal thyroiditis [12, 13]; however, in certain cases there is no increase; there is no correlation since thyroglobulin may leak from the thyroid gland with neutralization of circulating serum antibody.

Precipitin Test for Antithyroglobulin Antibody
This test is performed in agar gel with crude saline extract of postmortem thyroid glands or with thyroglobulin purified by salt fractionation. The thyroglobulin (concentration of approximately 1 mg/ml) is placed in one well of a gel diffusion plate; a precipitin line may form within 24 to 48 hours when reacted against precipitating antibodies to thyroglobulin. The precipitin test is a reliable index of diffuse thyroiditis and is negative in greater than one-half the cases of sera from patients with Hashimoto's disease.

Latex Agglutination Test for Antithyroglobulin Antibody
This test is commercially available with the use of thyroglobulin-coated particles and may be used as a quick screening test; however, the test is insensitive and will miss cases of Hashimoto's disease with low antithyroglobulin antibodies. The test should be performed with the patient's serum diluted 1:20. Undiluted serum will yield false positive reactions in the presence of rheumatoid factor or in the traces of human macroglobulins present in the thyroglobulin-coated particles [2].

Tanned Red Cell Agglutination Test for
Antithyroglobulin Antibody
This test is approximately 1,000 times more sensitive than the precipitin reaction [18]. Patients with thyroiditis may have a titer of 1,000 to 5,000 or greater, and the test should be run in conjunction with the complement fixation test. Both tests combined should diagnose 90% or more of the cases of Hashimoto's disease. In primary myxedema the tanned red cell test may be the only test showing positive results.

Complement Fixation Test for Antithyroid
Microsomal Antibody
With the immunofluorescence test the cytoplasmic fluorescence is concentrated toward the apical margin of the thyroid, and the procedure

is useful in the screening test for antimicrosomal antibody. The complement fixation test has been positive in 80% of cases with Hashimoto's disease, and the titers are frequently higher than 1 to 32 whereas in thyroid cancer and other diseases such as nontoxic nodular goiters, only 20% of the sera contains these complement-fixing antibodies, often in lower titer.

Immunofluorescence Studies of Thyroid Gland Biopsies from Thyroditis and Graves' Disease

Immunofluorescence studies with anti-human immunoglobulin antisera including anti-IgG, anti-IgA, anti-IgM, and anti-C3 can be used to study needle biopsies of various thyroid goiters. The antigen-antibody complexes have been demonstrated in Hashimoto's thyroiditis with immunofluorescence studies. The acinar cells of the thyroid gland may show fluorescence with anti-IgG conjugate. The fixed antibodies to colloid are usually non-complement fixing and do not stain with anti-C3 conjugates. The immunofluorescent stains may be negative in the presence of thyroiditis with many inflammatory cells, since the antibody may be phagocytized by the surrounding inflammatory cells [12].

In a study of thyroid glands from patients with Graves' disease, positive immunofluorescent staining was observed in focal areas of thyroid gland stroma with specific antiserum to human IgG, IgM, and IgE, and to C1q and C3 components of complement [41]. The connective tissue localization of complement and immunoglobulins provides evidence that Graves' disease may be an immune disorder, as described below.

Serum Immunoglobulins in Thyroid Disorders

Serum IgG immunoglobulins tend to be elevated in Graves' disease and Hashimoto's thyroiditis [21]. Twenty-one percent of patients with a first episode of thyrotoxicosis had elevated serum IgG levels and a high percentage of patients (80%) had elevated IgG levels (1930 $\pm$ 465 mg/100 ml) after relapse from Carbimazole treatment [21]. Eighteen (16.3%) of the patients with thyroiditis had high serum levels of IgG, and there was no correlation to metabolic thyroid status. The patients with thyroiditis and high IgG levels had a high titer of antithyroglobulin antibodies when compared to the case with thyroiditis without elevated IgG levels.

Very few patients with primary myxedema, nontoxic goiter, and adenoma had abnormal levels of immunoglobulins. No significant differences were noted in IgM or IgA immunoglobulin levels in any of the thyroid disorders studied [21].

Thyrotoxicosis

The Relationship of Thyroiditis and Thyrotoxicosis (Graves' Disease)

A large percentage of patients with thyrotoxicosis have evidence of antithyroglobulin antibody, and the majority of thyrotoxic glands removed in operations contain small areas of lymphoid infiltration. Thyrotoxicosis is usually associated with males and females equally, whereas Hashimoto's disease and myxedema are more common in women. The antithyroid antibody titers tend to be higher in patients with progressive exophthalmos.

Graves' disease is a multisystem disease of unknown cause consisting of one or both of the following conditions: (a) hyperthyroidism due to diffuse thyroidal hyperplasia, and (b) infiltrative ophthalmopathy, usually called localized orbital myxedema. The disease, in addition, shows one diagnostic laboratory finding, a titer of long-acting thyroid stimulator (LATS) sufficient to yield a response index of 250 or greater [4]. The LATS found in Graves' disease has been identified as an immunoglobulin in the IgG fraction, and observation has led to the speculation that Graves' disease may be an autoimmune disorder.

Role of LATS in Graves' Disease

LATS was originally described by Adams and Purves [1], who demonstrated that the serum of patients with Graves' disease exerted prolonged stimulatory effect on the radioiodine released from the thyroid of guinea pigs. In contrast to the maximal stimulation time of 2 to 4 hours caused by the thyroid-stimulating hormone (TSH), the peak stimulation of LATS was observed at 7 to 24 hours.

LATS has been definitely identified in the IgG fraction. The activity has been recovered with the heavy chain of IgG which has been separated from the light chain. The specific anti-human IgG antiserum neutralizes the biological effects of LATS [3, 23]. It is believed that the antigen is located on the plasma membrane of the thyroid cells; that the LATS reacts with the microsomal portion in the cell fraction; and that the reaction of LATS is an antigen-antibody reaction. It has been definitely shown that LATS does not react with thyroglobulin. There have been reports of detection of LATS in thyroid tissue by immunofluorescence techniques [5, 6], but the procedure has not had wide applicability because of the inconsistency in the results [4]. The most widely used assay for LATS is a bioassay which involves the release of radioiodine from the thyroid gland of an initially prepared mouse [1, 23, 28].

The present hypothesis is that LATS is the cause of hyperthyroidism in Graves' disease. The role of LATS in the production of exophthalmos and myxedema is unknown.

Associated Autoimmune Antibodies in Graves' Disease

Patients with Graves' disease often have sera of all of the other antithyroid antibodies discussed in the cases of thyroiditis. Precipitating antibodies to thyroglobulin are rarely found. However, 50% of patients have low titers of thyroid-agglutinating antibodies. A significant number of patients has positive antimicrosomal antibody detected by thyroid cytoplasmic immunofluorescence or complement fixation assays. Other antibodies such as that to gastric parietal cells are frequently present, and Graves' disease appears to demonstrate the overlap in the various auto-immune diseases [4].

Procedures

Combined Immunofluorescence Test for Detection of
Antibodies to Thyroglobulin and Thyroid
Microsomal Antigen
The procedure is performed similar to the combined immunofluorescence test described by Roitt and Doniach and others [14, 30] and Whittingham [43] previously described in Chapter 8. It is important to obtain human thyroid tissue, specifically fresh thyrotoxic glandular tissue, which has tall columnar epithelial cells and many small acini filled with colloid. The tall columnar cells will help in differentiating between the cytoplasmic fluorescence from nuclear fluorescence.

It is possible to perform the antithyroid antibody tests with the use of fixed and unfixed thyroid tissue mounted on the same slide. A section of thyroid tissue is mounted on a glass slide and then fixed in absolute methyl alcohol heated in a Coplin jar to 56° C in a 60° C water bath. The slide with the thyroid section is placed in the heated alcohol for 3 min and rapidly air dried with a fan. After application of the fixed thyroid section, an unfixed section from a composite block made up of thyroid, stomach, and kidney tissues is applied to a slide. By examination of the thyroid, kidney, and stomach tissues, one can differentiate whether the cytoplasmic fluorescence in the thyroid is due to antithyroid micro-somal antibodies or to antimitochondrial antibodies found in other autoimmune diseases.

Methods for Isolation of Human Thyroglobulin

SALT FRACTIONATION.   (Modified from methods described by Derrien et al. [11] and Shulman and Witebsky [34].)
1. Fresh thyroid gland tissue is obtained from autopsy and washed with saline solution. The thyroid gland tissue is minced into small pieces and extracted with a volume of isotonic saline solution which is ap-proximately 5 times the volume of the tissue.
2. The extraction is refrigerated for a period of 24 hours. The soluble extract is then salted with ammonium sulfate at a concentration of 1.4–1.8 M. The thyroglobulin is precipitated at this concentration of ammonium sulfate, which is between 30 and 50% saturation. The precipitate is dissolved in a small amount of saline solution and is subsequently dialyzed against large volumes of saline solution to re-move the ammonium sulfate. The dialysate is tested with acidification of the dialysate and addition of two drops of saturated solution of barium chloride to test for the insoluble precipitate of barium sul-fate.

3. The thyroglobulin solution is concentrated by vacuum dialysis and can be stored at 4° C with the addition of merthiolate 1:10,000.

COLUMN CHROMATOGRAPHY.   The saline extract of the thyroglobulin may also be isolated by a passage through a Sephadex G–200 (Pharmacia) [32] or Bio-Gel P–300 (BioRad) column [25]. The first peak of the void volume fraction will contain thyroglobulin.

Thyroglobulin isolation by either of the above methods will have trace amounts of contaminating serum macroglobulins.

Precipitin Test for Antithyroglobulin Antibody
An agar gel double-diffusion test may be performed with standard agar gel templates obtainable commercially.
1. The serum sample is placed in one well.
2. Purified thyroglobulin is placed in the opposite end in a concentration of 1 mg/ml.
3. Appropriate controls are set up, such as thyroglobulin vs. known antithyroglobulin antibody, to establish lines of identity, etc.
4. The materials are allowed to react for 48 hours at room temperature in a moist chamber.

INTERPRETATION.   Approximately one-half of the cases of Hashimoto's type of diffuse thyroiditis show evidence of precipitating antibodies to thyroglobulin [13]. The presence of precipitating antibodies to thyroglobulin is strong evidence in favor of the diagnosis of Hashimoto's thyroiditis. However, since the precipitin test is very insensitive, a negative test does not rule out thyroiditis.

Thyroglobulin Latex Slide Agglutination Test
(Hyland TA Test [2])
This test is a slide screening test for the detection of antithyroglobulin antibodies. The reagent consists of a polystyrene latex particle which has been coated with thyroglobulin and which will give a positive reaction to a serum specimen containing precipitating antibodies to human antithyroglobulin.

REAGENTS
1. The latex thyroglobulin-coated particles can be stored at 4° C. Glycine-saline buffer (pH 8.2) is used as the diluent.
2. Positive and negative control sera are provided with the test kit.

PROCEDURE
1. The patient's serum is heated at 56° C for 30 min to inactivate the components of complement which may give a false positive reaction.

2. The reagents are brought to room temperature prior to testing.
3. One drop of serum is added to 1 ml glycine-saline buffered diluent to make a serum dilution of 1:20. It is advisable to make this 1:20 dilution to avoid false positive reactions. The presence of rheumatoid factor can cause agglutination of the particles, since the thyroglobulin antigen may have contaminating macroglobulins.
4. One drop each of positive and negative control serum, along with one drop of undiluted test serum and one drop of diluted test serum, are tested separately. The thyroglobulin latex reagent is mixed to provide an even suspension, and one drop is applied to each serum sample. Next, the serum and latex reagent are mixed with a wooden applicator stick.
5. The slide is tilted slowly from side to side for 3 min. The slides are read over a dark background and examined by oblique reflected light.

Anderson and co-workers [2] have reported that, when a transmitted light is used, there may be a fine barely visible aggregate in serum specimens, which are negative for antithyroglobulin antibody. A positive test shows agglutination of the latex particles, and this is compared with the test specimens along with the control serum. A 1:20 dilution also may eliminate prozone reaction due to the inhibition by excess antibody. If titrations of positive sera are desired, the sera may be further tested after four-fold dilutions. However, the glycine-saline diluent should contain enough bovine serum albumin to establish a concentration of 1% protein. Without any protein there may be a visible aggregation of latex particles at a very dilute solution. The latex particles mixed with a glycine-saline diluent often show a fine aggregation within 3 min without evidence of protein.

The latex test is not as sensitive as the tanned red cell test for the detection of antithyroglobulin antibodies. The test may miss cases of Hashimoto's thyroiditis with low antithyroglobulin antibodies. However, a positive test will favor the diagnosis of Hashimoto's thyroiditis or a diffuse type of thyroiditis.

The serum samples should be tested at a 1:20 dilution to eliminate prozone reactions and false positive reactions due to rheumatoid factor, which reacts with the traces of macroglobulins present in the thyroglobulin-coated latex particles.

Tanned Red Cell Agglutination Method for
Antithyroglobulin Antibody
This test is an agglutination test for thyroglobulin and makes use of thyroglobulin-sensitized sheep cells according to the method described by Fulthorpe et al. [18]. Red cells are treated with tannic acid and the surface is altered and binds with the thyroglobulin protein. The stability of the thyroglobulin-coated tanned cells is achieved by formalin-

ization. The cells coated with thyroglobulin are agglutinated by the specific autoantibody and if positive yield a fine dispersion of cells in the bottom of a tube. The absence of agglutination is indicated by the cells settling in a tight button.

REAGENTS.   The reagent material is available from Wellcome: (a) thyroglobulin-sensitized cells, (b) uncoated control cells, and (c) 0.9% physiologic saline solution.

The sensitized cells and control cells can be kept at 4° C for at least 2 years. The cells are dispensed in volumes sufficient for approximately 50 tests with a 1% suspension in sodium borate-succinic acid buffer at pH 7.5, 0.05 M, containing 1% bovine serum albumin and 0.2% formalin. On standing, the cells settle and adhere firmly to the bottom of the container. They must be resuspended by shaking immediately before use.

PROCEDURE.   The tanned red cell test is carried out in the microtiter apparatus using plastic agglutination trays with V-type cups (Linbro). The tulip-like loops may be obtained from Cooke Engineering. With the use of the plastic trays, serum dilutions are made as follows:
1. 4 drops of saline solution are delivered in each cup of row 1 with the standard 0.025 ml dropper; 1 drop is placed in all remaining cups. 0.025 ml serum is taken up into a tulip-shaped wire loop and mixed with the saline solution in row 1 to give a 1:5 dilution.
2. The loop is then transferred to row 2 for the 1:10 control.
3. This is repeated for all 8 sera on the tray. With the first loop, another 0.025 ml of 1:5 serum is picked up from front row 1 and placed in row 3 to start the serial two-fold dilution from 1:10 to 1:5120.
4. Next, the standard drop of control cells is placed in each cup of row 2.
5. A standard drop of thyroglobulin-sensitized cell is added to each cup in rows 3 to 12.
6. The cells and sera are mixed by gentle shaking of the trays, which are covered to prevent evaporation. These cells are then allowed to settle at room temperature, where readings are taken at 2 to 3 hours.

INTERPRETATION OF TEST.   In the positive agglutination test, the cells are evenly distributed and form a carpet at the bottom of the cup. In the negative tests, the cells fall to the tip of the V and form a tight central button. Partial agglutination patterns are seen where both the carpet and the small central button can be distinguished. The agglutination titer is taken at the highest serum dilution producing a complete agglutination and the trace of ± results are discounted. If complete agglutination is present in a dilution of 1:5120, the original serum specimen is diluted to an appropriate dilution and retested so that the agglutination pattern does not exceed the one row of wells. This is important since there is a definite amount of carryover with the transfer loops. Titration techniques which utilize more than 1 longitudinal row of an agglutination tray may result in a significant dilution error. Heterophile sheep reactions are rarely found in dilutions of 1:10 or greater; however, if the control row shows agglutination, 0.1 ml of test serum is absorbed with packed cells from 1 ml of the control suspension, and the mixture is shaken and left in contact for 10 min and spun in the centrifuge. The test is then repeated after the absorption process.

Thyroid Complement Fixation Test for Microsomal Antibody
(Procedure of Roitt and Doniach [30])

The standard complement fixation test is used with commercial freeze-dried thyrotoxic thyroid microsomal antigen obtained from Wellcome. Serial dilutions of the patient's serum are incubated with the antigen and guinea pig complement. Individual complement is then detected by the addition of the indicator system, which consists of sheep red cells sensitized with rabbit antisera to sheep cell. If the patient's serum contains antimicrosomal antibodies, complement will be fixed by the antigen-antibody reaction and will not be available for lysis of the indicator red cell; thus, inhibition of hemolysis indicates a positive test for antithyroid antibody and the titer is expressed as a reciprocal of the highest dilution of the patient's serum giving these positive results. In this procedure the microtiter apparatus is used to make dilutions of the serum. Controls are set up to detect anticomplementary sera at the time of testing.

Guinea pig complement is standardized in terms of minimum hemolytic dose (MHD) needed to lyse a fixed amount of sensitized sheep red cells. Two MHD are used in the test. The complement in the patient's serum is inactivated by heating at 56° C for 30 min. Appropriate controls are set up to detect anticomplementary factors in the test serum.

REAGENTS

A. Thyroid complement-fixing antigen (freeze-dried thyrotoxic thyroid microsome). This antigen is dispensed in sealed bottles and may be kept at refrigerated temperatures for 1 year.
B. Each composite is reconstituted with 1 ml saline solution. Complement is guinea pig serum freeze-dried.
C. Hemolytic serum for sheep red cells (rabbit antiserum to sheep red cells).
D. Sheep red cells are collected in Alsever's solution. The collected cells are allowed to stabilize one week to give uniform results.
E. Complement fixation test (CFT) buffer is composed of a barbital buffer with saline solution and divalent calcium and magnesium ions.

Barbitone complement fixation test diluent tablets may be obtained from Consolidated Laboratories.

Oxoid Code No. BR 16 formula
Diethyl barbituric acid
   (Barbitone)   0.575 gm/liter
Sodium chloride   8.5   gm
Magnesium chloride   0.168 gm
Calcium chloride   0.028 gm
Sodium diethylbarbiturate
   (Barbitone soluble)   0.185 gm

One tablet is dissolved in 100 ml warm distilled water and the final pH should be 7.2.

APPARATUS.   The microtitration apparatus was obtained from Cooke Engineering. The tulip loop is standardized to pick up 0.025 ml of fluid by capillary attraction. For further comment, see Technical Precautions with Use of the Microtiter System for Serial Dilutions below.
A. The dilutions of serum are made in small disposable plastic plates, which are 8 × 12 with U-shaped cups, by successfully transferring the spiral-loop contents along the series of cups, each containing 0.025 ml diluent buffer.
B. The disposable plastic trays may be obtained from Cooke Engineering or Linbro.

PREPARATION OF SENSITIZED SHEEP CELLS.   To prepare 30 ml 3% sensitized sheep cells:
1. 4 ml sheep blood in Alsever's solution are placed in a 10 ml graduated centrifuge tube and spun lightly at 1,000 rpm for 3 min.
2. The supernatant is removed and the cells are washed 3 times in CFT buffer.
3. The washed cells are transferred into a 25 ml graduated cylinder with CFT buffer and the volume is adjusted to 15 ml.
4. 1 ml cell suspension is transferred to another graduated cylinder and made up to 25 ml with 0.04% ammonia solution to lyse the cells. This changes hemoglobin into oxyhemoglobin.
5. The oxyhemoglobin concentration is measured in the spectrophotometer at 541 μ against a distilled water blank. The reading should be between 0.48 and 0.50 for a 6% suspension of red cells.
6. If the reading is less than 0.48, the cell suspension is spun in the centrifuge, some buffer is discarded, and the cells are resuspended in a smaller volume and the reading repeated. If the reading is more than 0.50, each ml of cells should be diluted by the following factor:

$$\frac{\text{Reading obtained}}{0.49}$$

7. 15 ml CFT buffer are mixed in a conical flask with 0.1 ml of Wellcome hemolytic serum. To this are added 15 ml 6% cell suspension, giving a final 3% suspension of sensitized cells. These are incubated for 15 min in a 37° C bath and can be used for up to 24 hours.

COMPLEMENT TITRATION. Increasing dilutions of complement are made from a 1:10 dilution obtained by mixing 0.1 ml reconstituted guinea pig freeze-dried complement (C) with 0.7 ml distilled water in a set of 7 tubes.

Set 1

Tube No.	1	2	3	4	5	6	7
Final C dilution	1:20	1:30	1:40	1:50	1:60	1:70	1:80
Amount buffer ml	0.1	0.2	0.3	0.4	0.5	0.6	0.7
Amount 1/10 C	0.1	0.1	0.1	0.1	0.1	0.1	0.1

Set 2

Tube No.	1	2	3	4	5	6	7
ml buffer	0.2	0.2	0.2	0.2	0.2	0.2	0.2
ml C from set 1	0.1	0.1	0.1	0.1	0.1	0.1	0.1
ml red cell suspension	0.1	0.1	0.1	0.1	0.1	0.1	0.1

Incubate tubes of set 2 for 30 min in 37° C bath, then centrifuge lightly. The first tube showing a button of cells should be taken as the unit of complement. For the tests use two units; this usually works out at a 1:20 to 1:25 dilution. If preserved complement is employed, complement titration is necessary only when a new bottle is started.

PREPARATION OF THYROID TISSUE ANTIGEN
(Method of Roitt and Doniach [30])
Six grams of fresh human thyrotoxic gland tissue are weighed and finely minced. The tissue is homogenized with 4 vol CFT buffer in a Waring blender for 3 min. The homogenate is centrifuged at 1,300 rpm for 5 min and the supernatant is stored in 2 ml aliquots at −70° C. The antigen must be checked and titrated as certain preparations are not suitable.

ANTIGEN TITRATION. With the use of the Wellcome thyroid complement fixing antigen, weekly antigen titrations are not required. However, batches of antigen should be checked against a serum of known titer. The antigen control cups should show complete hemolysis; if the antigen is anticomplementary it cannot be used.

The antigen titration should be performed just after the complement titration. The stored 20% tissue homogenate is thawed and diluted 1:8 and 1:16. In a microtiter plate, 3 rows of serial dilutions of standard positive serum are made from 1:2 to 1:128; the last cup in the plate is left for the antigen control. Into each successive row of cups are placed (1) 1 drop of antigen diluted 1:8, (2) 1 drop of antigen diluted 1:16, and (3) 1 drop of buffer. The titration is carried out as for the serum test described below. If the antigen is anticomplementary, it cannot be used.

COMPLEMENT FIXATION PROCEDURE IN MICROTITER PLASTIC TRAYS
1. The sera are inactivated at 56° C for 30 min.
2. 1 drop (0.025 ml) CFT buffer is delivered into all the cups from the standard microtiter pipette.
3. The same amount of inactivated serum is picked up with the tulip loop for each row, and dilutions from 1:2 to 1:128 are made simultaneously. Serum dilution 1:2 is left without antigen and used as serum control, while the last cup of each row is left without serum and used as the antigen control.
4. 1 drop of 1:8 antigen is delivered from the standard pipette into cups 2 to 8 and 1 drop of buffer into the serum and antigen control cups.
5. This is followed by 1 drop of freshly prepared complement dilution equivalent to 2 MHD, added to all cups in the tray.
6. After mixing, the trays are stacked or covered with a glass plate to prevent evaporation and incubated for 1 hour at 37° C.
7. 1 drop of sensitized red cells is then added to all cups, the trays are agitated, and incubation continued for a further 30 min. To prevent undue cooling, each tray should be withdrawn from the incubator separately for the addition of the red cells, and immediately replaced.
8. After hemolysis, the trays are agitated again and left to stand on the bench for 20 min before reading the results. These are recorded as degrees of hemolysis assessed visually:

4 = no hemolysis; full button of cells, colorless supernatant
3 = smaller button and slightly colored supernatant, approximately 25% hemolysis
2 = approximately 50% hemolysis
1 = 75% hemolysis
0 = complete hemolysis, no cells visible

The complement fixation titer (CFT) is the highest serum dilution giving not more than 50% hemolysis. If the control cup does not show hemolysis, the serum is anticomplementary. When an organ specificity control is needed, as in certain connective tissue disorders and liver diseases, a second row of serum dilutions is added and tested with rat kidney or monkey liver antigen. If the titer is greater than 1:128, the test is repeated, using the 12 cup row, which gives dilutions up to 1:2048.

Technical Precautions with Use of the Microtiter
System for Serial Dilutions
The original microtiter system was first described by Takatsy in 1950 and has since been applied to complement fixation, hemagglutination, and the hemagglutination inhibition test [33]. With use of the microtiter system and plastic trays, certain precautions must be taken to obtain reproducible results [9].
A. The pipette droppers and transfer pipettes should be calibrated. This can be done with solutions containing radioactive albumin [9].
B. The plastic microtiter plate should be wiped on the undersurface with a damp cloth to remove the static charge, which can cause technical difficulties [20].
C. The metal transfer pipettes are first heated to incandescence in a flame, cooled in distilled water, and dried on a paper towel. The wetting ensures proper filling by capillary action. The pipettes are filled by touching only to the surface of the liquid or serum sample. Wetting of the outside of the pipette will deliver more than 25 μl volume to the first well. Each pipette should be examined after filling for defects, such as bubbles [9].
D. The transfer pipettes should be placed into the various wells without touching the sides of the wells or the surface of the plate.
E. The optimal speed and number of rotations of transfer pipettes were found to be 30 back-and-forth rotations in 8 sec [9]. Slow and fast speeds will result in improper mixing.

References

1. Adams, D. D., and Purves, H. D.   Abnormal responses in the assay of thyrotropin. *Proc. Univ. Otago Med. School* 34:11, 1956.
2. Anderson, J. R., Buchanan, W. W., Gondie, R. B., and Gray, K. G. Diagnostic tests for thyroid antibodies: A comparison of the precipitin and latex-fixation (Hyland TA) tests. *J. Clin. Pathol.* 15:462, 1962.
3. Beall, G. N., and Solomon, D. H.   On the immunological nature of the long acting thyroid stimulator. *J. Clin. Endocrinol. Metab.* 20:1382, 1966.
4. Beall, G. N., and Solomon, D. H.   Hashimoto's disease and Graves' disease. In M. Samter (ed.), *Immunologic Diseases.* Boston: Little, Brown, 1971, 2nd ed., p. 1198.
5. Blum, A. S., Greenspan, F. S., Hargadine, J. R., and Lowenstein, J. M. Simultaneous detection of thyroid stimulating hormone (TSH) and long acting thyroid stimulator (LATS). *Metabolism* 16:960, 1967.
6. Burke, G., and Yuan, L.   Immunofluorescent studies of long acting thyroid stimulator. *Clin. Rev.* 16:439, 1968.
7. Chiller, J. M., Habicht, G. S., and Weigle, W. O.   Cellular sites of immunologic unresponsiveness. *Proc. Natl. Acad. Sci. U.S.A.* 65:551, 1970.

8. Chiller, J. M., Habicht, G. S., and Weigle, W. O.   Kinetic differences in unresponsiveness of thymus and bone marrow cells. *Science* 171:813, 1971.

9. Cooper, H. A., Bowie, E. J. W., and Owen, C. A.   Pitfalls of the microtiter system for serial dilutions and standardization using radioiodinated albumin. *Am. J. Clin. Pathol.* 57:332, 1972.

10. Daniel, P. M., Pratt, O. E., Roitt, I. M., and Torrigiani, E.   The release of thyroglobulin from the thyroid gland into thyroid lymphatics; the identification of thyroglobulin in the thyroid lymph and in the blood of monkeys by physical and immunological methods and its estimation by radioimmunoassay. *Immunology* 12:489, 1967.

11. Derrien, Y., Michel, R., and Roche, J.   Recherches sur la preparation et les propriétés de la thyroglobuline pure. *Biochim. Biophys. Acta* 2:454, 1948.

12. Doniach, D.   Thyroid autoimmune disease. *J. Clin. Pathol.* 20:385, 1967.

13. Doniach, D., and Roitt, I. M.   Thyroid auto-allergic disease. In P. G. H. Gell and R. R. A. Coombs (eds.), *Clinical Aspects of Immunology.* Oxford: Blackwell, 1968, 2nd ed., chap. 35.

14. Doniach, D., Delhanty, J., Lindqvist, H. J., and Catterall, R. D.   Mitochondrial and other tissue antibodies in patients with chronic biological false positive reactions for syphilis. *Clin. Exp. Immunol.* 6:871, 1970.

15. Donnelley, M.   Studies in experimental immunology of influenza: VII. An improved complement fixation technique. *Aust. J. Exp. Biol. Med. Sci.* 29:137, 1951.

16. Dunning, E. J.   Struma lymphomatosa: Reports of three cases in one family. *J. Clin. Endocrinol. Metab.* 19:1121, 1959.

17. Eyland, E., Zmucky, R., and Sheba, C. H.   Mumps virus and subacute thyroiditis: Evidence of a causal association. *Lancet* 1:1062, 1957.

18. Fulthorpe, A. J., Roitt, I. M., Doniach, D., and Couchman, K.   A stable sheep cell preparation for detecting thyroglobulin autoantibodies and its clinical applications. *J. Clin. Pathol.* 14:654, 1961.

19. Gajdusek, D. C.   An "autoimmune" reaction against human tissue antigens in certain acute and chronic diseases: 1. Serological investigations. *Arch. Intern. Med.* 101:9, 1958.

20. Gavan, T. L., and Town, M. A.   A microdilution method for antibiotic susceptibility testing: An evaluation. *Am. J. Clin. Pathol.* 53:880, 1970.

21. Glynne, A., and Thomson, J. A.   Serum immunoglobulin levels in thyroid disease. *Clin. Exp. Immunol.* 12:71, 1972.

22. Hall, R., Owen, S. E., and Smart, G. A.   Evidence for genetic predisposition to formation of thyroid autoantibodies. *Lancet* 2:187, 1960.

23. McKenzie, J. M.   Humoral factors in the pathogenesis of Graves' disease. *Physiol. Rev.* 48:252, 1968.

24. Milgrom, F., and Witebsky, E.   Autoantibodies and autoimmune diseases. *J.A.M.A.* 181:706, 1962.

25. Nakamura, R. M., and Weigle, W. O.   In vivo behavior of homologous and heterologous thyroglobulin and induction of immunologic unresponsiveness to heterologous thyroglobulin. *J. Immunol.* 98:653, 1967.

26. Nakamura, R. M., and Weigle, W. O.   Passive transfer of experimental autoimmune thyroiditis from donor rabbits injected with soluble thyro-

globulin without adjuvant. *Int. Arch. Allergy Appl. Immunol.* 32:506, 1967.

27. Nakamura, R. M., and Weigle, W. O.   Transfer of experimental autoimmune thyroiditis by serum from thyroidectomized donors. *J. Exp. Med.* 130:263, 1969.

28. Ochi, Y., and De Groot, C. J.   Long acting thyroid stimulator of Graves' disease. *N. Engl. J. Med.* 278:718, 1968.

29. Roitt, I. M., and Torrigiani, G.   Identification and estimation of undegraded thyroglobulin in human sera. *Endocrinology* 81:421, 1967.

30. Roitt, I. M., and Doniach, D.   Immunofluorescent tests for the detection of autoantibodies. In *World Health Organization Manual for Autoimmune Serology.* Geneva: World Health Organization, 1969.

31. Roitt, I. M.   *Essential Immunology.* London: Blackwell, 1971.

32. Salvatore, G., Salvatore, M., Cahnmann, H. J., and Robbins, J.   Separation of thyroidal iodoprotein and purification of thyroglobulin by gel filtration and density gradient centrifugation. *J. Biol. Chem.* 239:3267, 1964.

33. Sever, J. L.   Application of a microtechnique to viral serologic investigations. *J. Immunol.* 88:320, 1962.

34. Shulman, S., and Witebsky, E.   Studies on organ specificity: XII. Fractionation of hog thyroid extract. Preparation of thyroglobulin and thyroid thyralbumin. *J. Immunol.* 88:221, 1962.

35. Shulman, S.   Thyroid antigens and autoimmunity. In F. J. Dixon and H. G. Kunkel (eds.), *Advances in Immunology.* New York: Academic, 1971, vol. 14, p. 85.

36. Sommers, S. C., and Meissner, W. A.   Basement membrane changes in chronic thyroiditis and other thyroid diseases. *Am. J. Clin. Pathol.* 24:434, 1954.

37. Stuart, A. E., and Allan, W. S. A.   Significance of basement membrane changes in thyroid disease. *Lancet* 2:1204, 1958.

38. Vickery, A. L., and Hamlin, E., Jr.   Struma lymphomatosa (Hashimoto's thyroiditis) observations on repeated biopsies in sixteen patients. *N. Engl. J. Med.* 264:226, 1961.

39. Weigle, W. O.   Recent observations and concepts in immunological unresponsiveness and autoimmunity. *Clin. Exp. Immunol.* 9:437, 1971.

40. Weigle, W. O.   Immunologic unresponsiveness. *Hosp. Practice* 6:121, 1971.

41. Werner, S. C., Wegelius, O., Frierer, J. A., and Hsu, K. C.   Immunoglobulins (E, M, G) and complement in the connective tissues of the thyroid in Graves' disease. *N. Engl. J. Med.* 287:421, 1972.

42. Whittingham, S., Irwin, J., MacKay, I. R., Marsh, S., and Cowling, P. C.   Autoantibodies in healthy subjects. *Aust. Ann. Med.* 18:130, 1969.

43. Whittingham, S.   Serological methods in autoimmune diseases in man. In J. B. G. Kwapinski (ed.), *Research in Immunochemistry and Immunobiology.* Baltimore: University Park Press, 1972, vol. 1, p. 121.

44. Witebsky, E., Rose, N. R., Terplan, K., Paine, J. R., and Egan, R. W.   Chronic thyroiditis and autoimmunization. *J.A.M.A.* 164:1439, 1957.

12

Immunologic Human Renal Diseases

Robert M. Nakamura and Ernest S. Tucker, III

There is abundant evidence to support the role of immunologic mechanisms in the pathogenesis of human renal disease [23, 26, 45]. The major forms of glomerulonephritis include (a) antiglomerular basement (GBM) glomerulonephritis and (b) immune complex glomerulonephritis.

Immunofluorescence studies of kidney biopsies have been of value in elucidating the pathogenesis of various diseases [27]. The studies are usually performed on kidney biopsies with labeled antisera to human IgG, IgM, IgA, IgE, C3 component of complement, fibrinogen, and albumin. The labeled antialbumin is used to evaluate nonspecific protein deposition in chronic glomerular disease. Characteristic staining patterns for immunoglobulin and complement are helpful in the diagnosis of various immunologic kidney diseases. On the other hand, deposits of immunoglobulin and complement are absent in other diseases such as toxemia of pregnancy and hemolytic uremic syndrome.

Antiglomerular Basement Membrane (GBM) Glomerulonephritis

Glomerular basement membrane (GBM) antibodies react directly with glomerular basement membrane [45], and complement usually participates in the reaction. The anti-GBM glomerulonephritis accounts for less than 5% of the various types of immunologically induced glomerular disease [51]. The anti-GBM antibody is found in Goodpasture's syndrome, and the resulting nephritis is diagnosed by detecting fixation of IgG in a linear pattern along the glomerular basement by immunofluorescence studies of a renal biopsy (Fig. 12–1).

The cause of formation of anti-GBM antibody is not exactly known. One popular explanation is that basement membrane antigens of vessels and lung may be altered by toxins or infections (see Chapter 4). The altered basement membrane becomes immunogenic and results in cross-

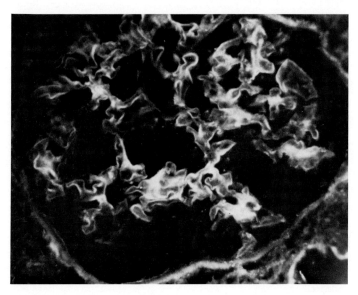

Figure 12-1
Goodpasture's syndrome. Lesion demonstrated a linear fluorescent staining pattern with localization of IgG and C3 characteristic of glomerular anti-basement membrane antibodies. (Approximately 440× before 20% reduction.)

reacting antibodies. It is well known that antilung antibodies will react with kidney basement membrane [51]. In support of the above concept a recent case of influenza A2 infection with anti-GBM nephritis was observed [52]. A second theory of spontaneous formation of anti-GBM antibodies is the possibility of exogenous antigens which cross react with GBM. Anti-GBM antibodies have been found in certain heterologous antilymphocyte globulin preparations [50], and most likely are antibodies formed to contaminant vascular membranes.

The most common pathway of injury in anti-GBM nephritis is through the pathway of complement fixation. Alternate pathways of injury are probably also involved because (a) duck anti-GBM antibodies can produce experimental glomerular injury without participation of complement or polymorphonuclear leukocytes [45]; and (b) one-third of patients with active anti-GBM antibody nephritis do not show C3 fixation when kidney biopsies are examined with immunofluorescence methods [51]. One can speculate that the kinin and coagulation proteins may be involved in the mediation of anti-GBM nephritis in which there is a lack of complement participation [37, 53].

In the diagnosis of anti-GBM disease, McCluskey [27] has enumerated three types of problems. First, finely granular deposits of immune

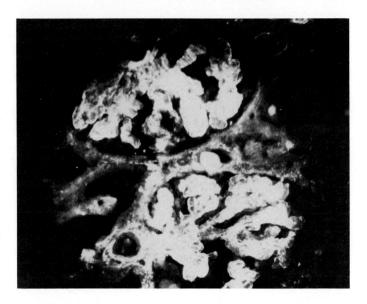

Figure 12-2
Chronic glomerulonephritis. Biopsy section showed large irregular deposits of IgG and C3 by fluorescent antibody test. The staining pattern is consistent with a chronic immune complex type of glomerulonephritis. (400× before 20% reduction.)

complexes in glomeruli may appear to present a "linear pattern" when reacted with labeled IgG. Usually if the so-called "linear pattern" is examined under a high power, some granularity can almost always be seen. Such cases may have actually been due to immune complex deposition. Second, in late stages of anti-GBM disease, one may see fibrin deposits with glomerular sclerosis and distortion with an irregular fluorescence pattern of the basement membrane which does not appear linear. Third, certain cases of linear staining of IgG by fluorescence studies are seen in kidney glomeruli which are not due to anti-GBM antibody. Koffler et al. [19] have described linear staining in cases of lupus nephritis and could not demonstrate anti-GBM antibody in eluates of kidney glomeruli. Also, Gallo [11] has reported linear staining of IgG in glomeruli of patients with diabetic glomerulosclerosis without evidence of anti-GBM antibody. Other cases of unclassified glomerular disease with bright linear fluorescent staining of IgG without evidence of anti-GBM antibody have been reported [27].

Immune Complex Glomerulonephritis

In this lesion, the antibodies react with circulating antigen, and immune complexes so formed can fix complement and deposit along the glomeru-

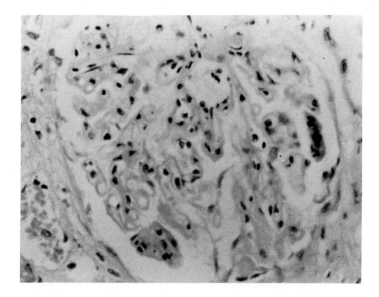

a

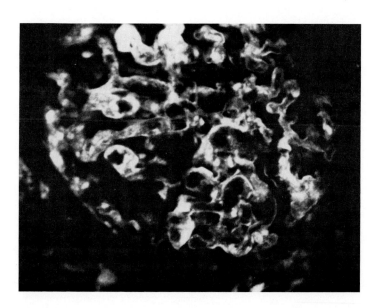

b

Figure 12-3
Kidney lesion of systemic lupus erythematosus. (a) H&E stained section of
glomerulus with irregular lobular lesions. (b) The irregular lumpy-bumpy
type of pattern of immune complex nephritis. There was localization of
IgG and C3. (Both 440× before 20% reduction.)

lar basement membrane. The deposits can be identified in the sub-epithelial layers and other sites along the basement membrane with an electron microscope [2]. The immune complexes appear on biopsy as granular and lumpy deposits in the kidney glomeruli when stained with fluorescence-labeled antibodies specific for the immunoglobulin, complement, or antigen involved (Fig. 12–2, 12–3, 12–4).

Numerous different types of antigen-antibody may be involved. However, only a few antigens are known in human cases of glomerulonephritis [27, 51]. The exogenous sources of antigen include (a) foreign proteins and drugs, (b) infectious agents such as streptococci, *Plasmodium malariae*, and Australia antigen, and (c) viruses such as Epstein-Barr, lymphocytic choriomeningitis, hepatitis, and B virus.

The endogenous antigens known in human glomerulonephritis are (a) DNA in lupus nephritis [20] (Fig. 12–3), (b) thyroglobulin in thyroiditis [18], and (c) cryoproteins [1, 29, 30].

In many human diseases, scanty focal deposits of IgG and C3 may be seen. Included in such diseases are end stage-sclerosing glomerulonephritis and unclassified glomerulonephritis. The presence of focal deposits of IgG and C3 may indicate immune complexes or nonimmunologic deposits of proteins in the glomeruli. The immunofluorescence

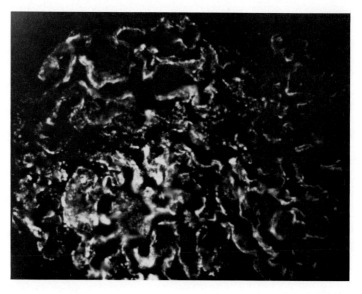

Figure 12-4
Nephrotic syndrome with immune complex glomerulonephritis. Examination of kidney biopsy showed a finely granular pattern of deposits of IgG and C3 along the basement membrane. (450× before 20% reduction.)

studies will have to be evaluated in conjunction with the histology and clinical picture. The absence of detectable IgG or C3 in sclerotic glomeruli does not exclude the possibility that immune complexes were not involved in the original glomerular injury [27].

Chronic Membranoproliferative Glomerulonephritis with Hypocomplementemia

This is an identifiable form of glomerulonephritis initially described by West et al. [48]. The disease is manifested in different states, as (a) asymptomatic proteinuria and hematuria, (b) nephrotic syndrome, (c) gross hematuria, or (d) an acute nephritic syndrome. The kidney lesion may be a form of nonimmune complement mediated glomerulonephritis.

Biopsy studies reveal extensive mesangial cell proliferation and increased matrix with thickening of the glomerular capillary [15, 48]. Deposits of C3 and properdin are uniformly seen in peripheral lobular distribution by immunofluorescence studies [32, 49]. The studies show granular deposits of C3 along the GBM with or without immunoglobulin [48]. The immunoglobulin may disappear upon serial studies while fixation of C3 is seen [15] (Fig. 12–5).

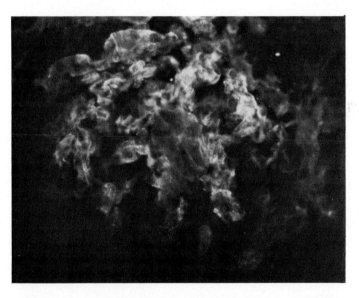

Figure 12-5
Chronic membranoproliferative glomerulonephritis. Fluorescent antibody studies of kidney biopsy showed localization of C3 mostly in the mesangial areas. Only a small amount of IgG was noted along the basement membrane of the glomeruli. The patient had a very low serum C3 level and other findings consistent with the diagnosis. (400× before 20% reduction.)

Properdin and Alternate Pathway of Complement Activation in Immunologic Renal Disease

Properdin

The properdin system was described by Pillemer and co-workers [36] in 1954. Properdin has been demonstrated to be a serum protein [35] distinct from the immunoglobulins and complement components. The properdin system inactivates C3 after activation by zymosan, inulin, or endotoxin without involvement of the earlier complement components.

Recent interest in properdin has been aroused by the demonstration of properdin in glomeruli of patients with acute poststreptococcal glomerulonephritis and chronic membranoproliferative glomerulonephritis [49]. The deposition of properdin and C3 were observed often without the presence of immunoglobulins in the kidneys of patients with acute glomerulonephritis or membranoproliferative glomerulonephritis [49].

Recent investigations of cases of systemic lupus erythematosus (SLE) revealed that properdin is commonly found along with IgG and C3 in lupus nephritis [39]. In addition properdin has been demonstrated at the dermal epidermal junction in the skin biopsy of one patient with SLE. Thus, it appears the properdin system participates in SLE nephritis and that both the classic pathway involving C1, C4, and C2 and the alternate pathway of complement activation (properdin system) are involved in the pathogenesis of the renal lesions.

Alternate Pathway of Complement Activation

It is now known that C3 can be activated by an alternate pathway through the C3 proactivator protein [13, 21, 40]. (See Chapter 4.) Götze and Müller-Eberhard [13] recently described a C3 proactivator which possesses C3 convertase activity when activated by another serum component, properdin factor D and which results in C3 to C9 consumption. This alternate pathway does not involve the C1, 4, 2 system. Aggregated IgA immunoglobulins as well as bacterial polysaccharide, yeast cell walls and inulin can activate the alternate system. This could explain the absence of IgG and presence of C3 and properdin in certain cases of poststreptococcal glomerulonephritis and membranoproliferative glomerulonephritis [49]. A virus or bacterial products may activate properdin and then activate C3, which subsequently produces chemotactic factors with resultant injury. Thus, glomerular injury can occur without participation of a specific antibody-antigen reaction.

It appears that two mechanisms may be operative in the lesions of glomerulonephritis. Terminal complement activation by the properdin system with properdin in the glomerular deposits suggests an alternate pathway of C3 activation as a cause of the injury. In addition, there is evidence for a component of immunologic injury by the classic complement pathway when glomerular deposits of immunoglobulins and earlier reacting components of complement are seen.

The mechanism of depression of the third component of complement (C3) was studied in 20 patients with SLE nephritis and 41 patients with chronic glomerulonephritis [16]. In patients with a low C3 serum level, catabolic rates of C3 were observed to be elevated. The study indicated that in hypocomplementemic mesangioproliferative glomerulonephritis, activation of the alternative pathway of complement was selective, whereas in the case of SLE with nephritis, both pathways of complement activation were involved in the pathogenesis of the lesions.

Nephrotic Syndrome and the Role of IgE Immunoglobulins

The nephrotic syndrome is characterized by edema, proteinuria, hyper-cholesterolemia, and hypoalbuminemia. It is a syndrome of multiple causes [9, 43].

In some cases IgE may play a role in the pathogenesis of the nephrotic syndrome [12]. In a study of nephrotic syndrome with minimal renal changes, IgE immunoglobulin was demonstrated in the capillary walls in a "comma like" fluorescent pattern in the absence of IgG, IgM, IgA, and complement in 7 of 9 patients [12]. The extent of IgE in the glomeruli corresponded to the degree of proteinuria. In 4 patients with nephrotic syndrome with evidence of either focal sclerosing glomerular lesions or membranous chronic glomerulonephritis, a prominent deposition of IgE immunoglobulin was observed in a granular or segmental linear fluorescent pattern along the capillary walls [12]. In 3 of these 4 patients IgG and complement were also detected in the glomeruli.

In a patient with nephrotic syndrome and bronchial carcinoma, immunologic studies suggested that deposition of anti-tumor specific antibody or antibody complexes in the glomeruli may be one mechanism in the development of the nephrotic syndrome in malignant disease [24]. Immunodiffusion studies showed that glomerular eluate and extract of the tumor revealed a line of identity between the patient's serum and the same tumor extract.

Nephropathy with Mesangial IgG-IgA Deposits

Berger [5] has described a glomerular disease in which patients show persistent or recurrent hematuria with mild proteinuria and normal renal function. He reported a series of 55 patients in which renal disease runs a chronic course; only one patient developed renal insufficiency. There is no associated systemic disease, and the disease has features of chronic immune complex disease of unknown etiologic factors.

The diagnosis is made by immunofluorescence studies of a kidney biopsy. The histologic findings are not clear cut, and a few cases show an increase in glomerular mesangial cells. Characteristically, the immunofluorescence studies show granular deposits of IgA, IgG, and C3 largely in mesangial areas of the glomeruli. A similar picture is seen only in anaphylactoid purpura and lupus nephritis [27].

Immune Complex Tubular Disorders

McCluskey [27] has reported 4 cases of a tubular disorder probably due to immune complexes which can be recognized only by immunofluorescence studies. Three patients had lupus nephritis, and 1 had idiopathic hematuria. They all showed bright granular deposits of IgG and C3 along basement membranes of proximal convoluted tubules. The deposits were associated with interstitial fibrosis and mononuclear cell infiltration. Similar deposits of immune complexes along tubular basement membrane have been seen in patients with membranous glomerulonephritis [4] and in renal allografts [3]. The tubular deposits have been noted in experimental kidney disease [17, 44]. The immune deposits may result from the union of autologous antigen of the proximal tubules combining with autoantibody.

Immunologic Aspects of Renal Allografts

Immunofluorescence studies have shown that there are 3 possible mechanisms of damage as outlined by Milgrom et al. [33]: (a) cellular and humoral reactions due to the allograft reaction itself, (b) recurrence of original glomerular disease, and (c) damage due to autoimmune reactions caused by altered tissue specific antigens in the graft. Andres et al. [3] have shown a diffuse linear staining pattern for IgG, and complement was noted in renal allografts. Immunoferritin studies demonstrated localization of immunoglobulins in the subendothelial space, rather than in the basement membrane proper of the glomeruli. The antibodies in the subendothelial space were probably transplantation antibodies and not anti-GBM antibodies.

Humoral and Cell-Mediated Immunity to Kidney Basement Membranes in Various Kidney Diseases

The lymphocytes of certain patients with glomerulonephritis are sensitized to soluble antigens of glomerular basement membrane and correlate with positive in vitro leukocyte migration tests and the presence of linear deposits of IgG and C3 on the renal glomeruli [38].

With use of a passive hemagglutination test in which sheep red cells are coated with human basement membrane antigens, 7% of 194 patients with renal disease had circulating antibodies with titers from 1:16 to 1:64 [34]. Normal controls were negative. The patients with positive results had focal and diffuse proliferative glomerulonephritis nephropathies with necrotizing vascular lesions [34]. Fourteen of 83 patients had evidence of cell-mediated immunity to kidney basement membrane [34] as assessed by the leukocyte migration test of Söborg and Bendixen [42]. One-half of the 14 patients did not demonstrate circulating antibodies to basement membrane by the passive hemagglutination test.

The cell-mediated and humoral immunity to basement membrane probably arise secondarily from alteration of the glomerular tissue and are not the primary cause of the lesions. In contrast, the anti-basement membrane antibodies with high affinity demonstrating strong linear fluorescent localization of IgG and C3 deposits play a dominant role in the pathogenesis of anti-basement membrane glomerulonephritis [31, 45].

Relationship Between Immunofluorescence Patterns and Type of Kidney Lesions

A. A linear pattern of fluorescence along glomeruli showing deposition of IgG and C3 is suggestive of antiglomerular basement membrane nephritis [45]. Linear fluorescent staining of IgG may be seen in cases of lupus nephritis [19], diabetic glomerulosclerosis [11], renal allografts [3], and other unclassified diseases [27].
B. A lumpy-bumpy irregular deposit of IgG or IgM and C3 along the epithelial side of the basement membrane indicates immune complex nephritis [26, 45, 51]. Nuclear localization of IgM and IgG is indicative of lupus nephritis [28].
C. Diffuse deposition of IgG in a granular pattern along the glomerular basement membrane appears characteristic of membranous glomerulonephritis [25].
D. Scattered deposits of C3 and IgG are found in acute proliferative glomerulonephritis [25].
E. Poststreptococcal glomerulonephritis may show scattered deposits of C3, properdin with or without IgG by immunofluorescence studies [49] (Fig. 12–6).
F. In addition to deposits of IgG and C3, significant deposits of fibrinogen are seen in rapidly progressive glomerulonephritis with epithelial crescents [25] (Fig. 12–7).
G. Deposits of C3 and properdin with or without immunoglobulins are noted in a peripheral lobular distribution along the glomerular basement membrane in chronic membranoproliferative glomerulonephritis with serum hypocomplementemia [49].
H. Nephrotic syndrome with membranous lesions may show fluorescent localization of IgE in a comma-like pattern, or IgE may be seen with deposits of IgG and C3 in a granular or segmented linear fluorescence pattern [12].

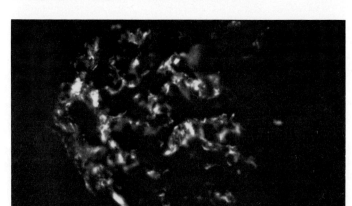

Figure 12–6
Poststreptococcal glomerulonephritis. Fluorescent antibody studies show focal deposits of C3 and IgG. (400× before 20% reduction.)

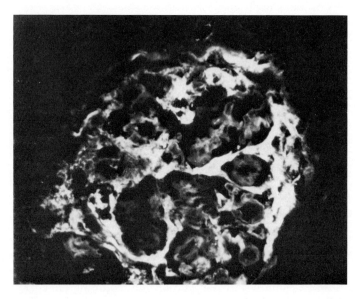

Figure 12–7
Rapidly progressive (subacute type) glomerulonephritis with epithelial crescent formation. Fluorescent antibody study shows dense deposits of fibrinogen. (400× before 20% reduction.)

I. Immunofluorescence patterns of granular IgA and IgG and C3 in mesangial areas of the glomeruli may be seen with focal glomerulonephritis [5, 27].

J. Granular deposits of IgG and C3 along the basement membrane of proximal convoluted tubules are seen in immune complex tubular disorders [27].

The Value of Immunofluorescence Study in Nonimmunologic Renal Disease

Negative immunofluorescence studies with absence of IgG and C3 deposits in the glomeruli are helpful in the diagnosis of lipoid nephrosis and toxemia of pregnancy [26, 27].

Immunofluorescence studies have provided evidence that fibrin and fibrinogen may play a pathogenic role in certain glomerular diseases [47]. In toxemia of pregnancy, fibrinogen and derivatives are found within and between glomerular cells [47]. In rapidly progressive glomerulonephritis, fibrin deposits have accelerated the glomerular sclerosis. In hemolytic uremic syndrome, fibrin-like material was noted along the capillary basement membrane of glomeruli, and fluorescent staining with anti-IgG antibody showed pale dots and streaks in the glomeruli [10].

Summary of Useful Laboratory Tests in the Diagnosis of Immunologic Renal Disease

The history is extremely important for selection of different laboratory tests:

A. Urinalysis and renal function tests

B. Protein electrophoresis of urine and serum.

C. Immunoelectrophoresis and immunoglobulin quantitative analyses when a serum protein abnormality is suspected

D. Antistreptolysin 0 and anti-DNAse antibody titers if poststreptococcal glomerulonephritis is suspected [8].

E. Test for serum immune complexes (see Chapter 6). If immune complex nephritis is suspected, rule out systemic lupus erythematosus, cryoglobulinemia, viral infections, etc. Other useful tests helpful in diagnosis and evaluation are for (a) antinuclear antibodies, (b) serum cryoglobulins, (c) rheumatoid factor, and (d) cold agglutinins.

F. Serum anti-basement membrane antibody test in suspected Goodpasture's syndrome [22, 31].

G. Tissue biopsy studies: (a) routine histology; (b) immunofluorescence studies with antibodies to IgG, IgM, IgA, IgE immunoglobulins, and anti-C3, antifibrinogen, and antialbumin antibodies. Evaluation of nonspecific diffusion of serum protein may be made by study of albumin fixation and distribution. Immunofluorescence studies for localization of properdin will be extremely helpful in certain kidney lesions [39, 49]; (c) electron microscopic studies [6, 41].

Renal Biopsy Studies

Immunofluorescence Studies

Percutaneous biopsy is useful in generalized extensive disease but is of less value in diseases with scattered lesions such as pyelonephritis. Wedge biopsies taken at the time of surgery have certain advantages in that areas with lesions may be selected. However, wedge biopsies may provide only superficial cortex and not contain deeper areas as the corticomedullary junction. Maximal information can be obtained from a wedge biopsy and a needle biopsy of the exposed kidney.

Two segments of tissue obtained by needle biopsy would be ideal for routine histologic, immunofluorescence, and electron microscopic studies. Immunofluorescence studies should be performed in most cases; but electron microscopy is of great value in the evaluation of glomerular lesions [6, 41]. Much information may be gained by evaluation of the 0.5–1 μ Epon embedded sections as foot processes, and fine glomerular deposits may be easily seen [41].

MATERIALS AND REAGENTS
A. Fresh needle core or wedge of renal biopsy
B. Onko Sponge (Histo-Med)
C. Thick glass-walled or plastic test tube with lid
D. Liquid nitrogen or dry ice and acetone bath
E. Frost-free freezer for storage
F. Microtome chuck
G. Cryostat
H. Acid-cleaned slides with coverslips
 I. Buffered saline solution (pH 7.0–7.2; phosphate 0.01 M)
J. Absolute alcohol
K. Dry ethyl ether
L. 95% alcohol
M. Fluorescein-conjugated antibody
N. Moist chamber
O. Buffered glycerol (for mounting slides)

PREPARATION OF RENAL BIOPSY
1. Fresh needle core of renal biopsy is placed on moistened Onko Sponge or a piece of cork.
2. The biopsy tissue with sponge or cork base is lowered into a thick glass-walled or plastic test tube so that it is straight and flush against the wall of the tube.

3. The uncapped tube is placed into liquid nitrogen or dry ice and acetone bath. The tissue is snap frozen through the wall of the tube.
4. Wedge biopsies can be handled by placing tissue directly against the wall of the test tube without sponge and snap frozen by immersion of the test tube into the liquid nitrogen bath.
5. The tubes are removed from the freezing bath, capped, and stored in dry ice or a frost-free freezer. The tissues are not allowed to thaw.

PROCEDURE
1. The tissue is carefully removed from the test tube, mounted on a microtome chuck, and placed in the cryostat. The tissue is handled quickly and not allowed to thaw.
2. 5 μ sections of the biopsy are cut and mounted on acid-cleaned slides.
3. The tissues are washed for 20 to 30 min in 3 changes of cold phosphate-buffered saline solution to remove extraneous protein.
4. The kidney sections may be processed with or without fixation.
5. For fixation, sections are placed in an equal mixture of absolute ethanol and dry ethyl ether at room temperature for 10 min and then in 95% alcohol for 15 min. The sections are then washed with two washes of phosphate-buffered saline solution with 5 min periods for each wash.
6. After drying the slide around the tissue, the wet tissue is covered with the fluorescein-conjugated antibody.
7. The fluorescein conjugate is incubated with the tissue for 30 to 40 min in a moist chamber to prevent evaporation and drying.
8. Then the excess fluorescein conjugate is initially rinsed off by dipping the slides in phosphate-buffered saline solution and then washed with two 8 min rinses in phosphate-buffered saline solution.
9. The sections are then mounted with buffered glycerol and coverslipped.

Peroxidase-Labeled Antibody Studies
(Modified from Davey and Busch [7])
This method is useful; however, it is difficult to obtain a wide spectrum of good reagents.

MATERIALS AND REAGENTS
A. Renal cryostat sections (see Immunofluorescence Studies)
B. Cold acetone
C. Buffered saline solution (pH 7.0; phosphate 0.01 M)
D. Peroxidase-labeled antisera
E. Moist chamber
F. 3,3 diaminobenzidine (Sigma)—75 mg
G. 0.001% peroxidase
H. Tris buffer (pH 7.6, 0.05 M)—100 ml

I. 2% osmium tetroxide
J. Distilled water
K. 70%, 95%, 100% alcohols
L. Xylol
M. Permount (for slides)

PROCEDURE
1. Renal cryostat sections are first fixed in cold acetone for 1 min.
2. The sections are then washed in three changes of phosphate-buffered saline solution with 5 min for each wash.
3. The tissue section is covered with peroxidase-labeled antisera and incubated in a moist chamber for 40 min.
4. Sections are then washed in phosphate-buffered saline solution for 3 times of 5 min each.
5. The sections are then incubated at room temperature for 30 min in a solution described by Graham and Karnovsky [43]: 75 mg 3,3 diaminobenzidine (Sigma) and 0.001% peroxidase in 100 ml tris buffer.
6. The tissues are washed for 10 min in tris buffer.
7. The sections are then reacted with 2% osmium tetroxide in distilled water for 30 min, washed in distilled water, dehydrated in 70%, 95%, 100% alcohols, cleared in 3 changes of xylol, and mounted with permount.

Test for Serum Anti-Basement Membrane Antibodies
(Modified from Lerner et al. [22].)
An indirect fluorescent antibody test may be performed with use of fresh human kidney substrate obtained at surgery or autopsy. It is preferable to obtain kidney from patients of type O blood group.

MATERIALS AND REAGENTS
A. Human kidney substrate
B. Aluminum foil paper
C. OCT (optimal temperature cutting compound) (Lab-Tek)
D. Liquid nitrogen
E. Cryostat
F. Acid-cleaned glass slides and coverslips
G. Phosphate-buffered saline solution 0.01 M, pH 7.0
H. Absolute ethyl alcohol
I. Ethyl ether
J. 95% ethyl alcohol
K. Test serum diluted 1:1
L. Fluorescein-labeled antihuman immunoglobulin
M. Moist chamber
N. Buffered glycerol (for mounting slides)

PROCEDURE

1. Human kidney substrate is collected in aluminum foil paper and covered with OCT (Lab-Tek) and snap frozen in liquid nitrogen.
2. 5–6 μ sections are cut in the cryostat.
3. Sections are washed in phosphate-buffered saline solution 2 times for 10 min each.
4. The kidney sections are then fixed in equal parts of absolute ethyl alcohol and ethyl ether for 10 min.
5. The sections are then placed in ethyl alcohol for 15 min.
6. Following the alcohol, the sections are placed in phosphate-buffered saline solution 2 times for 5 min each.
7. Sections are then reacted with test serum (diluted 1:1) for 30 min.
8. The sections are rinsed in phosphate-buffered saline solution and washed twice more for 10 min each in phosphate-buffered saline solution.
9. The sections are reacted with fluorescein-labeled antihuman immunoglobulin and incubated for 30 to 40 min in a moist chamber.
10. The slides are rinsed in phosphate-buffered saline solution and washed in phosphate-buffered saline solution 2 times for 10 min each, mounted in buffered glycerol, and coverslipped.

Appropriate control normal serum samples should be run concurrently. When examined with the fluorescence microscope, a linear pattern of glomerular fluorescence may be noted. A positive test serum may be titered and retested.

References

1. Agnello, V., Koffler, D., Eisenberg, J. W., Winchester, R. J., and Kunkel, H. G. Cl_q precipitins in the sera of patients with systemic lupus erythematosus and other hypocomplementemic states: Characterization of high and low molecular weight types. *J. Exp. Med.* 134:228s, 1971.
2. Andres, G. A., Accinni, L., Hsu, K. C., Zabriskie, J. B., and Seegal, B. C.   Electron microscopic studies of human glomerulonephritis with ferritin-conjugated antibody. *J. Exp. Med.* 123:399, 1966.
3. Andres, G. A., Accinni, L., Hsu, K. C., Penn, I., Porter, K. A., Kendall, J. M., Seegal, B. C., and Starzl, T. E.   Human renal transplants: III. Immunopathologic studies. *Lab. Invest.* 22:580, 1970.
4. Berger, J., and Galle, P.   Depots denses au sein des membranes basales du rein. Étude en microscopies optique et electronique. *Presse Méd.* 71:2351, 1963.
5. Berger, J.   IgA glomerular deposits in renal disease. *Transplant. Proc.* 1:939, 1969.
6. Churg, J., and Greshman, E.   Ultrastructure of immune deposits in renal glomeruli. *Ann. Intern. Med.* 76:479, 1972.
7. Davey, F. R., and Busch, G. J.   Immunohistochemistry of glomerulonephritis using horseradish peroxidase and fluorescein labeled antibody: A comparison of two technics. *Am. J. Clin. Pathol.* 53:531, 1970.

8. Dillon, H. C., Jr., and Derrick, C. W., Jr.   Streptococcal complications: The outlook for prevention. *Hosp. Practice.* 7:93, 1972.

9. Earley, L. E., Havel, R. J., Hopper, J., Jr., and Grausz, H.   Nephrotic syndrome. *Calif. Med.* 115:23, 1971.

10. Franklin, W. A., Simon, N. M., Potter, E. W., and Krumlovsky, F. A. The hemolytic-uremic syndrome. *Arch. Pathol.* 94:230, 1972.

11. Gallo, G.   Elution studies in kidneys with linear deposition of immunoglobulin in glomeruli. *Am. J. Pathol.* 61:377, 1970.

12. Gerber, M. A., and Paronetto, F.   IgE in glomeruli of patients with nephrotic syndrome. *Lancet* 1:1097, 1971.

13. Götze, O., and Müller-Eberhard, H. J.   The C3 activator system: An alternate pathway of complement activation. *J. Exp. Med.* 134:90s, 1971.

14. Graham, R. C., and Karnovsky, M. J.   The early stages of absorption of injected horseradish peroxidase in the proximal tubules of mouse kidney: Ultrastructural cytochemistry by a new technique. *J. Histochem. Cytochem.* 14:291, 1966.

15. Herdman, R. C., Pickering, R. J., Michael, A. F., Vernier, R. L., Fish, A. J., Gewurz, H., and Good, R. A.   Chronic glomerulonephritis associated with low serum complement activity (chronic) hypocomplementemic glomerulonephritis. *Medicine* (Baltimore) 49:207, 1970.

16. Hunsicker, L. G., Ruddy, S., Carpenter, C. B., Schur, P. H., Merrill, J. P., Müller-Eberhard, H. J., and Austen, K. F.   Metabolism of third complement component (C3) in nephritis. *N. Engl. J. Med.* 287:835, 1972.

17. Klassen, J., McCluskey, R. T., and Milgrom, F.   Nonglomerular renal disease produced in rabbits by immunization with homologous kidney. *Am. J. Pathol.* 63:333, 1971.

18. Koffler, D., Sandson, J., and Kunkel, H. G.   Elution studies on tissue from patients with Goodpasture's syndrome and other forms of subacute glomerulonephritis. *J. Clin. Invest.* 47:55a, 1968.

19. Koffler, D., Agnello, V., Carr, R. I., and Kunkel, H. G.   Variable patterns of immunoglobulins and complement deposition in the kidneys of patients with systemic lupus erythematosus. *Am. J. Pathol.* 56:305, 1969.

20. Koffler, D., Agnello, V., Thoburn, R., and Kunkel, H. G.   Systemic lupus erythematosus: Prototype of immune complex nephritis in man. *J. Exp. Med.* 134:169s, 1971.

21. Lepow, I. H., and Rosen, F. S.   Pathways to the complement system. *N. Engl. J. Med.* 286:942, 1972.

22. Lerner, R. A., Glassock, R. J., and Dixon, F. J.   The role of antiglomerular basement membrane antibody in the pathogenesis of human glomerulonephritis. *J. Exp. Med.* 126:989, 1967.

23. Lewis, E. J., and Couser, W. E.   The immunologic basis of human renal disease. *Pediatr. Clin. North Am.* 18:417, 1971.

24. Lewis, M. G., Loughridge, L. W., and Phillips, T. M.   Immunological studies in nephrotic syndrome associated with extrarenal malignant disease. *Lancet* 2:134, 1971.

25. Mahieu, P., Dardenne, M., and Bach, J. F.   Detection of humoral and cell mediated immunity to kidney basement membrane in human renal diseases. *Am. J. Med.* 53:185, 1972.

26. McCluskey, R. T., Vassali, P., Gallo, G., and Baldwin, D. S.   An im-

munofluorescent study of pathogenic mechanisms in glomerular diseases. *N. Engl. J. Med.* 274:695, 1966.

27. McCluskey, R. T.   The value of immunofluorescence in the study of human renal disease. *J. Exp. Med.* 134:242s, 1971.

28. McCoy, R. C.   Nuclear localization of immunoglobulins in renal biopsies of patients with lupus nephritis. *Am. J. Pathol.* 68:469, 1972.

29. McIntosh, R. M., Kaufman, D. B., Kulvinskas, C., and Grossman, B. J. Cryoglobulins: I. Studies on the nature, incidence and clinical significance of serum cryoproteins in glomerulonephritis. *J. Lab. Clin. Med.* 75:566, 1970.

30. McIntosh, R. M., and Grossman, B.   IgG, B_{1C}, fibrinogen in acute glomerulonephritis. *N. Engl. J. Med.* 285:1521, 1971.

31. McPhaul, J. J., and Dixon, F. J.   Characterization of antiglomerular basement membrane antibodies eluted from glomerulonephritic kidneys. *J. Clin. Invest.* 49:308, 1970.

32. Michael, A. F., Westberg, N. G., Fish, A. J., and Vernier, R. L.   Studies on chronic membranoproliferative glomerulonephritis with hypocomplementemia. *J. Exp. Med.* 134:208s, 1971.

33. Milgrom, F., Klassen, J., and Fuji, H.   Immunologic injury of renal homografts. *J. Exp. Med.* 134:193s, 1971.

34. Morel-Maroger, L., Leathem, A., and Richet, G.   Glomerular abnormalities in nonsystemic diseases—relationship between findings by light microscopy and immunofluorescence in 433 renal biopsy specimens. *Am. J. Med.* 53:170, 1972.

35. Pensky, J., Hinz, C. F., Jr., Todd, E. W., Wedgwood, R. J., Boyer, J. T., and Lepow, I. H.   Properties of high purified human properdin. *J. Immunol.* 100:142, 1966.

36. Pillemer, L., Blum, L., Lepow, I. H., Ross, O. A., Todd, E. W., and Wardlaw, A. C.   The properdin system and immunity: I. Demonstration and isolation of a new serum protein, properdin, and its role in immune phenomena. *Science* 120:279, 1954.

37. Ratnoff, O. D.   The interrelationship of clotting and immunologic mechanisms. *Hosp. Practice* 6:119, 1971.

38. Rocklin, R. E., Lewis, E. J., and David, J. R.   In vitro evidence for cellular hypersensitivity to glomerular basement membrane antigens in human glomerulonephritis. *N. Engl. J. Med.* 282:1340, 1970.

39. Rothfield, N., Ross, A., Minta, J., and Lepow, I. H.   Glomerular and dermal deposition of properdin in systemic lupus erythematosus. *N. Engl. J. Med.* 287:681, 1972.

40. Ruddy, S., Gigli, I., and Austen, K. F.   The complement system of man. *N. Engl. J. Med.* 287:489, 545, 592, and 642, 1972.

41. Seymour, A. E., Spargo, B. H., and Penksa, R.   Contributions of renal biopsy studies to the understanding of disease. *Am. J. Pathol.* 65:550, 1971.

42. Söborg, M., and Bendixen, G.   Human lymphocyte migration as a parameter of hypersensitivity. *Acta Med. Scand.* 3:247, 1967.

43. Smith, F. G., Gonick, H., Stanley, T. H., and McIntosh, R. M.   The nephrotic syndrome: Current concepts. *Ann. Intern. Med.* 76:463, 1972.

44. Unanue, E. R., and Dixon, F. J.   Experimental allergic glomerulonephritis induced in the rabbit with heterologous renal antigens. *J. Exp. Med.* 125:149, 1967.

45. Unanue, E. R., and Dixon, F. J.   Experimental glomerulonephritis: Immunological events and pathogenetic mechanisms. In F. J. Dixon, and J. H. Humphrey (eds.), *Advances in Immunology*. New York: Academic, 1967, vol. 6, p. 1.
46. Vallota, E. H., Forristal, R., Spitzer, R. E., Davis, M. D., and West, C. D.   Characteristics of a noncomplement dependent C3-reactive complex formed from factors in nephritic and normal serum. *J. Exp. Med.* 131:1306, 1970.
47. Vassalli, P., Morris, R. H., and McCluskey, R. T.   The pathogenic role of fibrin deposition in the glomerular lesions of toxemia of pregnancy. *J. Exp. Med.* 118:467, 1963.
48. West, C. D., McAdams, A. J., McConville, J. M., Davis, M. C., and Holland, M. H.   Hypocomplementemic and normocomplementemic persistent (chronic) glomerulonephritis: Clinical and pathological characteristics. *J. Pediatr.* 67:1089, 1965.
49. Westberg, H. E., Naff, G. B., Boyer, J. T., and Michael, A. F.   Glomerular deposition of properdin in acute and chronic glomerulonephritis with hypocomplementemia. *J. Clin. Invest.* 50:642, 1971.
50. Wilson, C. B., Dixon, F. J., Fortner, J. G., and Carilli, G. J.   Glomerular basement membrane reactive antibodies in antilymphocyte globulin. *J. Clin. Invest.* 50:1525, 1971.
51. Wilson, C. B.   Immunological mechanisms of glomerulonephritis. Medical Staff Conference, University of California, San Francisco, Calif. *Calif. Med.* 116:47, 1972.
52. Wilson, C. B., and Smith, R. C.   Goodpasture's syndrome associated with influenza A2 virus infection. *Ann. Intern. Med.* 76:91, 1972.
53. Zimmerman, T. S., and Müller-Eberhard, H.   Blood coagulation initiation by a complement mediated pathway. *J. Exp. Med.* 134:1601, 1971.

13

Laboratory Tests for Autoimmune Disorders of the Skin

S kin lesions may reflect a wide variety of systemic diseases. There are a group of skin diseases in which autoantibody to host tissue is present in the skin lesions as well as in the serum. In many skin diseases there is no definite evidence of an autoantibody; however, since there is evidence of immune pathogenesis, such diseases are called auto-allergies or autosensitizations to skin diseases [28]. Whitfield [28], in 1921, described 3 skin lesions which resulted in autosensitization of the patient to his own skin resulting from local trauma to intact skin or circumscribed area of dermatitis. The term *allergy* has been largely used in humans to designate the skin-sensitizing IgE antibody with anaphylactic and atopic skin reactions. Autosensitization dermatitis has remained as a clinical concept, and the term has been applied loosely to secondary dissemination of chronic eczema often involving the lower leg. However, the terms *autosensitization, autoallergy,* and *autoimmunity* are quite often used interchangeably.

The exact etiology is often unknown in the various skin diseases of either primary or secondary immune pathogenesis. Skin diseases with a primary immune pathogenesis are referred to as *autoimmune disorders of the skin* and include pemphigus and bullous pemphigoid. The primary diseases demonstrate autoantibodies which may play a role in the pathogenesis of the skin lesions. The inciting factor in the production of autoantibodies is unknown in most cases. In certain skin diseases, such as generalized eczema, one can speculate that the autoantibody may arise from the skin lesion with cross reactive properties. The resultant cross reactive antibody may be pathogenic and contribute to the lesions.

Autoimmune Disorders of the Skin

A. Pemphigus—two groups classified according to severity of the disease: (1) pemphigus vulgaris and pemphigus vegetans—this group is the most common and the disease is usually nonextensive and severe; and (2) pemphigus foliaceous: (a) Brazilian pemphigus and

    (b) pemphigus erythematosus—this group has a milder form of the disease than the first group
B. Bullous pemphigoid
C. Cicatricial or benign mucous membrane pemphigoid
D. Dermatitis herpetiformis
E. Lupus erythematosus
F. Behcet's syndrome
G. Cytotoxic antibody in exfoliative dermatitis and generalized eczema

Pemphigus

The diagnosis of pemphigus may be made when the skin lesions demonstrate acantholysis and the patients have specific serum autoantibodies reacting to intercellular substances of the prickle cells [5] (Fig. 13–1). These antibodies are mainly of the IgG type and are directed against the

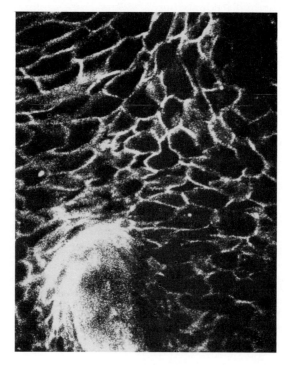

Figure 13-1
Positive indirect fluorescence test for antibodies to intercellular bridges of squamous epithelial cells in pemphigus vulgaris. Substrate is human skin from a normal blood group O patient and was first reacted with serum from a patient with pemphigus vulgaris. The section was then washed and reacted with fluorescein isothiocyanate-labeled rabbit anti-human IgG. Portion of hair follicle is seen in lower part of section. (400× before 20% reduction.)

intercellular substance of the prickle cell layer of the epidermis, and are nonspecies specific. The antibodies have been found to be fixed in vivo and can be demonstrated by direct fluorescence study of the skin lesion. The serum of pemphigus patients shows antibody which is detected by in vitro tests. Several preliminary reports suggested, in skin biopsies of patients with pemphigus, that complement is fixed in vivo in the intracellular areas of epidermis. However, more recent studies with different anti-human complement reagents have provided evidence that complement does not fix in vivo [3, 16]. The level of the antibody in serum is correlated with the progress of the disease and the severity and extent of the lesions. Experience to date indicates that there is localization of the immunoglobulin in the intracellular areas of epidermis in very early lesions from cases of pemphigus. Titers of antibodies are proportional to the severity of the disease in cases of pemphigus vulgaris and pemphigus vegetans.

Serum antibodies in pemphigus are nonspecies specific and can react with heterologous mucosal tissue and skin. The antibodies in pemphigus are usually IgG; however, IgM and IgA have been detected in some patients' sera [24]. Antibodies of the IgA type may occur in early cases of pemphigus in the absence of the IgG type. IgM antibodies have been found only in low titer [3]. IgG and IgA antibodies have also been detected in skin blister fluid [26]. The presence of pemphigus antibodies was demonstrated in the skin blister fluid of a patient whose serum did not contain demonstrable titer [3].

The question which needs to be answered is whether the antibody is the result of the skin lesion or is directly the primary cause of the skin lesions. In pemphigus and bullous pemphigoid it is believed that the antibody is the primary reactive material, since there is an absence of white cells in the early skin lesions. The etiology or inciting factors for the production of the antibodies is not known.

The existence of autoantibody has been documented in both cases by passive transfer of patients' sera from bullous pemphigoid antibodies by intradermal injection of rabbits and guinea pigs yielded in vivo binding of the antibody. Preliminary results demonstrated no subepidermal lesions [3]. However, when passive transfers were done with high titer sera from pemphigus patients, bullous skin lesions of pemphigus were induced in rabbits [2] and monkeys [29]. When skin was treated with a 1 to 2% solution of 2,4-dinitro-benzene immediately following intradermal injection of sera, the epidermal changes consisted of microbullae which resemble pemphigus lesions. The histologic picture and immunofluorescence pattern were both characteristic of pemphigus.

Bullous Pemphigoid

In this disease there are associated autoantibodies in the serum, and the lesions show in vivo fixation of IgG and other immunoglobulins. In bul-

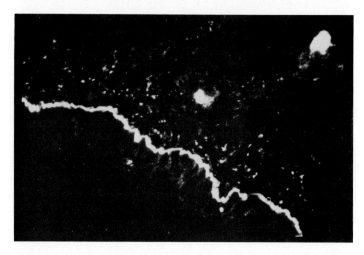

Figure 13-2
Positive indirect fluorescence test for antibody to epithelial basement membrane in bullous pemphigoid. Section consists of human skin from a normal blood group O patient and was first reacted with serum from a patient with bullous pemphigoid and then washed. The section was then reacted with fluorescein isothiocyanate-labeled rabbit anti-human IgG. Note intense fluorescence of epithelial basement membrane. (100× before 20% reduction.)

lous pemphigoid, the antibodies are directed toward the basement membrane of the epidermis and are also nonspecies specific (Fig. 13-2). In vivo and in vitro fixation of complement with antibody have been demonstrated [8]. There is a definite correlation of the level of the antibody with the extent and severity of the lesions. The anti-basement membrane antibodies of bullous pemphigoid do not cross react and fix with the basement membrane of kidney glomeruli. Experimental transfer of bullous pemphigoid antibody yields in vivo binding, but no definite lesions in experimental animals. There is speculation that the bullous disease may be due to a virus.

Cicatricial Pemphigoid
Cicatricial or benign mucous membrane pemphigoid is a distinctive entity which involves skin and mucous membranes. Mucous membrane lesions are characteristic of the disease, and the histopathology is similar to bullous pemphigoid. Recently immunofluorescence studies of 4 cases of cicatricial pemphigoid showed evidence of in vivo fixation of IgG immunoglobulin and complement in the basement membranes of squamous mucosal tissue [1]. The patients showed no evidence of circulating anti-basement membrane antibodies (Fig. 13-3).
These findings suggest a close relationship between cicatricial and

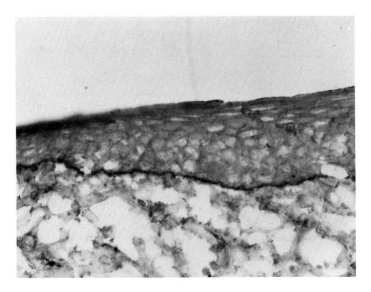

Figure 13-3
Positive direct immunoenzyme test for in vivo fixed IgG in cicatricial or mucous membrane pemphigoid. Frozen section of laryngeal mucosa was obtained at autopsy from a patient with cicatricial pemphigoid. The section was reacted with peroxidase-labeled goat anti-human IgG. After washing, the section was reacted with the substrate to demonstrate a dark brown precipitate along the epithelial basement membrane. (100× before 20% reduction.)

bullous pemphigoid. Cicatricial pemphigoid may be a variant of bullous pemphigoid which differs from bullous pemphigoid by having (a) characteristic mucous membrane lesion tending to form scars, and (b) no detectable serum autoantibodies.

Dermatitis Herpetiformis
In dermatitis herpetiformis there have been reports of IgA and complement in the dermal papillae and near the epidermal junction surrounding the bulla [7, 27]. The deposits show a granular staining pattern by direct immunofluorescence studies (Fig. 13-4). IgG immunoglobulin is less frequently seen in the skin of cases with dermatitis herpetiformis [7, 27]. Indirect immunofluorescence studies for evidence of antiserum antibodies reactive with skin are negative.

Dermatitis herpetiformis and pemphigoid appear somewhat related since there are cases which present features of both entities. One patient studied changed from a diagnosis of dermatitis herpetiformis to that of bullous pemphigoid [15].

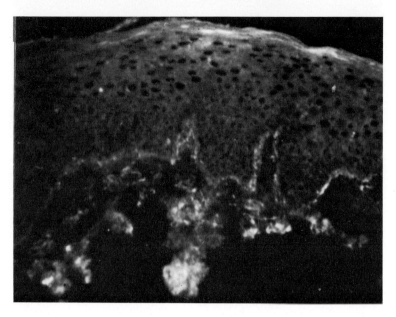

Figure 13-4
Positive direct fluorescence test for IgA immunoglobulin in section of skin adjacent to lesion in dermatitis herpetiformis. A frozen section is reacted with fluorescein isothiocyanate-conjugated rabbit anti-human IgA. Note irregular fluorescent reactions along epithelial basement membrane and upper portion of dermis. (Approximately 100×.)

The role of IgA in skin lesions of dermatitis herpetiformis is unknown. IgA immunoglobulins are found in intestinal mucosa. It is interesting to note that patients with dermatitis herpetiformis have a high incidence of intestinal lesions with coeliac syndrome [18, 22]. The cause of the skin lesions and enteropathy in dermatitis herpetiformis is unknown. Recent studies have indicated an immunological abnormality in dermatitis herpetiformis and adult coeliac disease [22]. A new IgG antibody which reacts with connective tissue reticulin in rat and human organs was found in 17% of patients with dermatitis herpetiformis and 36% of patients with adult coeliac disease [22]. The antibody is directed against reticulin and does not react with basement membrane.

Lupus Erythematosus
A fluorescence technique may be used for the detection of the presence of immunoglobulin at the epidermal junctions, and lupus erythematosus and dermatitis herpetiformis on skin biopsies. Immunoglobulin deposits in the epidermal junctions have been seen in lupus erythematosus [24]. In lupus erythematosus, disrupted nuclear fragments may combine with

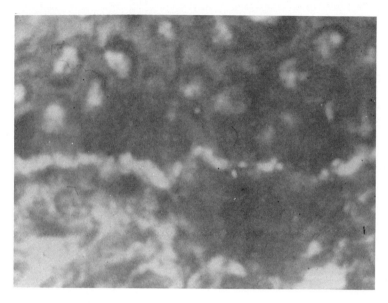

Figure 13-5
Positive direct fluorescence test for fixation of IgG in a skin lesion of patient with systemic lupus erythematosus. A frozen section of skin is reacted with fluorescein isothiocyanate-conjugated rabbit anti-human IgG.
Note fluorescence of squamous cell nuclei along with irregular fluorescence
along basement membrane and upper part of dermis. The nuclear fluorescence is due to antinuclear antibodies, while DNA–anti-DNA immune
complexes are responsible for fluorescence along the basement membrane and
upper dermis. (Approximately 200×.)

circulating antinuclear antibodies, and the resulting antigen-antibody
complexes are deposited near the epidermal junction and the upper
portion of the dermis [24]. (Fig. 13-5) The immunoglobulin found in
lupus primarily consists of IgG, some IgM, and less frequently IgA is
noted with fixation of complement [10].

Behcet's Syndrome [17]
This is a disease of the skin and mucous membranes associated with the
development of autoantibody. The condition consists of ulcers in the
mouth and genitals, arthritis, and in some cases, encephalitis. The
lesions show nonspecific inflammation of the dermis, and autoantibodies
against cells derived from oral mucous membranes are found in the
serum. The antibodies are not organ specific and cross-react with fetal
skin and colon. In certain cases of Behcet's syndrome infective agents
suggested as inclusion bodies have been seen which show herpetiform
lesions.

*Cytotoxic Antibody in Exfoliative Dermatitis
and Generalized Eczema*

Parris et al. [20, 21] have found in patients with chronic dermatitis, who later developed a generalized eczema, that certain numbers have shown specific cytotoxic antibody in their sera. Cytotoxic antibodies to IgG with the ability to fix complement in vitro were found in the sera of 5 or 6 patients. The antibody agglutinated red cells coated with skin extract It appeared in the patient's serum with eczema and disappeared during remission. The interesting thing about this antibody is that it reacts with cells in the subcorneal region and reacts only with homologous skin. The antigen is believed to be a protein in the cells of the stratum granulosum and those cells adjacent to it. The antibody will fix to homologous skin in vitro in the outer epidermis of the stratum granulosum, the hair follicles, and the sweat ducts.

Clinical Significance of Antibodies in Pemphigus and Bullous Pemphigoid [3, 5]

In pemphigus, the titer of antibodies to skin intracellular bridges is useful in following the course of the disease. Antibody titers correlate with the severity of the disease and with the presence and extent of skin and mucous membrane lesions. Pemphigus foliaceus patients may have very extensive skin lesions that have titers up to 10,000 by the immunofluorescence test. Pemphigus foliaceus lesions are more superficial and less severe than pemphigus vulgaris. It is important to study the presence of in vivo bound pemphigus antibodies. There may be some cases with in vivo bound antibodies without evidence of antibodies in the serum.

In bullous pemphigoid, the anti-basement membrane antibodies show in vivo and in vitro fixation along with fixation of complement. There is good correlation of the titer of antibody with the extent and severity of the disease.

*Immunologic Reactions Similar to Those to Antibodies to
Pemphigus and Bullous Pemphigoid*

In patients with Lydel's toxic necrolysis, extensive burns, and myasthenia gravis, there may be serum autoantibodies which react with intracellular bridges of the squamous cells [3]. The immunofluorescence staining reactions are usually weak, and the antibodies probably differ in the antigenic specificity from the true pemphigus antibodies.

The blood group A and B antigens in the intracellular areas of various epithelial cells may result in a false positive test, with individual serum showing a high titer of hyperimmune anti-A or anti-B antisera. Blood group antibodies differ from pemphigus antibodies not only in their response to absorption to their blood group antigens but also in their organ specificity [14].

The antibodies to glomerular basement membrane produced experimentally are nonspecies and non-organ specific and will react with all types of basement membrane.

There is an overlap among these autoimmune diseases, and patients with pemphigus may show a lupus-like syndrome with the presence of antinuclear antibodies and rheumatoid factor.

Diseases Associated with Pemphigus and Bullous Pemphigoid

Pemphigus erythematosus is a form of pemphigus that combines features characteristic of pemphigus and lupus erythematosus. This disease (Senear-Usher syndrome) reveals the presence of pemphigus antibodies and also antinuclear antibodies with other signs of autosensitization [23]. Direct immunofluorescence studies of the skin biopsies of lesions can show presence of antipemphigus antibodies and IgG in vivo bound complement along the dermal-epidermal junction consistent with the diagnosis of the two diseases. Pemphigus can co-exist with lupus erythematosus, thymoma, and myasthenia gravis. This characteristic not only speaks in favor of some common underlying autoimmune disturbances, but also distinguishes the entity from other forms of pemphigus [3].

The relationship between bullous pemphigoid and dermatitis herpetiformis has been discussed above [15]. Both diseases may be seen in association with a malignancy. The increased incidence of tumors in patients with bullous pemphigoid is well recognized [11].

Recommended Work-Up for Laboratory Diagnosis of Autoimmune Disorders of the Skin

A. Tissue biopsy for histopathologic studies. Characteristic histologic features of many of the bullous lesions are described in an excellent review by Graham [13].
B. Direct immunofluorescence studies. Localization of IgG, IgA, and IgM immunoglobulins and C3 complement on biopsy sections of early lesions which include the peripheral skin adjacent to the lesion.
C. Positive findings
   a. Pemphigus: (a) fixation of IgG or other immunoglobulins along intracellular bridges of squamous cells; and (b) no evidence of C3 fixation.
   b. Bullous pemphigoid and cicatricial pemphigoid: (a) fixation of IgG and C3 along epidermal basement membrane.
   c. Dermatitis herpetiformis: fixation of IgA immunoglobulin deposits near the epidermal-dermal junction of skin adjacent to bullae.
   d. Lupus erythematosus: fixation of granular deposits of IgG and other immunoglobulins and complement along the epidermal-dermal junction.

D. Indirect immunofluorescence studies for detection of serum autoanti-
    bodies to skin
    a. Pemphigus and bullous pemphigoid: positive test for in vitro
        fixation of antibodies is seen.
    b. Cicatricial pemphigoid or dermatitis herpetiformis: no serum
        antibodies are seen.
E. Tests for antinuclear antibodies and rheumatoid factor. Evidence of
    antinuclear antibodies may be present and high titers of anti-DNA
    would lead one to suspect a concomitant lupus erythematosus. A
    presence of significant levels of antinuclear antibodies may interfere
    with the detection of serum antiskin antibodies seen in pemphigus
    and bullous pemphigoid. Test for rheumatoid factor: rheumatoid
    factor often occurs in sera of patients with pemphigus and bullous
    pemphigoid.
F. Cases with positive evidence of autoantibodies. These should be
    examined for associated malignancy and other autoimmune diseases.

Practical Methods for Demonstration of Autoantibodies in Skin Disorders

By the direct immunofluorescence method, skin biopsies from patients
are directly studied to demonstrate in vivo fixation of immunoglobulin
and/or complement in cases of pemphigus and bullous pemphigoid.
Serum is tested for the presence of autoantibodies and reacted with
homologous or heterologous epithelial tissue by the indirect immunofluorescence method.

Direct immunofluorescent staining of skin lesions of bullous pemphigoid with labeled anti-human IgG is evidence for in vivo fixation of antibody. A failure to demonstrate IgG in some biopsies may be due to a
secondary change in the tissue due to infection and inflammatory reaction. Thus, a biopsy should be taken from a fresh edematous lesion
without evidence of bullae with a surrounding halo and include healthy-
appearing skin. From a practical point of view, both direct and indirect
staining with patient's serum and direct immunofluorescent staining and
biopsy of fresh lesions for in vivo bound IgG and of complement (C3)
should be carried out in suspected cases of bullous pemphigoid or
pemphigus.

Direct Immunofluorescence Method

MATERIALS AND REAGENTS
A. Skin biopsy from patient
B. Dry ice and acetone or liquid nitrogen
C. Cryostat
D. Clean glass slides
E. Buffered saline solution (pH 7.0; phosphate 0.01 M)

F. Fluorescein-conjugated anti-human IgG and C3
G. Moist chamber
H. Buffered glycerol (for mounting slides)
I. Fluorescence microscope

PROCEDURE
1. A skin biopsy from the patient is snap frozen in dry ice and acetone or liquid nitrogen.
2. Sections are cut at 5 μ in a cryostat and mounted on clean glass slides.
3. The tissue sections are then rinsed and washed in two 8-min changes of phosphate-buffered saline solution.
4. The saline solution is removed surrounding the sections without allowing them to dry out. Fluorescein-conjugated anti-human IgG and C3 are placed on different sections in a moist chamber for 30 min. Each section must be labeled with the type of conjugate it contains.
5. The sections are rinsed and placed in saline washes for two 8-min changes in phosphate-buffered saline solution.
6. The sections are mounted in buffered glycerol and examined under the fluorescence microscope.

Indirect Immunofluorescence Method for the Detection of Serum Autoantibodies to Skin

MATERIALS AND REAGENTS
A. Fresh skin (squamous epithelial tissue) from human with blood type O or guinea pig epithelium from lip or esophagus
B. Negative controls for all procedures (see Interpretation below)
C. Dry ice and acetone or liquid nitrogen (for snap freezing)
D. OCT (optimum temperature cutting compound) (Lab-Tek)
E. Aluminum foil
F. Bottle with screw cap
G. Freezer, $-70°$ C (for storage of tissue)
H. Acetone, ethanol, and methanol (for fixation of tissue if desired)
I. Cryostat
J. Clean glass slides
K. Patient's serum
L. Moist chamber
M. Buffered saline solution (pH 7.0; phosphate 0.01 M)
N. Fluorescein-conjugated anti-human IgG or C3 antibodies
O. Buffered glycerol (for mounting slides)
P. Fluorescence microscope
Q. Washed liver sediment (for absorbing interfering antibodies if necessary)

PROCEDURE
1. Convenient tissues are fresh skin from a human patient with blood type O or guinea pig epithelium from lip or esophagus. Squamous

mucosal tissue is preferred since certain pemphigus sera will react more strongly with a stratified squamous mucous membrane tissue than with epidermis [3]. The frozen tissue can be snap frozen with dry ice and acetone or liquid nitrogen with covering of OCT. The section may be wrapped in aluminum foil and placed in a bottle with a screw cap and stored at $-70°$ C in a nonfrost-free freezer. At present, the unfixed tissue sections afford the antigen of choice for demonstration of the antibodies in pemphigus and bullous pemphigoid. However, acetone-fixed tissue may enhance the staining reaction of pemphigus antibody. Ethanol and methanol fixation removes antigens reactive with pemphigus and bullous pemphigoid antibodies [3].

2. Tissue is cut into 5 μ sections in a cryostat and mounted on clean glass slides.
3. The patient's serum is diluted 1:10 before placing on section. As a recommended procedure, the sera are usually screened at 1:10, 1:40, and 1:160 to avoid prozone reaction. Prozones of negative staining may occur at low serum dilutions with fresh sera of certain patients [3].
4. The section with patient's diluted serum is placed in a moist chamber for 30 min, later rinsed with 2 washes of 8 min each in buffered saline solution.
5. The saline solution is removed surrounding the sections without allowing the sections to dry out, and fluorescein-conjugated anti-human IgG and anti-human C3 are placed upon separate sections and incubated in the moist chamber for 30 min.
6. The slides are rinsed and placed in buffered saline solution for 2 washes of 8 min each.
7. The sections are mounted in buffered glycerol and examined with a fluorescence microscope.

INTERPRETATION. The patient with pemphigus will demonstrate antibodies reactive with the intracellular areas of the prickle cells, while sera from patients with bullous pemphigoid will show a positive reaction in the basement membrane of the skin. The basic negative controls must be clearly distinguishable from the positive reaction patterns. Controls must be included with all experiments, and the staining patterns of pemphigus and bullous pemphigoid antibody should be readily distinguishable from the various controls.

The presence of other antitissue antibodies such as antinuclear antibodies may interfere with the detection of antibodies in pemphigus [3] by means of competitive consumption of the fluorescein-labeled antiglobulin reagent. In suspected cases of pemphigus in which the serum demonstrates antinuclear antibodies and no evidence of skin reactive antibodies, one may absorb the interfering antinuclear antibodies with washed liver sediment [3].

For reproducible fluorescence studies, it is important that the test procedure and reagents are carefully standardized. Beutner and coworkers [3, 6] have shown in their quantitative immunofluorescence studies that good results are seen when the fluorescent anti-human IgG conjugates have at least 4 units of antibody activity with a molar fluorescein-to-protein ratio of 3:5. A unit of precipitating antibody is that amount which will give a precipitin line when reacted with 1 mg IgG/ml by an agar gel double-diffusion technique [4]. Such conjugates may be used at a dilution containing ¼ to ⅛ unit of the conjugate per milliliter for the fluorescence studies.

Peroxidase-Labeled Antibody Method for Demonstration of Autoantibodies to Skin

The peroxidase-labeled antibody method described by Nakane and Pierce [19] has been utilized and reported by Fukuyama and co-workers for the demonstration of pemphigus and bullous pemphigoid antibodies [12]. The peroxidase label conjugate has been used in a similar fashion as the immunofluorescence technique. The reaction is localized by the insoluble products formed following reaction of the enzyme and substrate.

MATERIALS AND REAGENTS
A. Items A, C-M from Indirect Immunofluorescence Method immediately preceding
B. Sera from normal individuals as well as from patients
C. Peroxidase-labeled anti-human IgG antibody
D. Liver powder
E. Saturated solution of 3,3'-diaminobenzidine, 0.0025% hydrogen peroxide in tris buffer solution (pH 7.6; 0.05 M)
F. 2% osmium tetroxide solution
G. Alcohol
H. Xylol

PROCEDURE
1. Guinea pig lip and human skin are used as substrates, and the tissue is quick frozen and cut at 5–6 μ on a cryostat.
2. Sections are incubated with sera from patients and normal individuals for 30 min at room temperature, and then washed with 2 changes of phosphate-buffered saline for a total of 16 to 20 min.
3. Sections are overlaid with peroxidase-labeled anti-human IgG (the conjugate may be adsorbed with liver powder before use). The sections are incubated 30 min at room temperature.
4. The sections are again washed with phosphate-buffered saline solution as in step 2. They are then reacted with substrate solution of 3,3'-diaminobenzidine and hydrogen peroxide for 15 min.
5. The poorly reactive sections are then treated with 2% osmium tetrox-

ide solution, which is placed on the section for 1 hour to enhance the reaction product.
6. The section is then dehydrated in alcohol, cleared in xylol, and mounted.

Indirect Immunofluorescence Test for Detection of Antireticulin Antibody in Dermatitis Herpetiformis and Adult Coeliac Syndrome
(Method of Seah et al. [22])

MATERIALS AND REAGENTS.   See Indirect Immunofluorescence Method for the Detection of Serum Antibodies to Skin.

PROCEDURE
1. Rat kidney sections are cut at 5–6 μ with the use of a cryostat and mounted on clean glass slides.
2. The unfixed sections are reacted with test sera diluted 1:10 for 30 min at room temperature in a moist chamber.
3. The sections are rinsed of excess sera and washed in two 8-min changes of phosphate-buffered saline solution (pH 7.0–7.2).
4. The excess moisture is removed from the slide while keeping the section moist. The tissue is then reacted with the fluoresceinated anti-human IgG conjugate for 30 to 40 min.
5. The sections are rinsed of excess fluorescent conjugate and washed twice for 8 min each in phosphate-buffered saline solution.
6. The sections are mounted with buffered glycerol and coverslips are placed on the slides.
7. The sections are examined with a fluorescence microscope.

INTERPRETATION.   A positive test for antireticulin antibody will show fluorescent staining of the peritubular fibers, Bowman's capsule, and adventitia. The antibody was observed in 17% of 29 cases of dermatitis herpetiformis, and in 36% of 31 patients with adult coeliac disease [22]. In a significant number of cases of dermatitis herpetiformis, one will observe the presence of antinuclear antibodies.

References

1. Bean, S. F., Waisman, M., Michel, B., Thomas, C. I., Knox, J. M., and Levine, M.   Cicatricial pemphigoid. *Arch. Dermatol.* 106:195, 1972.
2. Beutner, E. H., Chorzelski, T. P., Jarzabek, M., Wood, G. W., Leme de Abreu, C., and Bier, O.   Passive induction of intraepidermal clefts in rabbits by transfer of sera from Brazilian pemphigus foliaceous patients. *Int. Arch. Allergy Appl. Immunol.* 42:545, 1972.
3. Beutner, E. H., Chorzelski, T. P., and Jordan, R. E.   *Autosensitization in Pemphigus and Bullous Pemphigoid.* Springfield, Ill.: Thomas, 1970.
4. Beutner, E. H., Holborow, E. J., and Johnson, G. D.   Quantitative studies of immunofluorescent staining: I. Analysis of mixed immuno-fluorescence. *Immunology* 12:327, 1967.
5. Beutner, E. H., Jordan, R. E., and Chorzelski, T. P.   The immuno-

pathology of pemphigus and bullous pemphigoid. *J. Invest. Dermatol.* 51:63, 1968.

6. Beutner, E. H., Sepulveda, M. R., and Barnett, E. V. Quantitative studies of immunofluorescent staining: II. Relationships of characteristics of unabsorbed anti-human conjugates to their specific and nonspecific staining properties in an indirect test for antinuclear factors. *Bull. W.H.O.* 39:587, 1968.

7. Chorzelski, T. P., Beutner, E. H., Jablonska, S., Blaszczyk, M., and Triftshauser, C. Immunofluorescence studies in the diagnosis of dermatitis herpetiformis and its differentiation from bullous pemphigoid. *J. Invest. Dermatol.* 56:373, 1971.

8. Chorzelski, T. P., and Cormane, R. H. The presence of complement, "bound" in vivo in the skin of patients with pemphigoid. *Dermatologica* 137:134, 1968.

9. Chorzelski, T. P., Jablonska, S., and Blaszczyk, M. Immunopathologic investigation in the Senear-Usher syndrome: Co-existence of pemphigus with lupus erythematosus. *Br. J. Dermatol.* 80:211, 1968.

10. Cormane, R. H., Ballieux, R. E., Kalsbek, G. L., and Hymans, W. Classification of immunoglobulins in the dermal-epidermal junction in lupus erythematosus. *Clin. Exp. Immunol.* 1:207, 1966.

11. Cormia, F. E., and Domonkos, A. W. Cutaneous reactions of internal malignancy. *Med. Clin. North Am.* 49:655, 1965.

12. Fukuyama, L., Douglas, S. D., Tuffanelli, D. L., and Epstein, W. L. Immunohistochemical method for localization of antibodies in cutaneous disease. *Am. J. Clin. Pathol.* 54:410, 1970.

13. Graham, J. H. Bullous and pustular dermatoses. In E. B. Helwig and F. K. Mostofi (eds.), *The Skin.* Monograph 10 of the International Academy of Pathology. Baltimore: Williams & Wilkins, 1971, chap. 18.

14. Grob, P. J., and Inderbitzen, T. M. Pemphigus antigen and blood group substances A and B. *J. Invest. Dermatol.* 49:285, 1967.

15. Honeyman, J. F., Honeyman, A., Lobitz, W. C., Jr., and Storrs, F. J. The enigma of bullous pemphigoid and dermatitis herpetiformis. *Arch. Dermatol.* 106:22, 1972.

16. Jordan, R. E., Sams, W. M., and Beutner, E. H. Complement fixing in bullous pemphigoid. *Clin. Res.* 17:275, 1969.

17. Lehner, T. Behcet's syndrome and autoimmunity. *Br. Med. J.* 1:465, 1967.

18. Marks, J., and Shuster, S. Small intestinal mucosa in pemphigoid and subcorneal pustular dermatosis. *Arch. Dermatol.* 100:136, 1969.

19. Nakane, P. K., and Pierce, G. B. Enzyme labeled antibodies for the light and electron microscopic localization of tissue antigens. *J. Cell Biol.* 33:307, 1967.

20. Parrish, W. E., and Rook, A. J. Skin autosensitization. In P. G. H. Gill and R. R. A. Coombs (eds.), *Clinical Aspects of Immunology.* Oxford: Blackwell, 1968, p. 895.

21. Parrish, W. E., Rook, A. J., and Champion, R. H. A study of auto-allergy in generalized eczema. *Br. J. Dermatol.* 77:479, 1965.

22. Seah, P. P., Fry, L., Hoffbrand, A. V., and Holborow, E. J. Tissue antibodies in dermatitis herpetiformis and adult coeliac disease. *Lancet* 1:834, 1971.

23. Shuster, S., Watson, A. J., and Marks, J.　Coeliac syndrome in dermatitis herpetiformis. *Lancet* 1:1101, 1968.
24. Tan, E. M., and Kunkel, H. G.　An immunofluorescent study of the skin lesions in systemic lupus erythematosus. *Arthritis Rheum.* 9:37, 1966.
25. Triftshauser, C., and Beutner, E. H.　IgA and IgM reactive antibodies in the serum from pemphigus patients. *Fed. Proc.* 28:770, 1969.
26. Triftshauser, C., Jordan, E. R., Fergus, A., and Beutner, E. H.　Pemphigus antibodies of the IgA type. Abstracts of the 46th International Association of Dermatology Research. Meeting, 1968, p. 105.
27. Van der Meer, J. B.　Granular deposits of immunoglobulin and the skin of patients with dermatitis herpetiformis: An immunofluorescent study. *Br. J. Dermatol.* 81:493, 1969.
28. Whitfield, A.　Some points on the aetiology of skin disease: Lecture II. *Lancet* 2:122, 1921.
29. Wood, G. W., Beutner, E. W., and Chorzelski, T. P.　Studies in immunodermatology: II. Production of pemphigus-like lesions by intradermal injection of monkeys with Brazilian pemphigus foliaceous sera. *Int. Arch. Allergy Appl. Immunol.* 42:556, 1972.

14

Laboratory Evaluation of Autoimmune Hemolytic Anemias

Carol A. Bell

Introduction

Classification of Hemolytic Anemias

Hemolytic anemias encompass a diverse group of biochemical and immunologic disorders (Table 14-1). Diagnosis of the specific type of hemolysis depends largely on the laboratory and has long-term effect on the clinical management of the patient and his ultimate prognosis.

Most congenital hemolytic anemias have a proven genetically controlled biochemical basis [16, 50, 65], whereas autoimmune hemolytic anemias are due to acquired autoantibodies to antigenic determinants on the red cell membrane [11, 13, 51]. These anemias have proven more difficult to classify than the congenital hemolytic anemias. For example, classic division into warm and cold types [11, 60] by the thermal range of autoantibody activity may appear inconsistent when hemolysins are encountered, which has led to expanded systems of classification [18, 62]. The autoantibody coating of the red cell usually gives rise to a positive direct antiglobulin test (AGT or Coombs test), which is an important part of the diagnosis. It is not the sine qua non, however [22], and classifications with regard to "Coombs positive" vs. "Coombs negative" types of hemolytic anemia may not be valid following acute hemolysis, since the direct AGT may then be negative. Furthermore, paroxysmal nocturnal hemoglobinuria (PNH), an acquired defect of the red cell membrane [23, 24], rather than a serum antibody, must frequently be considered in the diagnosis of immune hemolytic anemias.

Pathogenesis of Autoimmune Hemolytic Anemia (AIHA)

The pathogenesis of erythrocyte autoantibody production is unknown, although several hypotheses have been advanced [7, 14, 15, 19, 43, 51, 58, 59]. Theories regarding pathogenesis of autoimmune disease in

Table 14–1. Etiologic Classification of Hemolytic Anemias.

I. Congenital hemolytic anemias (intrinsic, Coombs negative)
  A. Defects in hemoglobin synthesis (Hgb S, Hgb Zurich, thalassemia)
  B. Defects in red cell enzymes (G-6PD, pyruvate kinase, triose isomerase)
  C. Defects in red cell membrane (hereditary spherocytosis)
II. Acquired hemolytic anemias (*usually* extrinsic, Coombs positive or negative)
  A. Physical trauma to red cell (burns, hemolytic-uremic syndrome)
  B. Chemical effects (direct, dose-related toxins; indirect, red cell enzyme related)
  C. Infections (protozoa, leptospira, virus, bacteria)
  D. Antibody
    1. isoantibody (incompatible pregnancy or transfusion)
    2. autoantibody
      a. primary (idiopathic)
      b. secondary
        (1) hematologic neoplasm: chronic lymphocytic leukemia, lymphosarcoma
        (2) collagen disease: SLE, RA, ulcerative colitis, Hashimoto's thyroiditis
        (3) drug induced: penicillin, alpha-methyldopa, stibophen
        (4) infections: virus, bacteria, Mycoplasma
        (5) epithelial neoplasm: thymoma, ovarian ca.
  E. Paroxysmal nocturnal hemoglobinuria (PNH)
  F. Miscellaneous or undetermined causes

---

general have been extrapolated to the red cell, as summarized in Fig. 14-1. Burnet [7] favors a "forbidden clone" of immunocytes (T-cells?) uncensored by thymus, producing a forbidden antibody in response to change in the target (RBC) cell. Dameshek [15] believes a "foreign clone" of otherwise unchanged antibody-producing cells (B-cells or plasma cells?) produces a monoclonal forbidden autoantibody. Fudenberg [19] has suggested that the defect may be one of immunodeficiency. Thus, normal mechanisms that would prevent "forbidden" or "foreign" clones from proliferating are absent. Weigle [58] has shown that alteration of a normal self antigen can break the normal immune tolerance to self, allowing production of autoantibody. Thus, destruction of T-cell tolerance leaves normal B-cells competent to produce autoantibody unmonitored. Alternatively the macrophage or antigen-recognition cell becomes supersensitive to previously tolerated self antigen and produces autoantibody [59]. Combining the immune deficiency and broken tolerance theories, Pirofsky [51] hypothesizes that somatic mutation of RBC antigen by virus, drug, metabolite, etc., creates a related antigen which terminates tolerance to the RBC, and autoantibody is formed.

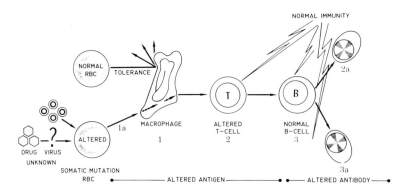

Figure 14-1
Theories of autoimmunity. 1. Increased macrophage responsiveness to previously tolerated (unprocessed) antigen; 1a. broken tolerance. 2. Forbidden clone (uncensored T-cell) among normal clones; 2a. production of forbidden antibody by normal plasma cells. 3. Foreign clone (B cells?); 3a. production of foreign antibody. 4. Immune deficiency unable to block 1, 2, or 3 products as a normal defense.

Chronic production of low levels of altered red cells permits continuation of hemolytic anemia. If the altered stimulus source is stopped, remission occurs. However, according to Weigle's experiments [58, 59], large numbers of normal RBC should block such a process. It is evident from all theories that there may be four levels of responsiveness in AIHA, the red cell, the macrophage, the lymphocyte (T-cell), and the lymphocyte (B-cell). It is evident also from the differences in antibody specificity of the warm and cold hemolytic anemias, and their clinical manifestations, that the pathogenesis for each type may differ and may be a combination of one or more theories. Aldomet, alpha-methyldopa, induced warm antibody hemolytic anemia may provide the model which solves the problem, but as yet it has not done so [41, 64].

MECHANISM OF ACTION. The mechanism of injury, whatever its pathogenesis, is cytolysis of the red cell by IgG or IgM molecules, rarely IgA. These immunoglobulins bind to red cells by means of antigen specific configurations on their Fab fragments. In the case of IgG antibody (Fig. 14-2), as in warm AIHA, the coated cell is vulnerable to macrophages which bind to the Fc portion of the IgG via their surface antigen receptors [43]. In the case of IgM antibodies (Fig. 14-3), as in cold hemolytic anemias, complement is also attached to the cell membrane. The IgM antibody can, and usually does, dissociate rather easily from antigenic receptors in response to temperature variation, but complement remains to coat the cell or to cause its eventual lysis.

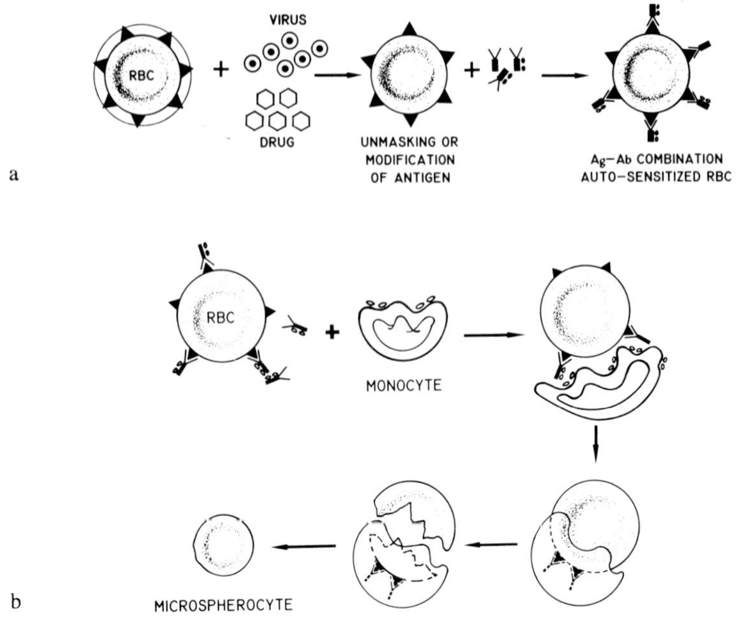

a

b   MICROSPHEROCYTE

Figure 14-2
Mechanism of cell destruction in warm antibody hemolytic anemia. (a) Antigen is unmasked and autoantibody produced. Ab combines via Fab fragment. (b) Macrophage membrane receptors bind to Fc determinants of IgG antibody. Macrophage engulfs RBC; residual fragment re-establishes membrane as somewhat smaller spherocyte.

Clinical Manifestations
Classic cases of warm autoantibody hemolytic anemia are clinically severe with abrupt onset, jaundice, splenomegaly; the peripheral smear contains many spherocytes [11]. It is associated with a high incidence of lymphocytic neoplasms, or with collagen disease, particularly systemic lupus erythematosus [13]. Due to the latter group, warm hemolytic anemias are somewhat more frequent in young age groups with slightly more females than males. Warm hemolytic anemias usually respond well to steroid therapy or to splenectomy [49]. Survival may be for prolonged periods of time depending on the underlying disease and on the side effects of steroid therapy.

Increasing numbers of cases of true warm AIHA are due to α-methyldopa (Aldomet) (Merck) therapy [41, 64] and occasionally other drugs such as mefenamic acid (Ponstel) (Parke-Davis) and indomethacin [4, 13]. The presence of the drug is not necessary once the process has begun, and the positive direct Coombs test may persist for many months

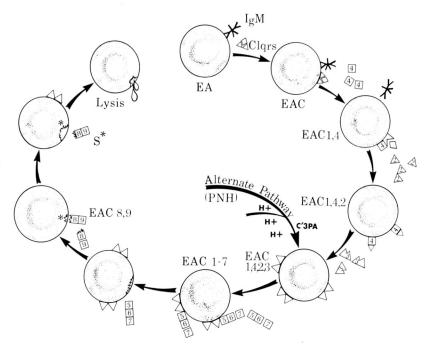

Figure 14-3
Mechanism of cell destruction in cold hemolytic anemia via classic complement pathway. IgM antibody (A) combines with erythrocyte (E). Sequential action of C' fractions proceeds to hemolysis. Antibody may detach to
sensitize other cells. Osmotic leak (S*) is produced in RBC membrane leading to hemolysis. The alternate pathway can be activated without antibody
by low pH, or aggregated globulin by activating C3 proactivator (C3PA)
as in PNH.

[13] before spontaneously subsiding. The mechanism of autoantibody
production is not understood [14, 15, 41], although incorporation of
the drug at the marrow level of development has been suggested [64].

Clinically, cold hemolytic anemias are usually insidious in onset, producing few symptoms, without splenomegaly, with subclinical jaundice;
few spherocytes are seen on the peripheral smear. However, post-viral
anemias may be abrupt and severe. Except for the acute onset type following viral infection, most others are idiopathic. When neoplasms appear they are usually reticulum cell sarcoma, or Hodgkin's disease. These
patients respond poorly to steroids or splenectomy, and survival is dependent on the underlying disease [11, 13].

Of the various types of hemolytic anemia, those due to autoantibodies
are the most complex and confusing, often studied under less than opti-

mum conditions due to pressures of time in acute hemolysis, or failure to recognize the clinical picture in chronic hemolysis. Information is, therefore, obtained in a fragmentary fashion increasingly obscured by steroid or transfusion therapy. The evaluation need not be confused or excessively complex if approached in a logical manner.

Serologic Evaluation of RBC Autoantibodies

The organized approach to laboratory testing in hemolytic anemia should encompass a battery of tests which characterize (a) cell and cell adsorbed antibody and (b) serum antibody (Fig. 14-4), as outlined below:

A. Direct antiglobulin tests with anti-γ and anticomplement reagents
B. Acid hemolysis (PNH) screening test, and if indicated: (1) extended tests; (2) sugar-water lysis test
C. Donath-Landsteiner hemolysin (PCH) screening test
D. Serum autoantibodies: (1) 37° C vs. untreated, vs. papain treated RBC; (2) 4° C vs. treated, vs. papain treated RBC
E. Isoantibody identification

From these tests a working diagnosis can be made which can direct therapy. Any other tests merely lend supportive evidence to the antibody classification and can be completed when time permits. Although transfusion is not recommended, if it becomes necessary, the sorting out of autoantibodies vs. isoantibodies will be critical in these baseline studies. Follow-up studies after steroid therapy become more meaningful as well.

Specimens
In order to perform all of the tests outlined, two 10 ml clots and a 7 ml EDTA Vacutainer tube (Becton-Dickinson) of blood are required. Defibrinated blood is useful for later follow-up tests, but it is not an absolute requirement.

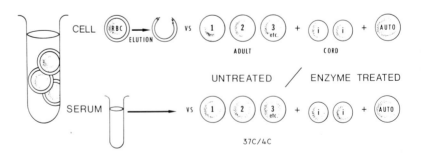

Figure 14-4
Serologic analysis of autoimmune hemolytic anemia.

Optimally, blood for hemolytic anemia work-up should be collected in a syringe warmed to 37° C and deposited in prewarmed tubes. Serum is separated from the clot while it remains at 37° C, and then is frozen if not tested immediately. These maneuvers are directed at preventing absorption of cold antibodies to the clot, thus lowering serum antibody titer and changing the red cell globulin coat. However, collection of specimens is not always under control of the laboratory, and clots are submitted for testing without fastidious collection. They should then be incubated 30 min at 37° C before serum is removed for testing. Once removed, serum can be refrigerated, or frozen if hemolysins are to be tested for. If sera are stored at −70° C they may be saved for several years.

Direct Antiglobulin Tests (Direct Coombs Tests)
Anti-human globulin reagents show considerable variability in the spectrum of globulins they detect [20] (Fig. 14-5). Many reagents are broad spectrum, adequately balanced, between γ and non-γ (complement) detection; others are distinctly γ oriented and will not detect complement. Anti-non-γ reagents for detection of the β globulins of complement may not be regularly available. However, they can be produced by precipitating the anti-γ fraction from a broad spectrum reagent with γ globulin [17, 33].

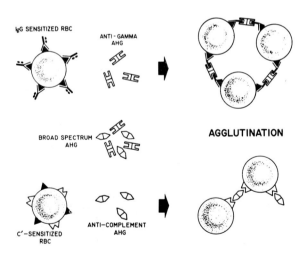

Figure 14-5
Broad spectrum antiglobulin reagent may be used as components specific for an immunoglobulin class, anti-γ G for usual IgG warm autoantibody, or anticomplement when IgM antibodies are involved as in cold hemolytic anemia.

γ-Globulin Neutralization (*Anti-non-γ Coombs reagent*) [17]
1. Dilute AHG 1:4 with saline solution.
2. Add equal volume of 1% pure γ globulin (7S) (Calbiochem) or 1:1000 anti-D Immune Globulin, Human.
3. Incubate 10 min at 37° C.
4. Reagent may be aliquoted and stored. However, to prevent dissociation of the neutralized 7S–anti-7S antibody, it is preferable to use the reagent in the first few days.
5. Control: complement coated cell [32]. (See below, Preparation of Control Coated Cells for Specific Antiglobulin Reagents.)

The direct antiglobulin test is performed with both anti-γ and anti-complement reagents. Anti-γ reactions show IgG antibody which is compatible with warm hemolytic anemia. Anti-complement reactions are compatible with complement absorption, implying previously adsorbed, but no longer present or not detectable, IgM antibody and cold hemolytic anemia. In some cases complement absorption may be associated with IgG antibody [6, 18].

More specific antiglobulin reagents may be obtained from immunodiffusion kits used for quantitation of immunoglobulins. Of particular value are anti-IgG, anti-IgM, anti-IgA, anti-β_{1C} (C3), and anti-β_{1E} (C4). They should not be used directly because the high concentration can cause prozones and false negative results. In addition, antispecies antibodies are still present which agglutinate all human red cells. These must either be absorbed out or the working dilution (1:16 or 1:32) chosen to avoid them. Usually the latter achieves both goals with one step. Control red cells with the appropriate globulin class absorbed to them are necessary to evaluate test results.

PREPARATION OF CONTROL COATED CELLS FOR SPECIFIC ANTIGLOBULIN REAGENTS
IgG Control Cell
1. Rh_0 positive cell, washed and packed. Add equal volumes of saline.
2. Dilute anti-D slide typing serum 1:4 in saline.
3. Add equal volume diluted anti-D to cell-saline mixture.
4. Incubate 45–60 min at 37° C and wash 3 times with normal saline. Use as 2–5% suspension.
IgM Control Cell [12]
1. Use serum with anti-Le^a previously identified, 10 volumes.
2. Add 1 volume EDTA neutralized to pH 7.0 (to block complement absorption)
   K_2EDTA .89 Gm
   1N NaOH 1.5 ml
   Water to make 20 ml.
3. 1 volume 50% saline suspension group O, Le a+ cells + 10 volumes of anti-Le^a serum − EDTA mixture is incubated 1–2 hours at 37° C.

4. Wash cells 3 times in normal saline solution and use as 2–5% suspension.

Complement Control Cell [33]
1. Prepare 6% solution of chemical grade sucrose and 0.15% NaCl in distilled water.
2. To 3 ml this solution add 2–3 drops of defibrinated fresh whole blood (NEVER anticoagulated).
3. Incubate 15 min at 37° C.
4. Wash cells 2 times in physiological saline. Use as 2–5% suspension.

A technique using trypsinized red cells [54] can be modified to provide a control cell.

ABSORPTION OF HETEROSPECIFIC ANTIBODIES FROM SPECIFIC ANTI-GLOBULIN REAGENTS [47]
1. Dilute antiserum 1:1 with 0.85% NaCl. Heat at 56° C for 30 min.
2. Pool equal volumes of group A_1, B, and O red cells. Wash 10 times in saline and pack.
3. Absorb diluted, inactivated antiserum with an equal volume of pooled cells for 1 hour at 4° C.
4. Centrifuge and remove absorbed serum.
5. Aliquot absorbed serum in 0.5 ml volumes and freeze.

In some cases, papain treatment of the red cells reduces neutralization of the antiglobulin reagent by nonspecifically absorbed globulins which may be present on the red cell membrane.

A sensitive estimate of globulin adsorbed to red cells using Coombs consumption has been described [6]. However, the most sensitive method uses ^{125}I-labeled anti-γ-globulin to measure bound antibody in micrograms [31]. Occasional cases of active immune hemolysis have been reported with a negative antiglobulin test [22]. These may be due to improper antiglobulin reagent [20], incredibly minute amounts of adsorbed antibody, or technical error in allowing the AGT to reverse as it stands on the red cells. All tests must be resuspended promptly and read macroscopically and microscopically.

Elution Techniques
The adsorbed globulin should give at least a 1+ reaction with antiglobulin reagents in order to yield enough eluted antibody for identification.

Various techniques have been employed for eluting antibody. Many involve lysis of the red cell with its antibody and/or complement and precipitation of the globulin by an organic solvent with subsequent mechanical separation from the red cell stroma by centrifugation. Some of the following techniques have been evaluated for ease, time, and antibody yield [36]. The cold alcohol precipitation method [61] is useful because complement is preserved, antibody yield is good, and eluates may be stored at $-70°$ C for several years. It requires 2 or 3 hours to prepare, however, and the eluate is hemoglobin stained. This is really no disadvantage when eluate identification tests are carried to antiglobulin phase, but direct readings cannot be interpreted with regard to hemolysis. The simplest technique is heat elution [39], useful in studying warm hemolytic anemia. However, unsuspected complement is lost and eluates store poorly if future comparative testing is to be done. These two methods each yield 33% of the antibody globulin [12].

The ether elution method [53] depends greatly on the anhydrous quality of the ether to precipitate globulin efficiently. It is difficult to use because its volatile nature may propel the eluate across the laboratory. The globulin yield is good (50–70%), but eluates tolerate storage poorly. For non-hemoglobin stained eluates with good storage properties the digitoxin method [37] is suggested. Its major disadvantage is the 16–20 hours needed to prepare the final globulin.

The eluate is tested against untreated and enzyme-treated panel cells at $37°$ C to determine specificity. Reactions should be carried to antiglobulin phase for greatest sensitivity. IgG antibodies usually show specificity for anti-e or other parts of the Rh-Hr complex, whereas eluted complement has no activity against red cells.

RED CELL ANTIGENS.   In order to understand the significance of cell-adsorbed globulin, particularly in warm hemolytic anemia, the cell should be typed for all pertinent antigens, which usually involves at least ABO grouping and the Rh phenotype. Saline typing sera should be used since any antiglobulin technique only duplicates the direct Coombs test. Mixed field appearance is present if the hemolytic process is recent in onset or if there have been recent transfusions. Typing cells for I may be of value in transfused cold AIHA since isoanti-I in the rare adult i can also cause hemolysis.

Serum Antibody Evaluation

Using standard identification panels, tests are conducted simultaneously at $37°$ C and at $4°$ C using an untreated and an enzyme-treated series of cells. An enzyme-treated series should be included since weak antibodies may be detected only by this technique [13]. This is particularly true for eluates. Standard identification panels usually include 8 or 9 group O adult cells, but they differ in the completeness with which the antigens are determined. Use panels where P, Lutheran, and Sutter groups are determined, and an Le(a-b-) cell is present. Some panels have U negative cells, which is a useful bonus [44]. To the panel add 2 group O cord blood samples and the patient's own cells. To screen the patient's serum for antibodies reacting optimally at 4° C, one may use a "short panel" of untreated and enzyme treated red cells. That is, select 3 panel members that include among them all of the major antigens (V, f, and Diego can be excluded). Use these panel members individually, not pooled. Add to the short panel at least one cord blood and the autologous cells. If results are negative, further testing at 4° C can be dispensed with. If positive, tests must be repeated with the full panel.

Enzyme Treatment of Red Cells
Enzyme treatment of red cells can use one of several proteolytic enzymes including bromelin, ficin, papain, and trypsin [56]. Pretreatment of the cells allows more reproducible results, and it is therefore helpful if 20–25% cell suspension identification panels are available rather than the standard 4–8%.

Papain pretreatment is easily accomplished by the Kuhns and Bailey method [38, 56]. The papain should be crude since refining it reduces its effectiveness. Although trypsin can be used for pretreatment, unspecific reversible agglutination on immediate centrifugation [30] can produce technical problems and difficulty in interpretation. The efficiency of cell treatment also varies with the preparation [27].

Papain Pretreatment of Red Cells [38]

SPECIMEN.   At least 0.15 ml red cells, washed and packed 2 times. Contaminating serum contains inhibitors of enzyme action and must be removed.

MATERIALS
37° C water bath

REAGENTS
A. Stock papain solution 1%
   Crude papain (Difco)—1 gm
   0.85% NaCl—100 ml
   1. Filter through Whatman No. 1 filter paper.
   2. Freeze in 1 ml aliquots. Good for six months if stored at −40° C.
B. Phosphate-buffered saline (pH 7.3)
   Normal saline 0.85%—90 ml
   Phosphate buffer (pH 7.3)—10 ml
   1. Keep refrigerated.

PROCEDURE
1. Immediately before use, an aliquot of 1% frozen papain stock is thawed and diluted 1:10 with phosphate-buffered saline.
2. Add 1 volume packed red cells to 2 volumes 0.1% papain solution. Mix.

3. Incubate exactly 30 min in 37° C water bath with frequent agitation.
4. Wash papain treated cells 3 times in fresh saline, carefully aspirating saline after each washing. Adjust red cell suspension to 3–4%.
5. Mark cells as papain treated. If refrigerated overnight, cells are good for approximately 48 hours, but should not be used after this. They may be left at 25–27° C during work day with no damage.
6. For use on 2nd day aspirate hemoglobin-tinged saline, wash once in saline and resuspend at 3–4%.

NOTES
A. Papain destroys M, N, S, Fy^a, Fy^b, and Sp_1 antigens.
B. 20–25% suspension red cell panels are the most useful. These are currently supplied by Hyland Laboratories and by special arrangement from Gamma Biologicals.

Trypsin Pretreatment of Red Cells [56]

SPECIMEN.   Use 2% suspension of red cells washed 2 times.

REAGENT
Stock trypsin solution 1%
Trypsin powder (Difco)—1 gm dissolved in phosphate buffer (pH 7.4) —100 ml
1. Filter through Whatman No. 1 filter paper.
2. Freeze in 1 ml aliquots. Good for 6 months if stored at −40° C.

PROCEDURE
1. Add 1 volume of stock trypsin solution to 10 volumes washed 2% suspension red cells.
2. Incubate 15 min at 37° C. Wash 3 times with saline and resuspend at 2%, labeled trypsin-treated.

NOTES
A. Fy^a antigens survive trypsin treatment.
B. May be kept 48 hours if refrigerated overnight. Wash once before using on second day.
C. For antibody testing use 2 drops trypsin-treated cells with 2 drops of serum. Incubate 1 hour at 37° C and read macroscopically and microscopically. Do NOT centrifuge. (Trypsin is subject to reversible false agglutination [30] by normal serum antitrypsin antibody.) Reaction can then be carried to antiglobulin phase.

Antibody identification utilizes standard techniques [33]. Antibodies are designated autoantibody or isoantibody by their reactivity with autologous cells, confirmed by determination of the specific antigen on the red cell. Retesting the serum after absorption may be necessary when both autoantibodies and isoantibodies are present.

The autoantibody may be titered against the autologous cells and R_2R_2 cells, both untreated and enzyme-treated, as a base line for following therapy in warm hemolytic anemia. In cold antibody hemolytic anemia, cold agglutinin titers serve this purpose. They may be titrated against self or against one of the identification panel cells.

Isoantibody Identification in AIHA

It is important to identify underlying isoantibodies which may have resulted from recent transfusion in clinically unrecognized AIHA or from transfusion in the more remote past. Although transfusion in AIHA should be avoided, if it becomes necessary, isoantibodies must be considered in donor selection. Certain isoantibodies to rare antigens are significant in that they occur only with autoimmune hemolytic anemia. Anti-Miltenberger (anti-Mi^a), anti-Wright (anti-Wr^a), anti-Sw^a, anti-By, anti-Vw (Verwyst), and anti-C^x fall into this group [47, 52].

Where transfusions have been recently administered it may be difficult to determine isoantibody and secondary positive direct AGT vs. autoantibody and primary positive direct AGT. Observance of mixed fields in red cell antigen testing as well as in the direct AGT may be helpful. In general the patient's own cells are dominant in the mixed field, and if those red cell antigens are of the same specificity as the antibody, the antibody should be considered autoantibody.

Absorption and Elution Studies

Combined absorption or elution can be helpful for the ultimate answer, but clinically useful information is available without these additional maneuvers. Sera may be absorbed of nonspecific background autoantibody and retested to determine other antibody specificities. Frequently absorption with enzyme-treated autologous cells is most efficient for this procedure. Absorption of sera with R_2R_2, R_1R_1, and rr cells can be useful, with subsequent elution of the absorbed globulin, testing of the eluate for specificity, and retesting the serum for residual activity.

If Rh null cells or other Rh-deleted cells are available, the eluate (and serum, if group compatible) should be tested against them. The "nonspecific" pan-agglutinin can then be further classified as anti-nl (all cells except Rh null or deleted cells), anti-pdl (all cells including deleted cells, but not the Rh null), and anti-dl (all cells including Rh null), indicating the degree of primitiveness to the autoantibody [57, 60].

Polyagglutinable Cells in AIHA

Polyagglutinable cells may occur in hemolytic anemia with more frequency than commonly realized, because it is a circumstance where it is difficult to recognize them. Failure to identify their presence may lead to unexplainable results either in the initial serologic evaluation or in follow-up studies after therapy has begun. In the absence of AIHA, polyagglutinable cells characteristically [5, 34, 35] are not agglutinated by the patient's own serum, nor are the cells Coombs positive, two points no longer applicable in AIHA. They may be recognized as an aberrant ABO typing, or as mixed field agglutinations in other typings or minor cross-matches. Agglutination is stronger at lower temperatures. Cord serums lacking the ubiquitous anti-T and anti-Tn do not agglutinate these cells.

Polyagglutinable cells have been divided into four major groups [5], those due to T activation, those due to Tn activation, Cad positive cells, and type III or acquired B antigen. As a matter of fact, Tn cells were first reported in AIHA [33]. Subgroups of nonconforming polyagglutinability are recognized with increasing frequency [5]. Polyagglutinability should be suspected when (a) unusual results are found in ABO typings, (b) all typing sera give positive results, or (c) mixed fields are prominent. Proof of polyagglutinability can be accomplished by noting agglutination of the patient's red cells by three adult AB serums known to be free of atypical red cell antibodies and cold agglutinins. Cord serums will not agglutinate them. A polybrene technique for differentiating polyagglutinable from normal cells is available for those who wish to pursue the serologic diagnosis [34]. Neuraminidase treatment of cells activates the T-antigen for absorption studies.

Neuraminidase-Treated Red Cells

SPECIMEN.   Red cells washed in saline 3 times and packed.

REAGENTS.   Neuraminidase, diluted 1:4 in normal saline with 0.4% $CaCl_2$ added (Behring).

PROCEDURE
1. Add 1 volume packed red cells to 1 volume neuraminidase solution.
2. Incubate 30 min at 37° C.
3. Wash cells 5 times in normal saline.

NOTES
A. Neuraminidase activates the T-receptor, and is useful in evaluation of polyagglutinability [5, 34, 35].
B. Neuraminidase destroys Sp_1 receptor [45].

HEMOLYSIS AND HEMOLYSINS
Intravascular hemolysis may be not only a feature of either warm or cold AIHA, but also a disease entity of its own as in PNH or PCH. Therefore, the hemolysins are a necessary part of any serologic evaluation. The diseases they represent are often confusing and can be easily overlooked if these tests are not included.

Acid Hemolysis (Test for PNH)
This test is indicated in all cases of intravascular hemolysis or aplastic anemia. It has been said that paroxysmal nocturnal hemoglobinuria (PNH) may not be paroxysmal, is seldom nocturnal, and may be without hemoglobinuria. Differing from the usual AIHA, the hemolysis is due to a red cell defect, not a serum antibody. It was hypothesized [23, 24] that a nocturnal decrease in respiratory rate with sleep allowed an increase in serum pCO_2 which lowered the serum pH. The hemolysis is due to abnormal sensitivity of the red cell membrane to complement in the presence of a factor found only in human serums and active at acid pH [28, 29]. It has been suggested that the ubiquitous serum factor is properdin B (C3 proactivator) [23]. At acid pH, properdin B and C3 are activated following the alternate complement pathway to proceed to hemolysis (see Fig. 14-3). An antigen-antibody reaction is not necessary to activate this pathway. Hence the direct AGT and serum antibody studies are usually negative even with anticomplement reagents. The cell defect is acquired and has been found frequently in aplastic anemias [40]. Not all red cells are uniformly affected. Therefore after a hemolytic crisis the diagnostic cell population may be absent for a time. Conflicting reports suggest that membrane acetyl-cholinesterase may be decreased. The acquired defect is not restricted to the red cell, for leukocyte alkaline phosphatase may be markedly decreased and acetyl-cholinesterase is decreased in leukocytes and platelets [1].

Acid Hemolysis (Ham's) Screening Test, Modified [66]
Ham designed the standard test for PNH [12, 24] to duplicate the in vivo characteristic of red cell hemolysis in the presence of human complement at an acid pH. If the screening test is positive the test is extended to show that hemolysis is complement dependent (heat inactivation of serum), is human complement dependent (substitution of guinea pig complement after heat inactivation), is reacting only at acid pH (using alkaline buffering), and is due to the patient's red cell (lyses in any normal serum) and not to his serum (which has no effect on a normal red cell). The most common false positive reaction is due to high titer cold agglutinins, which are enhanced at acid pH but which are serum, not cell, derived.

SPECIMEN.   Fresh serum separated from clot at 37° C. Save red cells and freeze serum if not used in 30–45 min.

MATERIALS
A. 13 × 100 mm tubes—8
B. Centrifuge
C. 37° C water bath

REAGENTS.   ⅓ N HCl (pH 6.5–6.8). Keep refrigerated.

PROCEDURE   (modified to accommodate small amounts of serum)

1. Wash patient's cells from clot 3 times in 37° C saline. Use as 5% suspension.
2. Acidify patient's serum and a fresh normal group compatible serum by adding 0.05 ml ⅓ N HCl to 0.95 ml serum.
3. Prepare four tubes as follows·
   a. Tubes 1 and 2: 0.5 ml 5% cell suspension from patient; 3—0.5 ml panel pooled cells; 4—0.5 ml cord cells. Centrifuge and remove saline to provide a dry cell button.
   b. Add 0.5 ml acidified *patient* serum to each of the 4 tubes. Set up duplicate series adding acidified *normal* serum to the dry cell buttons.
4. Incubate tubes 2, 3, 4 in 37° C water bath for one hour.
5. Centrifuge and examine serum for hemolysis compared to non-incubated tube 1, graded 0–4+ for complete hemolysis. Note any agglutination, graded 0–4+.

Modified Ham's Test Extended

MATERIALS

A. See preceding test
B. Additional 13 × 100 mm tubes—7

PROCEDURE

1. Prepare 5% cell suspensions and acidified patient and 3 control serums as above.
2. Inactivate 1.5 ml aliquots of patient serum and control serums by incubating for 30 min at 56° C.
3. Set up 7 13 × 100 mm tubes as follows:

Volume	1	2	3	4	5	6	
Cell button*	P cells	P cells	P cells	P cells	P cells	P cells	C
0.5 ml	P serum	C inactive serum	C inactive serum	C serum	C serum	C serum	P
0.5 ml	—	⅓ N HCl	⅓ N HCl	⅓ N HCl	PO₄ buffer pH 8.0	—	⅓
0.1 ml	—	—	1:10 gp. compl.	—	—	—	

* Cells are dry buttons after centrifuging and decanting saline.
P = patient
C = control

4. Incubate tubes 1 hour at 37° C. Centrifuge 4 min and compare supernatant with an unincubated sample. Grade hemolysis 0–4+.

INTERPRETATION
A. For a positive test, tube 4 should show hemolysis. Tubes 1 or 6 may show lesser degrees or no hemolysis.
B. Hemolysis in tube 7 demonstrates a serum acid hemolysin often associated with high titer cold agglutinins.

Sugar-Water Lysis Test
The sugar-water test of Hartmann-Jenkins [26] is easily performed on defibrinated blood and is said to be more specific, or at least more sensitive [25, 26], than Ham's test for PNH. The defibrinated blood is incubated in a 10% sucrose solution. The sucrose solution is of low ionic strength, which causes nonspecific absorption of complement from the serum of the defibrinated whole blood to absorb to the red cells. PNH cells will lyse because of their increased complement sensitivity, whereas a normal RBC will not. Chemical grade sucrose has some advantages over table sugar [25], and the patient's red cell suspension may be obtained from clot sources with blood group compatible serum added as a complement source [26].

Positive results have been seen in myelofibrosis [25], which may be paralleling experience with acid hemolysis in aplastic anemias. A technical difficulty is agglutination rather than hemolysis of red cells, which is of apparently no diagnostic significance but which happens more often when the red cells are clot derived [4].

Other tests less readily performed are the adsorption of IgM high titer cold agglutinins [10] or the thrombin test [9]. Dacie has shown that high titer cold agglutinins can cause hemolysis of PNH red cells by virtue of their complement binding. The hypersensitive cell is then lysed. The addition of thrombin to serum has been shown to cause hemolysis of PNH cells possibly due to heterospecific antibodies contaminating the bovine thrombin, rather than to any specific effect on the PNH cell.

Due to its paroxysmal and often obscure clinical course, PNH may be difficult to document. Other laboratory tests that are helpful are urinary sediments stained for hemosiderin, and leukocyte alkaline phosphatase studies for which most laboratories have a standard procedure.

Donath-Landsteiner Test for Biphasic Hemolysins in PCH
Biphasic hemolysins either occur in clinically overt paroxysmal cold hemoglobinuria (PCH) or may be idiopathic [13] as part of the spectrum of cold AIHA, or follow multiple transfusions in AIHA. In PCH there is gross intravascular hemolysis with resultant hemoglobinuria due to antibody adsorbed to red cells at 4° C in the presence of complement fraction C1q [29], followed by hemolysis at 37° C, hence biphasic (Fig. 14-6). The hemolysin originally associated with syphilis is now more commonly postviral [51]. The antibody is usually 7S and often has specificity in the P system [63]. However, examples of 19S biphasic hemolysins with specificity of HI [2, 60], I [3, 18], and i [4, 18] have

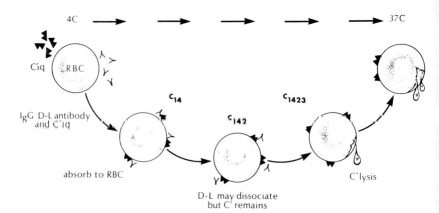

Figure 14-6
Donath-Landsteiner (biphasic) hemolysis. Optimum temperature for D–L antibody fixation is 4° C. Optimum temperature for C′ lysis is 37° C. C1q requires 4° C for fixation to RBC, C4 warm or cold temperatures, and C2, C3 cause hemolysis at 37° C.

been noted. These less usual specificities result from routine examination of sera for biphasic hemolysins using adult, cord, and autologous cells.

Serologic characterization duplicates in vitro the in vivo behavior of the hemolysin. In the presence of complement, serum is allowed to react with autologous or other test cells at 4° C and then the mixture is incubated at 37° C. If hemolysis occurs, a biphasic hemolysin has been demonstrated. Tests are then extended to demonstrate temperature variables, red cell stability, and effects of complement. Reaction mixtures are observed at each temperature alone to demonstrate that both are necessary and in the sequence cold-warm. Cell controls are necessary to exclude excessive cell fragility as the cause of any hemolysis. A complement control is used to exclude heterospecific hemolysins where guinea pig complement is used. Once the screening test has identified a biphasic hemolysin, repeat the biphasic procedure using an untreated full cell panel including cord bloods, to determine specificity. If possible include Tj^a negative cells.

The direct AGT of the patient's cells is usually negative unless anticomplement reagents are used. Following acute hemolysis no sensitized cells may remain.

Hemolysin, Biphasic (Donath-Landsteiner) Screening Test [66]
SPECIMEN.   Venous blood drawn and allowed to clot at 37° C. Serum separated and used in 1 hour or frozen. Control serums obtained and prepared similarly. Save the clots.

MATERIALS
A. 37° C water bath
B. 13 × 100 mm tubes—3
C. Ice cubes or melting ice
D. Refrigerator
E. Centrifuge
F. Pasteur pipettes

REAGENTS
A. Kolmer normal saline
B. Guinea pig complement: reconstitute and prepare 5 ml as 1:10 dilution in Kolmer saline. Keep cold and use immediately.

PROCEDURE
1. Warm the saline and tubes to 37° C.
2. Cells from clots are 3 times warm (37° C) saline washed, and resuspended to 5%.
3. Set up 3 13 × 100 mm tubes, as indicated below. Add the 1:10 dilution of guinea pig complement last, keeping it cold until use.

Reagent	1	2	3
Saline (ml)	0.1	0.1	0.1
Serum (ml)	0.5 P	0.5 P	0.5 P
5% RBC (ml)	0.2 P	0.2 C	0.2 cord
1:10 gp C' (ml)	0.2	0.2	0.2

P = patient   0.1 ml = 5 drops Pasteur pipette
C = control

4. Place tubes in glass of melting ice and place in refrigerator for 60 min.
5. Then warm in 37° C water bath for 60 min. Centrifuge.
6. Record supernatant hemolysis, graded 0–4+.
    If test is positive use extended tests to document. If Tj[a] negative cells can be obtained they may prove useful.

Hemolysin, Biphasics Extended Test [12, 66]
Specimen and reagents as above.

MATERIALS
A. As above
B. 13 × 100 mm tubes—6

PROCEDURE
1. Warm syringes, tubes, and saline to 37° C.
2. Prepare 5% warm saline washed cell suspensions.
3. Set up 13 × 100 mm tubes 1–6 as below. Add gp C' 1:10 dilution last, keeping it cold.

Reagent	1	2	3	4	5	6
Saline (ml)	0.1	0.1	0.1	0.1	0.6	0.6
Serum (ml)	0.5 P	0.5 C	0.5 P	0.5 C	—	—
5% RBC (ml)	0.2 P	0.2 C	0.2 C	0.2 P	0.2 P	0.2 C
1:10 gp C' (ml)	0.2	0.2	0.2	0.2	0.2	0.2

4. Refrigerate tubes in a melting ice bath for 60 min. Then incubate at 37° C for 60 min. Record supernatant hemolysis, graded 0–4+.

INTERPRETATION
A. Hemolysis in tubes 1 and 3: positive test
B. Hemolysis in tube 4: suggests hemolysin in control serum, repeat test using another control; or fragile patient's cell, confirm with osmotic fragility test and exclude PNH
C. Hemolysis in tube 2 and any other tube: invalid control
D. Hemolysis in tube 5: excessively fragile RBC or one sensitive to gp complement. Consider spherocytes.

Ancillary Tests
The serologic evaluation of hemolytic anemia may show a mixed pattern of warm and cold, γ and non-γ antiglobulin tests, with hemolysins, making it difficult to define which is the dominant process in order to assess prognosis. Ancillary tests may clarify the picture.

Osmotic fragility is increased in warm AIHA due to the presence of microspherocytes, but remains normal in cold AIHA. However, the test is a nonspecific indicator of spherocytosis, so that hereditary spherocytosis should be excluded. Hemolysis of normal cells in hypotonic saline solutions usually begins at 0.45% saline becoming maximal at 0.30%. If the numbers of spherocytes are not great or if the jaundice of anemia has produced target cells resistant to osmotic stress, the test may not be clearly abnormal. It can be exaggerated by incubating the blood specimen at 37° C for 24 hours and repeating the test. Normal values for nonincubated and incubated tests are recorded [12].

AUTOHEMOLYSIS.   A standard sterile clot may withstand incubation at 37° C for several days. In cases of red cell enzyme or membrane defects, red cell metabolism proceeds beyond the limits of the glycolytic pathway, and the cell, its sodium-potassium pump failing, imbibes water and hemolyses. The same process occurs whenever spherocytes are present since they lack any volume reserve [8]. Hemolysis begins in 24 hours and may be gross at 48 hours by visual inspection. The test is otherwise nonspecific. It can be quantitated with Dacie's method [12] if defibrinated blood is obtained.

SERUM COMPLEMENT.   Normal in warm AIHA, serum complement is decreased in cold AIHA due to binding in the antigen-antibody reaction. It may be decreased in PCH and PNH as well. Measurement of serum complement is usually performed by the method of Mayer [46], which is determined by 50% hemolysis of an amboceptor sensitized sheep cell suspension, reported as $C'H_{50}$ units.

IMMUNOGLOBULIN DEFICIENCIES.   IgG, IgA, and IgM immunoglobulin deficiencies may be present in warm AIHA, particularly in cases associated with chronic lymphocytic leukemia or lymphosarcoma. They should be quantitated by radial immunodiffusion rather than by relying on standard protein electrophoresis, since only single globulins may be decreased. Similarly, M proteins may be seen in either cold or warm hemolytic anemia when it is part of Waldenstroem's macroglobulinemia. The M protein characteristic skewing is best seen by immunoelectrophoresis rather than by relying on quantitation.

COLD AGGLUTININ TITERS.   Cold agglutinin titers are elevated by definition in cold antibody hemolytic anemia. For uniformity titers should be performed using group compatible cells or group O panel cells. To avoid trailing end points, ± to astronomic levels, pipettes must be changed after the first tube and every third or fourth tube thereafter. Titrations can be two-fold or arithmetic, whichever seems most useful dependent on the ultimate titer.

SERUM HAPTOGLOBIN.   Haptoglobin, the α_2-globulin that binds free hemoglobin, can be measured by spectrophotometic optical density, by radial immunodiffusion, or by electrophoresis. The latter technique is preferred because it allows (a) visual detection of free serum hemoglobin migrating with the β-globulin transferrin; (b) detection of methemalbumin; and (c) detection of haptoglobin hemoglobin-bound but not absent (Fig. 14-7). The half-life of haptoglobin is 4 to 5 days. Thus, it is possible to estimate that hemolysis is continuing if methemalbumin is present, or is an acute one-time event if haptoglobin is present but bound to hemoglobin. Results may be inaccurate when hemolytic anemia follows pneumonia or other inflammation, since all α_2-globulins increase, masking significant hemoglobin binding. Rare individuals are genetically without haptoglobin. Haptoglobin bound to hemoglobin will

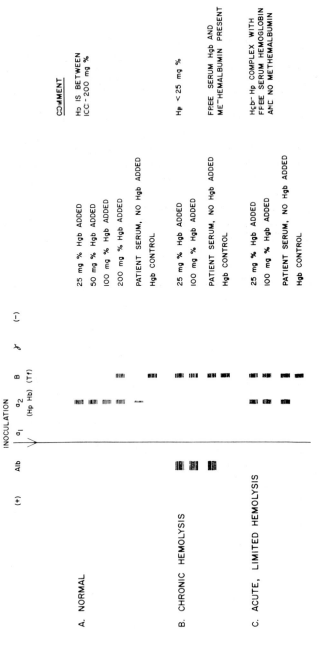

Figure 14-7
Patterns of haptoglobin-hemoglobin binding. Dark bands are benzidine positive indicating heme binding. Point of inoculation is indicated by the arrow. Albumin migrates to the (+) pole; the remaining proteins due to endosmosis migrate to (−) pole.

be measured by immunodiffusion methods as haptoglobin alone [4], which limits the usefulness of this technique. This is apparently due to the presence of three antigenic determinants on the haptoglobin molecule, of which only two are bound by hemoglobin, leaving the third to be recognized by polyvalent antisera [21].

INTERPRETATION AND REPORTING OF RESULTS
The serologic summary should include a succinct statement of hemolytic anemia type such as "autoimmune hemolytic anemia, warm (or cold) antibody type" with specificity of the autoantibody, if this can be determined. Fig. 14-8 illustrates a report form which is useful in listing test results from cell to serum, followed by the pathologist's statement.

Serologic findings sufficient to diagnose an autoimmune cause for hemolysis depend primarily on finding a positive direct antiglobulin test with a serum antibody of compatible immunoglobulin class. In some cases the serum antibody may be weak, detectable only with enzyme-treated cells. Absence of any serum antibody raises the possibility of drug etiology.

Direct Coombs reactions should be more than just weakly positive, i.e., $2+$ or greater, to consider active hemolysis. Direct AGT with broad

Blood group: Rh phenotype:	IC tests: + or − Papain tests: + or −	Direct Coombs, γ: + or − anti-C′: + or −

Other antigens: (determined as necessary)
Serologic findings:
    Eluate specificity:
    Serum autoantibody specificity:
        at 37° C: Titer:
        at 4° C: Titer:
    Serum isoantibody specificity:
    Acid hemolysis (PNH): Positive or negative
    Biphasic hemolysis (PCH): Positive or negative
    Other significant findings:

                                                ————————————————————, serologist

Comment:

Date: ————————————————————, pathologist

Figure 14-8
Format for immunohematology report.

spectrum or anticomplement reagents alone may be weakly (1+) posi-tive in as many as 8% of normal patients [13]. Cases of AIHA with negative direct AGT have been reported [22], but are difficult to evaluate without very sensitive antiglobulin techniques.

Criteria for classifying AIHA as warm antibody type usually require a direct AGT with anti-γ reagents, occasionally with anticomplement reagents as well. Strength of the reaction does not correlate with clinical severity of hemolysis, although degree of spherocytosis may do so [6]. The eluted antibody should agglutinate red cells at 37° C by antiglobu-lin or enzyme antiglobulin techniques. Cases in which both anti-γ and anticomplement Coombs tests are positive are usually seen when anti-bodies of more than one globulin class are present, one of them comple-ment binding [6, 12, 60]. Such is generally seen with warm agglutinins (7 S) and warm hemolysins (19 S), or when warm autoantibody (7 S) and nonspecific cold agglutinins (19 S) coexist. Only one of the anti-bodies may be the clinically important autoantibody. Serum antibody should react parallel to eluates, compatible with cell and serum antibody being the same immunoglobulin class. Reactions are marginal or absent at 4° C. If the temperature of major activity is not obvious, titrating the antibody against R_2R_2 cells at both temperatures will usually clarify the point. Specificity can be shown to be Rh-Hr in 25% of cases, particu-larly if Rh null or other Rh-deleted cells are available [13].

AIHA cold antibody type has a positive direct AGT with anticomple-ment reagents. The eluted globulin will not react with red cells since it is complement. The serum antibody may show reactivity at 37° C, but it is weaker and often with an incomplete pattern compared to tests at 4° C. Bovine albumin or enzyme treatment of red cells enhances ac-tivity detected in saline extending the thermal range. If activity is de-creased with enzyme-treated cells, anti-Sp_1 should be considered [45]. Titration will clearly indicate the temperature of optimum reactivity and may be necessary to clarify specificity as to I or i where antibodies are exceptionally strong. In some cases specificity I vs. i remains un-clear, and serum absorption with adult or cord cells must be used [33]. The antibodies often become monophasic hemolysins particularly at pH 6.5–6.8, giving rise to false positive Ham's tests.

At this point the question arises of when do cold agglutinins, the nemesis of all blood bankers, become the cause of hemolytic anemia. All people have very low titers of cold agglutinins. These may increase slightly with any viral infection, usually respiratory, but titers remain low (128 or less); agglutination occurs only at 20° C or less, more often at 4° C; and the agglutinins do not attach to the patient's red cells, i.e., the direct antiglobulin test, even with anticomplement reagent, is negative. After some infections and particularly those due to *Myco-plasma pneumoniae,* cold agglutinin titers rise sharply and their thermal range increases to 30–35° C. The bond to red cell becomes less tenu-ous, the avidity for red cells is increased, and antibody coats red cells, binding complement. Thus, the direct antiglobulin test with broad spectrum or anticomplement reagents is now positive. At this point hemolysis may begin. Amazingly, in rare patients it does not, nor does the cold agglutinin titer correlate with degree of hemolysis [4, 55]. Extreme titers in the hundreds of thousands raise the possibility of technical error due to trailing end-points. Titers above 50,000 suggest cold agglutinin disease, as a manifestation of dysproteinemia, rather than the cold hemolytic anemia typically seen in elderly women.

Once it has been determined that the hemolytic anemia is autoimmune, and the antibody type classified, screening studies to determine the underlying cause, if any, should be suggested if these are not already in progress.

For warm AIHA the commonest secondary causes are (a) lymphosarcoma or chronic lymphocytic leukemia; (b) collagen disease, SLE, RA, ulcerative colitis; (c) alpha-methyldopa (rarely Indocin or Ponstel); (d) myeloproliferative disorders; and (e) carcinoma, thymomas, or ovarian cystomas—rarely. The lymphosarcomas may be occult, are often retroperitoneal, and are difficult to document. The AIHA may precede them by many years.

Of the collagen diseases, SLE is most common. Therefore antinuclear factors and rheumatoid factor should be looked for. Serologic tests for syphilis will give biologic false reactions, and complement fixation technics will be anticomplementary due to IgG–anti-IgG aggregates. This alone is useful in diagnosing autoimmune disease, but the FTA-Abs test should be done to exclude syphilis.

Aldomet effects persist for many months after the drug is withdrawn, so details of the clinical history must be specific regarding past as well as current therapy. Although 10–35% of patients taking the drug develop positive AGT, only 1% or less hemolyze [41]. The drug does not have to be present to have positive serologic findings, nor does it neutralize the autoantibodies. The positive AGT appears in 3–6 months and is followed eventually by serum antibody. When serum antibody appears, transfusion may be unsafe. This fact should be kept in mind for the long range management of the patient and, if possible, the drug withdrawn. With removal of the drug the process reverses, although this may take 18 months to 2 years [13]. Restarting of the drug apparently has the same lag period as it did originally with no acceleration in return of the autoantibody [64]. Other drugs creating true warm AIHA are mefenamic acid (Ponstel), flufenamic acid [10], indomethacin [4, 10], and levodopa.

For cold AIHA secondary causes may be difficult to find. There are two types and the clinical onset will indicate whether the disease is (a) post-viral or (b) chronic cold agglutinin disease. Post-viral cases may be diagnosed retrospectively by drawing acute and convalescent sera, 10 to 14 days apart, for viral serologic studies by local or state agencies. Commonest virus involved is *M. pneumoniae,* but CMV virus can be involved. Respiratory infection with gram negative rods may be responsible, but superimposed *Mycoplasma* infection should be excluded. Rarely cold AIHA, due to anti-i, follows infectious mononucleosis [13].

Chronic cold agglutinin disease is usually idiopathic but may be associated with lympho-histiocytic lesions, reticulum cell sarcoma, or Hodgkin's disease. In mild climates the classic symptoms of Raynaud's phenomenon and acrocyanosis are absent [55]. Since extremely high titer cold agglutinins may be closer akin to dysproteinemias, protein electrophoresis should be done.

Donath-Landsteiner hemolysins may be associated with (a) syphilis, (b) viral infections, or (c) remain idiopathic. The clinical history may indicate the viral etiology. Serologic tests for syphilis should be done, but biologic false reactors (BFR) are often encountered and should be excluded by appropriate tests. Post-viral cases have acute onset with classic symptoms. However, idiopathic D–L antibodies may be found in the course of other hemolytic anemias or with myeloproliferative-aplastic disorders [2].

PNH is usually not associated with other types of AIHA. It may be seen as part of myelofibrosis or aplastic anemia [13]. Slow hemolysis may produce iron deficiency. Urinary sediment hemosiderin is present, and leukocyte alkaline phosphatase levels are similar to those of chronic granulocytic leukemia. There may be BFR to serologic tests for syphilis.

Transfusion Therapy

Transfusion should be avoided in all cases of autoimmune hemolytic anemia [13]. However, when clinical complications of gastrointestinal hemorrhage, or myocardial and cerebral ischemia supervene, donors will have to be selected. Transfused units in the presence of warm autoantibodies have a $T_{1/2}$ approximating the patient's own cells, but in cold antibody AIHA donor survival may be reduced to hours [47]. At best, transfusion becomes a temporizing measure of only short-term benefit.

Donor Selection

In warm AIHA if specificity of the autoantibody is sufficiently narrow and identified, for example anti-e (anti-hr″), donors should be selected to avoid the (hr″) antigen. These donors are expected to have normal survival [47]. Where auto-anti-hr″ appears with antibody to the Rh complex, donor survival will probably be poor.

Serum compatibility tests at 37° C, using saline cell suspensions carried to antiglobulin phase, will usually make major cross-matches appear satisfactory, although the minor cross-matches are incompatible by virtue of the positive direct antiglobulin test. In cases of warm AIHA, where eluate specificity differs from serum, eluates can be used for compatibility testing. Usually donor selection is more efficient if typing sera are used to select donors, or if donor red cells are pretreated with enzymes before crossmatching with eluate or serum [56]. If necessary, recipient sera may be diluted before crossmatch in order to find the weakest (or least incompatible) reaction.

In cold AIHA the complement-binding capacity of antigen and antibody raises the real risk of intravascular hemolysis rather than sequestration of the donor cells. The characteristic anti-I limits donors to rare i adult cells. Where these have been tried, donor survival is said to be normal [42], but they may be as poor as I+ donors, i.e., 1–3 days [4].

In PNH stable complement fractions remaining in the anticoagulant of a donor unit may cause further hemolysis. Hence, washed cells or frozen blood is indicated. In PCH keeping the patient warm prevents further episodes of hemolysis and transfusion can be avoided.

Biologic crossmatch is recommended despite the manufactured compatibility of serologic testing. In cold AIHA it is advisable to administer the unit through a warming coil. The donor unit and 1/6M Ringer's lactate are infused using a Y arrangement of intravenous tubing. Baseline blood pressure, pulse, and temperature are recorded. Urine output must be monitored. A 30 ml bolus of blood, which includes the estimated capacity of the I.V. tubing, blood filter, etc., is infused over a 5 to 10 min period and the I.V. switched to Ringer's lactate. Infusion of smaller amounts may not be sufficient to give visible hemolysis, leading to a false sense of security. After 10 min a venous sample of blood is atraumatically collected in heparin from the opposite arm and plasma is inspected for free hemoglobin. Comparisons can be made with visual standards or quantitated. Visual standards for 0, 25, 50, 75, 100, and 200 mg per 100 ml free hemoglobin made in saline, or their dye equivalents using dilutions of nuclear red dye or dichromate, are satisfactory. This limits laboratory delay in estimating hemolysis and may be supervised by the blood bank personnel. Levels of 25 mg per 100 ml or less are permissible. The unit is then continued to completion, another plasma specimen drawn, and the evaluation repeated. The Ringer's lactate should be used to maintain the intravenous portal for at least two hours following transfusion. Unless there is active bleeding, transfusions should be limited to one or two per day and given as sedimented cells. No more blood should be infused than is necessary to achieve the primary objective, i.e., increase blood volume to maintain blood pressure or to relieve hypoxic symptoms. Bilirubin levels may be obtained at 6 hours for retrospective evidence of cell destruction, if desired. Since hemolysis is ongoing, serum haptoglobin levels are absent and not useful in following biologic crossmatches.

If facilities are available, [51]Chromium survival of an aliquot of prospective donor blood can be performed. The disadvantage is that multiple venipunctures are necessary, and red cell survival is likely to be dismal in any case. Blood samples are obtained at 3, 10, and 60 min. If

^{51}Cr counts at 60 min are 99% of those at 3 min, the unit has a probable slow rate of destruction and may prove beneficial [32].

Complications result from decreased red cell survival with secondary effects on the kidney, and from the assault of foreign antigens on an immune system already too willing to produce antibody. Hydration must be maintained to avoid renal consequences of the expected donor cell demise. If this appears to be in the form of acute intravascular hemolysis, 20 ml of 50% mannitol can be infused followed by 500 ml of 5% mannitol in Ringer's lactate solution to ensure diuresis. The patient is usually already on steroids, useful only in suppressing symptoms, but not the actual hemolysis. Fever and muscular aching can be controlled with aspirin or Tylenol (McNeil).

The serum must be restudied between each series of transfusions, usually every 24 or 48 hours. This is necessary to detect the stimulation of previous isoantibodies or of new ones. Unfortunately, these may be multiple, and future units must be selected to avoid them. It is possible to elicit iso-anti-E in a patient with auto-anti-e rendering further transfusion essentially impossible. In such situations the autoantibody may prove the lesser of two evils.

In general patients maintain and tolerate hemoglobin levels of 7–8 gm% quite well once in remission and transfusion is not necessary. Proper serologic evaluation can allow the willing laboratory and pathologist some control over good transfusion therapy, management, and follow-up of the patient.

References

1. Aster, R. H., and Enright, S. E.   A platelet and granulocyte membrane defect in paroxysmal nocturnal hemoglobinuria: Usefulness for the detection of platelet antibodies. *J. Clin. Invest.* 48:1199, 1969.
2. Bell, C. A., and Zwicker, H.   Donath-Landsteiner hemolysin with anti-HI specificity. In *Proceedings of the 20th Annual Meeting* of the American Association of Blood Banks, New York, 1967. See also, *Transfusion* 7:384, 1967 (Abstr.).
3. Bell, C. A., Zwicker, H., and Rosenbaum, D.   PCH following Mycoplasma infection: Anti-I specificity of the biphasic hemolysin. *Transfusion* 13:138, 1973.
4. Bell, C. A.   Unpublished data.
5. Berman, H. J., Smarto, J., Issitt, C. H., Issitt, P. D., Marsh, W. L., and Jensen, L.   Tn-activation with acquired A-like antigen. *Transfusion* 12:35, 1972.
6. von dem Borne, A. E. G. Kr., Engelfriet, C. P., Beckers, Do., and van Loghem, J. J.   Some aspects of autoimmune hemolytic anemia with incomplete warm hemolysins. *Bibl. Haematol.* 29:479, 1968.
7. Burnet, F. M.   *The Concept of Autoimmunity.* Proceedings of the 11th Congress of the International Society. Blood Transfusion, Sydney 1966; *Bibl. Haematol.* 29:423 (New York and Basel: S. Karger), 1968.

8. Chapman, S. J., Allison, J. V., and Grimes, A. J.   Factors affecting the autohemolysis of normal human red cells and the mechanisms of lysis in vitro. *Scand. J. Haematol.* 8:347, 1971.
9. Crosby, W. H., and Benjamin, N. R.   Paroxysmal nocturnal hemoglobinuria. The role of antibodies in the diagnostic thrombin test. *Blood* 15:505, 1960.
10. Dacie, J. V., Lewis, S. M., and Tillis, D.   Comparative sensitivity of the erythrocytes in paroxysmal nocturnal hemoglobinuria to hemolysis by acidified normal serum and by high titer cold antibody. *Br. J. Haematol.* 6:362, 1960.
11. Dacie, J. V.   *The Hemolytic Anemias, Part II.* New York: Grune & Stratton, 2nd ed., 1963.
12. Dacie, J. V., and Lewis, S. M.   *Practical Hematology.* New York: Grune & Stratton, 1968, 4th ed., p. 204.
13. Dacie, J. V., and Worlledge, S. M.   Autoimmune hemolytic anemias. *Prog. Hematol.* 6:82, 1969.
14. Dameshek, W.   Theories of autoimmunity. In R. W. Cumley et al. (eds.), *Conceptual Advances in Immunology and Oncology.* New York: Harper & Row, 1963.
15. Dameshek, W.   Alpha-methyldopa red cell antibody: Cross-reaction or forbidden clones? *N. Engl. J. Med.* 276:1382, 1967.
16. Dausset, J., and Contu, L.   Drug induced hemolysis. *Ann. Rev. Med.* 18:55, 1967.
17. Dorner, I.   Warm autoantibodies. In *A Seminar on Problems Encountered in Pre-Transfusion Tests. Proceedings 25th Annual Meeting* of the American Association of Blood Banks, Washington, D.C., 1972.
18. Engelfriet, C. P., von dem Borne, A. E. G. Kr., Moes, M., and van Loghem, J. J.   Autoimmune hemolytic anemia, serologic studies in. *Bibl. Haematol.* 29:472 (New York and Basel: S. Karger), 1968.
19. Fudenberg, H.   Immunologic deficiency, autoimmune disease and lymphoma: Observations, implications, and speculations. *Arthritis Rheum.* 9:464, 1966.
20. Garratty, G., and Petz, L. D.   An evaluation of commercial antiglobulin sera with particular reference to their anticomplement properties. *Transfusion* 11:79, 1971.
21. Giblett, E. R.   *Genetic Markers in Human Blood.* Philadelphia: Davis, 1969.
22. Gilliland, B. C., Baxter, E., and Evans, R. S.   Red cell antibodies in acquired hemolytic anemia with negative antiglobulin serum tests. *N. Engl. J. Med.* 285:252, 1971.
23. Götze, O., and Müller-Eberhard, H. J.   Paroxysmal nocturnal hemoglobinuria. Hemolysis initiated by the C3 activator system. *N. Engl. J. Med.* 286:180, 1972.
24. Ham, T. H.   Chronic hemolytic anemia with paroxysmal nocturnal hemoglobinuria: Study of the mechanism of hemolysis in relation to acid-base equilibrium. *N. Engl. J. Med.* 217:915, 1937.
25. Hansen, N. E.   The sucrose hemolysis test in paroxysmal nocturnal hemoglobinuria. *Acta Med. Scand.* 184:543, 1968.
26. Hartman, R. C., and Jenkins, D. E.   The "sugar-water" test for paroxysmal nocturnal hemoglobinuria. *N. Engl. J. Med.* 275:155, 1966.
27. Heisto, H., Jensen, L., and Knuds, F.   Studies on trypsin treatment of

red cells with special reference to differences between trypsin preparations. *Vox Sang.* 21:115, 1971.

28. Hinz, C. F., Jr., Jordan, W. S., Jr., and Pillemer, L.   The properdin system and immunity. IV. Hemolysis of erythrocytes from patients with paroxysmal nocturnal hemoglobinuria. *J. Clin. Invest.* 35:453, 1956.

29. Hinz, C. F., Jr., and Mollner, A. M.   Studies on immune hemolysis. III. Role of 11S component in initiating the Donath-Landsteiner reaction. *J. Immunol.* 91:512, 1964.

30. Hoyt, R. E., and Zwicker, H   The role of enzyme in reversible agglutination of red cells. *J. Immunol.* 71:325, 1953.

31. Hughes-Jones, N. C.   The estimation of the concentration and equilibrium constant of anti-D. *Immunology* 12:565, 1967.

32. International Committee for Standardization in Hematology.   Recommended methods for radioisotopic erythrocyte survival studies. *Am. J. Clin. Pathol.* 58:71, 1972.

33. Issitt, P. D.   *Applied Blood Group Serology.* Oxnard, Calif.: Spectra Biologicals, 1970.

34. Issitt, P. D.   Polyagglutination. In *A Seminar on Problems Encountered in Pre-Transfusion Tests. Proceedings of the 25th Annual Meeting* of the American Association of Blood Banks, Washington, D.C., 1972.

35. Issitt, P. D., Issitt, C. H., Moulds, J., and Berman, H. J.   Some observations on the T, Tn, and Sd[a] antigens and the antibodies that define them. *Transfusion* 12:217, 1972.

36. Jensen, K. G.   Elution of incomplete antibodies from red cells: A comparison of different methods. *Vox Sang.* 4:230, 1959.

37. Kochwa, S., and Rosenfield, R. E.   Immunochemical studies of the Rh system. I. Isolation and characterization of antibodies. *J. Immunol.* 92:682, 1964.

38. Kuhns, W. J., and Bailey, A.   Use of red cells modified by papain for detection of Rh antibodies. *Am. J. Clin. Path.* 20:1067, 1950.

39. Landsteiner, K., and Miller, C. P.   Serologic studies on the blood of primates: II. The blood groups in anthropoid apes. *J. Exp. Med.* 42:853, 1925.

40. Lewis, S. M., and Dacie, J. V.   The aplastic anemia-paroxysmal hemoglobinuria syndrome. *Br. J. Haematol.* 13:236, 1967.

41. LoBuglio, A. F., and Jandl, J. H.   The nature of the alphamethyldopa red-cell antibody. *N. Engl. J. Med.* 276:658, 1967.

42. van Loghem, J. J., Peetoom, F., van der Hart, M., van der Veer, M., van der Giessen, M., Prins, H. K., Zurcher, C., and Engelfriet, C. P.   Serological and immunochemical studies in hemolytic anemia with high titer cold agglutinins. *Vox Sang.* 8:33, 1963.

43. Mackay, I. R.   Autoimmune disease in humans. *Bibl. Haematol.* 29:463, 1968.

44. Marsh, W. L., Reid, M. E., and Scott, E. P.   Autoantibodies of U blood group specificity in autoimmune hemolytic anemia. *Br. J. Haematol.* 22:625, 1972.

45. Marsh, W. L., and Jenkins, W. J.   Anti-Sp$_1$: The recognition of a new cold antibody. *Vox Sang.* 15:177, 1968.

46. Mayer, M. M.   Complement and complement fixation. In E. A. Kabat and M. M. Mayer, *Experimental Immunochemistry.* Springfield, Ill.: Thomas, 1967, 2nd ed., p. 149.

47. Mollison, P. *Blood Transfusion in Clinical Medicine.* Philadelphia: Davis, 1967, 4th ed.
48. Mollison, P. L., and Polley, M. J.   Uptake of γ-globulin and complement by red cells exposed to serum at low ionic strength. *Nature* (Lond.) 203:535, 1964.
49. Nightingale, D., Prankard, T. A. J., Richards, J. D. M., and Thompson, O.   Splenectomy in Anemia. *Q. J. Med.* 41:261, 1972.
50. Oski, F. A.   The metabolism of erythrocytes and its relation to hemolytic anemias of the newborn. *Pediatr. Clin. North Am.* 12:687, 1965.
51. Pirofsky, B.   *Autoimmunization and the Autoimmune Hemolytic Anemias.* Baltimore: Williams & Wilkins, 1969.
52. Race, R. R., and Sanger, R.   *Blood Groups in Man.* Philadelphia: Davis, 1968, 5th ed.
53. Rubin, H.   Antibody elution from red blood cells. *J. Clin. Pathol.* 16:70, 1963.
54. Rubin, H.   Preparation of rabbit antihuman complement reagent. *Transfusion* 11:36, 1971.
55. Schubothe, H.   The cold hemagglutinin disease. *Semin. Hematol.* 3:27, 1966.
56. American Association of Blood Banks. *Technical Methods and Procedures.* Chicago: American Association of Blood Banks, 1970, 5th ed.
57. Vos, G. H., Petz, L., and Fudenberg, H. H.   Specificity and immunoglobulin characteristics of autoantibodies in acquired hemolytic anemia. *J. Immunol.* 104:1172, 1971.
58. Weigle, W. O.   *Natural and Acquired Immunologic Unresponsiveness.* Cleveland: World, 1969.
59. Weigle, W. O.   Immunologic unresponsiveness. *Hosp. Practice,* 6:121, 1971.
60. Weiner, W.   The specificity of the antibodies in acquired hemolytic anemia. *Proceedings of the 10th Congress of the International Society of Blood Transfusion, Stockholm, 1964.* (New York and Basel: S. Karger), 1965, p. 24.
61. Weiner, W.   Eluting red cell antibodies: A method and its application. *Br. J. Haematol.* 3:276, 1957.
62. Weiner, W.   Classification of immune hemolytic anemias. *10th Congress of the European Society of Hematology, Strasbourg, 1965.* (New York and Basel: S. Karger), 1967, part 2, p. 327.
63. Worlledge, S. M., and Rousso, C.   Studies on the serology of paroxysmal cold hemoglobinuria (P.C.H.) with special reference to its relationship with P blood group system. *Vox Sang.* 10:293, 1965.
64. Worlledge, S. M.   Immune drug induced hemolytic anemias. *Semin. Hematol.* 6:181, 1969.
65. Zarkowsky, H. S., Oski, F. A., Sha'afi, R., Shohet, S. B., and Nathan, D. G.   Congenital hemolytic anemia with high sodium, low potassium red cells. *N. Engl. J. Med.* 278:573, 1968.
66. Zwicker, H., and Bell, C. A.   Unpublished method.

15

Serologic Evaluation of Drug-Induced Immune Hematologic Disorders

Carol A. Bell

D rug destruction of the formed elements of the blood can occur by direct toxic effect to bone marrow, through biochemical interaction in the peripheral blood, or by immune (allergic) mechanisms. Drug-induced autoantibodies are less common than direct toxic effects or interaction with red cell enzymes, but this circumstance may be due to lack of widely available, simple methods of approaching the problem that yield a serologic proof. At present, most of the serologically proven drug-induced autoantibodies have been studied with regard to their effects either on red cells [9, 37] or on platelets [24, 35], although certain drugs are known to induce antibodies to more than one blood element [32].

Pathogenesis

The way in which drugs foment immune damage depends upon the drug, its macromolecular support, the antibody globulin produced, and the target cell [9]. In general, the drug must first combine with some macromolecule, but just what that macromolecule is gives rise to differing theories.

Ackroyd [1] believes that the macromolecule may be the target cell, either red cell or platelet. Antibody is then induced to the drug, to the carrier, or to both, combines with the carrier-drug, and with or without complement, destroys it. Shulman [32] hypothesizes that drug as a hapten on a macromolecular carrier (e.g., plasma proteins) induces antibody. Antigenic drug combines with its antibody, forming soluble immune complexes which adhere to an "innocent-bystander" target cell, binding complement. Alternatively, these soluble complexes cause fixation of complement to target cells without remaining attached themselves; they can, therefore, skip from cell to cell, causing extensive involvement with relatively few complexes. Hemolysis results from complement membrane damage. However, the red cell membrane may participate as somewhat more than an absolutely "innocent" bystander, since there is some variability in membrane susceptibility to the lytic action of complement [25].

The ease with which specific drugs induce antibody is apparently a function of bond strength between drug and its protein carrier, whatever that carrier might be [9, 37], and between drug and target cell. The relative rarity of drug-induced immune hemolysis is probably due to generally low binding constants. The stronger these bonds are in vitro, however, the easier the serologic proof becomes.

There appears to be little constancy in the pathogenesis of drug antibody. Thus, differing immune globulin classes have been induced by the same drug, and the same immunoglobulin by different drugs, for the same target cell [3, 10, 32]. Both 7 S and 19 S antibodies have been shown to be complement binding [25, 32], although this is not necessary for cytopenia. Finally, the ability of the inciting drug to neutralize its antibody appears to be a point in favor of the hapten mechanism [1] when it can be demonstrated.

Mechanism of Action

The final pathway to cell destruction is the same regardless of the method of antibody production. In some cases, complement is so completely bound that actual intravascular hemolysis occurs by either osmotic colloid defects or actual membrane holes. More often sublytic amounts of complement or subagglutinating levels of antibody lead to extravascular destruction following reticuloendothelial sequestration.

Drug-Induced Red Cell Antibodies

Where the RBC is the target cell there are four major mechanisms for drug interaction. These are hapten formation (e.g., penicillin); adsorption of immune complexes (e.g., stibophen, quinine); nonspecific adsorption of any and all globulins following nonimmune membrane damage (e.g., cephalothin); and true warm antibody hemolytic anemia (e.g., alpha-methyldopa). In each case, globulin attaches to the red cell. Therefore, the possibility of drug-induced antibody should be considered whenever there is a positive direct antiglobulin test in the absence of any demonstrable serum antibody. The majority of cases will be due to penicillin or α-methyldopa, but conscientious investigation can expand the current list of drug autoantibodies [9, 25, 37] (Fig. 15-1).

Screening for drug-induced red cell autoantibodies requires:
A. Direct antiglobulin test (AGT) with anti-γ and anticomplement reagents
B. Eluates of globulin positive cells, preferably using a cold alcohol technique [36]

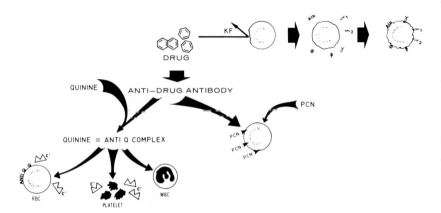

Figure 15-1
Mechanisms of drug-induced hemolytic anemia. Three drug prototypes are illustrated. In quinine (Q) type, the anti-drug antibody complexes to quinine. The immune complex and C′ bind to the innocent bystander target cell, RBC, WBC, or platelet, and destroy it. Penicillin (PCN) is firmly bonded to the RBC; anti-penicillin antibody attacks the inciting hapten. Cephalothin (KF) modifies the RBC membrane, and nonimmune adsorption of serum proteins follows.

C. Screening the serum to exclude the possibility of atypical red cell antibodies (using enzyme-treated as well as untreated RBC)
D. Treatment of a test RBC with the drug(s) in question
E. Testing serum and eluate against these treated RBC
F. Neutralization of the serum or eluate with dilutions of drug solution

Hapten (Penicillin)
Penicillin, and its cogeners methicillin, ampicillin, and oxacillin, form firm covalent bonds with the red cell in vivo, as well as in vitro [22]. The antibody induced is usually IgG and is directed at the haptenic drug, or rather the benzyl penicillinoyl moiety of the drug (Fig. 15-2). The process is dependent on dose, route of administration, and time. The route is always intravenous, usually 10–20 million units or more per day, and requires at least 8 days of such therapy to induce antibody. However, only occasional patients on such a regimen will produce an IgG antibody and develop hemolytic anemia [22, 23]. The direct AGT is strongly positive with anti-γ reagents. Complement does not seem to be involved. The serum contains no antibody by standard screening procedures, but use of a penicillinized red cell shows the antibody in serum and in red cell eluates. Both the serum anti-penicillin antibody

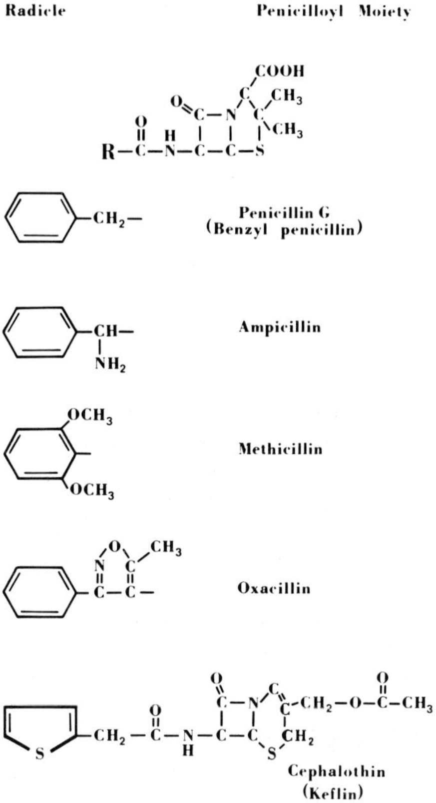

Radicle   Penicilloyl Moiety

Penicillin G
(Benzyl penicillin)

Ampicillin

Methicillin

Oxacillin

Cephalothin
(Keflin)

Figure 15-2
Penicillin analogues.

and the same antibody eluted from the red cell can be neutralized by solutions of penicillin. Anti-penicillin antibody may not cross react with cells treated with methicillin or ampicillin, although it usually does so with Keflinized cells [13, 15, 16]. Finding anti-penicillin antibodies does not mean hemolytic anemia unless the clinical history is compatible, since 90% of people will have an IgM penicillin antibody, presumably due to dietary exposure. Penicillin antibodies associated with hemolytic anemia (high titer IgG antibodies) usually differ in globulin class from those causing skin and other manifestations of penicillin allergy [22], which may be IgM or IgE. Hemolytic anemia and atopic symptoms are usually unrelated.

Penicillin Treatment of Red Cells
(Method of A. B. Ley et al. [23])
The ease with which red cells absorb penicillin makes almost any concentration of penicillin above 3,000 μ/ml and any incubation time or temperature satisfactory, as shown by Ley et al. [23]. The most conve-

nient form of the drug is the powdered penicillin G 600,000 units intended for intravenous administration.

1. Draw 4 ml whole blood into 4 ml Alsever's solution. (Alternatively, any anticoagulated whole blood specimen is satisfactory.)
2. Add the 8 ml whole blood-Alsever's mixture to the powdered penicillin G.
3. Incubate at 37° C for 1 hour.
4. Remove a 1 ml aliquot of the treated RBC and wash in 0.85% saline 3 times.
5. Resuspend penicillinized cells at 4% for testing with patient sera.
6. Treated cells may be refrigerated for 1–3 weeks. Aliquots are removed and saline washed as needed.

Methods of penicillin treatment using less concentrated solutions of reconstituted penicillin G powder have been devised, but require overnight refrigeration before the cells are used [5]. Such methods appear to have no advantage over Ley's technique.

Antibody will agglutinate the pretreated red cells only, and not those of the untreated identification panel unless it has been preserved in penicillin [23]. Prior to neutralization studies the antibody should be titered against penicillinized cells.

Other drug antibodies can be shown to act by haptenic mechanisms if the treated red cells are prepared by incubation with any drug. If the binding constant is so weak that this does not prove successful, chemical binding in the presence of chromium chloride may prove useful [14].

General Treatment of Red Cells with Drug

MATERIALS AND REAGENTS
A. Soluble form of drug preferred if possible
B. 0.85% saline
C. 37° C water bath
D. Centrifuge
E. Whatman No. 1 filter paper
F. Washed and packed fresh group O blood cells
G. Refrigerator

PROCEDURE
1. Use a soluble form of the drug if it is available despite the fact that the patient may be taking tablet forms (e.g., quinidine gluconate for injection rather than the less soluble quinidine sulfate powder).
2. If no soluble form is available, dissolve 1 tablet or empty 1 capsule into 5 ml 0.85% saline, and incubate 1 hour in 37° C water bath with occasional agitation. (a) Centrifuge the tube and use clear supernatant. (b) If centrifugation does not yield a clear supernatant, filter the solution through Whatman No. 1 filter paper.

3. Add 0.5 ml aliquots of washed and packed fresh group O cells to equal volumes of drug solution undiluted, 1:10 dilution and 1:40 dilution, hopefully to obtain an optimum concentration for cell combination.
4. Incubate red cells in drug solution for 1 hour at 37° C. Wash red cells 3 times in saline and store in refrigerator.
5. When drug-treated cells are tested with the patient's eluate or serum, a cell control must be carried to antiglobulin phase since many drugs or the tablet binders tend to alter red cell membranes nonspecifically (e.g., cephalothin, Quinaglute [Cooper]), which negates the test.

Neutralization Studies

In general, antibodies to haptens can be neutralized by the drug in question using direct or indirect techniques. The serum or red cell eluates are incubated at 37° C for 30 min with an equal volume of drug solutions (as prepared above). These solutions are used saturated (undiluted) and in 1:10, 1:40, 1:100, or 1:200 dilutions for most drugs. Greater dilutions may be necessary for penicillin, e.g., 1:250, 1:2500, 1:25,000, 1:50,000, etc. [5]. In the direct agglutination method of neutralization, one volume of 4% suspension of penicillinized red cells or other drug-treated cells is added to the 2 volumes of serum-drug dilution mixture and incubated at 37° C for 1 hour. The reaction mixture is centrifuged and agglutination graded 0−4+. For some drugs an indirect method is necessary to show neutralization. The red cells are then saline washed and carried to antiglobulin phase. Record the dilution at which agglutination reappears to determine the degree of neutralization (Table 15-1). Saline-serum dilutions and tests vs. untreated cells are needed as controls.

Immune Complexes (Quinine, Quinidine)

Most drug antibodies will probably fall into this class. Drug–drug antibody complexes and complement absorb loosely to red cells. The drug antibodies are usually IgM [7, 32], but may be IgG [3, 11, 25], with variable degrees of complement binding. The direct AGT will be positive with anticomplement reagents only, and eluates of the red cell will generally have no reactivity with drug-treated red cells because either (a) the drug–drug antibody complex, being weakly bound to red cell, is no longer present, or (b) the in vitro attempts to bind drug to the test red cell have been unsuccessful. Neutralization studies are usually unsuccessful in this class since antibody is already bound to drug in vivo. Furthermore, preparation of drug-treated red cells meets with only limited success since covalent bonds are weak.

Method for Demonstrating Quinine Type
1. Incubate drug dilutions (see General Treatment of Red Cells with Drug above), patient's serum, and an equal volume of RBC simul-

Table 15-1. Drug Neutralization of Penicillin Antibody Demonstrated by Hemagglutination Inhibition.

Concentration of Penicillin (units/ml)	+	Serum[a]	4% Suspension Penicillinized RBC	Direct Agglutination[b]
		Incubate at 37° C for 30 min	Incubate at 37° C for 60 min and centrifuge	
0.1 ml	0 (saline)	0.1 ml	0.1 ml	+++
0.1 ml	3000	0.1 ml	0.1 ml	+++
0.1 ml	6000	0.1 ml	0.1 ml	+++
0.1 ml	25,000	0.1 ml	0.1 ml	++
0.1 ml	50,000	0.1 ml	0.1 ml	+
0.1 ml	100,000	0.1 ml	0.1 ml	±[c]
0.1 ml	200,000	0.1 ml	0.1 ml	0
0.1 ml	Saline	0.1 ml	Untreated RBC	0

SOURCE: Zwicker, H, and Bell, C. A. [40] derived from Ley, A. et al. [23]
[a] Anti-penicillin antibody, titer 256 in neat serum.
[b] If agglutination is negative, carry reaction to antiglobulin phase, i.e., indirect method.
[c] Neutralizing dilution 100,000–200,000 units/ml.

taneously at 37° C for 1 hour. Agitate occasionally. Centrifuge and examine macroscopically for hemolysis or agglutination.
2. After washing the RBC 3 times with saline, test with anticomplement Coombs as well as anti-γ reagents. In general, only the anticomplement reagent is positive.

In rare cases, even with immune complexes, eluates of red cells may have activity against drug-treated cells [3, 11].

Nonspecific Protein Adsorption (Cephalothin)
Drugs in this class include cephalothin and cephaloridine. These drugs alter the red cell membrane in vivo and in vitro, causing nonimmunologic adsorption of all protein fractions to the injured red cell membrane. Approximately 3% of patients on cephalothin will develop a positive direct AGT. This effect is dose and time related. The positive direct AGT appears as soon as 5–6 days after the drug is begun in doses of 6 gm daily [13, 34]. Incubation of red cells with even the most dilute solutions of drug can yield red cells agglutinating in the cell control. This may be a function of inadequate buffering, and it is best to maintain a pH above 7. Positive cell controls have made it difficult to prove cases of true hemolytic anemia due to cephalothin antibody [15, 16] or to penicillin antibodies cross-reacting with Keflinized cells. The artifact of nonspecific adsorption of serum proteins will be minimized if an eluate is used for testing instead. Note that there are similarities in molecular structure between cephalothin and the benzylpenicillinoyl molecule which accounts for the cross-reactivity [34] (see Fig. 15-2).

Since albumin to γ-globulin can be adsorbed to the cell [28], any and all antiglobulin reagents may produce a positive direct AGT. Consequently, eluates of this nonspecific globulin should have no activity against drug-treated cells; this point is difficult to evaluate if the red cell membrane is altered and agglutinates spontaneously. However, eluates occasionally show activity directed toward Keflinized cells [16]. A satisfactory method of cephalothin treatment follows.

Keflinized Red Cells
(Method of H. R. Gralnik et al. [15])

REAGENT
A. Sodium cephalothin (Keflin) (Lilly) 1 gm for I.M. injection to be reconstituted with 4 ml sterile water for injection or 0.85% NaCl
B. Phosphate-buffered saline (pH 7.4)

MATERIALS
A. Packed and washed fresh group O red cells
B. 37° C water bath
C. Patient's serum or red cell eluate
D. Controls: negative, 3 normal sera; positive, serum containing anti-penicillin antibody (if available)

PROCEDURE

1. Add 1 ml reconstituted cephalothin to 39 ml phosphate-buffered saline (dilution 1:40).
2. To one volume packed, washed, fresh group O red cells add 10 volumes 1:40 cephalothin solution.
3. Incubate 60 min at 37° C.
4. Wash 4 times in saline and use as 2–5% suspension.
5. For test add patient's serum or red cell eluate to an equal volume of cephalothin-treated red cells (2 drops). Incubate at 37° C for 20 min and carry to antiglobulin phase.
6. Controls: (a) Negative control. To rule out Keflin-induced polyagglutinability, test 3 normal sera in parallel. No agglutination should be present with these sera. (b) Positive control. If available, incubate serum containing antipenicillin antibody with Keflinized cells. They should agglutinate by cross reaction.

True Warm Antibody Hemolytic Anemia (α-Methyldopa)

Drugs in this class now include mefenamic acid (Ponstel; Parke, Davis), flufenamic acid, indomethecin (Indocin) (Merck) and levodopa [8]. Some of the chemical structures are seen in Fig. 15-3. Along with penicillin the most frequent cause of drug-associated immune hemolytic anemia is α-methyldopa. Unlike the other classes of drugs, however, a true hemolytic anemia, warm antibody type, is produced, often with anti-Rh specificity of autoantibodies [38]. The drug does not have to be present for the process to continue. The production of a positive AGT and serum antibody appears to be dose related since patients taking 2 gm/day develop a positive AGT in 19–36% of cases, whereas when patients are on doses of 1 gm/day only 11% develop a positive AGT.

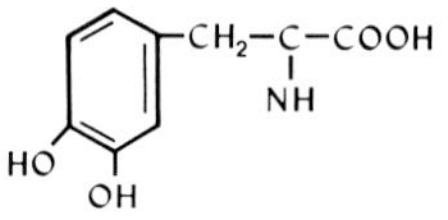

L–dopa

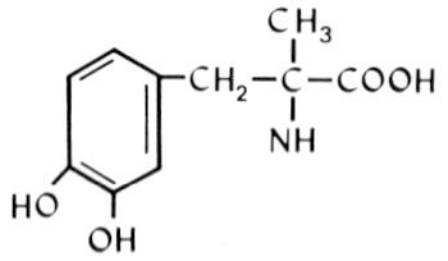

a–methyl dopa
(Aldomet)

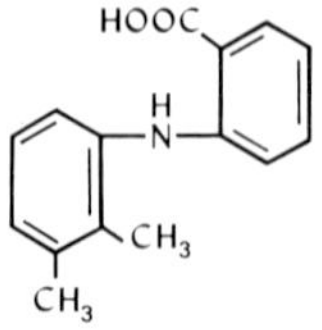

mefenamic acid
(Ponstel)

Figure 15-3
Chemical structures of levodopa, α-methyldopa, and mefenamic acid.

The positive test persists for as long as 24 months after the drug is discontinued [4].

The mechanism of action is still unknown [24]. Worlledge and associates [38] have suggested that the drug may somehow be incorporated into the red cell stroma in the bone marrow, and that this explains the persistence of a positive antiglobulin test for so many months after the drug has been discontinued. However, Schwartz and Costea [31] have shown that for any particular autoantibody, avidity may be great enough to allow it to transfer from red cell to red cell, remaining essentially sequestered from normal protein catabolism able to persist for many months. They also showed that serum rather than cell-adsorbed antibody indicated the current autoantibody production. Such sequestered autoantibody may explain more satisfactorily the persistence of the positive direct AGT. Their theory regarding the significance of serum vs. cell-adsorbed antibody correlates well with the fact that these patients often do not have serum autoantibody, and overtly hemolyze infrequently, maintaining hemoglobin levels of 14 gm% [8]. Platelet and leukocyte antibodies in the presence of α-methyldopa have been reported [26] but may be the result of a different mechanism than for red cells since the drug presence was necessary for their demonstration.

The serologic evaluation of α-methyldopa hemolytic anemia has been described under warm antibody hemolytic anemias. Briefly, the direct antiglobulin test is positive with anti-γ reagents only, since the autoantibody is IgG. The red cell eluates are active against normal red cells *without* the drug being present. The IgG serum antibody, if present, acts at 37° C against untreated and enzyme-treated cells by antiglobulin technique. About half the cases show definite antibody specificity within the Rh-Hr system [36], anti-e, anti-C plus anti-e appearing commonly. If Rh null or Rh-deleted cells are available for testing, many cases can be shown to react with the Rh complex.

As in all warm hemolytic anemias, transfusion in the presence of serum autoantibody should be avoided, although it is apparently harmless where only a positive direct AGT is present.

The major points of drug-induced red cell antibody and transfusion risk for each category are summarized in Table 15-2. When the drug must be present to show the antibody, transfusion is not contraindicated, since donor cells are not drug coated.

Platelet Antibodies, Drug Induced and Autoimmune

General Remarks

Many of the theories on pathogenesis of red cell drug autoantibody were derived from work with platelets [1, 32]. Indeed, in some cases antibody of one immunoglobulin class may react with the red cell and a second immunoglobulin class with the platelet [32].

Table 15-2. Serologic Summary of Immunologic Drug Anemias. Comparison with Warm Autoimmune Hemolytic Anemia (AIHA).

	DRUG				AIHA
	The drug must be present			drug not present	
	Penicillin	Quinine	Keflin	Aldomet	
Mechanism of Action	Hapten	Immune Complex	Nonspec Ads Protein	Warm AIHA	Warm Autoantibody
Direct AGT[a]	+ (IgG)	var. (C')	+ (all)	+ (IgG)	+ (IgG)
Serum Antibody[b]:	IgG	IgM	not-spec.[c]	IgG	IgG
vs. normal RBC	0	0	0	+	+
vs. penicillinized RBC	+	0	+/0	0	0
vs. Keflinized RBC	+	0	+ rare	0	0
vs. Aldomet RBC	0	0	0	0	0
RBC eluate	aggl. Pen RBC	no activity	normal globulin	aggl. normal RBC	aggl. normal RBC
Hemolytic anemia	Yes	Rare	Rare	Yes	Yes
Transfusion permitted	Yes	Yes	Yes	No	No

[a] AGT = antiglobulin test. Reagent type appears in parenthesis.
[b] Antibodies of the immune complex type can only rarely be shown to have RBC activity against the appropriate drug-treated RBC.
[c] In one documented case of true hemolytic anemia [16], anti-cephalothin antibody was IgG.

Methods for Detection
Any method of platelet antibody detection, whether post-transfusion iso-antibody, autoantibody as in ITP, or drug antibody, is limited by technical problems of spontaneous platelet aggregation; and the correlation to clinical response of increasing platelet count on withdrawal of the drug is never 100% [6, 35].

Techniques have included inhibition of clot retraction [2], complement fixation [32], platelet lysis [10, 35], antiglobulin consumption [6], indirect agglutination [16], and immunofluorescence [33]. Some techniques are better suited for isoantibodies, some for complete antibodies, and a few are adaptable to drug antibodies. The subject has been extensively reviewed by Maupin [27] (Table 15-3).

Most methods require a test platelet suspension freshly shed into an EDTA-citrated solution, to prevent nonspecific complement absorption. For complement fixation or antiglobulin consumption techniques, the suspension is washed free of all contaminating globulin. Siliconized tubes and intravenous tubing should be used. All materials must be washed scrupulously clean, preferably not with other laboratory glassware since the silicon spreads. The platelets should be group O or group compatible with test serums. The serum specimens are obtained from clots and can be stored at $-25°$ C for 6 months. They should be drawn at least 5 days after the offending drug has been stopped. Drugs such as quinine or quinidine bind to plasma proteins, and it takes several days for them to elute or be catabolized from the protein carrier. Since all tests are conducted such that serum is incubated with platelet suspensions with and without added drug, no residual unexpected drug can be present for a valid result.

Table 15-3. Application of Techniques for Detection of Platelet Antibodies.

Technique	Drug Antibody	ITP Autoantibody	Isoantibody
Direct agglutination [17]	Fair–Good[a]	Poor	Fair
Clot retraction inhibition [2]	Fair	0	Fair
Complement fixation [32]	Good	0	Fair–Good
Antiglobulin consumption [6]	Fair	Fair–Good	Poor
Fluorescent technique [33]	0	Poor	Poor
Platelet lysis [10]	Good	Fair	0

[a] If the procedure has been shown to work it is rated on scale of poor-fair-good. No procedure can be considered excellent.

Preparation of Platelet Rich Plasma
(Method of W. J. Harrington et al. [17])

REAGENT.   Fresh blood from group O donor

EQUIPMENT
A. One 15-ml plastic centrifuge tube containing 0.3 ml 5% EDTA
B. Siliconized needles (19 gauge)
C. Blood donor set
D. Plastic 2 ml syringes
E. Plastic 13 × 100 mm tubes or 12 × 75 mm
F. 0.2 ml pipettes, serologic
G. Parafilm
H. Horizontal head centrifuge
 I. Phase microscope
J. Refrigerator

PROCEDURE
1. Use siliconized 19 gauge needle and donor set. Apply tourniquet only long enough to enter vein. By gravity allow 10 ml venous blood to flow into plastic centrifuge tube containing EDTA.
2. Agitate tube as blood flows to prevent clotting.
3. Cap tube with parafilm. Invert gently to mix.
4. Centrifuge in horizontal head centrifuge at 1,000 rpm for 30 min.
5. Remove supernatant platelet rich plasma with siliconized needle and 2 ml plastic syringe.
6. Do platelet count using phase microscopy.
7. Keep platelet rich plasma, needle, and syringe in refrigerator until ready to use. Must be used within 6 hours.

Direct Agglutination
(Method of W. J. Harrington et al. [17])
Direct agglutination is studied after incubation of platelets, washed in EDTA, and serum containing the drug antibody, first in the presence of the offending drug, and then in its absence. Several serum dilutions are tested which allows quantitation of the drug antibody and permits subtracting any aggregation artifacts in the base line. This method is satisfactory only for "complete" antibodies, usually leaving undetected "incomplete" antibodies which may occur. However, the test can be modified with regard to temperature in an attempt to detect all antibody classes [6]. The method has been adapted for drug and ITP autoantibody, but isoantibodies are often better detected than the autoantibody of ITP possibly due to the more superficial location of the haptenic or other antigen [18, 35] for isoantibodies.

Platelet antibody must be tested for with and without drug, which requires both parts I and II.

SPECIMEN.   Serum for 5 ml clot drawn at least 5 days after offending drug has been discontinued.

EQUIPMENT
A. Serologic pipettes
B. Plastic 13 × 100 or 12 × 75 mm tubes—24
C. 2 ml syringe
D. Siliconized needles (19 gauge) or siliconized pipette
E. Parafilm
F. 37° C water bath
G. Refrigerator
H. Centrifuge, horizontal head
 I. Phase microscope with 40 × magnification
 J. Whatman No. 1 filter paper
K. Pasteur pipettes

REAGENTS
A. Platelet rich plasma prepared in previous 6 hours
B. ⅓ N citric acid
C. AB plasma collected in ACD or CPD (usual source, blood bank)
D. 5% solution EDTA

PROCEDURE FOR PLATELET AGGLUTINATION WITHOUT DRUG (I)
1. Acidify 0.9 ml patient's serum with 0.1 ml ⅓ N citric acid. Acidify AB plasma in same manner. Acidified sera must be prepared fresh.
2. For titrations dilute patient's acidified serum with acidified AB plasma 1:1, 1:10, 1:40, and 1:160.
3. Add 0.06 ml (1 drop) 5% EDTA for each ml acidified serum.
4. Pipette 0.1 ml acidified EDTA serum or serum dilutions into plastic 13 × 100 mm tubes.
5. Add 0.1 ml platelet rich plasma using 2 ml syringe and needle from Preparation of Platelet Rich Plasma above. (Alternative: dispense from 1 ml siliconized pipette.)
6. Mix. Cap with parafilm. Place in 37° C water bath 1 hour. Then refrigerate at least 2 hours; may leave overnight.
7. Centrifuge at 1,600 rpm for 2 min.
8. Tap tube gently 10 times. Record agglutination read microscopically under 40× magnification using phase microscope.

PROCEDURE FOR DRUG-INDUCED PLATELET AGGLUTINATION (II)
1. Dissolve drug in 5 ml acidified EDTA AB plasma at 37° C. Filter through Whatman No. 1 filter paper.
2. Prepare dilutions of drug solution in acidified EDTA, AB plasma (1:10, 1:50, 1:100).

3. Make dilutions of patient's acidified serum in acidified EDTA, AB plasma (1:1, 1:10, 1:40, 1:160).
4. Using Pasteur pipette add 1 drop serum dilution to 1 drop drug solution. Add 1 drop platelet rich plasma. Mix. Cap with parafilm.
5. Place in 37° C water bath 1 hour followed by refrigeration at least 2 hours or overnight.
6. Control tubes
   a. Serum acidified EDTA + platelet rich plasma (PRP).
   b. AB plasma acidified EDTA + PRP.
   c. AB plasma acidified EDTA + PRP + drug solution.
   Incubate control tubes as in step 5.
7. Centrifuge at 1,600 rpm for 2 min.
8. Tap gently 10 times. Read microscopically under 40× phase. Record agglutination 0–4+.
9. Interpretation: (a) Control (without drug): negative or ± agglutination; (b) Positive: agglutination 1–4+. Record titer of last dilution showing 1+ agglutination.

Clot Retraction Inhibition
(Method of J. F. Ackroyd [2])
Clot retraction inhibition is the simplest but least sensitive measure of alteration in platelet function; however, it is particularly adaptable to screening for drug-induced antibodies [2]. Blood is shed into centrifuge tubes containing saline or saline solutions of the drug in question and allowed to clot. The clot should then retract if platelet function is unaltered. Inhibition of clot retraction suggests platelet injury. The major disadvantage is that the antibody must be high titer in order to show inhibition [27]. The technique has been made more sensitive by conducting the test on fibrin clots without red cells [39].

MATERIALS AND REAGENTS
A. Graduated centrifuge tube with cork closure and spring inserted into cork—2
B. Saturated solution of drug or dilutions
C. Saline
D. 37° C incubator

PROCEDURE
1. Place 0.5 ml saturated solution of drug or dilutions into graduated centrifuge tube.
2. Control tube contains 0.5 ml saline.
3. Add 2 ml blood to each tube and cork. Spring should contact surface of blood.
4. Mix by repeated inversion. Note height of column of blood.
5. Allow to clot at room temperature, then place in 37° C incubator.

Examine at 1 hour. If adherent to wall of tube loosen cork and gently rim clot to allow more complete retraction.
6. Incubate 3 more hours at 37° C, then overnight at room temperature. Remove cork with clot attached to spring. Measure height of serum and note consistency of clot.
7. Calculation: $\% \text{ retraction} = \dfrac{\text{ht of serum}}{\text{ht of whole blood}} \times 100$

Normal: 48–63% (Range for 3 S.D.)

Complement Fixation

Complement fixation [32] can detect only agglutinating antibodies. It has been most helpful in detecting isoantibodies following pregnancy or transfusion, but can be applied to drug antibodies, many of which are complement fixing. Autoantibodies of ITP are not detected. Microtechniques for complement fixation are available [18]. Technical difficulties arise as a result of prozones; therefore several serum dilutions should be tested. The pH of the reaction mixture and adequate density of the platelet suspension determine the sensitivity of the test. For weak antibodies, incubation time usually requires 1–2 hours. A major disadvantage is that, for incomplete type antibody, as in ITP, indirect methods of detection are necessary. This requires the use of a known complement-fixing platelet antibody to demonstrate the competition by the test serum for platelet antigenic sites. If incomplete antibody is binding the sites, the known complement-fixing antibody will then be unable to bind, and complement remains unfixed.

Antiglobulin Consumption

Both direct and indirect techniques using antiglobulin serum with thoroughly washed platelet suspensions have been devised [6, 35] (Fig. 15-4). A direct AGT with in vivo-sensitized platelets is generally not satisfactory because the bond between platelet and drug–antibody complex is a weak one [32], and the globulin coat is thus not detectable in vitro. The indirect method of "Coombs consumption" requires attention to detail and some serologic experience. It can detect only 50–79% of antibodies due to the requirements of the indicator system [6] and is poorly adaptable for drug antibody. Because the visible indicator is usually an Rh_o positive red cell coated with anti-Rh_o, which is 7 S globulin, only 7 S antibodies will cause a decreased titer in the AHG reagent. In order to detect the incomplete antibodies, the indicator system should be coated with IgM antibody and complement, and an anti-complement reagent titered for use.

Platelet Lysis

Measurement of platelet lysis can be adapted to detection of drug antibody, but is said to be too weak without radical alteration of the test platelet [21, 35]. Also, platelet lysis is complement dependent, which

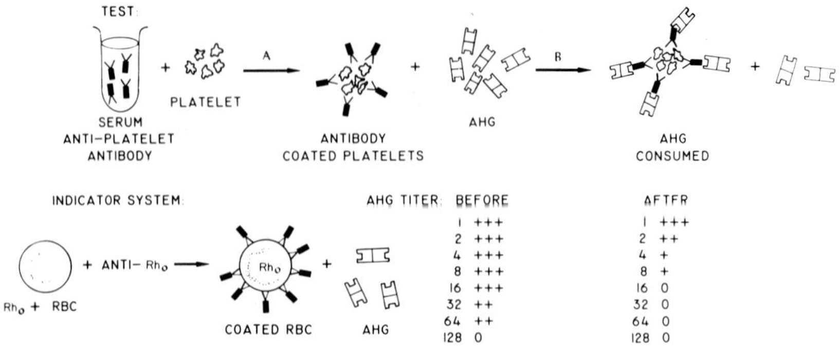

Figure 15-4
Antiglobulin consumption. Indirect method (A) requires sensitizing platelets with antiplatelet antibody in vitro. Titered AHG is consumed in the second step of the reaction. If sensitization has already occurred in vivo (B), only one step will be required, the addition of AHG. Both methods require titration of AHG against appropriately coated red cell before and after the test as an indicator system.

must be taken into account. The process of platelet lysis can be measured by released thromboplastin and a shortened Russel viper venom time; this procedure has proven satisfactory in detection of quinine [10] and quinidine [19] antibodies.

Immunofluorescence
Fluorescence methods [33] lack sensitivity if platelet washing is adequate, possibly due to elution of the immune complex during washing, and are plagued by nonspecific background fluorescence if washing has been inadequate.

If the serologic test selected fails to document what is clinically obvious, a few points must be kept in mind. In general, all tests lack sensitivity because antibody that can cause significant thrombocytopenia need be only 1/10 that required for in vitro detection [32]. Furthermore, no one technique will be applicable for all drugs, so that in cases where documentation is important, a second procedure should be tried. Sensitivity of the test appears to bear an inverse relationship to the ease with which it is performed.

Drug-Induced Leukocyte Antibodies

Other than direct effects drugs may exert on bone marrow precursors, there have been only rare cases of serologically proven drug-induced leukocyte antibodies [20, 35]. This may be due, in part, to failure to document drug causes for leukopenia because techniques are too time consuming and difficult for the general laboratory. Furthermore, interpretation of results has been confused by the possibility of nonspecific, possibly nonantibody, reactions, and spontaneous antibodies of undetermined etiology [21, 35]. However, methods similar to those used for platelets can be used, e.g., direct agglutination, complement fixation, and antiglobulin consumption with the addition of leukocyte migration inhibition [35] (see Chapter 3).

Leukocytes can be obtained using a micromethod [12] or macromethod [29]. The leukocyte of interest is usually the granulocyte rather than the lymphocyte. A rosette test using the patient's lymphocytes and drug-coated tanned sheep red cells has been proposed [29], but it raises the possibility of nonspecific reaction due to interaction with sheep cell membrane-bound globulins and the patient's B-lymphocytes. This drawback can be avoided if the test is modified to use tanned human group O red cells with complexing of the drug in question to the red cell membrane.

Conclusion

From the foregoing it can be seen that demonstration of drug-induced antibodies may require perseverance and ingenuity, but it is not impossible. A negative result should never be considered final, and clinical correlation is absolutely necessary.

References

1. Ackroyd, J. F.   Sedormid purpura: An immunological study of a form of drug hypersensitivity. *Prog. Allergy* 3:531, 1952.
2. Ackroyd, J. F.   Pathogenesis of sedormid purpura. *Clin. Sci.* 7:250, 1949.
3. Bell, C. A., and Zwicker, H.   Quinidine hemolytic anemia in the abscence of thrombocytopenia. *Transfusion* 13:100, 1973.
4. Carstairs, K.C., Breckenridge, A., Dollery, C. T., and Worlledge, S. M. Incidence of a positive direct Coombs test in patients on α-methyldopa. *Lancet* 2:133, 1966.
5. Clayton, E. M., Altshuler, J., and Bove, J. B.   Penicillin antibody as a cause of positive direct antiglobulin tests. *Am. J. Clin. Pathol.* 44:648, 1965.
6. Colombani, J.   Auto- and isoimmune thrombocytopenia. *Semin. Hematol.* 3:74, 1966.
7. Croft, J. D., Jr., Swisher, S. N., Jr., Gilliland, B. C., Bakemeier, R. F., Leddy, J. P., and Weed, R. I.   Coombs test positivity induced by drugs. Mechanisms of immunologic reactions and red cell destruction. *Ann. Intern. Med.* 68:176, 1968.
8. Dacie, J. V., and Worlledge, S. M.   Autoimmune hemolytic anemias. *Prog. Hematol.* 6:82, 1969.

9. Dausset, J., and Contu, L.   Drug-induced hemolysis. *Ann. Rev. Med.* 18:55, 1967.
10. Eisner, E. V., and Korbitz, B. C.   Quinine-induced thrombocytopenic purpura due to an IgM and an IgG antibody. *Transfusion* 12:317, 1972.
11. Faulk, W. P., Tomsovic, E. J., and Fudenberg, H. H.   Insulin resistance in juvenile diabetes mellitus. *Am. J. Med.* 49:133, 1970.
12. Fotino, M., Merson, E. J., and Allen, F. H., Jr.   Instant lymphocytes. *Vox Sang.* 21:469, 1971.
13. Garratty, G.   Drug-related problems. In *A Seminar on Problems Encountered in Pre-Transfusion Tests. Proceedings 25th Annual Meeting,* American Association of Blood Banks, Washington, D.C., 1972.
14. Gold, E. R., and Fudenberg, H. H.   Chromic chloride: A coupling reagent for passive hemagglutination reactions. *J. Immunol.* 99:859, 1967.
15. Gralnick, H. R., Wright, L. D., and McGinniss, M. H.   Coombs positive reactions associated with sodium cephalothin therapy. *J.A.M.A.* 199:725, 1967.
16. Gralnick, H. R., McGinniss, M., Elton, W., and McCurdy, P.   Hemolytic anemia associated with cephalothin. *J.A.M.A.* 217:1193, 1971.
17. Harrington, W. J., Sprague, C. C., Minnick, V., Moore, C. V., Ahlvin, R. C., and Dubach, R.   Immunologic mechanisms in idiopathic and neonatal thrombocytopenic purpura. *Ann. Intern. Med.* 38:433, 1953.
18. Heinrich, D., and Muller-Eckhardt, Ch.   Micro-complement fixation with platelets. *Vox Sang.* 21:251, 1971.
19. Horowitz, H. I., Rappaport, H. I., Young, R. C., and Fujimoto, M. M.   Change in platelet factor 3 as a means of determining immune reactions involving platelets: Its use as a test for quinidine-induced thrombocytopenia. *Transfusion* 5:336, 1965.
20. Huguley, C. M., Lea, J. W., and Butts, J. A.   Adverse hematologic reactions to drugs. *Prog. Hematol.* 5:105, 1966.
21. Lalezari, P.   Clinical significance of leucocyte iso- and autoantibodies. *Semin. Hematol.* 3:87, 1966.
22. Levine, B. B., Redmond, A. P., Fellner, M. J., Voss, H. F., and Levytska, V.   Penicillin allergy and the heterogeneous immune responses of man to benzyl penicillin. *J. Clin. Invest.* 45:1895, 1966.
23. Ley, A. B., Harris, J. P., Brinkley, M., Liles, B., Jack, J. A., and Cahan, A.   Circulating antibody directed against penicillin. *Science* 127:1118, 1958.
24. LoBruglio, A. F., and Jandl, J. H.   The nature of the alpha-methyldopa red cell antibody. *N. Engl. J. Med.* 276:658, 1967.
25. Logue, G. L., Boyd, A. E., and Rosse, W. F.   Chlorpropamide-induced immune hemolytic anemia. *N. Engl. J. Med.* 283:900, 1970.
26. Manohitharajah, S. M., Jenkins, W. J., Roberts, P. D., and Clarke, R. C.   Methyldopa and associated thrombocytopenia. *Br. Med. J.* I:494, 1971.
27. Maupin, B.   *Blood Platelets in Man and Animals.* New York: Pergamon Press, 1969, p. 344.
28. Molthan, L., Reidenberg, M. M., and Eichman, M. F.   Positive direct Coombs tests due to cephalothin. *N. Engl. J. Med.* 277:123, 1967.
29. Payne, R., and Rolfs, M. R.   Fetomaternal leucocyte incompatibility. *J. Clin. Invest.* 37:1756, 1958.

30. Perrudet, B. A., and Frei, P. C.   Detection of antibodies on blood lymphocytes in drug hypersensitivity using a rosette technique. *Int. Arch. Allergy Appl. Immunol.* 41:149, 1971.
31. Schwartz, R. S., and Costea, N.   Autoimmune hemolytic anemia. *Semin. Hematol.* 3:2, 1966.
32. Shulman, N. R.   A mechanism of cell destruction in individuals sensitized to foreign antigens and its implications in autoimmunity. *Ann. Intern. Med.* 60:506, 1964.
33. Silber, R., Benitez, R., Eveland, W. C., Ackroyd, J. H., and Dunne, C. J. Fluorescent antibody methods and study of platelets. *Blood* 16:958, 1960.
34. Spath, P., Garratty, G., and Petz, L. D.   Studies on the immune response to penicillin and cephalothin in humans. II. Immunohematologic reactions to cephalothin administration. *J. Immunol.* 107:860, 1971.
35. Tullis, J.   Leucocyte and thrombocyte antibodies. Current concepts of their origin, identity and significance. *J.A.M.A.* 180:958, 1962.
36. Weiner, W.   Eluting red cell antibodies: A method and its application. *Br. J. Haematol.* 3:276, 1967.
37. Worlledge, S. M.   Immune drug induced hemolytic anemias. *Semin. Hematol.* 6:181, 1969.
38. Worlledge, S. M., Carstairs, K. C., and Dacie, J. V.   Autoimmune hemolytic anemia, associated with α-methyldopa therapy. *Lancet* 2:135, 1966.
39. Zucker, M. B., Ley, A. B., Borrelli, J., Mayer, K., and Firmat, J. Thrombocytopenia with a circulating platelet agglutinin, platelet lysin and clot retraction inhibitor. *Blood* 14:148, 1959.
40. Zwicker, H., and Bell, C. A.   Unpublished data.

16

Laboratory Tests for the Evaluation of Rheumatoid Arthritis and Related Disorders

Rheumatoid arthritis may be defined as a chronic inflammatory disease of an unpredictable course characterized in such a way that it mainly involves the joints and connective tissues throughout the body (Fig. 16-1). The disease is most common in females aged 30 to 40 years. In general, the disease may consist of bilateral symmetrical arthritis, which mainly involves the peripheral joints and possibly affects other more centrally located joints. The presence of subcutaneous rheumatoid nodules with a characteristic histologic pattern is diagnostic (Fig. 16-2). The diagnosis of rheumatoid arthritis is a *clinical diagnosis,* and x rays and laboratory work are useful (a) to confirm the clinical diagnosis and (b) to evaluate the severity and prognosis of an individual case.

The American Rheumatism Association (ARA) proposes arbitrary criteria [91, 92] which have gained general acceptance. The patient often gives a history of morning stiffness with signs and symptoms characteristic of chronic synovitis in bilaterally symmetrical joints. Other features are (a) bilateral involvement, predominantly of the proximal metacarpophalangeal and wrist joints of the hand. In contrast, the peripheral phalangeal joints may be affected by osteoarthritis; (b) the synovitis begins in several joints simultaneously rather than involving one joint at a time, in stepwise fashion, such as in osteoarthritis; (c) the larger joints may be affected along with the peripheral joints; (d) the chronically inflamed synovial tissue may be palpated in the joints; (e) in the late stages there is interosseous muscle atrophy and ulnar deviation of the hands; (f) rheumatoid nodules may occur near pressure points of the joint, and a rheumatoid nodule in the eye is referred to as scleromalacia perforans.

Immune Complexes in the Pathogenesis of Rheumatoid Arthritis

The etiology of rheumatoid arthritis is still unknown; however, there has been much investigation on the pathogenesis of the condition. There

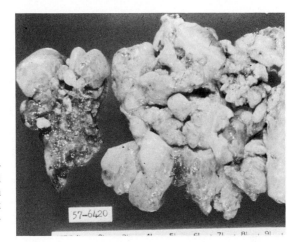

Figure 16-1
Rheumatoid synovi-
tis. Villous synovial
tissue removed from
knee joint of patient
with chronic rheu-
matoid arthritis.

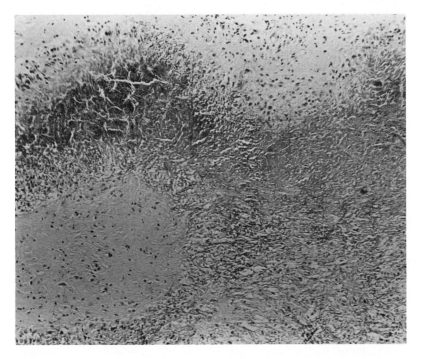

Figure 16-2
Section of subcutaneous rheumatoid nodule. The lesion has a zone of
necrosis with fibrinoid material demarcated by a zone of fibroblasts and
fibrocystic cells, which are oriented with the long axis radially to form a
palisade. At the periphery of the nodule there are aggregates of mononuclear
inflammatory cells and swollen vascular endothelial cells. (H&E stain; 40×
before 5% reduction.)

is evidence that immune complexes are involved in the pathogenesis of synovial lesions. The antigen-antibody complexes form soluble complexes and activate complement, which in turn release chemotactic factors. The chemotactic factors will attract granulocytes which are involved in the release of lysosomal enzymes and vasoactive amines and cause inflammatory destruction of tissue.

The rheumatoid synovial membrane is characterized by proliferation of the lining cells and infiltration of the deeper layers with mononuclear cells. The lining layer consists of two types of cells [135]. (a) Synovial cells resembling macrophages are called type A cells and have a phagocytic function in the joint space. (b) The type B cells are rich in endoplasmic reticulum and are responsible for the synthesis of the synovial fluid constituents.

There is hypertrophy of the lining cells with increased vascularity and mononuclear cells. There is also pannus formation with increased villous folds and large lymphoid follicles. Many alterations have been observed as follows [23, 131, 139]:

A. Deposits of IgG and IgM have been identified in the synovial tissue by fluorescent staining.

B. Localization of the complement has been demonstrated along the synovial tissues in the area of the IgG and IgM deposits.

C. Active synthesis of rheumatoid factor has been shown with the use of the fluorescent antibody technique, and rheumatoid factor has been found in the plasma cells of the synovium.

D. Inflammatory cells with intracytoplasmic inclusion bodies containing 7 S and 19 S immunoglobulins and complement have been identified in the neutrophils of the synovial fluid [22, 118].

E. There is a marked depression in complement [22, 95, 97] in rheumatoid arthritis relative to other inflammatory conditions such as gout, spondylitis, psoriatic arthritis, colitic arthritis, and Reiter's syndrome.

F. Immunoconglutinins have been observed to bind to synovial tissue from patients with rheumatoid arthritis [78]. The immunoconglutinin reaction will increase complement fixation and activation.

G. In a 20 ml effusion of a rheumatoid joint with 10,000 cells/mm^3, there are 200,000,000 white blood cells in the joint fluid with a 4 to 5 hour turnover time. Thus, there are approximately one-half billion white cells entering the joint daily, and many of the cells have been shown to produce significant amounts of the immunoglobulin [103, 139].

H. Anti-IgG–IgG complexes, cryoprecipitate, and various antiglobulin agglutinators such as pepsin agglutinators are present [79, 130, 131].

I. Complexes of cell nuclear fragments with anti-DNA antibodies contribute to joint inflammation in rheumatoid arthritis [39, 73, 138]. Antinuclear factors are often present in joint fluid and absent in the serum [44].

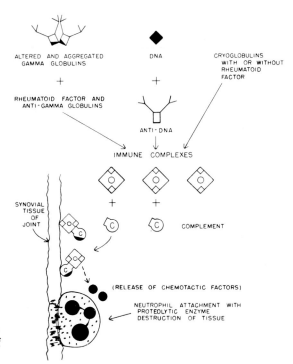

Figure 16-3
Various immune com-
plexes in joint lesions of
rheumatoid arthritis.

J. Cryoprecipitable complexes of varying amounts of IgG and IgM
   have been detected in joint fluid from seropositive rheumatoid patients and not in the serum of these patients [11, 75].
K. Anti-γ-globulins including IgG, IgA, and IgM immunoglobulins are
   detected in significant amounts in the joint fluid in cases of adult
   rheumatoid arthritis and juvenile rheumatoid arthritis [14, 84, 113,
   114, 115].

Thus, there seems to be indisputable evidence that immune complex
plays a role in the pathogenesis of joint lesions in rheumatoid arthritis
(Fig. 16-3). The immune complexes of RF and aggregated immunoglobulins, nuclear-antinuclear antibody, and cryoglobulins are able to
fix complement and initiate neutrophil infiltration. The antigen-antibody
complex can, in turn, activate plasma kallikrein and lead to kinin
formation and initiate synovial inflammation [82].

Reactivity of Immune Complexes at the Molecular Level in Rheumatoid Arthritis

Rheumatoid arthritis patients have γ-globulin complexes in both sera
and joint fluid. The rheumatoid factor involved is usually polyclonal

and combines with γ-globulin to form immune complexes. The complexes found in the serum and joint fluid differ in their immunochemical properties. The γ-globulin complexes from joint fluid of patients react readily in vitro with C1q, polyclonal or monoclonal RF to form a precipitate [130, 131]. The joint fluid complexes are pathogenic and contribute to the inflammatory destruction of the joint space.

Winchester et al. [130, 131] demonstrated that the γ-globulin complexes in the sera and joint fluid of rheumatoid arthritis differ in their reactivity to C1q and monoclonal RF. Serum complexes from patients with rheumatoid arthritis consist in large part of high molecular weight but acid-dissociable 7 S γ-globulin molecule. The exact nature of the complex is unknown, although 7 S γ-globulin rheumatoid factors play a role. The serum complexes do not precipitate with C1q but are able to demonstrate an in vivo precipitin in gel diffusion with monoclonal RF. The serum complexes in rheumatoid arthritis are not usually associated with an in vivo depression of complement, and their different properties help explain the low incidence of glomerulonephritis in patients with rheumatoid arthritis (Fig. 16-4). Although the serum immune complexes in rheumatoid arthritis may not induce a severe glomerulonephritis, they may play a role in the reduced glomerular function observed in cases of rheumatoid arthritis [25]. Patients who had rheumatoid disease with articular erosions and subcutaneous nodules had significantly lower endogenous creatinine clearance which had no correlation to therapy and medications [25].

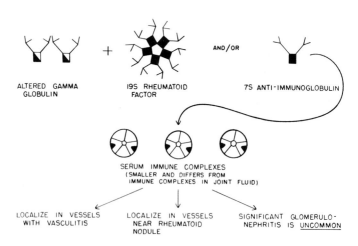

Figure 16-4
Serum immune complexes in rheumatoid arthritis.

Etiology and Role of Rheumatoid Factor

The etiology is unknown. Currently, viruses have been suspected; however, there is no evidence of virus infection by a variety of methods [55, 87]. There may be genetic as well as dietary factors involved in the disease. A rheumatoid-like arthritis has been induced in pigs by a protein rich diet influencing the growth of *Clostridium perfringens* in the intestinal tract [74] or by infection with *Erysipelothrix insidiosa* [52].

The main hypotheses are that rheumatoid arthritis currently may be an autoimmune disease, or may have a large genetic component, or is an infection. There are probably at least two phases to the disease [52]:

1. Systemic infection by some organism with a tendency to settle in the synovial membranes, and host immune response initiating the chronic inflammation. This phase may last several months and may subside.
2. The second phase may be a reinfection with another agent, or auto-immunization to various antigens (initiated by alteration of tissue antigens by the first infecting agent and host inflammatory response). The autoimmune response will perpetuate the injury.

Rheumatoid factor probably does not play a primary role in the etiology of rheumatoid arthritis. The following evidence is given:

A. Rheumatoid factor is not always present in patients with rheumatoid arthritis even in the presence of severe disease.
B. Normal subjects may show rheumatoid factor in low titers in their serum.
C. The strongest argument against a primary role of RF stems from the observation that one-third of children with agammaglobulinemia develop a disease which is very similar to rheumatoid arthritis; the children lack both IgG and IgM and have no demonstrable rheumatoid factor in their serum [53].

Other investigators have confirmed the coexistence of rheumatoid-like arthritis and immunodeficiency [10, 77]. The coexistence of arthritis and immunodeficiency is consistent with the theory of an infectious process. Some of the agammaglobulinemic patients show a clearing of the arthritic symptoms after treatment with exogenous γ-globulin.

Despite the strong evidence against a primary role of RF in the pathogenesis, it is implicated in a secondary way. It is well known that patients with high titers of rheumatoid factor have a severe joint disease and a poor prognosis. The systemic manifestations such as subcutaneous nodules, arteritis, peripheral neuropathy, and Felty's syndrome are all associated with high titers of rheumatoid factor. It is possible that rheumatoid factor in IgG complexes is present in high concentrations and may become insoluble and deposit in the vascular endothelium of blood vessels, subcutaneous tissue, and peripheral nerves, producing vascular disease, subcutaneous nodules, dermal infarction with ulcers, and peripheral neuritis [45].

Another secondary role of rheumatoid factor is perpetuation of established joint inflammation. This hypothesis ascribes a pathogenic role to rheumatoid factor only when it is in synovial fluid, and it reacts with synovial fluid with altered or denatured IgG, resulting in complexes which fix complement and attract leukocytes by chemotaxis. Phagocytosis with release of leukocyte lysosomal enzyme causes tissue inflammation and further denaturation of IgG.

Types of Rheumatoid Factor in the Pathogenesis of Rheumatoid Arthritis

In the past, rheumatoid factor (RF) has been generally assumed to be 19 S IgM antibodies [50, 66]. However, the rheumatoid factor reactivity includes both 7 S [35] and 19 S immunoglobulins with antibody specificity to determinant on the γ-globulin molecule [50, 66]. Production of antibodies directed against host IgG probably results from antigen stimulation by IgG which has undergone in vivo structural change through [90] (a) abnormal physical conditions, (b) proteolytic enzyme action of inflammatory cells, or (c) complexing of IgG with an antigen.

The antiglobulins have been found in the IgG, IgA, and IgM classes of immunoglobulins, and show reactivity against a number of specificities on the IgG molecule [14, 84, 113, 114, 115]. However, although the affinity of the antiglobulins (rheumatoid factors) is weak, it is greater with aggregated IgG.

The RF in rheumatoid arthritis is usually polyclonal in nature and may be produced as an antibody to an antigen-antibody complex. The γ-globulin may be altered in the reaction with a specific bacterium or virus, and RF is produced as hidden γ-globulin determinants become exposed in the host.

Notkins and co-workers have shown that RF will interact with viral-antiviral complexes and increase susceptibility to neutralization by interaction with complement [83]. The herpes simplex viral-antibody complexes will not be neutralized by the interaction of RF alone, but the RF allows fixation of complement, which in turn will help neutralize the virus infectivity. Thus, RF may be produced in the host to play a protective role.

Relationship of IgG, IgA, and IgM Antiglobulins to Adult and Juvenile Rheumatoid Arthritis

Rheumatoid factor (RF) is usually measured in the clinical laboratory by the latex fixation test (LFT) and sensitized sheep cell agglutination tests (SSC). These tests, in general, are more sensitive for the detection of 19 S IgM RF. When the agglutination tests for RF are negative or positive, rheumatoid arthritis patients are called seronegative or seropositive. Normal people may show evidence of RF by the agglutination test. RF is usually found in low titers, and the frequency of positive reactions increases with age [42]. An interesting finding is that there is a higher prevalence of RF in the sera of relatives and spouses of patients with rheumatoid arthritis [126]. The prevalence of RF in the spouses of probands suggests that environmental factors are involved.

The agglutination tests are often negative in cases of juvenile rheumatoid arthritis [6, 17], and milder forms of adult rheumatoid arthritis (RA). Adult seropositive RA cases have a worse prognosis with active disease.

With the use of more sensitive methods as immunoadsorbents for the isolation of the antiglobulins, it has been well established that there can be various IgG, IgA, and IgM antiglobulins in seropositive and seronegative groups of both juvenile and adult rheumatoid arthritis [2, 3, 14, 15, 58, 84, 113, 114, 115].

Increased levels of IgG, IgA, and IgM immunoglobulins were associated with clinical findings of active and severe adult and juvenile rheumatoid arthritis [14, 84, 113, 114, 115]. In adult rheumatoid arthritis, IgM immunoglobulins were elevated only in seropositive patients. Increased levels of serum and synovial fluid IgG and IgM anti-γ globulins were each associated with diminished serum and synovial fluid complement levels. In acute self-limited juvenile rheumatoid arthritis, elevated levels of IgG antiglobulins were observed with a negative latex fixation test [14].

There are "cold reactive" RF's belonging to the 19 S IgM class of antibodies in the sera of patients with infectious mononucleosis and reticulum sarcoma [29]. Such "cold reactive" RF's were found to be associated with serum active cases of juvenile rheumatoid arthritis, and were not observed in cases of seronegative adult RA [14].

7 S IgM immunoglobulins have been noted in rheumatoid arthritis and a wide variety of diseases [107, 112]. Stage and Mannik [105] used a double diffusion technique with 4% polyacrylamide gel to detect 7 S IgM, as 19 S IgM will penetrate only slightly into the gel under these conditions. The 7 S IgM was quantitated by a radial immunodiffusion method following sucrose density ultracentrifugation. The 7 S IgM was associated with severe articular disease and subcutaneous nodules.

Systemic Manifestations of Rheumatoid Arthritis, Vasculitis, and Rheumatoid Nodules

The complications of rheumatoid nodules and vasculitis are associated with the presence of RF. Although RF may be present without nodules, the nodules occur only in seropositive rheumatoid arthritis patients

[27]. Digital vasculitis and vascular lesions affecting the viscera usually occur only in seropositive patients. Vasculitis and rheumatoid arthritis are first seen to affect the fingers with an initial obliterative change, and later the viscera are involved. Different forms of vasculitis are seen in rheumatoid arthritis. There are two types of vascular lesions [52]: (a) an obliterating endarteritis which often involves the arteries of the finger, and (b) a necrotizing arteritis characterized by fibrinoid necrosis of the intima and media with disruption of the elastic lamina.

The inflammatory reactions of the small vessels may play a role in the development of the rheumatoid nodule, lesions of synovial membranes [27], and peripheral neuritis [52]. The subcutaneous nodules are often found near the elbows and other points of friction or pressure. The lesion shows a zone of necrosis with fibrinoid material demarcated by a zone of fibroblasts and fibrocytic cells which are oriented with the long axis radially to form a palisade [52]. Peripherally, the rheumatoid nodule contains vessels with swollen endothelial and perivascular aggregations of lymphocytes and plasma cells.

Heart and Lung

Rheumatoid nodules may appear in the lung, usually subpleurally [76], and virtually always associated with a positive test for rheumatoid factor. A diffuse chronic interstitial pneumonitis with diffuse fibrosis is a less frequent complication. Cardiovascular lesions which have been shown to be part of the rheumatic process [47, 89] are (a) valvular rheumatoid nodules, (b) granulomatous myocarditis, and (c) aortitis.

Juvenile Rheumatoid Arthritis

Juvenile arthritis (Still's disease) is a syndrome with polyarthritis with or without systemic involvement. The disease has a variable course from mild seronegative arthritis to a more severe disease resembling the adult disease. It is more common in girls than boys, and the onset develops before 16 years of age. Certain symptoms occur more often in children than adults and are as follows [28, 71]:
A. High fever with afternoon or evening spikes to 103° F and reverting to normal by morning.
B. Frequent monoarticular onset of arthritis.
C. Leukocytosis over 12,000 in 50% of the patients.
D. Low grade eosinophilia and moderate anemia may be present.

The incidence of positive tests for anti-γ-globulin varies with the test employed, age of the child, and activity of the disease. With the latex fixation test, positive results have been reported to be from 20 to 29.5% [28, 67]. The sheep cell agglutination test was found to be positive in 31.5% of 142 children with rheumatoid arthritis [26]. By a special method with the use of immunoadsorbent polymers, IgG, IgA, and

IgM anti-γ-globulins were found to be elevated in juvenile rheumatoid arthritis [14, 114].

The incidence of anti-γ-globulins is more common in children whose onset of the disease occurs after age 10. Patients with evidence of serum anti-γ-globulins have a higher incidence of fever, rheumatoid nodules [28], and antinuclear antibodies [94]. The antistreptolysin O titer is elevated often in juvenile arthritis and is of value in ruling out the possibility of acute rheumatic fever when the level of antistreptolysin antibody is low [71].

Arthritis Associated with General Systemic Diseases

Cases of arthritis often associated with other systemic lesions are spondylitis (Marie-Strümpell disease), Reiter's syndrome, colitic arthritis, and psoriatic arthropathy. These conditions have certain features in common. The arthritis is associated with other lesions such as prostatitis, urethritis, ileitis, sacroileitis, spondylitis, and ocular involvement. Ziff [136] has suggested that the joint lesion may arise from an antigen or inflammatory agent absorbed into a common circulation which communicates the spinal joints and the eye. The venous circulation system discovered by Batson [12], which drains the urethra and prostate and connects with the venous drainage of the spinal and sacroiliac joints, may explain the interrelationships. The variants of rheumatoid arthritis are usually negative for serum RF, and the joint fluid does not show depression of complement components.

Polymyalgia Rheumatica

Polymyalgia rheumatica, a syndrome which affects elderly persons, is infrequently seen in persons under the age of 50 and is more commonly seen in women. The following clinical features should be observed [54, 57, 63, 88, 119]:

A. Shoulder or pelvic girdle pain which is primarily muscular
B. Absence of evidence of rheumatoid or other inflammatory arthritis
C. Marked elevation of erythrocyte sedimentation rate, and slight anemia and increased α_2-globulin
D. Absence of objective sites of muscle disease
E. Prompt and dramatic response to corticosteroids

The etiology of this condition is unknown; however, the typical polymyalgia rheumatica syndrome is often complicated by other separate underlying diseases such as (a) temporal giant cell arteritis, (b) rheumatoid arthritis, (c) other connective tissue disorders, (d) infections, and (e) neoplasms.

The syndrome is most frequently associated with temporal giant cell arteritis. There is no evidence of degenerative or inflammatory changes in the muscle. The giant cell arteritis occurs in the medium and large size arteries. There is a panarteritis with pronounced internal proliferation, producing symmetrical narrowing of long portions of the major arteries. Microscopically, the findings consist of panarteritis with giant cell granuloma and fragmented elastic fibers in the media as well as internal thickening producing a narrowed lumen with thrombus formation or internal swelling. Biopsies from arteries other than temporal arteries have shown that of 250 patients, 19 or 7.6% had positive tests for rheumatoid factor [63]; the remainder tested in a number of series showed only nonspecific changes. The highest incidence of positive rheumatoid factor, 14 of 34, was reported by Bagratuni [8], and 1 of 14 later developed rheumatoid arthritis.

There is some evidence linking polymyalgia rheumatica with temporal arteritis as a variant of rheumatoid arthritis with vasculitis. Waaler and Milde [119] described a patient with polymyalgia rheumatica and giant cell (temporal) arteritis in which a 19 S rheumatoid factor was eluted from the site of the vascular lesion. Repeated serum tests on the patient were negative for rheumatoid factor. At the present time, polymyalgia rheumatica should be considered a syndrome distinct and separate from rheumatoid arthritis, which differs in its clinical course and response to therapy. In the evaluation of a patient suspected of having a polymyalgia rheumatica syndrome, one should always consider the possible existence of other underlying associated lesions.

Histochemical studies of muscle biopsies in cases of polymyalgia demonstrate type 2 muscle fiber atrophy with moth-eaten and whorled fibers [24]. In mild rheumatoid arthritis, similar changes are seen with focal inflammatory response primarily of lymphocytes.

Sjögren's Syndrome

Sjögren's syndrome, also known as Mikulicz's disease, is a chronic inflammatory disease characterized by diminished tear and salivary secretions resulting in keratoconjunctivitis sicca and xerostomia [16, 102]. The etiology of the disease is unknown but probably is influenced by a number of factors such as genetic, viral, and immunologic [41]. The diminished secretions are due to chronic inflammatory cells in the lacrimal and salivary glands. Approximately 30 to 50% of the patients have rheumatoid arthritis [16, 41, 104]. Other diseases, such as systemic lupus erythematosus, progressive systemic sclerosis, and dermatomyositis or polyarteritis nodosa are also frequently associated with the syndrome [41, 104]. The term *sicca syndrome* is used when keratoconjunctivitis sicca and xerostomia are present.

The disease, usually seen in females about 50 years of age, is often present with the development of keratoconjunctivitis sicca and xerostomia, and in patients with preexisting rheumatoid arthritis. In 10% of the cases, the sicca complex may affect the patient before the collagen disease [16]. Of the systemic manifestations, the most striking one is a renal tubular acidosis present as hyperchloremic acidosis, which is seen in 20% of the cases [111]. Renal biopsy shows a chronic interstitial infiltration of lymphocytes with fibrosis, as well as periglomerular fibrosis. Glomerulonephritis is uncommon; if it is present it is usually associated with cryoglobulinemia [111]. Patients with Sjögren's syndrome do not usually have anti-DNA antibodies in their serum and thus are unlikely to develop an immune complex glomerulonephritis as seen in systemic lupus erythematosus.

Diseases Associated with Sjögren's Syndrome
A wide spectrum of diseases is associated with Sjögren's syndrome, and all have certain autoimmune manifestations with lymphocytic infiltration. The following diseases have been noted [41, 104]: (a) rheumatoid arthritis, (b) scleroderma, (c) lupus erythematosus, (d) polymyositis, (e) chronic hepatitis, (f) Hashimoto's thyroiditis, (g) pulmonary fibrosis, and (h) lymphoproliferative neoplastic disorders.

LYMPHOPROLIFERATIVE NEOPLASMS. The incidence of lymphomas, macroglobulinemias, and hyperglobulinemias is extremely high [109, 110]. The associated abnormalities range from benign lymphocytic infiltration of glandular structures to a malignant lymphoid neoplasm such as reticulum cell sarcoma. The increased incidence of malignancy in cases of autoimmune disorders has been well established. Monoclonal macroglobulinemia may be noted with the presence of cryoglobulins, and the rheumatoid factor may be a monoclonal type.

Tests for Diagnosis of Sjögren's Syndrome
ROSE BENGAL DYE TEST [116]. The patients may in the late stages of the disease begin to show evidence of keratitis filiformis, and the devitalized corneal epithelium may be shown to take up the rose bengal dye.

SCHIRMER OCULAR TEST [116]. This is a crude test not sensitive or specific enough for a definitive diagnosis. Filter paper strips are placed under the eyelids at the inner canthus, and the quantity of tears produced to irritation in a 5 min period is measured. A normal person usually wets 15 mm or more of paper strips. One-third of elderly persons may wet only 10 mm of the paper in 5 min. When wetting of 5 mm or less is used as the end point, approximately 15% of normal patients and patients with Sjögren's syndrome are misclassified [104].

TESTS TO ASSESS SALIVARY GLAND FUNCTION
Secretory Sialography. Radiopaque material is injected directly into the parotid ducts by catheter, so the procedure carries the risk of parotitis.

Salivary Flow Rates [18].   The flow rates can be measured and are characteristically depressed.

Sequential Salivary Scintigraphy with $^{99m}T_c$ [96].   This test is free of side effects and correlates well with the degree of abnormality in the parotid gland and with the severity of xerostomia.

SALIVARY GLAND BIOPSY.   Often a biopsy of the minor salivary labial gland is taken for study. The lesions usually show (a) massive lymphoid tissue infiltration with atrophy of acinar glands, and (b) alteration of ductal epithelial cells with proliferation of intraductal cells and formation of epimyoepithelial islands or nests [80].

Immunologic Findings

Sjögren's syndrome is of particular interest, for it provides a wide spectrum of autoimmune phenomena and seems to be the central point, interrelating various diseases such as systemic lupus erythematosus and rheumatoid arthritis.

A. Rheumatoid factor is present in 90% of the cases where human γ-globulin is used as a reactant and 75% in which rabbit γ-globulin is used [16].

B. Antinuclear factors can be detected in approximately 75% of the patients. The LE cell phenomenon is present in 15–20% of the patients [46]. Antibodies to native DNA are not usually present in patients with Sjögren's syndrome.

C. There is an increased incidence of thyroid, smooth muscle, and antimitochondrial antibodies [41, 104].

D. Anti-salivary duct and anti-epithelial cell antibody reactive with the cytoplasm of these cells may be present in 70–75% of the cases. This antibody is seen in only 10–20% of cases of Sjögren's disease with the sicca complex alone [16, 127] and in 25% of the cases of rheumatoid arthritis without evidence of Sjögren's syndrome. The presence of antisalivary duct antibody probably reflects a subclinical lymphocytic sialadenitis in the major and minor salivary glands [127].

E. Cell-mediated immune responses are impaired in Sjögren's syndrome [70, 129]. An impaired lymphocyte transformation to phytohemagglutinin, streptolysin O, and a diminution in delayed hypersensitivity to dinitrochlorobenzene has been seen in 50% of the cases [70, 129]. The lack of cellular immunity and defective T-cell function would be in accordance with the increased incidence of autoimmune antibodies and malignancy. Twenty-eight of 30 patients showed reactivity to parotid extract antigen in the leukocyte migration test [13]. The cell sensitivity to parotid extract antigen was also noted in rheumatoid arthritis without evidence of Sjögren's disease and with autoimmune liver disease with and without evidence of a keratoconjunctivitis sicca syndrome.

Laboratory Tests in the Diagnosis of Rheumatoid Arthritis and Related Conditions

A. Nonspecific tests for inflammatory diseases
   a. Complete blood count and urinalysis
   b. Serum C-reactive protein (CRP)
   c. Sedimentation rate
   d. Antistreptococcal antibodies, antistreptolysin O, antideoxyribo-nuclease, and antihyaluronidase
B. X ray studies
C. Serum rheumatoid factor (RF) by conventional agglutination tests
D. Analysis of joint fluid
   a. Appearance, mucin test, and protein content
   b. White blood count and differential
   c. Examination for crystals
   d. Determination of complement levels
   e. Analysis of rheumatoid factor
   f. Culture
   g. Immunofluorescent studies for localization of IgG, IgM, and C3
   h. Other tests
E. Biopsy of synovium and subcutaneous nodules
F. Secondary serum tests

Nonspecific Tests for Inflammatory Diseases
A. Complete blood count and urinalysis
B. Serum C-reactive protein
C. Sedimentation rate
D. Antistreptococcal antibodies, antistreptolysin O, antideoxyribonu-clease, and antihyaluronidase

Patients with classic rheumatoid arthritis may have eosinophilia ranging from 20 to 89% [85]. In one series of 45 cases of rheumatoid arthritis, 40% showed unexplained eosinophilia of 5% or greater [132]. The patients with eosinophilia were often associated with cases having extra-articular manifestations such as pleuropericarditis, pulmonary fibrosis, and subcutaneous nodules [132].

The nonspecific tests help differentiate the inflammatory type from the noninflammatory type of rheumatic disease. A negative erythrocyte sedimentation test will help rule against the diagnosis of rheumatoid arthritis. The C-reactive protein (CRP) level correlates with the inflammatory response of the host and returns to normal levels with cessation of inflammation. It is primarily of value in following cases of acute rheumatic fever [48]. There are many different tests for the detection of CRP, and one should be aware of the possible differences in reactivity and specificity of anti-CRP antisera [81].

The antistreptolysin O titer is elevated frequently in juvenile rheumatoid arthritis; and the test is of major value in eliminating the diagnosis of acute rheumatic fever when the titer is low [71]. However, a negative antistreptolysin O does not necessarily rule out a recent streptococcal infection. In cases of recent streptococcal infections, one antibody, such as antistreptolysin O, is elevated in 80% of the cases and 2 or more antibodies are elevated in 90%; and if three antibodies are measured, more than 95% will show an increase in titers of at least one antibody [108].

X Ray Studies

These tests are helpful in the confirmation of the clinical diagnosis and evaluation of the severity of the joint lesions. In active cases of rheumatoid arthritis, there is a gradual loss of continuity of the bone and narrowing of the cartilage, surface erosion, and pocket erosion with cyst formation. There is destruction with very little evidence of healing. X rays of the neck should be taken in a neutral position and also in flexion, as the atlanto-axial joint may show subluxation of the cervical vertebra because of ligamentous changes.

Serum Rheumatoid Factor (RF) by Conventional
Agglutination Methods

Laboratory testing for rheumatoid factor is not of a diagnostic nature but is helpful in the prognosis, since patients with active and more severe disease tend to have high levels of rheumatoid factor. The RF test is positive in 70% of clinical cases of rheumatoid arthritis [117]. In the early stages, a rheumatoid factor may not be seen in 15–25% of the cases, and the test for RF is negative [99]. As stated above, sensitive techniques will demonstrate IgM, IgA, and IgG rheumatoid factors with antiglobulin activity in so-called seropositive and seronegative cases of rheumatoid arthritis. The quantitative levels of the antiglobulins have been noted to correlate with disease activity. Thus, in a strict sense, the term *seronegative* does not mean a complete absence of existing antiglobulins.

Patients with rheumatoid arthritis and high titers of RF will have (a) a higher incidence of complications, and (b) good response to therapy in only 20% of cases. On the other hand, rheumatoid arthritis patients who are seronegative for rheumatoid factor tend to have (a) a milder course, (b) less frequent complications, and (c) better response to therapy.

The prognostic value of the rheumatoid factor is increased if the test is done on several occasions. The prognosis in seropositive patients is much the same irrespective of whether the serologic reactions are consistently positive or swing between positive and negative. Of every 6 patients with early disease destined to be seropositive at some time, one will have a negative result when first tested [60]. By the end of one year of continuous disease, the patients usually fall into a seropositive or seronegative category. Spontaneous or clinical remissions by treatment are often accompanied by a fall in the titer or the disappearance of rheumatoid factor from the serum [62]. Visceral complications of rheumatoid arthritis are associated with high titers of rheumatoid factor. On the other hand, there are examples of a relatively benign course in patients, especially in men, with consistently high titers of rheumatoid factor [60].

There are many diseases in which the rheumatoid factor is usually *absent*. The following diseases usually show absence of rheumatoid factor: (a) osteoarthritis, (b) ankylosing spondylitis, (c) gout, (d) rheumatic fever, (e) suppurative arthritis, (f) psoriatic arthritis, (g) colitic arthritis, (h) Reiter's syndrome, (i) palindromic arthritis.

The rheumatoid factor test is usually positive in a high percentage of the following diseases [51, 62]: (a) rheumatoid disease, (b) adult rheumatoid arthritis, (c) Sjögren's syndrome, (d) systemic lupus erythematosus, (e) scleroderma, (f) juvenile rheumatoid arthritis, (g) Still's disease.

It is present in other infectious diseases as follows [51, 62]: (a) subacute bacterial endocarditis, (b) tuberculosis, (c) syphilis, (d) infectious hepatitis, (e) kala azar, (f) leprosy, (g) sarcoidosis, (h) other conditions in which there is a chronic hypergammaglobulinemia, such as Waldenström's hypergammaglobulinemia.

Analysis of Joint Fluid

The fluid from a synovial joint is suitable for examination, and the most common site of aspiration is the knee joint. Aseptic precautions are essential. The following tests are useful:

A. Appearance, mucin test, and protein content
B. White blood count and differential
C. Examination for crystals
D. Determination of complement levels
E. Analysis for rheumatoid factor
F. Culture
G. Immunofluorescent localization studies for IgG, IgM, and C3
H. Other tests such as for antinuclear antibodies, cryoglobulins, and immune complexes

APPEARANCE, MUCIN TEST, AND PROTEIN CONTENT. Normal joint fluid is straw colored, clear, and viscous. The viscosity of joint fluid depends on the concentration and degree of polymerization of the hyaluronic acid. The inflammatory changes affect the viscosity by dilution of the hyaluronic acid and by causing depolymerization. Normal fluid is highly viscous, but in contrast the fluid may be quite watery in rheumatoid arthritis.

The addition of acetic acid to a final concentration of 1% in normal or near normal synovial fluid produces a firm mucin clot. Fluid from acutely inflamed joints gives a scanty and flocculant mucin clot. This test is usually not regarded as worth performing routinely, and other tests should be performed first if the amount of fluid aspirate is limited. In degenerative joint disease, a protein value of 2 to 3 gms/100 ml is common, while in rheumatoid arthritis the concentration of proteins is elevated and may be 4 to 7 gms/100 ml. The normal level of protein is approximately 2 gms/100 ml [37].

WHITE BLOOD COUNT AND DIFFERENTIAL.   In order to perform cell counts, synovial fluid is immediately mixed with EDTA anticoagulant. The viscosity of the fluid makes this examination rather inaccurate. The degree of turbidity of fluid provides a rough index of the cell count. Degenerative joint disease may produce synovial leukocyte counts of 0 to 5,000 cells/mm^3. Rheumatoid arthritis counts are of the order of 5,000 to 50,000 cells/mm^3. The synovial fluid leukocytes can be studied by smears with Wright's stain or by phase contrast microscopy.

Rheumatoid effusion usually contains about 90% neutrophilic leukocytes and the remainder of the cells are usually mononuclear in type. In degenerative joint disease, the percentage of mononuclear cells may be somewhat higher, while in septic arthritis and crystal synovitis, the predominant cell is the neutrophil. The multiple dark inclusion in cytoplasm of leukocytes is seen in a wide variety of circumstances, and the ragocytes or RA cells [61] are common in rheumatoid arthritis but not diagnostic of the condition.

EXAMINATION FOR CRYSTALS.   This procedure is absolutely essential for a definite diagnosis of gout or pseudogout. In gout, one can see extracellular or intracellular long thin urate crystals which exhibit a negative birefringence when examined with a polarizing microscope [37]. Pseudogout will show intracellular and extracellular calcium pyrophosphate crystals which are 8 to 10 μ in length and which have a broader width than urate crystals. The calcium pyrophosphate crystals have a faintly discernible line along the long axis and do *not* show a negative birefringence when examined under a polarizing microscope.

DETERMINATION OF COMPLEMENT LEVELS.   Determination of complement levels is extremely helpful in differentiating rheumatoid arthritis from other diseases. Complement levels in the joint fluid are depressed in active cases of rheumatoid arthritis, juvenile RA, and SLE, and reflect the active immune complex deposition and injury. On the other hand, complement levels are either normal or elevated in various other conditions such as (a) gout, (b) spondylitis, (c) psoriatic arthritis, (d) colitic arthritis, and (e) Reiter's syndrome.

Normally the complement levels in joint fluid are greater than 33% of the serum level, and the normal level of total serum complement in

200 $\pm$ 50 units/ml is determined as CH_{50} units [97]. In the analysis of joints, Ruddy and Austen [95] had expressed the total hemolytic complement in CH_{50} units/gm protein, and their results are as follows:
A. Rheumatoid arthritis patients' serum with positive serum test for RF = 11.6 $\pm$ 1.0 CH_{50} units/gm
B. Rheumatoid arthritis patients with negative serum test for RF = 27.7 $\pm$ 1.3 CH_{50} units/gm
C. Cases of degenerative joint disease = 24.3 $\pm$ 1.5 CH_{50} units/gm

It is important to assay for total hemolytic complement and/or C4 levels, since such measurements are more sensitive for the detection of active utilization of complement. The determination of C3 is not a sensitive indicator of complement activity; however, when C3 levels are depressed, the results are significant. In synovial fluids of seronegative patients, only C4 may be depleted to a significant extent as compared to the findings in the fluids of patients with degenerative joint disease [22]. In other inflammatory conditions, such as septic arthritis, the protein and complement concentrations are increased or normal.

ANALYSIS FOR RHEUMATOID FACTOR.   In active cases of rheumatoid factor, one often can detect the presence of RF in synovial fluid. Early cases of RF may show RF in the synovial fluid before it becomes detectable in the serum.

CULTURE.   A culture should be taken, especially in cases of suspected bacterial infections. One should suspect a complicating bacterial inflammation superimposed on a rheumatoid synovitis in cases where the patient gives a history of unusual progressive pain, particularly in one of the joints.

IMMUNOFLUORESCENCE LOCALIZATION STUDIES FOR IGG, IGM, AND C3. Immunofluorescence studies can be done to determine sites of localization of IgG, IgM, and C3 in cells containing large inclusion bodies or ragocytes [22].

OTHER TESTS SUCH AS FOR ANTINUCLEAR ANTIBODIES, CRYOGLOBULINS, AND IMMUNE COMPLEXES.   In severe cases, one can detect antinuclear factors and cryoglobulins in the joint fluid. As discussed above, these complexes are able to fix complement and initiate tissue injury similar to Ig–IgM complexes.
Immune complexes of Ig–IgM may be detected in the joint by an agar gel double diffusion, by interaction with the C1q component of complement [4]. The IgG–IgM complexes in joint fluid are large and react with C1q to form a precipitin line in the in vitro test. However, there are smaller γ-globulin complexes found in the serum in rheumatoid arthritis which will not form a precipitin line by interaction with

C1q, but will react with a monoclonal RF. Thus, one can see that the complexes in the joint and serum in cases of rheumatoid arthritis differ in their size and immunochemical properties [131].

Biopsy of Synovium and Subcutaneous Nodules

Biopsy studies of synovium will show hypertrophy of synovium with hyperplasia of synovial lining cells. There will be a villous proliferation of the synovial tissue with large lymphoid follicles showing prominent reactive germinal centers. The histologic findings in synovial tissue are characteristic, but not diagnostic for rheumatoid arthritis. Immuno-fluorescence studies of synovial tissue may be done for evidence of localization of IgG, IgM, and C3 immune complexes in intracellular and extracellular areas of the synovial tissue.

The subcutaneous nodule may show a pattern characteristic of a rheumatoid nodule. Granulomatous nodules usually occur only in seropositive rheumatoid arthritis patients [27]. Subcutaneous nodules seen in cases of agammaglobulinemia associated with polyarthritis resemble those of rheumatoid arthritis except for a paucity of mononuclear cells and the absence of plasma cells [10].

Secondary Serum Tests

SERUM URIC ACID. The normal uric acid level in men is 7.5–8.0 mg/ 100 ml and in women it is 6.5–7.0 mg/100 ml. A large percentage of patients with a uric acid level of greater than 9 mg/100 ml will develop clinical gout. Most clinical laboratory determinations of uric acid are not performed with the specific enzymatic method employing uricase. The elevated uric acid should be reassayed with a specific enzymatic method [72]. In the diagnosis and differentiation of gout from rheumatoid arthritis, the uric acid test is not diagnostic. The definite diagnosis of gout is made by the identification of characteristic uric acid crystals in joint fluid. The complement levels in joint fluid are usually normal.

SERUM ANTINUCLEAR ANTIBODIES. Although many cases of rheumatoid arthritis may have a positive test for antinuclear antibodies and positive LE cell test, the determination of type and titer of antinuclear antibodies will help differentiate rheumatoid arthritis from SLE and other collagen diseases. In active SLE, the antinuclear antibodies usually have much higher titers and the patients often show (a) more severe anemia, leukopenia, or thrombocytopenia, (b) false positive serologic tests for syphilis, and (c) glomerulonephritis and pericarditis.

SERUM CRYOGLOBULINS. RF is commonly found in many other diseases besides rheumatoid arthritis, and a disease with cryoglobulinemia may have a monoclonal type of RF associated with the cryoglobulinemia.

Methods for the Detection of Rheumatoid Factor (Anti-γ-Globulins)

The methods for detection of γ-globulin or altered γ-globulin should be distinguished from the anti-Fab antibodies known as serum agglutinators which are found in normal sera [122], acute and chronic infections [125], and in patients with rheumatoid arthritis. The specificity of these antibodies is determined by the modification of the Fab fragment characteristic of the proteolytic enzyme used for hydrolysis, for example, papain, pepsin, and trypsin agglutinators [123]. Various methods for the detection of γ-globulins are:

A. Human FII latex agglutination test
B. Human FII bentonite flocculation test
C. Automated charcoal coated human FII test
D. Sensitized sheep cell (SSC) agglutination test (Waaler-Rose)
E. Agglutination and inhibition by serum globulin in the sensitized sheep cell (SSC) agglutination test
F. Sensitized human OD (Rh+) cell agglutination (SHC) test
G. Human FII tanned red cell test
H. Detection and quantitation of IgG, IgA, and IgM antiglobulins with use of immunoadsorbent
 I. Rheumatoid rosette test
J. Other methods for detection and quantitation of anti-γ-globulins

Human FII Latex Agglutination Test

This test, first described by Singer and Plotz [100], used latex particles coated with human γ-globulin and reacted against various dilutions of test serum (Fig. 16-5). The initial test, a tube dilution test, has been adapted to a slide screening test. There are certain technical problems,

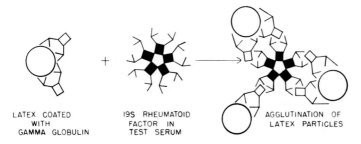

LATEX COATED   19S RHEUMATOID   AGGLUTINATION OF
     WITH   FACTOR IN   LATEX PARTICLES
GAMMA GLOBULIN   TEST SERUM

Figure 16-5
Latex agglutination test for rheumatoid factor.

such as (a) fibrinogen causes agglutination of latex so plasma should not be used; (b) a good buffer system must be used since the γ particles will agglutinate at the isoelectric point of γ-globulins; and (c) latex particles may spontaneously agglutinate if the protein concentration in the test system is markedly decreased.

However, the greatest problem with this test—and all tests—is a lack of standardization. Lea and Ward made a comparative study of different latex tests for rheumatoid factors [68]. Their conclusions were that there were wide differences among commercial latex reagents which were attributed to inadequate standardization. This may be due to the fact that two tests which use the same IgG antigen may occasionally give different results, if the orientation of this antigen on the particle surface differs in the two cases. The latex test should be standardized with a panel of reference sera in which the sheep cell agglutination or latex fixation titers are known, rather than by repeated reference to clinical information.

In a quantitative study of the latex fixation test, Cats and Klein [32] noted that male and female patients with 5 or more of the ARA (American Rheumatoid Association) criteria [91, 92] often had titers greater than 1:160.

The "cold reactive" RF belongs to the 19S IgM class of antibodies and was first observed in the sera of patients with infectious mononucleosis and reticulum cell sarcoma by Capra et al. [29]. These "cold reactive" factors were found in certain cases of juvenile rheumatoid arthritis and associated with a more severe disease. The "cold reactive" factors were not detected in patients with adult rheumatoid arthritis with negative agglutination tests. The determination of "cold reactive" rheumatoid factors is performed by a modification of the latex fixation test of Singer and Plotz [100]. Serum which is first inactivated at 56° C for 30 min is incubated with human γ-globulin-coated latex particles at 4° C for 18 hours. Titers greater than 1:20 are considered positive.

Human FII Bentonite Flocculation Test

The FII bentonite flocculation test is basically a modification of the FII latex fixation test in that clay particles of uniform sized bentonite have been used instead of latex [20]. The test has a comparable degree of sensitivity to the FII latex test, but has an advantage that titration end points can be read more accurately under the microscope.

Automated Charcoal-Coated Human FII Test

A continuous flow method with use of an autoanalyzer has been developed for the detection and quantitation of RF. The reactivity and sensitivity of the automated procedure is comparable to manual latex particle fixation test. The test utilizes sensitized charcoal particles instead of latex for the indicator reagent.

Sensitized Sheep Cell (SSC) Agglutination
Test (Waaler-Rose)
Sheep cells are coated with subagglutinating amounts of *rabbit* anti-
sheep red cell antibody and are the test reagent for rheumatoid factor
[93, 120]. The test does not have the sensitivity of the latex test and
probably is more specific for detection of RF (Fig. 16-6). It is not a
popular test in the clinical laboratory because of the necessity of pre-
absorption of serum with uncoated sheep cells. Other investigators
avoided the absorption procedure by the use of alligator cells [38]. Reagents for a slide test modification of this procedure is commercially
available [64].

Agglutination and Inhibition by Serum Globulin in the
Sensitized Sheep Cell (SSC) Agglutination Test
This procedure involves extraction of the euglobulin fraction from the test
serum sample, and SSC agglutination reactions are performed with both
the whole serum and globulin fractions. In the inhibition test, dilutions
of the euglobulin fraction to be tested are added to a fixed amount of
positive-reacting rheumatoid serum and then reacted with sensitized
sheep cells.

By this procedure, Ziff et al. [134] have increased the percentage of
positive tests from 78% in whole serum to 92% with the use of euglobulin fraction. In addition, the incidence of false positive reactions fell
from 13% to 2% [134]. The inhibition test was first performed to attempt to determine the presence of a serum inhibitor to explain the
significant number of negative reactions in patients with rheumatoid
arthritis. However, the serum euglobulin of 105 patients with rheumatoid arthritis did not show inhibition of SSC, whereas over 96% of
euglobulin fractions of the control subjects caused inhibition of SSC
when reacted with positive-reacting rheumatoid serum.

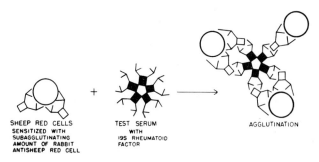

SHEEP RED CELLS
SENSITIZED WITH
SUBAGGLUTINATING
AMOUNT OF RABBIT
ANTISHEEP RED CELL

TEST SERUM
WITH
19S RHEUMATOID
FACTOR

AGGLUTINATION

Figure 16-6
Sensitized sheep cell agglutination test for rheumatoid factor.

This test is not popular because of the time and delay caused by the required extraction of euglobulin from the test sera.

Sensitized Human OD (Rh+) Cell Agglutination (SHC) Test

This test requires a rare serum containing an incomplete antibody to Rh+ which will coat Rh+ cells but leave the coated sensitized cells still capable of reacting with most of the rheumatoid factors [121]. Grubb and Laurell [56] were the first to note that certain antiglobulins (RF) will agglutinate Rh+ red cells coated by selected anti-Rh antibodies and will not agglutinate Rh+ cells coated by other anti-Rh antibodies. Further they noted the reaction could be inhibited by serum of certain individuals and this led to the identification of Gm, a genetic determinant of human immunoglobulins. Similar to the system described by Grubb and Laurell [56], there are rare patients who have incomplete anti-Rh antibodies which will detect almost all types of RF.

The SHC test is as sensitive and specific as the FII latex fixation test and the FII bentonite flocculation test. The test is not widely used because of a restricted supply of serum. Also, the procedure is more difficult to standardize since the anti-Rh+ antibody is obtained from human donors.

Human FII Tanned Red Cell Test

This test is performed in a manner similar to the sensitized sheep cell agglutination test [59]. Tanned sheep red cells are coated with human γ-globulin and used as the reactant to detect RF. The method has greater sensitivity than the SSC test and equal or greater sensitivity than the FII latex or bentonite test. Waller [124], in her study of comparing different methods for the detection of RF, found that the FII tanned cell test was the most sensitive test. The disadvantage of the method is that the sera must be adsorbed with uncoated sheep cells.

Detection and Quantitation of IgG, IgA, and IgM
Antiglobulins with Use of Immunoadsorbent (Fig. 16–7)

Various methods have been used to demonstrate IgG, IgA, and IgM anti-γ-globulins in the sera of patients with rheumatoid arthritis. Immunoadsorbents have been used to isolate the different antiglobulins. The following types of immunoadsorbents have been used by different investigators: (a) heat-denatured human FII [58], (b) bisdiazotized benzidine rabbit γ-globulin [113, 114], (c) bisdiazotized benzidine horse γ-globulin [115], (d) human γ-globulin cross-linked with glutaraldehyde [14, 84], and (e) bromacetyl cellulose coupled with human IgG [2].

Torrigiani and co-workers [113, 114] have developed a method in which serum containing anti-γ-globulins is reacted with insoluble immunoadsorbent containing rabbit γ-globulin. The various anti-γ-globulins from patients' serum will adhere to the immunoadsorbent and the other serum proteins are removed by washing. The adsorbed anti-γ-globulins are then eluted and quantitated by radial immunodiffusion in agar gel containing antibody to human IgG, IgA, or IgM immunoglobulin. This method will enable the detection of all three immunoglobulin classes, whereas the various agglutination procedures will primarily detect IgM rheumatoid factors.

Torrigiani and associates observed that IgG, IgA, and IgM anti-γ-globulins were seen in cases of rheumatoid arthritis and were not elevated in normal patients [113]. Elevated IgG antiglobulins were seen in cases of juvenile rheumatoid arthritis and were associated with disease activity [114].

By the use of insoluble cross-linked horse γ-globulin as an immunoadsorbent, Torrigiani et al. [115] found that the seronegative rheumatoid arthritis patients had increased concentrations of IgG antiglobulins. The patients had negative tests for rheumatoid factors by the conventional tests. By the more sensitive method, IgM antiglobulins were found in 6 and IgA in 4 of the 40 seronegative patients. In the adult cases of rheumatoid arthritis, a definite correlation between disease activity and elevated levels of IgG antiglobulins could not be established with the limited number of cases studied.

With use of an immunoadsorbent made up of cross-linked human γ-globulins, Bianco, Panush, Stillman, and Schur [14] have studied cases of juvenile rheumatoid arthritis and adult rheumatoid arthritis. In juvenile rheumatoid arthritis, they noted one group of patients with active disease had (a) elevated levels of IgG, IgA, and IgM antiglobulins and (b) relative depression of complement and complement components in the sera and synovial fluid. A second group of patients with juvenile rheumatoid arthritis had acute self-limited disease with (a) elevated levels of IgG and IgA anti-γ-globulins and (b) negative serum complement and latex fixation tests for rheumatoid factor. Abnormal test values returned to normal with clinical remission.

In patients with adult rheumatoid arthritis, Panush et al. [84] used an immunoadsorbent consisting of cross-linked human γ-globulin to quantitate the serum and synovial fluid IgG, IgA, and IgM anti-γ-globulins. They found that serum IgG and IgA and synovial fluid IgG anti-γ-globulin levels were significantly higher in patients with rheumatoid arthritis, and that the highest levels occurred in patients with positive latex fixation test [84]. Increased levels of IgG, IgA, and IgM anti-γ-globulins were each associated with the clinical findings of severe rheumatoid arthritis. The increased IgG and IgM levels in serum and synovial fluid were inversely proportional to the decreased complement levels.

In additional experiments, IgG, IgA, and IgM anti-γ-globulins were isolated in large amounts from patients with positive RF, negative RF, osteoarthritis, and normal patients [84]. After isolation of the various immunoglobulins with use of an immunoadsorbent, the individual immunoglobulins were separated by column chromatography methods.

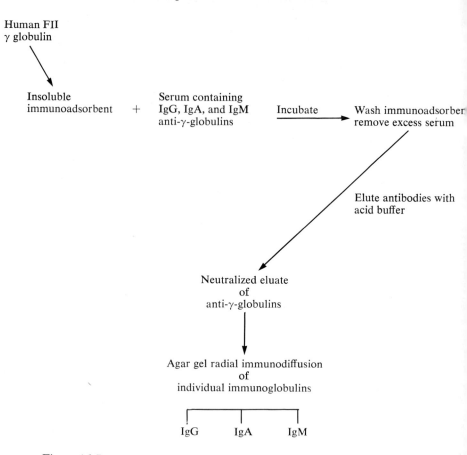

Figure 16-7
Quantitation of various anti-γ-globulins with use of immunoadsorbent and radial immunodiffusion.

The isolated IgG, IgA, and IgM anti-γ-globulins derived from patients with seronegative rheumatoid arthritis, when concentrated several times, each gave positive latex fixation tests.

Rheumatoid Rosette Test
Bach et al. [7] have developed a technique in which rheumatoid rosettes were obtained in vitro by mixing lymphocytes isolated from patients with rheumatoid arthritis and human O Rh− erythrocytes coated with rabbit immunoglobulin (Fig. 16-8). The rosette is defined as an agglutination of more than 4 erythrocytes around the lymphocyte. The results are expressed in a number of rosettes/1,000 lymphocytes. In a large study, more than 6 rheumatoid rosettes/1,000 lymphocytes were

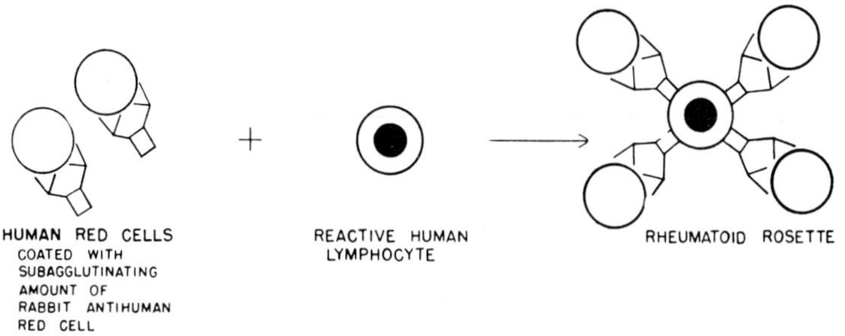

Figure 16-8
Rheumatoid rosette test.

found in 70% of 138 patients with rheumatoid arthritis, including gouty arthritis, and 5% of 158 control subjects. No direct correlation was observed between the number of rheumatoid rosettes and the serum titer of rheumatoid factor.

In the studies of Bach et al. [7], several tests for RF were compared. A Waaler-Rose reaction was performed with human O Rh erythrocyte coated with subagglutinating amounts of rabbit anti-human erythrocytes, and a latex reaction was performed according to the procedure of Singer and Plotz [100]. The results of these tests were considered positive when the titers exceeded 1:16 for the Waaler-Rose reaction and 1:180 for the latex reaction. The results showed the proportion of positive rosette tests were 76% of the seropositive and 64% of the seronegative groups of rheumatoid arthritis patients. A positive rheumatoid rosette test was significantly more frequent in patients with rheumatoid arthritis of recent onset than in those with long-standing rheumatoid arthritis; in patients with pain than in those without pain. A similar correlation was not found with the serum levels of rheumatoid factor. The rheumatoid rosette-forming cells are probably observed principally during the onset or during the active phase of rheumatoid arthritis; whereas high levels of serum rheumatoid factor are more typical of the chronic phase of the disease.

The rheumatoid rosette has been proposed as a new test bridging the seropositive and seronegative cases of rheumatoid arthritis. If this test is combined with serum agglutination reactions, the rheumatoid factor is demonstrated in more than 90% of patients with rheumatoid arthritis. A negative rosette test in a patient not treated with corticosteroids would suggest that the disease has become inactive. Rheumatoid rosette-forming cells are probably rheumatoid factor-producing cells or antigen sensitive cells involved in immunoglobulin recognition.

Lee and Ward [69] investigated rosette formation by circulating lymphocytes from rheumatoid and nonrheumatoid subjects. These investigators performed experiments slightly different from Bach et al. [7] and used (a) sheep red cells coated with rabbit and (b) human O Rh+ red cells coated with human antibody (Ripley anti-CD serum). With the use of these cells, they noted antiglobulin activity in both rheumatoid and nonrheumatoid subjects alike, and further noted that many rosettes were seen in various patients with the use of normal sheep cells. Thus, they did not provide additional evidence to support the observation of Bach et al. [7] that patients with rheumatoid arthritis will form rosettes with human 0 cells coated with rabbit antibody to human red cells.

In the rosette test, one should use human 0 cells coated with a rabbit or other heterologous antibody. It is well known that sheep cells will tend to form spontaneous rosettes with human lymphocytes which are probably T-cells [65, 133]. Human red cells coated with human γ-globulin may also give rise to artifacts since aggregated human γ-globulin will react with human peripheral surface bearing Ig lymphocytes of B-cell origin [43]. Further, Dickler and Kunkel [43] have noted that the site on the lymphocyte membrane responsible for binding aggregated γ-globulin was distinct from surface Ig.

Other Methods for Detection and Quantitation of Anti-γ-Globulins

A radioimmunoassay procedure has been reported by Franchimont and Suteanu [49]. With the use of ^{131}I-labeled aggregated γ-globulin, evidence has been presented that anti-γ-globulin and binding factors are present in most patients with rheumatoid arthritis and can be occasionally seen in normal persons.

An indirect immunofluorescence procedure for the detection of anti-γ-globulins has been reported [86]. Human 0 red cells are coated with rabbit anti-human red cell antibodies and fixed to a slide. Heat-inactivated test serum containing anti-γ-globulins is reacted with the substrate in different dilutions with the substrate. The slide is washed and reacted with fluoresceinated rabbit anti-human globulin. Anti-γ-globulins were detected in a significant percentage of sera which were negative by the sensitized sheep cell agglutination test.

IgA and IgG antiglobulins were detected by the use of the hemagglutination augmentation method [3]. In this method, human γ-globulin-coated red cells are used as the test reagent; the serum anti-γ-globulin will bind to coated red cells and give a titer of agglutination. The sensitized red cells with adherent IgA or IgG anti-γ-globulins are then reacted with specific heterologous anti-human IgA or IgG antisera, and the basic agglutination titer will be augmented many-fold depending upon the presence of IgA or IgG anti-γ-globulins.

Procedures

Problems on Selection of Tests for Use in the Clinical Laboratory

There is considerable controversy over the standardization, reproducibility, sensitivity, and specificity of the various tests for rheumatoid arthritis and the detection of the rheumatoid factor [9, 30, 32]. Waller [124] has done a considerable amount of work and compared several methods involved in the measurement of rheumatoid factor. In this study, the same technologist with 10 years of experience in serologic testing for rheumatoid factors compared various methods on 74 blood samples. The various tests compared were as follows:

A. Sensitized sheep cell test with the sheep erythrocyte sensitized at 1:5 and 1:10 dilutions of the basic agglutination titer of the rabbit anti-sheep cell antibody (SSC test) [93, 120]
B. Sensitized human cell test (SHC test) [121]. A special patient serum with anti-Rh antiserum is used to coat the human red cells in this method
C. Two different commercially available slide test reagents and three different commercially available tube latex reagents
D. Human FII tanned cell test [59]

The conclusions of the study were as follows:

A. Neither the sensitized sheep cell agglutination (SSC) test, with its unusual high degree of specificity, nor the FII tanned cell test, with its marked sensitivity, is suitable as a standardized test for clinicians.
B. It was not possible to single out any test as the most specific and at the same time the most sensitive.
C. The tube latex test is the most suitable titration test when time and skill are considered. This test needs to be better standardized since different reagents presently available differ in their performance, readability, and results.
D. Both the SSC and FII test require time-consuming inactivation and adsorption of sera prior to testing.

Waller believed that the tube latex test is probably the most practical and easy to use on a wide-scale basis [124].

The World Health Organization Committee on biological standardization requested the National Institute for Medical Research, London, England, to arrange a study to determine the suitability of establishing a reference preparation of rheumatoid arthritis serum [5]. When the serum was assayed by various laboratories, the results of the latex method varied more widely than those of other methods. The laboratories were asked to assay the samples with a recommended technique for sheep cell agglutination [5]. The international unit of rheumatoid arthritis serum has been defined as the activity contained in 0.171 mg of the international reference preparation.

It has been found that the specificity of slide latex test for the detection of rheumatoid factor can be increased by heat-inactivating the serum at 56° C for 30 min [34]. 48% of serum from patients with rheumatic diseases other than rheumatoid arthritis had a 1+ or greater positive latex fixation in the unheated state, and 9% of these were positive after heating. The thermal agglutinator in serum found to affect each of the 5 different slide test reagents reacted in the same manner as the C1q component of complement [34].

Recommendations in the Use of the Latex Fixation Test

Many commercial test kits are available as well as basic reagents to perform the test by the original Singer and Plotz procedure [100]. Most clinical laboratories are using some latex agglutination procedure for the detection of rheumatoid factor. The test has helped more in evaluating the severity and prognosis of rheumatoid arthritis than as a diagnostic tool. The following recommendations are given to improve the reproducibility and performance of the latex test:

A. Use the same reagent for the rapid slide and tube dilution test [124].
B. Use colored latex particles so the reactions are easy to read [124].
C. Heat inactive serum at 56° C for 30 min—probably best done after a 1:20 dilution of serum since the C1q component of complement probably causes false positive reactions [34].
D. Standardize the test with batches of reference sera of known titers [32].
E. Standardize the procedures with a short incubation period and elimination of overnight procedures [124].

Sensitized Sheep Agglutination Test

(Method of National Institute for Medical Research of England and World Health Organization Committee on Biological Standardization [5])

MATERIALS
A. Tubes for containing reagents
B. Refrigeration to 4° C; −20° C
C. Centrifuge
D. Water bath
E. Heat to 56° C
F. Incubator

REAGENTS

Alsever's solution

Dextrose	20.5 gm
Sodium citrate	8.0 gm
Citric acid	0.552 gm
Sodium chloride	4.2 gm
Water to	1 liter
Seitz filter	pH 6.1

Phosphate-buffered saline solution (PBS).   Prepare as 3 separate solutions
A. Sodium dihydrogen phosphate 24. 6 g/liter
B. Disodium hydrogen phosphate 22.4 g/liter
C. Sodium chloride 8.5 gm/liter

Mix (A) and (B) to pH 7.4 and then mix 1 part of (A + B) with 9 parts of (C).

SHEEP CELLS.   Store sheep cells in Alsever's solution at 4° C. Wash 3 times, each time make up to 5% in PBS pH 7.4, and centrifuge at 500 g for 15 min. The supernate should be clear after 3 washings. (Discard cells if, after 3 washings, supernate is not clear.) Make up as 1% and as 25% cells suspensions in PBS. 1% cells = 2×10^8 cells/ml.

AMBOCEPTOR.   Rabbit anti-sheep red cell antibody. One can dilute the original stock and store in aliquots at $-20°$ C; do not refreeze after thawing.

TEST RHEUMATOID SERUM.   Clot blood at 37° C for 1 hour, centrifuge at 500 g for 20 min, and store serum at $-20°$ C. Thaw serum in a water bath at room temperature and then heat at 56° C for 30 min before testing.

ADSORPTION OF SERUM
1. Centrifuge 1 ml 25% sheep cells at 500 g for 15 min and remove supernatant.
2. Add 0.75 ml 1:4 dilution of serum in PBS.
3. Shake and leave at room temperature for 60 min, then at 4° C for 60 min.
4. Centrifuge at 500 g for 15 min at 4° C; the supernatant is considered as a 1:4 dilution.

TITRATION OF AMBOCEPTOR
1. Dilute amboceptor in doubling dilutions of PBS (0.2 ml each).
2. Add equal volumes or 0.2 ml 1% sheep cells.
3. Leave at room temperature for 15 min.
4. Shake and leave at 4° C for 2 hours.
5. Read patterns of agglutination.

Use amboceptor as one-quarter of the concentration of the end point.

SENSITIZATION OF RED CELLS
1. Mix equal volumes of 1% cells and amboceptor at the determined dilution, both in PBS.

2. Incubate at room temperature for 15 min. If desired to store longer, for example an additional 15 min, this should be done at 4° C.

TITRATION OF TEST SERUM
1. Set up doubling dilutions of test serum in PBS at each dilution.
2. Include positive and negative control sera with each run.
3. Add an equal volume of 0.5% unsensitized cells to the first tube of each serum dilution.
4. Add an equal amount of 0.5% sensitized cells to all but the first tube of each dilution.
5. Leave at 4° C for 18 hours.

INTERPRETATION.   Read end point as the initial dilution of serum in the tube showing a + pattern of agglutination (initial dilution of serum before the addition of red cells). The unsensitized cells should show no agglutination. A positive agglutination of greater than 1:16 is usually considered to be significant.

Rheumatoid Rosette Test
(Modified from Bach [7])

MATERIALS AND REAGENTS
A. 20 ml blood
B. Heparinized syringe (Lipo-Hepin) (Riker)
C. Pigskin gelatin (Eastman Kodak)
D. Hanks' balanced saline solution
E. Incubator at 37° C
F. Centrifuge
G. Nylon column (Leucopak filter) (Fenwal)
H. Distilled water
 I. Agitator
J. Human O Rh− erythrocytes
K. Rabbit anti-human erythrocyte serum
L. Physiologic saline solution
M. Pipette
N. 10 test tubes
O. Water bath at 37° C
P. Refrigerator
Q. Hemocytometer chamber
R. Positive and negative controls

COLLECTION OF BLOOD AND ISOLATION OF LYMPHOCYTES
1. 20 ml blood is collected in a heparinized syringe.
2. One-half volume of 3% (w/v) pigskin gelatin in Hanks' balanced salt solution (BSS) is added to the blood and the mixture allowed to sediment for 1 hour at 37° C.

3. The leukocyte rich supernatant is collected and centrifuged at 1,000 rpm for 15 min and the cells are washed with Hanks' BSS.
4. The cells are passed through a nylon column to remove granulocytes.
5. The cells are washed 2 times in Hanks' BSS and centrifuged at 200 g for 5 min. Cells are then subjected to hypotonic shock by quickly mixing packed cells with 4 ml distilled H_2O and agitating for 20 sec, then 30 ml Hanks' BSS is added. (The exposure time of 20 sec is important, for prolonged exposure will be harmful to the lymphocytes.) Isotonicity of the solution is obtained with the third washing.
6. The lymphocyte cell suspension is adjusted to 15×10^6 lymphocytes/ml.

SENSITIZED ERYTHROCYTES
A. Human O Rh− erythrocytes are sensitized with rabbit anti-human erythrocyte serum. The rabbit anti-human erythrocyte serum is first titered with O Rh− erythrocytes to determine the subagglutinating concentration for sensitization, as in the Waaler-Rose reaction [93, 120].
B. Only a narrow range of concentration of rabbit anti-human erythrocytes may be used. Three different suspensions of sensitized erythrocytes are prepared by using hemagglutination concentrations 2, 4, and 8 times lower than those used in the Waaler-Rose reaction (this is the first subagglutinating concentration for sensitization).

TITRATION OF RABBIT ANTI-HUMAN RED CELL ANTIBODY AMBOCEPTOR
1. Prepare progressive dilutions of amboceptor in physiologic saline solution 1:100 to 1:1,000.
2. Pipette 0.2 ml from each dilution in a row of 10 test tubes.
3. Add 0.2 ml 1% human O Rh− red cell suspension to each tube.
4. Place the tubes in a water bath and let stand at 37° C for 1 hour.
5. Transfer the tubes to a refrigerator and leave overnight (18 hours).
6. The basal agglutination titer is the highest amboceptor dilution showing agglutination.

SENSITIZATION OF HUMAN O RH− RED CELLS
1. Mix equal volumes of amboceptor and 1% red cells in various dilutions. Use 1:4, 1:8, 1:16, and 1:32 dilutions of basal agglutinating dose determined in amboceptor titration.
2. With occasional shaking allow mixtures to stand at room temperature for 1 hour before use.

READING OF RESULTS [31].   Invert each tube 6 times to resuspend the cells. Inspect the tubes with the naked eye against the light of an electric bulb for the presence of sedimented agglutination.
(+) = positive

($\pm$) = partial
  0 = negative

The different cell suspensions are tested against positive serum and negative serum controls to determine proper rabbit antibody dilution to sensitize the red cells. A fresh suspension of sensitized erythrocytes should be prepared on each day of testing.

TEST PROCEDURE
1. Mix in test tube 0.5 ml lymphocyte suspension (4 $\times$ 10^6 cells) with 0.2 ml 1% suspension of sensitized cells and 0.3 ml Hanks' BSS.
2. The mixture is centrifuged for 5 min at 200 g at room temperature and then resuspended by gentle agitation for 10 min (vertical rotation at 10 rpm).
3. The hemocytometer chamber is filled with an aliquot of the suspension.
4. Lymphocytes and rosettes are counted separately. Two chambers are read for each test, and results are expressed as the number of rosettes/1,000 lymphocytes. A rosette is identified as an agglutination of more than 4 erythrocytes around a lymphocyte.
5. Positive and negative controls should be incubated in each analysis.

RESULTS
Normal subjects: 0–6 rosettes/1,000 lymphocytes
Positive: more than 6 rosettes/1,000 lymphocytes

A positive rosette test was more frequent in cases of rheumatoid arthritis of recent onset than in those of long-standing disease. The rosette test did not correlate with serum levels of rheumatoid factor. The rosette test in combination with a serum agglutination test for rheumatoid factor will be positive in more than 90% of the cases of rheumatoid arthritis [7].

References

1. Abraham, G. N., Clark, R. A., Kacaki, J., and Vaughan, J. H.   The character and specificity of an IgA rheumatoid factor. *Arthritis Rheum.* 13:300, 1970.
2. Abraham, G. N., Clark, R. A., and Vaughan, J. H.   Characterization of an IgA rheumatoid factor: Binding properties and reactivity with the subclasses of human γG globulin. *Immunochemistry* 9:301, 1972.
3. Adachi, M., Atsumi, T., Saito, N., Nakamura, M., and Horiuchi, Y. Detection of IgA and IgG rheumatoid factors by antiglobulin augmentation technique. *Int. Arch. Allergy Appl. Immunol.* 35:77, 1969.
4. Agnello, V., Koffler, D., Eisenberg, J. W., Winchester, R. J., and Kunkel, H. G.   C1q precipitins in the sera of patients with systemic lupus erythematosus and other hypocomplementemic states: Char-

acterization of high and low molecular weight types. *J. Exp. Med.* 134: 228s, 1971.

5. Anderson, S. G., Bentzon, M. W., Houba, V., and Krage, B.   International reference preparation of rheumatoid arthritis serum. *Bull. WHO* 42:311, 1970.

6. Ansell, B. M., Holborow, J. H., Zutski, D. E., and Reading, A.   Comparison of three serological tests in adult rheumatoid arthritis and Still's disease (juvenile rheumatoid arthritis). *Ann. N.Y. Acad. Sci.* 168:21, 1969.

7. Bach, J. F., Delrieu, F., and Delbarre, F.   The rheumatoid rosette: A diagnostic test unifying seropositive and seronegative rheumatoid arthritis. *Am. J. Med.* 49:215, 1970.

8. Bagratuni, L.   Prognosis in the anarthritic rheumatoid syndrome. *Br. Med. J.* 1:513, 1963.

9. Ball, J., DeGraaff, R., Falkenburg, H. A., and Westenborp Boerma, F.   Comparative studies of serologic tests for rheumatoid disease. I. A comparison of a latex test and two erythrocyte agglutination tests in a random population sample. *Arthritis Rheum.* 5:55, 1962.

10. Barnett, E. V., Winkelstein, A., and Weinberger, H.   Agammaglobulinemia with polyarthritis and subcutaneous nodules. *Am. J. Med.* 48: 40, 1970.

11. Barnett, E. V., Bluestone, R., Cracchiolo, A., Goldberg, L. S., Kantor, G. L., and McIntosh, R. M.   Cryoglobulinemia and disease. *Ann. Intern. Med.* 73:95, 1970.

12. Batson, O. V.   The function of the vertebral veins and their role in the spread of metastases. *Ann. Surg.* 112:138, 1940.

13. Berry, H., Bacon, P. A., and Davis, J. D.   Cell mediated immunity in Sjögren's syndrome. *Ann. Rheum. Dis.* 31:298, 1972.

14. Bianco, N. E., Panush, R. S., Stillman, S., and Schur, P. H.   Immunologic studies of juvenile rheumatoid arthritis. *Arthritis Rheum.* 14:685, 1971.

15. Bienenstock, J., Goldstein, G., and Tomasi, T. B.   Urinary γA rheumatoid factor. *J. Lab. Clin. Med.* 73:389, 1969.

16. Block, K. J., Buchanan, W. W., Wohl, M. J., and Bunim, J. J.   Sjögren's syndrome. A clinical, pathological, and serological study of sixty-two cases. *Medicine* (Baltimore) 44:187, 1965.

17. Bluestone, R., Goldberg, L. S., Katz, R. M., Marchesano, J. M., and Calabro, J. J.   Juvenile rheumatoid arthritis: A serologic survey of 200 consecutive patients. *J. Pediatr.* 77:98, 1970.

18. Bluestone, R., Gumpel, J. M., Goldberg, L. S., and Holborow, E. J.   Salivary immunoglobulins in Sjögren's syndrome. *Int. Arch. Allergy Appl. Immunol.* 42:686, 1972.

19. Boyle, J. A., and Buchanan, W. W. *Clinical Rheumatology.* Philadelphia: Davis, 1971.

20. Bozicevich, J., Bunim, J. J., Ward, S. B., and Freund, J.   Appendixes: III Serologic Techniques. In J. H. Kellgren, M. R. Jeffrey, and J. Ball (eds.), *The Epidemiology of Chronic Rheumatism.* Philadelphia: Davis, 1963, p. 399.

21. Brewer, E. J., Jr. *Juvenile Rheumatoid Arthritis.* Philadelphia: Saunders, 1970.

22. Britton, M. C., and Schur, P. H.   The complement system in rheumatoid synovitis. II. Intracytoplasmic inclusions of immunoglobulins and complement. *Arthritis Rheum.* 14:87, 1971.
23. Broder, I., Urowitz, M. B., and Gordon, D. A.   Appraisal of rheumatoid arthritis as an immune complex disease. *Med. Clin. North Am.* 56:529, 1972.
24. Brooke, M. H., and Kaplan, H.   Muscle pathology in rheumatoid arthritis, polymyalgia rheumatica and polymyositis. *Arch. Pathol.* 94:101, 1972.
25. Burry, H. C.   Reduced glomerular function in rheumatic disease. *Ann. Rheum. Dis.* 31:65, 1972.
26. Bywaters, E. G. L., Carter, M. E., and Scott, F. E. T.   Differential agglutination titer (DAT) in juvenile rheumatoid arthritis. *Ann. Rheum. Dis.* 18:225, 1959.
27. Bywaters, E. G. L.   Vasculitis and rheumatoid nodule. In J. J. R. Duthie and W. R. M. Alexander (eds.), *Rheumatic Diseases.* Baltimore: Williams & Wilkins, 1968.
28. Calabro, J. J., and Marchesano, J. M.   Juvenile rheumatoid arthritis. *N. Engl. J. Med.* 277:696, 1967.
29. Capra, D. B., Winchester, R. J., and Kunkel, H. G.   Cold reactive rheumatoid factors in infectious mononucleosis and other diseases. *Arthritis Rheum.* 12:67, 1969.
30. Cathcart, E. S., and O'Sullivan, J. B.   Standardization of sheep cell agglutination test. The use of pooled reference sera and hemagglutination trays. *Arthritis Rheum.* 8:530, 1965.
31. Cathcart, E. S.   Rheumatoid factors. 13. Serologic techniques. In A. S. Cohen (ed.), *Laboratory Diagnostic Procedures in the Rheumatic Diseases.* Boston: Little, Brown, 1967.
32. Cats, A., and Klein, R.   Quantitative aspects of the latex fixation and Waaler-Rose test. *Ann. Rheum. Dis.* 29:663, 1970.
33. Chayen, J., and Bitensky, L.   Lysosomal enzymes and inflammation with particular reference to rheumatoid disease. *Ann. Rheum. Dis.* 30:522, 1970.
34. Cheng, C. T., and Persellin, R. H.   Interference by C1q in slide latex test for rheumatoid factor. *Ann. Intern. Med.* 75:683, 1971.
35. Chodirker, W. B., and Tomasi, T. B.   Low molecular weight rheumatoid factor. *J. Clin. Invest.* 42:876, 1963.
36. Christian, C. L.   Rheumatoid arthritis. In M. Samter (ed.), *Immunologic Diseases.* Boston: Little, Brown, 1971, p. 1014.
37. Cohen, A. S.   *Laboratory Diagnostic Procedures in the Rheumatic Diseases.* Boston: Little, Brown, 1967.
38. Cohen, E., Nisonoff, A., Hermes, P., Norcross, B. M., and Lockie, L. M.   Agglutination of sensitized alligator erythrocytes by rheumatoid factor(s). *Nature* 190:552, 1961.
39. Cracchiolo, A., III, and Goldberg, L. S.   Elution of antiglobulins and antinuclear antibody from rheumatoid synovial membranes. *Ann. Rheum. Dis.* 31:186, 1972.
40. Cummings, N. A.   Oral manifestations of connective tissue disease. *Postgrad. Med.* 49:134, 1971.
41. Cummings, N. A., Schall, G. L., Asofsky, R., Anderson, L. G., and

Talal, N.   Sjögren's syndrome—newer aspects of research, diagnosis, and treatment. *Ann. Intern. Med.* 75:937, 1971.
42. Dequeker, J., Van Noyen, R., and Vandipitte, J.   Age related rheumatoid factors: Incidence and characteristics. *Ann. Rheum. Dis.* 28:431, 1969.
43. Dickler, H. B., and Kunkel, H. G.   Interaction of aggregated γ-globulin with B-lymphocytes. *J. Exp. Med.* 136:191, 1972.
44. Elling, P., Graudal, H., and Faber, V.   Granulocyte specific antinuclear factors in serum and synovial fluid in rheumatoid arthritis. *Ann. Rheum. Dis.* 27:225, 1968.
45. Epstein, W. B., and Engleman, E. T.   The relation of rheumatoid factor content of serum to clinical neurovascular manifestations of rheumatoid arthritis. *Arthritis Rheum.* 2:250, 1959.
46. Feltkamp, T. E., and Van Rossum, A. L.   Antibodies to salivary duct cells, and other autoantibodies in patients with Sjögren's syndrome and other idiopathic autoimmune diseases. *Clin. Exp. Immunol.* 3:1, 1968.
47. Ferguson, R. H., and Worthington, J. W.   Recent advances in rheumatic diseases: 1967 through 1969. *Ann. Intern. Med.* 73:109, 1970.
48. Fischel, E. C.   The C-reactive protein. In A. S. Cohen (ed.), *Laboratory Diagnostic Procedures in the Rheumatic Diseases.* Boston: Little, Brown, 1967, p. 3.
49. Franchimont, P., and Suteanu, S.   Radioimmunoassay of rheumatoid factor. *Arthritis Rheum.* 12:483, 1969.
50. Franklin, E. C., Holman, H. R., Müller-Eberhard, H. J., and Kunkel, H. G.   An unusual protein component of high molecular weight in the serum of certain patients with rheumatoid arthritis. *J. Exp. Med.* 105:425, 1957.
51. Freyberg, R. H.   Differential diagnosis of rheumatoid arthritis. *Postgrad. Med.* 51:20, 1972.
52. Glynn, L. E.   Pathology, pathogenesis, and aetiology of rheumatoid arthritis. Occasional Survey, Roy Cameron Lecture, 1971. *Ann. Rheum. Dis.* 31:412, 1972.
53. Good, R. A., and Rotstein, J.   Rheumatoid arthritis in agammaglobulinemia. *Bull. Rheum. Dis.* 10:203, 1960.
54. Goodman, M. A., and Pearson, C. M.   Polymyalgia rheumatica and associated arteritis: A review. *Calif. Med.* 111:453, 1969.
55. Grayzel, A. I., and Beck, C.   Rubella infection of synovial cells and the resistance of cells derived from patients with rheumatoid arthritis. *J. Exp. Med.* 131:367, 1970.
56. Grubb, R., and Laurell, A. B.   Hereditary serological human serum groups. *Acta Pathol. Microbiol. Scand.* 39:390, 1956.
57. Healey, L. A., Parker, F., and Wilske, K. R.   Polymyalgia rheumatica and giant cell arteritis. *Arthritis Rheum.* 14:138, 1970.
58. Heimer, R., and Levin, F. M.   On the distribution of rheumatoid factors among immunoglobulins. *Immunochemistry* 3:1, 1966.
59. Heller, G., Jacobson, A. S., Kolodny, M. H., and Kammer, W. H.   The hemagglutination test for rheumatoid arthritis. II. The influence of human plasma fraction II (gamma globulin) on the reaction. *J. Immunol.* 72:66, 1954.
60. Hill, A. G. S.   Diagnostic and prognostic significance of the rheuma-

toid factor. In J. J. R. Duthie and W. R. M. Alexander (eds.), *Rheumatic Diseases*. Baltimore: Williams & Wilkins, 1968.
61. Hollander, J. L., McCarty, D. J., Astorga, G., and Murillo, E. C. Studies on the pathogenesis of rheumatoid joint inflammation. I. The R.A. cell and a working hypothesis. *Ann. Intern. Med.* 62:271, 1965.
62. Hollingsworth, J. W. *Local and Systemic Complications of Rheumatoid Arthritis*. Philadelphia: Saunders, 1968.
63. Hunder, G. G., Disney, T. F., and Ward, L. E. Polymyalgia rheumatica. *Mayo Clin. Proc.* 44:849, 1969.
64. Janeff, J. A new slide test for rheumatoid arthritis: Comparison with Waaler-Rose and latex slide tests. *Arthritis Rheum.* 13:193, 1970.
65. Jondal, M., Holm, G., and Wigzell, H. Surface markers on human T and B lymphocytes. I. A large population of lymphocyte forming non-immune rosettes with sheep cells. *J. Exp. Med.* 136:207, 1972.
66. Kunkel, H. G. The structure of rheumatoid factors. *Arthritis Rheum.* 6:414, 1963.
67. Laaksonen, A. L. A prognostic study of juvenile rheumatoid arthritis: Analysis of 544 cases. *Acta Paediatr. Scand.* 166 (Suppl.), 1966.
68. Lea, D. J., and Ward, D. J. A comparison of latex test for rheumatoid factors. *Ann. Rheum. Dis.* 31:132, 1972.
69. Lea, D. J., and Ward, D. J. Rosette formation by circulating lymphocytes from rheumatoid and nonrheumatoid subjects. *Ann. Rheum. Dis.* 31:183, 1972.
70. Leventhal, B. G., Waldorf, D. S., and Talal, M. Impaired lymphocyte transformation and delayed sensitivity in Sjögren's syndrome. *J. Clin. Invest.* 46:1338, 1967.
71. Levinson, J. E. Juvenile rheumatoid arthritis. *Postgrad. Med.* 51:88, 1972.
72. Liddle, L., Seigmiller, J. E., and Laster, L. The enzymatic spectrophotometric method for determination of uric acid. *J. Lab. Clin. Med.* 54:903, 1959.
73. MacSween, R. H. M., Dalakos, T. G., Jasani, M. K., Boyle, J. A., Buchanan, W. W., and Goudie, R. B. A clinicoimmunologic study of serum and synovial fluid antinuclear factors in rheumatoid arthritis and other arthritis. *Clin. Exp. Immunol.* 3:17, 1968.
74. Mansson, I., Norberg, R., Olhagen, B., and Björklund, N. E. Arthritis in pigs induced by dietary factors. *Clin. Exp. Immunol.* 9:677, 1971.
75. Marcus, R. L., and Townes, A. S. The occurrence of cryoproteins in synovial fluid, the association of a complement fixing activity in rheumatoid synovial fluid with cold precipitable protein. *J. Clin. Invest.* 50:282, 1971.
76. Martel, W., Abell, M. R., Mikkelsen, W. M., and Whitehouse, W. M. Pulmonary and pleural lesions in rheumatic disease. *Radiology* 90:641, 1968.
77. McLaughlin, J. F., Schaller, J., and Wedgwood, R. J. Arthritis and immunodeficiency. *J. Pediatr.* 81:801, 1972.
78. Mellbye, O. J., and Munthe, E. Specific binding of immunoconglutinin in tissue and synovial fluid from patients with rheumatoid arthritis. *Clin. Exp. Immunol.* 8:713, 1971.
79. Mellbye, O. J., and Natvig, J. B. Evidence for immune complexes

containing antibody to the pepsin site of IgG in rheumatoid synovial fluids. *Clin. Exp. Immunol.* 8:889, 1971.
80. Morgan, W. S., and Castleman, B.   A clinicopathological study of "Mikulicz's disease." *Am. J. Pathol.* 29:471, 1953.
81. Nakamura, R. M., Magsaysay, R., Ford, J., and Kunitake, G.   Significant variations in commercial C-reactive protein antiserums. *Am. J. Clin. Pathol.* 44:290, 1965.
82. Nies, A. S., and Melmon, K. L.   Kinins and arthritis. *Bull. Rheum. Dis.* 19:512, 1968.
83. Notkins, A. L.   Infectious virus-antibody complexes: Interaction with anti-immunoglobulin, complement and rheumatoid factor. *J. Exp. Med.* 134:41s, 1971.
84. Panush, R. S., Bianco, N. E., and Schur, P. H.   Serum and synovial fluid IgG, IgA, and IgM antiglobulins in rheumatoid arthritis. *Arthritis Rheum.* 14:737, 1971.
85. Panush, R. S., Franco, A. E., and Schur, P. H.   Rheumatoid arthritis associated with eosinophilia. *Ann. Intern. Med.* 75:199, 1971.
86. Peltier, A. P., Atra, E., and Haim, T.   Detection of serum rheumatoid factor by immunofluorescence (IF). *Arthritis Rheum.* 14:179, 1971.
87. Phillips, P. E.   Virologic studies in rheumatoid arthritis and other connective tissue diseases. *J. Exp. Med.* 134:313s, 1971.
88. Plotz, C. M., and Spiera, H.   Polymyalgia rheumatica. *Bull. Rheum. Dis.* 10:578, 1969.
89. Roberts, W. C., Kehoe, J. A., Carpenter, D. F., and Golden, A.   Cardiac valvular lesions in rheumatoid arthritis. *Arch. Intern. Med.* 122:141, 1968.
90. Roitt, I. M.   Immunological phenomena in rheumatoid arthritis. In B. Amos (ed.), *Progress in Immunology.* 1st International Congress of Immunology. New York and London: Academic Press, 1971, p. 689.
91. Ropes, M. W., Bennett, G. A., Cobb, S., Jacox, R. F., and Jessar, R. A.   Proposed diagnostic criteria for rheumatoid arthritis. *Bull. Rheum. Dis.* 7:121, 1956.
92. Ropes, M. W., Bennett, G. A., Cobb, S., Jacox, R. F., and Jessar, R. A.   Proposed diagnostic criteria for rheumatoid arthritis. *Bull. Rheum. Dis.* 9:175, 1958.
93. Rose, H. M., Ragan, C., Pearce, E., and Lipman, M. O.   Differential agglutination of normal and sensitized sheep erythrocytes by sera of patients with rheumatoid arthritis. *Proc. Soc. Exp. Biol. Med.* 68:1, 1948.
94. Rothfield, N. F.   Diagnosis of lupus erythematosus and rheumatoid arthritis in children. *Pediatr. Clin. North Am.* 18:39, 1971.
95. Ruddy, S., and Austen, K. F.   The complement system in rheumatoid synovitis. I. An analysis of complement components active in rheumatoid synovial fluids. *Arthritis Rheum.* 13:713, 1970.
96. Schall, G. L., Anderson, L. G., Wolf, R. O., Herdt, J. R., and Tarpley, T. M., Jr.   Xerostomia in Sjögren's. Evaluation by sequential salivary scintigraphy. *J.A.M.A.* 216:2109, 1971.
97. Schur, P. H., and Franco, A. E.   Hypocomplementemia in rheumatoid arthritis. *Arthritis Rheum.* 14:231, 1971.
98. Schur, P. H., and Austen, K. F.   Complement in rheumatic diseases. *Bull. Rheum. Dis.* 22:666, 1971–72.

99. Sharp, J. T., Calkins, E., Cohen, A. S., Schubart, A. F., and Calabro, J. J. Observations on the clinical, chemical, and serological manifestations of rheumatoid arthritis, based on the course of 154 cases. *Medicine* 43:41, 1964.
100. Singer, J. M., and Plotz, C. M. The latex fixation test. I. Application to the serologic diagnosis of rheumatoid arthritis. *Am. J. Med.* 21:888, 1956.
101. Singer, J. M., Plotz, C. M., and Goldberg, R. The detection of antiglobulin factors utilizing precoated latex particles. *Arthritis Rheum.* 8:194, 1965.
102. Sjögren, H. Zur Kenntnis der Keratoconjunctivitis sicca (Keratitis filiformis bei Hypofunktion der Tränendrüsen). *Acta Ophthalmol.* (Kbh) 11:1, 1933.
103. Sliwinski, A. J., and Zvaifler, N. J. In vivo synthesis of IgG by the rheumatoid synovial membrane. *J. Lab. Clin. Med.* 76:304, 1970.
104. Smith, L. H., Watts, D., and Shearn, M. A. Clinical Spectrum of Sjögren's Syndrome. Medical Staff Conference, University of California at San Francisco. *Calif. Med.* 117:63, 1972.
105. Stage, D. E., and Mannik, M. 7S γM globulins in rheumatoid arthritis. *Arthritis Rheum.* 14:440, 1971.
106. Stevens, R. W., Stroebel, E., and Gaafer, H. An automated test for rheumatoid factor. *Arthritis Rheum.* 13:257, 1970.
107. Stobo, J. D., and Tomasi, T. B., Jr. A low molecular weight immunoglobulin antigenically related to 19S IgM. *J. Clin. Invest.* 46:1329, 1967.
108. Stollerman, G. H. Streptococcal antibodies in the diagnosis of rheumatoid fever. In A. S. Cohen (ed.), *Laboratory Diagnostic Procedures in the Rheumatic Diseases.* Boston: Little, Brown, 1967.
109. Talal, M., and Bumin, J. J. The development of malignant lymphoma in the course of Sjögren's syndrome. *Am. J. Med.* 36:529, 1964.
110. Talal, M., Sokoloff, L., and Barth, W. F. Extra salivary lymphoid abnormalities in Sjögren's syndrome. (Reticulum cell sarcoma, "pseudolymphoma," macroglobulinemia). *Am. J. Med.* 43:50, 1967.
111. Talal, M., Zisman, E., and Schur, P. H. Renal tubular acidosis, glomerulonephritis, and immunologic factors in Sjögren's syndrome. *Arthritis Rheum.* 11:774, 1968.
112. Tomasi, T. B., and Zigelbaum, S. D. The selective occurrence of γ1A globulins in certain body fluids. *J. Clin. Invest.* 42:1552, 1963.
113. Torrigiani, G., and Roitt, I. M. Antiglobulin factors in sera from patients with rheumatoid arthritis and normal subjects. Quantitative estimation of indifferent immunoglobulin classes. *Ann. Rheum. Dis.* 26:334, 1967.
114. Torrigiani, G., Ansell, B. M., Chown, E. E. A., and Roitt, I. M. Raised IgG antiglobulin factors in Still's disease. *Ann. Rheum. Dis.* 28:424, 1969.
115. Torrigiani, G., Roitt, I. M., Lloyd, K. N., and Corbett, M. Elevated IgG antiglobulins in patients with seronegative rheumatoid arthritis. *Lancet* 1:14, 1970.
116. van Bijsterveld, O. P. Diagnostic tests in the sicca syndrome. *Arch. Ophthalmol.* 82:10, 1969.

117. Vaughan, J. H.   Serum responses in rheumatoid arthritis. *Am. J. Med.* 26:596, 1959.
118. Vaughan, J. H., Jacox, R. F., and Noell, P.   Relation of intracytoplasmic inclusions in joint fluid leucocytes to antigammaglobulins. *Arthritis Rheum.* 11:135, 1968.
119. Waaler, E., and Milde, E. J.   Is there a relationship between giant cell arteritis with polymyalgia rheumatica and rheumatoid arthritis? *Acta Pathol. Microbiol. Scand.* 72:347, 1968.
120. Waaler, E.   On the occurrence of a factor in human serum activating the specific agglutination of sheep blood corpuscles. *Acta Pathol. Microbiol. Scand.* 17:172, 1940.
121. Waller, M. V., and Vaughan, J. H.   Use of anti-Rh sera for demonstrating agglutination activating factor in rheumatoid arthritis. *Proc. Soc. Exp. Biol. Med.* 92:198, 1956.
122. Waller, M., and Blaylock, K.   Further studies on the antiglobulin factors in human serum to the pepsin digested fragments of the Ri anti Rh antibody. *J. Immunol.* 97:438, 1966.
123. Waller, M., Curry, M., and Mallory, J.   Immunochemical and serological studies of enzymatically fractionated human IgG globulins. I. Hydrolysis with pepsin, papain, ficin, and bromelin. *Immunochemistry* 5:577, 1968.
124. Waller, M.   Methods of measurement of rheumatoid factor. *Ann. N.Y. Acad. Sci.* 168:5, 1969.
125. Waller, M., Duma, R. J., Farley, E. D., and Atkinson, J.   The influence of infection on titers of antiglobulin antibodies. *Clin. Exp. Immunol.* 8:451, 1971.
126. Wasmuth, A. G., Veale, A. M. O., Palmer, D. G., and Highton, T. C.   Prevalence of rheumatoid arthritis in families. *Ann. Rheum. Dis.* 31:85, 1972.
127. Whaley, K., Chisolm, D. M., Goudie, R. B., Downie, W. W., Dick, W. C., Boyle, J. A., and Williamson, J.   Salivary duct autoantibody in Sjögren's syndrome: Correlation with sialadenitis in the labial mucosa. *Clin. Exp. Immunol.* 4:273, 1969.
128. Whaley, K., and Buchanan, W. W.   Clinical aspects of autoimmunity. *Triangle* 9:61, 1969.
129. Whaley, K., Glen, A. C. A., MacSween, R. N. M., Deodhar, S., Dick, W. C., Nuki, G., Williamson, J., and Buchanan, W. W.   Immunological responses in Sjögren's syndrome and rheumatoid arthritis. *Clin. Exp. Immunol.* 9:721, 1971.
130. Winchester, R. J., Agnello, V., and Kunkel, H. G.   Gamma globulin complexes of synovial fluids of patients with rheumatoid arthritis: Partial characterization and relationship to lowered complement levels. *Clin. Exp. Immunol.* 6:689, 1970.
131. Winchester, R. J., Kunkel, H. G., and Agnello, V.   Occurrence of γ-globulin complexes in serum and joint fluid of rheumatoid arthritis patients: Use of monoclonal rheumatoid factors as reagents for their demonstration. *J. Exp. Med.* 134:286s, 1971.
132. Winchester, R. J., Litwin, S. D., Koffler, D., and Kunkel, H. G.   Observations in the eosinophilia of certain patients with rheumatoid arthritis. *Arthritis Rheum.* 14:650, 1971.
133. Wybran, J., Carr, M. C., and Fudenberg, H. H.   The human rosette

forming cell as a marker of a population of thymus derived cells. *J. Clin. Invest.* 51:2537, 1972.

134. Ziff, M., Brown, P., Lospalluto, J., Badin, J., and McEwen, C. Agglutination and inhibition by serum globulin in the sensitized sheep cell agglutination reaction in rheumatoid arthritis. *Am. J. Med.* 20:500, 1956.

135. Ziff, M. Summary of immunology of rheumatoid arthritis. In J. J. R. Duthie and W. R. M. Alexander (eds.), *Rheumatic Diseases.* Baltimore: Williams & Wilkins, 1968.

136. Ziff, M. Arthritis associated with systemic disease. *Postgrad. Med.* 51:99, 1972.

137. Zvaifler, N. J. Further speculation on the pathogenesis of joint inflammation in rheumatoid arthritis. *Arthritis Rheum.* 13:895, 1970.

138. Zvaifler, N. J., and Martinez, N. M. Antinuclear factors in synovial fluid leucocytes. *Clin. Exp. Immunol.* 8:271, 1971.

139. Zvaifler, N. J. Immunoreactants in rheumatic synovial effusions. *J. Exp. Med.* 134:276s, 1971.

III

Transplantation and Tumor Immunology

17

Transplantation Immunology

Stephan E. Ritzmann, Theona M. Vyvial,
Jerry C. Daniels, Courtney M. Townsend, Jr., and
Gerald A. Beathard

The historic blood transfusion of Pope Innocent VIII in 1491 [164] (Figure 17-1) ushered in the eras of transfusion and, more recently, organ transplantation. This event dramatized the triad of problems—ethical, technical, and immunologic—confronting the physician engaged in blood transfusions and organ transplantation. Presently, more than 4.5 million blood transfusions are administered annually in the United States. Additionally, since the first renal allotransplantation was performed about 20 years ago, more than 12,500 kidney, 200 heart, 180 liver, 120 bone marrow, 30 lung, and 30 pancreas and intestine transplants have been carried out throughout the world [1, 2, 62, 110].

The immunologic factors which facilitate successful blood transfusions and organ transplantations are threefold: appropriate donor selection, effective immunosuppression, and induction of immunologic tolerance. The immunologic aspects of donor selection for organ transplantation are essential for allograft acceptance. The well-known fact that grafts from identical twins are not subject to immunologic rejection emphasizes the importance of tissue compatibility. With each step away from this immunogenetic identity (i.e., from the closest, the related individuals with genetic identity, progressing to the most removed, the genetically unrelated donors), there is a "quantum jump" in tissue incompatibility, and rejection episodes occur in an increasing percentage of cases with these expanding genetic differences. This widening gap between organ acceptance and rejection, paralleling the increasing immunogenetic disparity, can partly but not entirely be explained by the role of certain ubiquitous antigens, including the ABO blood groups, HL–A tissue antigens, and mixed lymphocyte culture (MLC) antigenic determinants.

Histocompatibility Antigens

The factors thus far identified which are known to be responsible for histocompatibility are the ABO blood group antigens, the HL–A system antigens, and the MLC determinants.

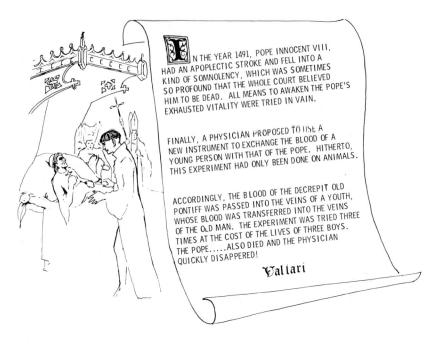

IN THE YEAR 1491, POPE INNOCENT VIII, HAD AN APOPLECTIC STROKE AND FELL INTO A KIND OF SOMNOLENCY, WHICH WAS SOMETIMES SO PROFOUND THAT THE WHOLE COURT BELIEVED HIM TO BE DEAD. ALL MEANS TO AWAKEN THE POPE'S EXHAUSTED VITALITY WERE TRIED IN VAIN.

FINALLY, A PHYSICIAN PROPOSED TO USE A NEW INSTRUMENT TO EXCHANGE THE BLOOD OF A YOUNG PERSON WITH THAT OF THE POPE. HITHERTO, THIS EXPERIMENT HAD ONLY BEEN DONE ON ANIMALS.

ACCORDINGLY, THE BLOOD OF THE DECREPIT OLD PONTIFF WAS PASSED INTO THE VEINS OF A YOUTH, WHOSE BLOOD WAS TRANSFERRED INTO THE VEINS OF THE OLD MAN. THE EXPERIMENT WAS TRIED THREE TIMES AT THE COST OF THE LIVES OF THREE BOYS. THE POPE.....ALSO DIED AND THE PHYSICIAN QUICKLY DISAPPEARED!

Vallari

Figure 17-1
An artist's conception of the first recorded blood transfusion. (Reproduced from Ritzmann and Daniels [118].)

The *ABO blood group antigens* are ubiquitous antigens present on erythrocytes and practically all tissues, with the exception of lymphocytes and, possibly, the brain and spinal cord [141]. Currently, more than 10 major blood group systems are known, in addition to the ABO and Rh systems. These include the common "public" blood groups (e.g., I, Vel, etc.) and the very rare "private" blood groups (see Table 17-1). Incompatibility at the ABO group loci poses a threat of hyperacute rejection [133]; therefore, ABO incompatibility must be avoided in organ transplantation.

The *HL–A system* (also termed histocompatibility locus-A [12]), human leukocyte antigens, or lymphocyte A-system (human leukocyte locus-A [33]), consists of widely distributed antigenic determinants [158], representing the transplantation antigens in the strict sense of the term. HL–A antigens are present on all tissues with the exception of erythrocytes and, possibly, the brain and spinal cord. Presently, more than 20 HL–A antigens have been generally accepted, and at least 20 additional proposed antigens are now under investigation. The HL–A antigens are controlled by a complex genetic locus (i.e., positions on a chromosome occupied by a gene), with two "segregant series" of anti-

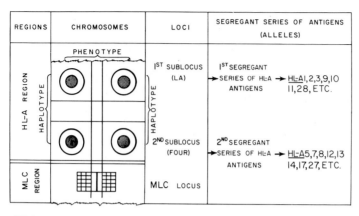

REGIONS	CHROMOSOMES	LOCI	SEGREGANT SERIES OF ANTIGENS (ALLELES)
HL-A REGION — HAPLOTYPE (PHENOTYPE)		1ST SUBLOCUS (LA)	1ST SEGREGANT SERIES OF HL-A ANTIGENS → HL-A1,2,3,9,10 11,28,ETC.
		2ND SUBLOCUS (FOUR)	2ND SEGREGANT SERIES OF HL-A ANTIGENS → HL-A5,7,8,12,13 14,17,27,ETC.
MLC REGION		MLC LOCUS	

Figure 17-2
Diagrammatic representation of the histocompatibility complex (HL–A and MLC regions). Relationships between components within the histocompatibility complex are as follows: *regions* refer to specific sites on chromosomes; *locus*: position on a chromosome occupied by a gene; *sublocus*: specific portion of a gene; in the case of HL–A, either the first or second segregant alleles; *segregant series*: allelic groups representing constellations of genetic characteristics at one of the two known HL–A subloci; *allele*: alternative form of a series of genetic units which can occupy a single locus or sublocus on either of a pair of homologous chromosomes; *haplotype*: two HL–A antigens of an individual, one each from the first and second sublocus; *phenotype*: sum of the individual's two haplotypes; *genotype*: physical expression of the phenotype; in the case of HL–A typing, defined by the phenotype derived from each parent and demonstrated by the typing procedure.

gens (i.e., mutually exclusive subsets), which are termed the first (LA) and second (Four) series (see Fig. 17-2). The HL–A antigen system is the most complex immunogenetic system thus far identified in man.

The *mixed lymphocyte culture (MLC) reaction* may reflect yet other histocompatibility antigens which are important for the immunological selection of donors in clinical allotransplantation. The MLC antigenic sites are controlled by genetic loci which appear to be distinct from those controlling the ABO, Rh, and HL–A loci [16, 27].

The ABO System
The numerous blood group antigens (Table 17-1) are regulated by several genetic loci. However, only two of these loci, those of the ABO and Rh blood group systems, play a major role in blood transfusion reactions or in maternal-fetal reactions (neonatal hemolytic disease). Of these antigenic systems, only the ABO system is of major importance in organ allotransplantation [48, 136].

Table 17-1. Blood Group Systems and Antigens.

Systems	Antigens
ABO	A_1, A_2; B; O (H)
Rh	C, c; D, d; E, e
P	P_1, P_2
I	I, i
MN	M, N
Ss	S, s
Kell	K, k
Lewis	Le[a], Le[b]
Duffy	Fy[a], Fy[b]
Kidd	Jk[a], Jk[b]
Lutheran	Lu[a], Lu[b]
Xg	Xg[a] (sex linked)

Unfortunately, the nomenclature of the blood group systems is confusing. Allelic antigens may be designated by different letters (A and B; M and N), or capital and lower-case letters (S and s; K and k; D and d), by symbols with superscripts (Lu[a] and Lu[b]; Fy[a] and Fy[b]; Jk[a] and Jk[b]), or by symbols with subscripts (A_1, A_2; P_1, P_2).

ABO ANTIGENS.   There are four major ABO phenotypes, termed the O (or H), A, B, and AB types (Table 17-2 [171]). There are also numerous subgroups of the ABO system (e.g., A_1, A_1B, etc.), but these subgroups do not appear to play a significant role in organ allotransplantation [6, 26, 32].

BIOCHEMISTRY OF ABO BLOOD GROUP SUBSTANCES.   The ABO blood group substances of erythrocytes are similar chemically; they consist of glycolipids (liposaccharides) which differ from each other mainly in the nature of the terminal sugar on their molecules (see Table 17-3).

The synthesis of ABO (H) and Lewis (Le) blood group substances results probably from the sequential action of the products of different blood group genes on a common precursor glycoprotein ("primitive substance"), leading to three-dimensional patterns of sugar residues which are responsible for the serologic specificities of such molecular species [73, 141, 142]. The "common precursor" theory suggests that the specificity of the blood group substances resides primarily in the terminal sugar residues of the macromolecules. The allelic ABO blood group genes appear to operate by producing enzymes which modify a common precursor substance into their respective "gene products" [143]. In vitro enzymatic degradation of A and B blood group substances yields H, Le, and Le[a] substances and a polysaccharide resembling a type XIV pneu-

Table 17-2. ABO Blood Group Systems.

Phenotypes: ABO Blood Groups	Genotypes	% Distribution in U.S. Population	Antigens on Red Blood Cells (Agglutinogens)	Antibodies in Serum (Isoagglutinins)
O	OO	44	H ("none")	Anti-A(α) and Anti-B(β)
A	AA AO	42	A	Anti-B(β)
B	BB BO	10	B	Anti-A(α)
AB	AB	4	A and B	none

mococcal substance [170], reflecting a gradual alteration of the sugar moieties from the pneumococcal type XIV "core" substance to H substance to Le substance to A blood group substance, and, finally, to B blood group substance.

ANTI-A AND ANTI-B ISOHEMAGGLUTININS.   The O gene is thought to reflect an inactive gene, allelic to the A and B genes, which regulates the enzymes converting a glycolipid (H substance) into similar glycolipids (A and B substances) (Table 17-3). Since persons of the genotype AB cannot have an O gene, the substance on group O cells detectable by "anti-O" reagents is not a direct product of the O gene; therefore, this substance was termed H substance [91]. H substance is present on almost all *human* erythrocytes and serves as a substrate for the production of A and B antigens under the control of the A and B genes.[1] Since A and B substances are widespread in nature (including ABO-like substances present in food and various other exogenous sources), constant low-level immunologic stimulation occurs throughout life, and *natural antibodies* usually develop to those ABO blood group substances which the individual does not possess (e.g., a person with blood group A would possess antibodies to blood group B).

DEGREES OF ABO COMPATIBILITY.   Transfused erythrocytes may be identical, compatible, or incompatible with the recipient's ABO system. Donor erythrocytes with ABO phenotypes identical with those of the recipient's are termed *identical;* those in which the donor has no antigens that are not also present in the recipient are termed *compatible;* and

[1] Antibodies to the H substance are not ordinarily found in persons of the ABO phenotypes. The H gene gives rise to the H Character; the very rare alelle h, when present in double dose, results in the absence of this character, the so-called "Bombay" phenotype. This phenotype is characterized by the total absence of ABH substances from the cells, and by the presence of antibodies to A, B, and H substances.

Table 17-3. Genes, Gene Products, and Antigenic Structures Responsible for ABH and Lewis Specificities. The proposed additions of sugar moieties to the glycolipid chain terminals controlled by the H, Le, A, and B genes, and the resulting serologic specificities of these structures, are shown. (Adapted from Fudenberg, Pink, Stites, and Wang, *Basic Immunogenetics,* Oxford University Press [45].)

Gene	Gene Product	Substance Transferred	Antigenic Structures
O (H)	Fucosyl transferase	Fucose	Gal β_1-3 GlcNAc 2 or | 4 Fuc α_1
A	N Acetyl galactosamine transferase	N Acetyl galactosamine	Gal NAc α_1-3Gal β_1-3GlcNac 2 or | 4 Fuc α_1
B	Galactosyl transferase	Galactose	Gal α_1-3Gal β_1-3GlcNAc 2 or | 4 Fuc α_1
Le^a	Fucosyl transferase	L Fucose	Gal β_1-3GlcNAc | Fuc α
Le^b	Fucosyl transferase	L Fucose	Gal β_1-3GlcNAc 2 4 | | Fuc α_1 Fuc α_1

donor erythrocytes possessing antigens which are not present in the recipient are termed *incompatible* (Table 17-4).

BLOOD TRANSFUSIONS.   Only erythrocytes with identical ABO blood groups should be transfused whenever possible. The first rule of blood transfusion is that the donor's red cells must not be given to any person who possesses antibodies which would react against them (e.g., avoid

Table 17-4. Blood Groups—Degrees of Compatibility.

Donor	Recipient	Classification
A	A	Identical
A	AB	Compatible
A	O	Incompatible

transfusions of A cells into recipient with B blood group and presence of anti-A isoagglutinins). The second rule of blood transfusion is that donor cells must not possess the Rh factor if it is absent from the cells of the proposed recipient (e.g., avoid transfusion of D red cells (i.e., Rh+) into Rh− recipient). To satisfy these two rules, both donor and recipient must be grouped with regard to ABO and Rh, and a cross-matching test must be done using the recipient's serum and the donor's cells [169].

The immunologic risks of blood transfusions. Of the more than 4.5 million blood transfusions administered annually in this country, there occurs approximately 1 reaction per 50 transfusions (i.e., 90,000), and there is one death for every 3,000 transfusions (i.e., 1,500 deaths). Therefore, precise assays for immunological donor selections are mandatory.[2]

The most important clinical immunologic transfusion reactions are as follows:

A. Febrile reactions (often due to lysis of HL–A incompatible leukocytes and platelets)
B. Allergic reactions (e.g., anaphylactic reactions due to anti-IgA antibodies in patients with selective IgA deficiency)
C. Hemolytic reactions, including (a) ABO blood group incompatibilities due to clerical or laboratory errors, (b) minor blood group antigenic incompatibility, especially Kell or Duffy, (c) A or AB subgroup incompatibility or Rh incompatibility, (d) minor incompatibility due to anti-ABO or anti-Rh antibodies, and (e) transfusion of outdated or hemolyzed blood.

ORGAN ALLOTRANSPLANTATION. For organ allotransplantation (e.g., kidney transplantation), organs from compatible ABO donors are acceptable (see Table 17-5), although organs from ABO identical donors are preferable.

ABO SYSTEM AND IMMUNOLOGIC DONOR SELECTION FOR ALLOTRANSPLANTATION. Organs from compatible ABO donors are acceptable (Table 17-5) but ABO blood group incompatibility has been shown to result in rapid tissue rejection [181, 182]. For instance, skin grafts from group A or group B donors to group O recipients [32, 182], or renal allografts in patients with major donor-recipient blood group incompatibilities [133], can be expected to undergo rapid rejection. *ABO incompatibility must be avoided because of the almost certain risk of hyperacute rejection of grafts* [136, 137].

THE RH SYSTEM. The Rh blood group system consists of factors present on human erythrocytes which were discovered in sera of rabbits and

---

[2] In addition to the typing and cross-matching procedures, blood must also be screened for the presence of hepatitis-associated antigens (HAA, Australian (Au) antigens, HB–Ag).

Table 17-5. Direction of Acceptable Mismatched Blood Group Antigens. O is universal donor, AB is universal recipient of allografts (Modified from Starzl and Putnam [137].)

Transfusion		Risk
O	to non-O	Safe
Rh	to Rh+	Safe
Rh+	to Rh−	Relatively safe
A	to non-A	Dangerous
B	to non-B	Dangerous
AB	to non-AB	Dangerous

guinea pigs after immunization with red cells from Rhesus monkeys. These anti-Rh antisera agglutinate erythrocytes of the majority of the U.S. population (Rh positive), whereas the remainder do not react (Rh negative) [116].

Rh antigens.   The distribution of Rh antigens is much more restricted than that of the ABO antigens. There exist three sets of allelic genes, designated C, D, and E, with allelic forms c, d, e, allowing the combinations: CDE, cde; CDe, etc. It is the D antigen which determines whether an individual is Rh positive or negative (phenotype DD or Dd: Rh positive; dd: Rh negative). Anti-D antiserum is used synonymously with anti-Rh antiserum. It reacts with approximately 70–80% of Caucasian and 90–95% of Negro Americans, who are therefore Rh positive. Rh antigens do not appear to play a significant role in organ allotransplantation [48, 137].

Anti-Rh antibodies.   These antibodies (specifically the anti-D antibodies) can be a cause of hemolytic transfusion reactions, and Rh incompatibility between mother and child. It is the most frequent cause of erythroblastosis fetalis. For instance, an Rh-negative (D-negative) mother with an Rh-positive (D-positive) fetus produces anti-D antibodies, often of the IgM class, to which the placenta is impermeable. However, restimulation (secondary or anamnestic response) due to additional pregnancies results in anti-D antibodies of the IgG class, which can cross the placenta into the fetal circulation, resulting in hemolysis of the fetal erythrocytes (hemolytic disease of the newborn). This can now be prevented by the prophylactic use of anti-D antiserum [29, 44, 90].

DISEASES ASSOCIATED WITH ABO BLOOD GROUPS.   A correlation between specific ABO blood groups and certain diseases has been postulated, but a convincing correlation is difficult to document. An association of peptic ulcers with the ABO antigens has been claimed; such ulcers are said to occur much more frequently in association with type O blood groups

[4, 19, 122, 173]. An interesting observation is the loss of A, B, and H determinants in primary carcinoma of the gastrointestinal tract [176].

The HL–A System

HL–A ANTIGENS.   Leukocytes, including neutrophilic, basophilic, and eosinophilic granulocytes, and lymphocytes (but not erythrocytes) possess antigens on their surfaces which belong to the HL–A system. Antigens which have been definitely characterized and internationally recognized and accepted by a Committee of the World Health Organization are termed HL–A antigens. Those antigens which are in the process of being completely characterized but are not yet accepted by the WHO Committee are termed Workshop (W) antigens.

Nature of HL–A antigens [27, 117, 144].   The HL–A antigens represent glycoproteins of approximately 30,000 to 50,000 daltons, but the antigenic determinants themselves are polypeptide in nature. Inheritance of the large number of known HL–A antigens is controlled by two series of multiple allelomorphic genes at two subloci on an unknown chromosome which are termed either *first segregant series* and *second segregant series;* or, alternatively, *LA-series* and *Four Series* (see Fig. 17-2). The antigenic determinants inherited from a single parent comprise one-half of an individual's phenotype (e.g., HL–A 1, 5 or 3, 7). This "genetic package," inherited from each parent, is called a *haplotype.* One HL–A antigen from each segregant series is transmitted to the offspring. The *HL–A phenotype* is the sum of an individual's two haplotypes; it consists of two HL–A antigens from each segregant series. Each individual can have no more than two of the alleles at each sublocus, one contributed by the paternal chromosome and the other by the maternal chromosome. The full determination of these 4 antigens in an individual has been referred to as a saturated or "full house" phenotype (see Figs. 17-2 and 17-4). In case of homozygosity, there is only one HL–A antigen expressed in a segregant series instead of two. Haplotyping is important for the immunologic selection of organ donors, since haplotype identity appears to carry with it a higher degree of allograft acceptance than phenotype identity [182]. Conversely, haplotype mismatches appear to be associated with a particularly unfavorable graft prognosis [9].

HL–nomenclature and equivalencies.   The HL–A and W nomenclature is summarized in Table 17-6.

Cross-reactivity of HL–A antigens.   A high frequency of cross-reactivity exists between certain HL–A antigens of the same segregant series [27, 30, 34, 36, 56, 59, 163] (i.e., CREGs—Cross Reacting Groups) [30] (Tables 17-6 and 17-7). Cross-reactions appear to reduce the immunogenicity of certain donor antigens after transplantation into a recipient. The practical result is that certain donors with an "incompatible" HL–A pattern may become "compatible" after correction for cross-reactivity (see Fig. 17-4).

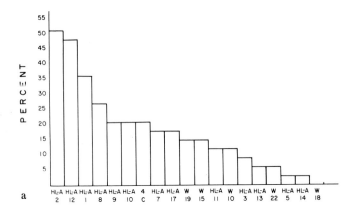

a

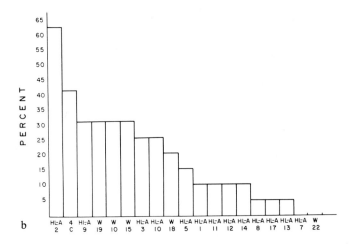

b

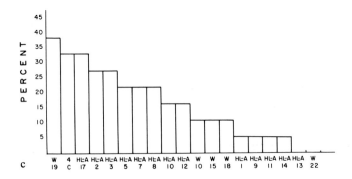

c

Table 17-6. HL–A System*—Nomenclature and Equivalencies.

1st Segregant Series (1st sublocus)		2nd Segregant series (2nd sublocus)	
HL–A 1		HL–A 5	= Tell
HL–A 2		W5	
HL–A 3		W18	= Te58, Da20
HL–A 9	= Te4	HL–A 7	
W23	= HL–A 9.1		
W24	= HL–A 9.2	HL–A 8	
HL–A 10	= Te12	HL–A 12	= Te9
W25	= HL–A 10.1		
W26	= HL–A 10.2	HL–A 13	= Te26
HL–A 11	= Te13	W14	= Ma Ki, Te54, Da18, To27
W28	= Ba*, Te40	W17	= Ma Pi, Te57, SL
W19 "Complex"	= W29, Te63, AO77	W27	= Te52, FJH, To29
	W30	W10	= BB, Te60, To23
	W31, Te66	W15	= Te55, LND, Da23
	W32, AO28, Te59	W16	= Te64, U18
		W21	= Te58, Da20
		W22	= Te51, AA*
		(4C "Complex"	= HL–A5, W5, W18, Te50, Te58)

* HL–A may be abbreviated A (e.g., HL–A 1 = A 1).

Population distribution of HL–A antigens. The HL–A frequency distribution differs for the various ethnic groups throughout the world [5, 6, 71, 151]. Any comparison of HL–A types must take this basic genetic fact into account, and each transplantation center needs to establish its own ethnic HL–A distribution profiles. Fig. 17-3 depicts the frequency of 19 HL–A and W antigens for 3 ethnic groups as determined in our laboratories.

Figure 17-3
Frequency distribution of 19 HL–A and W antigens among 3 control populations. (a) Caucasian; "full house" phenotypes found in 52% of this population; (b) Latin-American; "full house" phenotypes found in 57% of this population; (c) Negro; "full house" phenotypes found in 42% of this population.

Figure 17-4

Names	1	2	3	4	5	6
Recipient (R) or Donor (D)	R	D	D	D	D	D	D
Blood Group	O	O	O	O	O	O	O

First Segregant Series							
HL–A 1	+	+	−	−	+	−	−
HL–A 2	+	+	+	+	−	−	+
HL–A 3	−	−	−	⊕	−	−	⊕
HL–A 9	−	−	−	−	−	−	−
W23	−	−	−	−	−	−	−
W24	−	−	−	−	−	−	−
HL–A 10	−	−	−	−	−	−	−
W25	−	−	−	−	−	−	−
W26	−	−	−	−	−	−	−
HL–A 11	−	−	−	−	−	−	−
W28	−	−	−	−	⊕	⊕	−
W19	−	−	−	−	−	−	−
W29	−	−	−	−	−	⊕	−
W30	−	−	−	−	−	−	−

Second Segregant Series							
HL–A 5	+	+	−	+	−	−	+
HL–A 7	−	−	−	−	−	−	−
HL–A 8	−	−	−	−	−	−	−
HL–A 12	+	+	+	+	+	−	−
HL–A 13	−	−	−	−	−	⊕	−
W5	−	−	−	−	−	−	−
W10	−	−	−	−	−	−	−
W14	−	−	−	−	−	−	−
W15	−	−	−	−	−	−	−
W16	−	−	−	−	−	−	−
W17	−	−	−	−	−	−	−
W18	−	−	−	−	−	⊕	−
W22	−	−	−	−	−	−	−
W27	−	−	−	−	−	−	−
4C	−	−	−	−	⊕	−	⊕

	1	2	3	4	5	6
Cross Match	Neg	Neg	Neg	Neg	Neg	Pos
Match Grade	A/A*	B/B*	C/B*	D/B*	E/C*	F/F*

Table 17-7. Cross-Reactivity Among Various HL–A Antigens of the Same Segregant Series.

1st Segregant Series	2nd Segregant Series
A1, A3, A11, A10, W19	W18, A5 → W5 ⟷ W15 ⟷ W17
May cross react with one another	
A9 ⟷ A2 ⟷ W28	W22, W27 → A7 ⟷ A8 ⟷ W14
May cross react only in direction of arrows	
	A12 ⟷ A13 ⟷ W10
	May cross react only in direction of arrows

CORRELATION OF HL–A GRADES WITH SURVIVAL OF ALLOGRAFTS AND TRANSFUSED BLOOD CELLS. The results of histocompatibility typing (see Chapter 18) are based upon the grading of the results of the cytotoxicity assay, as estimated by the degree of cell death in the lymphocytotoxicity tests. The A–F classification of Terasaki [77] is based upon estimation of the number of mismatched HL–A antigens (Fig. 17-4) between a recipient and donor.

Allotransplantation. 1. In living related donor-recipients, a definite correlation among the degree of HL–A matching grades, mixed lymphocyte culture reactions (MLC), and the survival of the renal allografts has been documented [9, 36, 68, 70, 95, 105, 133, 138, 139, 157, 175] (Fig. 17-5).

2. Until recently in unrelated cadaveric donor-recipients, a precise relationship between the HL–A matching grades and renal allograft function and survival has eluded a clear-cut evaluation. Several early studies failed to show a definite correlation [69, 93, 102]. There are some failures of allograft survival in spite of good HL–A matches, and vice

Figure 17-4
HL–A match grades and cross-reactivity. Note: Circled antigens are mismatched to recipient. A = Identical, no mismatch; B = compatible, no group mismatch [homozygosity occurring in HL–A 2]; C = 1 group mismatch; D = 2 or more group mismatches; E = 2 allele difference [2 mismatches in one allele.]; F = positive cross-match. In donor situations 3, 4, and 5, the mismatched antigens are also cross-reacting antigens and the match grade might be considered "compatible." However, in situation 6, the positive cross match overrules any possible "corrections" for cross-reacting antigens. * = Match grade after correction for cross-reacting antigens.

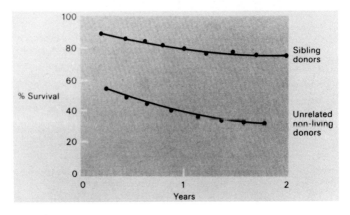

Figure 17-5
Survival rates after kidney transplantation since January 1967 (B. A. Barnes
& J. E. Murray, in 7th Report of Kidney Transplant Registry). (Reproduced
from I. M. Roitt [123].)

versa. Recently, however, data obtained from larger series, based upon
more homogeneous ethnic populations and more "full house" HL–A
matching results, have yielded evidence of a direct relationship [18, 36,
41, 68, 70, 94, 95, 111]. These new findings led Dausset [36] to postulate that the HL–A assays are extremely useful, if not indispensable, for
immunologic donor selection. In the case of related donors, "it makes it
possible to choose the 'ideal' donor, and in the case of unrelated donors,
it gives the patients about a 67% chance of a two-year survival (against
33% when the donor is incompatible)." He concluded that "no surgeon
has the right to refrain from giving his patient an additional one of two
chances of surviving at two years." (Fig. 17-6).

The relative importance of specific HL–A antigens (i.e., "strong" vs.
"weak" antigens) has been suggested by several studies [99, 156]. A
better survival of cadaveric renal allografts is seen when donors and recipients are matched for 3 or more of the HL–A antigens, and the graft
survival is better when matching has been accomplished for the second
locus antigens alone than for the first locus antigens alone. Such a relationship of allograft survival with matched HL–A antigens of the second
segregant series is particularly striking when the recipient has preformed
cytotoxic antibodies against leukocytes from individuals other than the
actual organ donor.

Blood transfusions.   The survival of transfused granulocytes and
platelets in polytransfused patients appears to depend upon the degree of
HL–A compatibility (Fig. 17-7). The rapid destruction of transfused incompatible platelets and granulocytes often results in febrile transfusion
reactions. This aspect is of clinical importance in patients with granulocytopenia or thrombocytopenia requiring frequent blood transfusions.

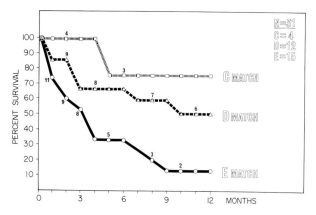

Figure 17-6
Cadaveric renal allotransplantation (HL–A types vs. renal survival). Relationship between the HL–A matching grades C, D, and E vs. the survival of 31 renal allotransplants performed at UTMB, Galveston, Texas. There is a tendency for the E-matching grades to be associated with less favorable survival rates than the D, and in particular the C, grades. This difference of survival rates becomes obvious during the first 3 months after allotransplantation.

RULES FOR IMMUNOLOGIC SELECTION OF ALLOGRAFT DONORS.   Certain guidelines have emerged for immunologic donor selection. The general rules are summarized in Table 17-8 and Fig. 17-8. The specific rules of the Scandiatransplant [56] are as follows:

1st PRIORITY: ABO GROUPS must be identical or compatible.
A. Blood group O donor grafts can be used for recipients of all other groups (i.e., universal donor).

Figure 17-7
Transfusion response to platelets. A = HL–A identical family member; B = HL–A nonidentical family members; C = random donors. Only the well-matched platelets from Donor A survive well in the host, whereas the mismatched platelets (B, C) are rapidly eliminated (immune elimination). (Adapted from Yankee, Grumet, and Rogentine [178] and Walford [167].)

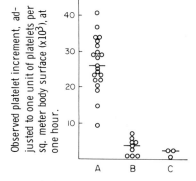

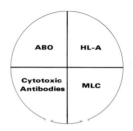

Figure 17-8
Immunologic donor selection based upon the evaluation of the ABO and HL–A types and cytotoxic antibodies (and MLC reactions in related donors). In general, the higher the degree of HLA and MLC incompatibility, the more immunosuppression is required, and vice versa. Recent data support the contention of major and minor HL–A antigens: matching for the 2nd segregant series alone may be more important for graft survival than matching for the 1st segregant series alone [99, 156].

B. Group O and B recipients, however, should receive priority before A and AB recipients; otherwise, the group O recipients would be less well-supplied than the other blood groups.

2nd PRIORITY: HL–A TYPES

A. First choice is given to A and B matches (i.e., identical or compatible).

B. Second choice is given to C matches (i.e., one HL–A antigen mismatched). Ranking of priorities is given to the following 3 categories of patients:

1. Recipients with anti-HL–A antibodies (i.e., preformed cytotoxic antibodies) but not reacting with the donor's lymphocytes (i.e., negative crossmatch between donor and recipient);

Table 17-8. Immunologic Donor Selection.

Procedure	Test System	Importance
1. ABO-typing[a,b]	Erythrocytes	Mandatory
2. Erythrocyte cross-matching	Erythrocytes-Serum	Desirable
3. HL–A typing[b]	Lymphocytes	Mandatory
4. Lymphocyte cross-matching[a]	Lymphocytes-Serum	Mandatory
5. MLC	Lymphocytes	Desirable

[a] Incompatibility by *either* of these two procedures (i.e., ABO typing or lymphocyte cross-matching) is an *absolute contraindication* to allotransplantation.
[b] For rules regarding the priorities of the various ABO and HL–A matching grades, see the rules of Scandiatransplant [56].

2. Recipients with cross-reacting HL–A antigens (i.e., compatible HL–A antigens in donor-recipient pair, which will "disappear" after "cleaning up" for cross reaction);
3. Recipients with calculated small probability of obtaining an A, B, or C match [56]. Under these circumstances, even D matches are given priority.

C. Third choice is given to D or E matches.

DONOR POOLS REQUIRED FOR ALLOTRANSPLANTATION.   Recently, quantitative data have been developed which allow an estimate of the number of potential donors required for the selection of compatible donors for allotransplantation. In order to increase the pool size, several international cooperative ventures have been formed for organ sharing (e.g., Scandiatransplant, Eurotransplant). The recipient pool size and the probability of finding an HL–A identical donor have been estimated [160] (Table 17-9).

The probability of obtaining acceptable HL–A matches depends in large measure upon the frequencies of the HL–A types to be matched [55] (see Fig. 17-3). For instance, the probability of obtaining an A match is about 10 per 1,000 for only two phenotypes (HL–A 1,3; 7,8 and HL–A 1,2; 8,12), and above 1 per 1,000 for 187 possible phenotypes, whereas as many as 3,518 possible phenotypes have a probability for an A match below 0.1 per 1,000 [56]. A different picture emerges if the sum of A, B, and C matches is considered. Half of all possible phenotypes have a probability above 10 per 1,000 for a C match or better, whereas only a small fraction (< 10%) has a probability below 1 per 1,000 [56].

The need for a large donor pool, and therefore, a regional and national organization, is emphasized by the following statement by Van Rood et al. [161]: "When donors are matched against a large recipient pool almost 20% of our patients can be provided with a perfect match and the majority of the remainder will be mismatched for, at most, one antigen. It is here that we can expect a significantly improved prognosis. . . ."

Table 17-9. Pool Size Required vs. Frequency of HL–A Phenotypes

Number in Pool	Frequency of Compatible HL–A Phenotypes		
	0.5%	1.0%	2.0%
200	0.63	0.87	0.98
500	0.92	0.99	1.0
1,000	0.99	1.0	1.0
2,000	1.0	1.0	1.0

Appendix. The first sublocus contains at least 14 different genes, and the second sublocus at least 27 genes, resulting in a complex polymorphism of the HL–A system. Since these genes behave as mutually exclusive alleles at the two loci, the following frequencies have been calculated [72]:

A. 378 (14 × 27) different haplotypes (i.e., different combinations of the first and second subloci genes on one chromosome);

B. 71,631 different genotypes: $(\dfrac{378 \times (378 + 1)}{2})$;

C. a. 92 different first sublocus phenotypes for the 14 different first sublocus genes: $(\dfrac{14 \times (14 - 1)}{2} + 1)$;

    b. 352 different second sublocus phenotype for the 27 different second sublocus genes: $(\dfrac{27 \times (27 - 1)}{2} + 1)$;

D. 32,384 different HL–A phenotypes or tissue types for these different first and second sublocus phenotypes: (92 × 352).

HL–A TYPES AND DISEASE ASSOCIATIONS.   Certain disorders appear to be associated with abnormal HL–A profiles [84]. The significance of such relationships is difficult to assess because of the vagaries of the

Table 17-10. HL–A Types and Disease States.

Disease States	HL–A Preponderance	References
1. Lupus erythematosus	W 15	[53]
2. Chronic glomerulonephritis	HL–A 2	[104]
3. Gluten-sensitive enteropathy	HL–A 8	[40]
4. Multiple sclerosis	HL–A 3, 7	[65, 97]
5. Breast cancer[a]	HL–A 7	[107]
6. Hodgkin's disease[a]	HL–A 1, 5, 8, 4C	[7, 21, 43, 180]
7. Acute lymphoblastic leukemia[a]	HL–A 2, 12	[108, 168]
8. Monoclonal gammopathies[a]	W 18, 4c; W 19; W 22	[21, 120, 121]
9. Combined B–T cell immunodeficiency disorders	Supernumerary HL–A Antigens (7–15 antigens)	[121, 140, 150]

[a] The possible significance of abnormal HL–A distribution patterns in certain diseases remains to be elucidated; however, a relationship analogous to the chromosomal abnormalities in certain disease states must be considered (e.g., Ph_1 positive vs. Ph_1 negative cases of chronic myelocytic leukemia, which represent different clinical variations).

populations involved and the tenuous basis for the comparison of results obtained in the various laboratories. For these reasons, the most stringent statistical criteria must be applied in these situations. Thus, results obtained by the X^2 test, with or without Yates' corrections [53] from at least 20 comparisons, need further "corrections" by multiplying the normal significance level by the number of antigens tested, to obtain a true significance level (Bodmer corrections). Additionally, an independent follow-up survey has been recommended to see whether the association that was indicated initially remains significant on follow-up [35, 85]. Table 17-10 summarizes some of these associations between HL–A profiles and certain clinical disorders [35].

Preformed Cytotoxic Antibodies

Nature of Cytotoxic Antibodies

Cytotoxic antibodies are found in a high percentage of recipients of multiple blood transfusions [25], previous renal [113] or skin [166] allotransplantation, and in multiparous women [67]. Cytotoxic autoantibodies have been demonstrated in patients with certain autoimmune disorders [147]. The nature of these cytotoxic antibodies varies; usually they are of the IgG class [66], traverse the placenta, fix complement, and may be characterized by unusual properties [3, 47, 92, 106]. The presence of preformed cytotoxic antibodies predisposes to hyperacute rejection of allografts [39, 113, 145, 146, 172].

Conditions Associated with Cytotoxic Antibodies

BLOOD TRANSFUSIONS. Cytotoxic antibodies are often directed toward the HL–A antigens of lymphocytes, granulocytes, and platelets [49] in transfused blood. They do not appear to be directed against other ubiquitous antigens, such as the I, $P + P_1$, and heterophile antigens [165]. Immunization of the recipient to HL–A incompatible antigens is expected, since blood transfusions require only ABO and Rh typing. In this sense, a blood transfusion, which must be considered to constitute the first allotransplantation, presensitizes the recipient to subsequent organ allografts, and may pave the way for a second set, or accelerated rejection of such grafts [113]. A high percentage of patients on chronic hemodialysis possesses cytotoxic antibodies. In one study, between 16% and 32% of prospective kidney recipients have been found to carry detectable lymphocytotoxic antibodies [137]. We have found cytotoxic antibodies in 20 of 38 (52.6%) of our transfused patients with chronic renal failure [120]. Attempts at minimizing the risk of presensitization consist of the administration of buffy-coat-poor blood or frozen blood resulting in the elimination of most HL–A-bearing cellular elements [9, 28, 56, 60, 152].

ALLOTRANSPLANTATION.   Previous renal or skin allotransplants likewise may sensitize the recipient to second allografts, by virtue of the incompatible HL–A antigens on the graft tissue [92, 137, 159, 172].

PREGNANCIES.   During pregnancy, fetal lymphocytes may enter the maternal circulation and evoke cytotoxic antibodies to HL–A antigens not present on maternal tissues [15, 149].

Clinical Significance of Cytotoxic Antibodies

In order to avoid hyperacute rejection episodes, tests for the presence of cytotoxic antibodies are performed prior to allotransplantation. Such cross-match tests, between the recipient's serum and the prospective donor's lymphocytes, must be considered to constitute an integral part of the immunologic donor selection process [103]. These cross-match tests should be performed as closely to the transplantation date as possible [8, 25]. The presence of cytotoxic antibodies to lymphocytes of a prospective donor (i.e., positive cross-match test, grade F in Terasaki's grading scheme), constitutes an *absolute contradindication to allotransplantation* [9, 103]. Cytotoxic antibodies in recipients which do not react with the donor's lymphocytes also pose a threat to the allograft, since there appears to be a poorer graft survival than in recipients without such antibodies [100, 148] (Fig. 17-9). Furthermore, such cytotoxic antibodies may decrease with time and become undetectable by presently available techniques. Following allotransplantation, therefore, an anamnestic response of such antibodies may then result in hyperacute rejection [106].

In 1969, Patel and Terasaki [103] reported that 24 of 30 kidneys transplanted across a positive cross match failed immediately, in contrast to 8 of 195 transplanted across a negative cross match. The authors'

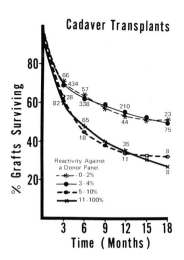

Figure 17-9
Survival rates of transplants into patients with cytotoxins. The number of patients in the 4 categories of reactivity against the random donor panel was 566 in 0% : 2% cytotoxins; 98 in 3% : 4%; 41 in 5% : 10%; and 124 in 11% : 100%. The figures on the lines denote the number of patients at risk. (By permission Opelz and Terasaki, *Transplant. Proc.* 4:433–437, 1972 [100].)

conclusions have subsequently become a guideline for immunologic donor selection: "The ethics of transplanting kidneys without the prior knowledge of the results of the cross-match test, or across a known positive cross-match result, can reasonably be expected to be questioned in the light of this evidence."

Mixed Lymphocyte Cultures (MLC)

Principle
The principle of MLC is based upon the fact that specific antigens (e.g., HL–A or related antigens) stimulate lymphocytes to undergo blastoid transformation. Specifically, HL–A transplantation antigens on the surfaces of lymphocytes can stimulate allogeneic lymphocytes possessing different antigens. In general, the magnitude of stimulation reflects the degree of histoincompatibility. The genetic locus which controls the MLC reaction is closely related to, but probably independent from, that of the HL–A system [17, 27]. Lymphocytes can thus stimulate, as well as respond to, nonidentical allogeneic lymphocytes. Bach introduced a one-way MLC technique which allows the separation of these two (stimulating and responding) parameters [11] (Fig. 17-10). In this test, the stimulating cells are treated with mitomycin C, which inhibits DNA synthesis (response mechanism) but not the stimulatory ability of these cells. The response capacity of lymphocytes can be assayed by using untreated, responding lymphocytes, and mitomycin C-treated stimulating

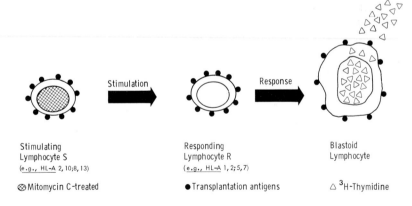

Stimulating
Lymphocyte S
(e.g., HL–A 2, 10;8, 13)

Responding
Lymphocyte R
(e.g., HL–A 1, 2;5,7)

Blastoid
Lymphocyte

⊗ Mitomycin C-treated   ● Transplantation antigens   △ ^{3}H-Thymidine

Figure 17-10
One-way mixed lymphocyte culture (MLC). The response capacity of histoincompatible lymphocytes can be assayed by treatment of lymphocyte S with mitomycin C (stimulating lymphocyte); culture with the untreated lymphocyte R, and subsequent determination of the degree of blastoid transformation by the assay of radiolabeled precursors of DNA. The response capacity of lymphocyte S can be assayed by the reverse sequence, rendering it the R lymphocyte. (From Sakai, Groves, Townsend, and Ritzmann [126].)

cells; DNA synthesis observed in this test is due to the responding cells only.

Unfortunately, the MLC reactions are time consuming (usually 5–7 days) and are therefore applicable only to living-related donors. Recently, however, a rapid MLC test has been developed which may be used in the immunologic selection of cadaveric donors [127].

Application and Interpretation of MLC

APPLICATION.   MLC is increasingly applied in clinical immunology, including histocompatibility assays and the detection of immunocompetent cells [51, 127], as described below:

1. Histocompatibility matching: (a) selection of donors for organ allotransplantation; (b) prediction of GvH reaction in bone marrow transplantation

2. Detection of immunocompetent lymphocytes: (a) detection of tolerance after allotransplantation; (b) diagnosis of immunodeficiency syndromes affecting T-lymphocytes; (c) evaluation of effectiveness of immunosuppressive therapy.

INTERPRETATION.   MLC results obtained from normal control persons show a wide range of both stimulatory and responding activity (see Chapter 18). In general, the higher the MLC results, the greater the antigen disparity or histoincompatibility between potential allograft donors and recipients, and vice versa. For instance, lymphocyte combinations with HL–A matching grades of D or E usually lead to a strong (i.e., positive) MLC response, whereas lymphocyte combinations with A or B grades usually produce negligible (i.e., negative) MLC responses [51].

These MLC differences are less pronounced in relatives than in unrelated dono-recipient pairs [27]. In identical twins, for example, neither set of cells stimulates the other, whereas in unrelated pairs there is almost always mutual stimulation [51]. Family studies have shown that the MLC reactions correlate with histocompatibility, as determined by HL–A genotyping and by skin graft survival. Exceptions occur, however. For instance, a positive MLC response is observed in about 1% of HL–A identical siblings [27]. This may be due to some degree of independence of the gene controlling the MLC locus, from the gene controlling the HL–A loci, from incomplete results of HL–A antigens obtained by serotyping, or from other determinants possibly related to the immune response (Ir) genes.

Clinical Significance of MLC Reactions

CLINICAL ALLOTRANSPLANTATION.   A correlation appears to exist between the degree of MLC reactions and renal functions after kidney allotransplantation [14]. Enhanced survival is associated with low levels of MLC reactivity between donor and recipient lymphocytes, and vice versa. This is exemplified by the following case report:

D. B., an 11-year-old female, had chronic pyelonephritis. She received a living related renal allotransplant from her father on January 3, 1973. The HL–A match grade was C and the MLC was positive (i.e., 48,343 DPM/culture). Postoperatively, she produced only small amounts of urine. Four days after transplantation, she developed a large, tender perinephric mass and surgical exploration was carried out. The renal transplant was mottled in color and bleeding from its entire surface. The diagnosis of rejection was made and a transplant nephrectomy was performed. Histologic examination demonstrated acute cellular rejection. This event occurred in spite of standard immunosuppressive therapy with azathioprine and prednisone and additional "pulses" of intravenous methyl-prednisolone.

The degree of GvH reactions following bone marrow allotransplantation is also correlated with the degree of MLC reaction between the donor and recipient.

OTHER CLINICAL DISORDERS
A. Immunodeficiency syndromes associated with decreased MLC reactions
   Congenital immunodeficiencies: (a) DiGeorge's syndrome [81]; (b) Swiss type agammaglobulinemia (i.e., combined B/T-cell immunodeficiency) [13]; (c) partial combined immunodeficiencies: ataxia-teleangiectasia [101]; Wiscott–Aldrich syndrome [83]
   Acquired immunodeficiencies: (a) Acquired agammaglobulinemia [80]; (b) Hodgkin's disease [75]
B. Granulomatous colitis. Lymphocytes from patients with Crohn's disease respond normally to the nonspecific mitogen phytohemagglutinin (PHA), but the ability of lymphocytes from these patients to respond to normal allogeneic lymphocytes or to stimulate these cells in one-way MLC, however, is significantly decreased when compared to normal controls [153, 154, 155].
C. Acute thermal burns. In patients with acute thermal burns, profound suppression of cellular immunity is reflected by decreased delayed skin hypersensitivity skin tests; reduced rejection potential of allografts; depletion of lymphocytes in thymus dependent areas of peripheral lymphoid tissues; and susceptibility to fungal, viral, and gram-negative bacterial infections. The MLC response and stimulation capacity in such patients is suppressed during the early postburn period [119].

APPENDIX: CELL-MEDIATED LYMPHOCYTOLYSIS (CML) [87]. The lymphocyte response in MLC is usually assayed by the synthesis rates of DNA, reflecting the incorporation rates of radiolabeled thymidine. Recently, however, another parameter for the lymphocyte activity in MLC has been developed, namely, the cell-mediated lymphocytolysis (CML) [87]. The principle of CML is based upon the fact that lymphocytes specifically sensitized by allogeneic lymphocytes in MLC can lyse allogeneic cells (i.e., target cells) in vitro. The lysis is reflected by Cr^{51}-release from the labeled surfaces of these target cells.

CML allows the assay of killer-cell functions of lymphocytes in MLC. Lymphocytes stimulated by allogeneic lymphocytes release mediator substances (i.e., lymphokines) [38, 76]. One of these lymphokines, lymphotoxin, can destroy target allogeneic lymphocytes. The MLC reaction, determined by DNA synthesis rates, however, does not always parallel the activity of CML. For this reason, Bach has suggested that CML is mediated by antibody-producing B-lymphocytes, whereas DNA synthesis in MLC reactions reflects the action of thymus dependent T-lymphocytes. It was further suggested that the CML may represent an in vitro model of allograft rejection, while the MLC reaction may reflect the in vitro analogue of the graft versus host reactions.

The specificity of this CML test is considerable, and the CML activity generally parallels the degree of HL–A compatibility (e.g., marked degree of CML activity between siblings with different HL–A haplotypes, but little or no CML activity between siblings with identical haplotypes). Although the precise mechanism of the CML phenomenon is not known, the high degree of specificity and sensitivity of this test provides a new tool for the evaluation of cellular immunity in various clinical areas.

Immunosuppression

Transplantation antigens, in general, represent substances which elicit specific immunologic recognition by the host. This recognition may result in complex reactions aimed at the immunologic elimination of substances bearing such foreign antigens. HL–A incompatibility thus often leads to allograft rejection in humans [98, 115, 132, 157] and animals [131], unless the immunologic consequences of the incompatibility at the HL–A and MLC loci can be overcome by immunosuppressive therapy (Fig. 17-11; see Fig. 17-8).

Modes of Immunosuppression

Most of the immunosuppressive agents used in allotransplantation (e.g., glucocorticosteroids, 6-mercaptopurine and its derivative azathioprine, cyclophosphamide) [114, 128, 130, 135] (see Fig. 17-11), represent the application of drugs developed in conjunction with cancer chemotherapy. Their universal immunosuppressive effects result in severe impairment of the host's defenses, which normally exist in a delicate equilibrium with his own indigenous bacterial, fungal, and viral flora.

Complications of Immunosuppression

Many patients who die following transplantation do so with obvious clinical infections which contribute to various extents to their deaths

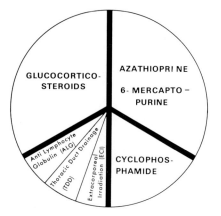

Figure 17–11
Modes of immunosuppression used in clinical allotransplantation, including glucocorticosteroids, 6-mercaptopurine and its derivative, azathioprine, cyclophosphamide, antilymphocyte globulin (ALG), thoracic duct drainage (TDD), and extracorporeal irradiation (ECI).

[125, 145]. Therefore, more specific forms of immunosuppressive therapy (e.g., antilymphocyte globulin (ALG), lymphocyte depletion by thoracic duct drainage (TDD), and extracorporeal irradiation (ECI) [10, 74, 96, 129, 174] have been developed in an attempt to affect more selectively those cells involved in allograft rejection. Immunosuppressive therapy, however, may also suppress the immunologic surveillance mechanisms [24, 86], a circumstance which may interfere with immunologic self-integrity and which may allow the emergence of neoplasia [78, 109, 134, 135].

Statistics show that the general risk of developing cancer in transplant recipients is about 80 times greater than that in the general population [110], and that reticulum cell sarcomas occur 4,000 times more frequently among transplant recipients than in the general population of similar age [78].

Allograft Rejection

When a transplant is performed between two histoincompatible individuals, an immunologic process of considerable complexity is initiated. This process will lead to destruction of the allograft if not suppressed. In such a recipient, even though clinical tolerance may be apparent, some degree of immunologic intolerance resulting in graft rejection can generally be detected by appropriate studies. Often, the first clinical clue of incomplete tolerance is the appearance of a rejection crisis, represented by acute deterioration of the function of the allograft. In others, progressive changes occur which lead to an insidious destruction of the allograft. The dynamic sequence of immunologic events leading to such destruction is referred to as allograft rejection.

Much that is currently understood concerning the mechanisms of allograft rejection has been gained from its study in relation to the kidney. This information, however, has been found to apply to the transplantation of other organs. Although the basic underlying principles governing allograft rejection are universal, their final modes of expression vary according to the structure and function of the organ involved, and the type and degree of immunosuppression applied.

Modes of Rejection

Allograft rejection represents a continuous spectrum involving both cellular and humoral immune reactions. Even though somewhat artificial, this process has been divided into several categories depending in part upon the primary mechanism involved and in part upon the time at which it occurs. These categories are referred to as *hyperacute, acute,* and *chronic* rejections.

HYPERACUTE REJECTION (HAR).   This term refers to the acute, fulminating reaction that occurs within minutes to hours after allotransplantation. The process is generally caused by an antibody-mediated reaction [67, 88, 133], although cell-mediated instances of HAR may occur [162]. The antibodies involved may be anti-A, anti-B, or anti-AB isohemagglutinins in the ABO incompatible recipient (e.g., anti-A antibodies in B blood group donor directed at A blood group antigens in A blood group recipient), or anti-HL–A antibodies (i.e., preformed cytotoxic antibodies to the donor's HL–A antigens) in the recipient's circulation. These latter antibodies in the allograft recipient are generally the result of multiple pregnancies, blood transfusions, or previous allografts [106, 148, 177, 179]. They may also be related to the patient's primary renal disease, or they may occur secondary to infection with certain types of bacteria [20].

When the preformed antibodies in the recipient's circulation react with the vascular surfaces of the transplanted organ, activation of the complement system occurs, leading sequentially to increased vascular permeability, leukocyte chemotaxis, and, ultimately, activation of the coagulation system with vascular thrombosis [20]. Morphologically, the manifestations of this reaction are interstitial edema, variable numbers of polymorphonuclear leukocytes marginating within glomerular and peritubular capillaries, and localized thrombosis of peritubular and glomerular capillaries. (Fig. 17-12). This reaction progresses to focal necrosis of tubular epithelial cells with focal interstitial hemorrhage and eventually widespread cortical necrosis of the allograft. Fluorescent antibody staining of biopsy material reveals the localization of immunoglobulin and complement within the glomerular and peritubular capillaries, and often, widespread deposition of fibrin.

Hyperacute Rejection Due to ABO Incompatibility—Case Report

J.B., a 22-year-old female with polycystic kidney disease, received thoracic duct lymphocyte depletion for 45 days prior to cadaveric renal allotrans-

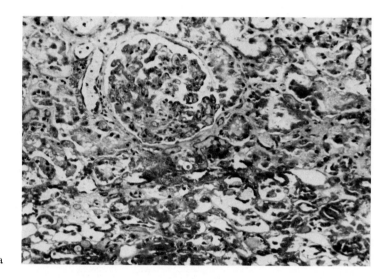

a

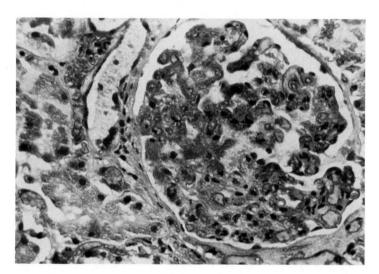

b

Figure 17-12
Hyperacute rejection. (a) Severe tubular necrosis is evident. In some areas, thrombosis of peritubular capillaries can be seen. In scattered areas, poly-morphonuclear leukocytes (PMNs) are present within peritubular capillaries as well. The glomerulus shows thrombosis and presence of PMNs within the capillary lumina. (250 × before 20% reduction.) (b) Within the glomerulus there is thrombosis of peritubular capillaries. A number of PMNs can be seen within the capillary lumina. Necrosis is evident within the tubules surrounding the glomerulus. (400× before 20% reduction.)

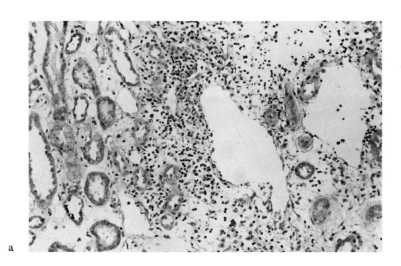

a

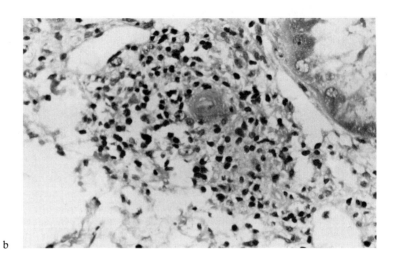

b

Figure 17-13
Acute rejection. (a) A venule surrounded by lymphocytes. A considerable
degree of interstitial edema is evident (250 × before 20% reduction). (b)
An arteriole surrounded by lymphocytes. Interstitial edema is also evident
(550 × before 20% reduction). (c) The glomerulus is normal except for
the presence of a few lymphocytes within the glomerular capillaries. The
glomerulus is surrounded on one side by a dense infiltrate of lymphocytes

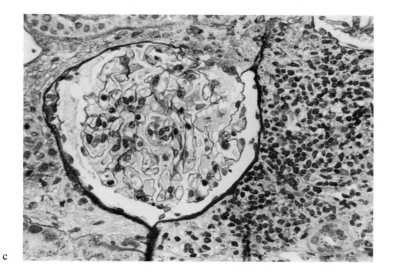

c

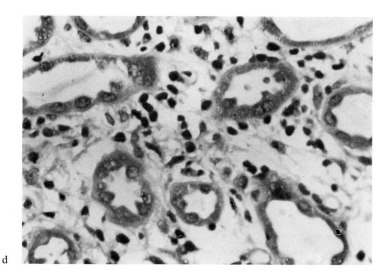

d

(400 × before 20% reduction). (d) Pronounced interstitial edema is demonstrated. Within the interstitium are scattered lymphocytes; lymphocytes can also be seen adhering to the endothelial lining of peritubular capillaries (740 × before 20% reduction).

plantation. Her blood type was 0+ and the blood type of the renal donor was A+. The kidney was apparently rejected within the first 2 hours after revascularization (Fig. 17-12). A fatal cardiac arrest secondary to hyperkalemia occurred 24 hours after operation.

ACUTE REJECTION.   This term refers to a type of rejection that occurs within the first few days following transplantation; it may either fulminate severely or smolder subclinically for prolonged periods of time. This form of allograft rejection may also occur as an acute exacerbation referred to as a *rejection crisis* which can threaten destruction of the transplanted organ even after relatively long periods of apparent immunologic tolerance.

Acute rejection is chiefly cell mediated. Actually, a spectrum of histologic and clinical reactions may exist in these patients, overlapping both with the HAR and with the chronic rejection categories. Morphologically, the reaction may begin within a few hours after transplantation in the immunologically modified recipient. This is recognized by the margination of lymphocytes in the peritubular capillaries (Fig. 17-13d), leading to damage of these structures and eventually to interstitial infiltration by lymphocytes. This lymphocytic infiltration is generally diffuse, but perivascular and periglomerular accumulations are often apparent (Fig. 17-13). In this process, glomeruli are relatively uninvolved. If the process is not controlled by immunosuppressive therapy [31], the terminal stages of this reaction ensue, which are characterized by interstitial edema, hemorrhage, and infiltration with polymorphonuclear leukocytes. Vascular necrosis and thrombosis can occur, and fibrin degradation products may be found in the urine [23, 61]. Occasionally, small amounts of immunoglobulin and complement may be demonstrated within the glomeruli by immunofluorescence techniques.

The presence of large numbers of lymphocytes, the sparsity of immunoglobulin deposition, and the time period after transplantation at which the rejection process occurs all distinguish this acute form from the hyperacute form of allograft rejection [20, 115].

Reversible Acute Rejection Crisis—Case Report
W. N., a 52-year-old male with chronic renal failure due to glomerulonephritis, underwent thoracic duct lymphocyte depletion for 61 days prior to cadaveric renal allotransplantation. Lymph flow was maintained for only 5 days post-transplantation. No immunosuppressive drugs were employed until day 50 post-transplantation. At that time, an increase of blood urea nitrogen (BUN) (from 25 mg to 45 mg/100 ml) occurred, and a renal biopsy was performed. It demonstrated mild perivascular lymphocytic infiltration (Fig. 17-13). Azathioprine (2 mg/kg per day) and prednisone (20 mg per day) were begun. A prompt return of the BUN to normal levels was noted and no other adverse changes in renal function occurred. A follow-up renal biopsy 7 months later revealed no evidence of rejection.

CHRONIC REJECTION.   This type of rejection is primarily mediated by humoral immune mechanisms. The process can begin quite early following transplantation, but it is usually a slow, insidious type of reaction leading to a gradual deterioration in transplant function. Morphologically, three types of lesions can be recognized in this category of rejection: progressive interstitial fibrosis, arterial lesions, and glomerular lesions [20]. These three lesions are generally seen in combinations. It is likely that the interstitial fibrosis (Fig. 17-14a, b) occurs on an ischemic basis and is secondary to the arterial lesions. These arterial lesions, a result of the action of antibody directed against their endothelial surfaces, consist of varying degrees of intimal proliferation which ultimately produce extreme narrowing of the vessel lumina and eventually ischemic changes within the transplant (Fig. 17-14b). The glomerular changes associated with chronic rejection generally consist of thickening of the glomerular capillary basement membrane associated with varying degrees of mesangial changes (Fig. 17-14a, b), both sclerosis and cellular proliferation. Immunofluorescent staining usually reveals a linear deposition of immunoglobulin and complement [82] along the glomerular capillary basement membranes, as well as mesangial deposition in some cases (Fig. 17-14c, d). It is not unusual to see varying degrees of cellular rejection (acute rejection) existing in combination with chronic rejection.

Chronic Rejection—Case Report
E. K., a 36-year-old male with familial nephritis, had lymphocyte depletion by continuous thoracic duct drainage for 61 days. Twenty-one days after transplantation, immunosuppressive drugs were begun because of histologic evidence of cellular rejection. A creatinine clearance of 103 ml/min eight months post-transplantation was found, and he maintained good to excellent renal function until 50 months post-transplantation. At that time his BUN was 30 mg/100 ml, serum creatinine 2.5 mg/100 ml, and creatinine clearance 38.5 ml/min. This degree of renal dysfunction did not preclude his working daily. However, he required maintenance hemodialysis in early December, 1972 (65 months post-transplantation), and on December 26, 1972, he received a second cadaveric renal allotransplant.

Mechanisms of Allograft Rejection
The immunologic mechanisms of cell-mediated acute allograft rejection, probably the most prevalent type, are depicted diagrammatically in Fig. 17-15.

In the acute forms of rejection, circulating small virgin lymphocytes (T_2-cells) encounter the circulating antigen liberated from the graft; they also "visit" the transplant via the bloodstream, recognize the incompatible HL–A antigens (e.g., recipient: HL–A 1,2; 5,7; donor: HL–A 2,10; 8,13) and become sensitized as a result. These lymphocytes migrate to the regional lymph nodes [52] where they undergo a

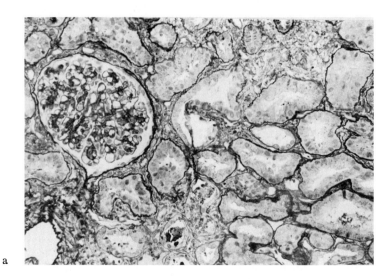

a

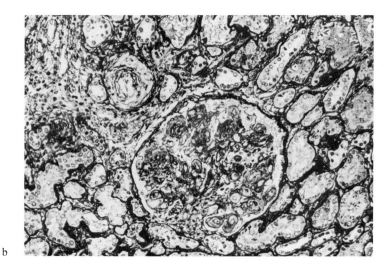

b

Figure 17-14
Chronic rejection. (a) The glomerulus shows a moderate degree of mesangial sclerosis. There is also a moderate degree of interstitial fibrosis (400 × before 20% reduction). (b) The glomerulus shows thickening of the glomerular capillary walls. In this silver stain, splitting of some of the capillary basement membranes is evident. A mild to moderate degree of mesangial sclerosis is present. The arteriole shows evidence of intimal proliferation, splitting, and reduplication of the internal elastic lamina. A mild degree of interstitial

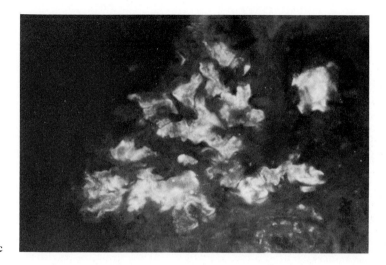

c

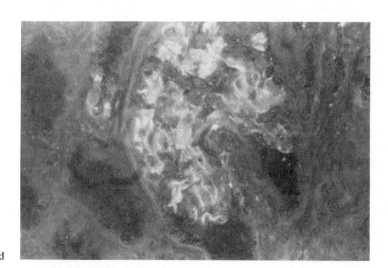

d

fibrosis and early tubular atrophy are present (400 × before 20% reduction). (c) Photomicrograph of the immunofluorescence stain for IgG showing extensive deposition of this immunoglobulin within the glomerulus. Some of the IgG is distributed in a linear pattern. Considerable mesangial staining is evident (600 × before 20% reduction). (d) Photomicrograph of the immunofluorescence stain for IgG showing a linear staining pattern corresponding to the deposition of IgG along the glomerular basement membrane (600% before 20% reduction).

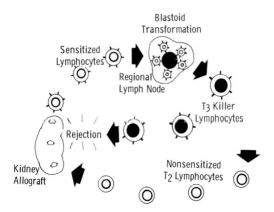

Figure 17-15
Role of lymphocytes in the mechanism of acute allograft rejection. (Adapted from Ritzmann and Daniels [118].)

process of morphologic enlargement and intense biochemical activity known as *blastoid transformation* (Fig. 17-16).

Following this process, activated specific killer cells (T_3-cells) emerge which are directly or indirectly involved in allograft destruction. The large activated T_3 lymphoid cells divide and return to the allografts, destined to initiate and mediate the chain of events which terminates in allograft rejection and graft destruction. Such activated T_3 killer cells elaborate a number of humoral factors (lymphokines), including macrophage migration inhibition factor (MIF), which serves to attract numerous macrophages to the attack sites [22, 37, 38]. Once these T_3 killer cells have defined the situation immunologically, a complex effector system (or *amplification system*) becomes involved in the task of actual graft destruction. This system consists of a cascade of reactions involving the complement system, certain clotting factors, the kinin and op-

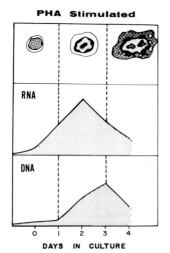

Figure 17-16
Blastoid transformation following lymphocyte stimulation by nonspecific antigens (mitogens such as phytohemagglutinin [PHA]), or by specific antigens (PPD, HL–A antigens, etc.). Correlation of morphological changes (top) with function changes, i.e., increased RNA synthesis (center) and increased DNA synthesis rates (bottom). (From Fischer et al. [42].)

sonin systems, and others [50, 63]. The process by which specifically sensitized T_3 killer cells are produced also gives rise to *memory cells* (T_4-cells), which respond to rechallenge with an exaggerated, anamnestic response to the same antigens.

Lymphocytes possess a dual function. They detect and identify antigenic (e.g., HL–A) differences, and are also endowed with the biologic means to attack such foreign cells, and directly or indirectly, eliminate them. This dual function (described above in connection with allograft rejection) enables the lymphocytes to provide an immunologic surveillance for microorganisms, neoplastic cells, and other manifestations of "non-self" antigenic structures [24, 86], such as histoincompatible allografts.

Survival of allografts and the degree of clinical complications in allotransplanted patients are strongly linked with the ABO and HL–A histocompatibility systems. For this inescapable reason, the selection of donors on a sound immunologic basis is of utmost importance and ultimately determines the degree of success of a given allotransplant program.

Graft versus Host (GvH) Reactions

Definition
GvH reactions [131] result from an immunological situation in which the graft "rejects" its host. Such a situation occurs (a) when significant histocompatibility differences between host and donor exist, and (b) when the immune capacity of the recipient is sufficiently decreased, so that the recipient host is unable to reject immunologically competent allogeneic cells.

This combination of circumstances is fulfilled when HL–A mismatched lymphocytes are transfused into a recipient with compromised cellular immunity (T-cell deficiency). Thus, transfused allogeneic lymphocytes or transplantation of bone marrow cells can produce fatal GvH reactions in patients with certain immune deficiency diseases [54, 58, 64, 79, 89].

Clinical Features
The clinical features of severe GvH reactions in man consist of fever, rash, diarrhea, hepatosplenomegaly, pancytopenia, and rapid death [57]; but in milder cases, the symptoms are less severe and recovery may occur [79].

Clinical Significance
It has been proposed [57] that not only patients with primary immunodeficiencies (diGeorge syndrome; lymphocytopenic Swiss type agammaglobulinemia or combined B/T-cell deficiency; Wiskott-Aldrich syndrome) are at risk, but patients with secondary T-cell deficiencies as

well (induced immunosuppression for control of transplant rejection, Hodgkin's disease, chronic lymphocytic leukemia). The latter group of patients may also include those suffering from T-cell deficiencies associated with acute thermal burns, chronic uremia, and other conditions.

Prevention of GvH Reactions

Blood Transfusions

To minimize the possibility of GvH reactions in immunologically compromised patients, the blood cells must be matched for ABO, Rh, HL–A, and MLC antigens. The number of blood transfusions, and most importantly, the number of transfused lymphocytes, granulocytes, and platelets should be limited to the absolute minimum in order to protect such patients, so far as possible, from the risk of GvH reactions. This may be accomplished by using buffy coat cell-free stored or frozen blood [60]. It should be kept in mind, however, that lymphocytes may cause GvH reactions even after 12 days of storage [46], and may survive more than 3 weeks in citrated stored blood [112].

Bone Marrow and Thymic Allotransplantation

In order to avoid GvH in these systems, it is mandatory to apply strict criteria for immunological donor selection. This includes the compatibility or identity of the ABO, HL–A types, negative MLC tests, and negative cross-match tests for cytotoxic antibodies.

Appendix

Definitions and Nomenclature (Modified from Russell and Monaco [124]).

Currently Preferred Nouns	Previous Nouns	Currently Preferred Adjectives	Previous Adjectives	Modes of Transplants
Autograft	Auto-graft	Autologous	Autologous	Tissue transplants within one individual
Isograft	Iso-graft	Isogeneic (syngeneic)	Isologous	Transplants between identical twins
Allograft	Homo-graft	Allogeneic	Homologous	Transplants between genetically non-identical individuals of the same species
Xenograft	Hetero-graft	Xenogeneic	Heterologous	Grafts between individuals of different species

References

1. ACS/NIH Organ Transplant Registry. Second scientific report. The tenth report of the Human Renal Transplant Registry. *J.A.M.A.* 221: 1486, 1972.
2. ACS/NIH Organ Transplant Registry. Human organ transplantation—world total. Personal communication, March 1, 1973.
3. Ahrous, S. Cytotoxic HL–A antibodies, methodological considerations. *Scand. J. Haemat.* 7:498, 1970.
4. Aird, I., Derek, R. L., and Fraser Roberts, J. A. ABO blood groups and cancer of oseophagus, cancer of pancreas and pituitary adenoma. *Br. Med. J.* 1:1163, 1960.
5. Albert, E. D., Mickey, M. R., and Terasaki, P. I. Genetics of four new HL–A specifications in the Caucasian and Negro populations. *Transplant. Proc.* 3:95, 1971.
6. Albert, E. D., Mickey, M. R., and Terasaki, P. I. Histocompatibility testing: Serology and genetics of the HL–A system. In J. S. Najarian and R. L. Simmons (eds.), *Transplantation.* Philadelphia: Lea & Febiger, 1972, pp. 388–403.
7. Amiel, J. L. Study of the leukocyte phenotypes in Hodgkin's disease. In E. S. Curtoni, P. L. Matting, and R. M. Tosi (eds.), *Histocompatibility Testing.* Copenhagen: Munksgaard, 1967, pp. 79–81.
8. Amos, D. B. Hyperacute rejection. *N. Engl. J. Med.* 280:48, 1969.
9. Amos, D. B., Anderson, E. E., Glenn, J. R., Gunnells, J. C., Lancaster, S. L., Mac-Queen, J. M., Robinson, R. R., Seigler, H. F., Stickel, D. L., and Ward, F. E. Selection of donors for kidney transplantation. In F. T. Rapaport and J. Dausset (eds.), *Tissue Typing Today.* New York and London: Grune & Stratton, 1971, pp. 15–25.
10. *Antilymphocyte globulin* [separate articles]. *Transplant. Proc.* 4:477–479; 481–485; 487–490; 491–495; 497–499; 501–505; 1972.
11. Bach, F. H., and Voynow, N. K. One-way stimulation in mixed leukocyte cultures. *Science* 153:545, 1966.
12. Bach, F. H. Transplantation: Problems of histocompatibility testing. *Science* 159:1196, 1968.
13. Bach, F. H., Meuwissen, H. J., Albertini, R. J., and Good, R. A. "Agammaglobulinemic Leukocytes"—their in vitro reactivity. In W. O. Reike (ed.), *Proceedings of the Third Annual Leukocyte Culture Conference.* New York: Appleton, 1969, pp. 709–723.
14. Bach, J. F., Debray-Sachs, M., Crosnier, J., Kreis, H., and Dormont, J. Correlation between mixed lymphocyte culture performed before renal transplantation and kidney function. *Clin. Exp. Immunol.* 6:821, 1970.
15. Bach, M. L., and Bach, F. H. The genetics of histocompatibility. *Hosp. Practice* 5:33, 1970.
16. Bach, F. H. The immunogenetics of histocompatibility with special reference to the HL–A locus: General anthropological considerations. *Transplant. Proc.* 5:23, 1973.
17. Bach, F., and Bach, M. Revised mixed lymphocyte culture test. In J. G. Ray, R. C. Scott, D. B. Hare, C. E. Harris, and D. E. Kayhoe (eds.), *Manual of Tissue Typing Techniques.* Bethesda, Md.: Trans-

plantation and Immunology Branch. National Institute of Allergy and Infectious Diseases, National Institutes of Health, 1972, pp. 64–66.

18. Batchelor, J. R., and Josey, V. C.   Influence of HL–A incompatibility on cadaveric renal allotransplantation. *Lancet* 2:790, 1969.

19. Beasley, W. H.   Blood groups of gastric ulcer and carcinoma. *Br. Med. J.* 1:1167, 1960.

20. Beathard, G. A.   Renal transplantation and rejection: A review. *Tex. Rep. Biol. Med.* 27:715, 1969.

21. Bertrams, J., Kuwert, U., Böhme, U., Reis, H. E., Galtmeier, W. M., Wetter, O., and Schmidt, C. G.   HL–A antigens in Hodgkin's disease and multiple myeloma. Increased frequency of W–18 in both diseases. *Tissue Antigens* 2:41, 1972.

22. Bloom, B. R., and Bennett, B.   Migration inhibitory factor associated with delayed type hypersensitivity. *Fed. Proc.* 27:13, 1968.

23. Braun, W. E., and Merrill, J. P.   Urine fibrinogen fragments in human renal allografts: possible mechanism of renal injury. *N. Engl. J. Med.* 278:1366, 1968.

24. Burnet, Mac F.   *Immunological Surveillance.* Oxford: Pergamon Press, 1970.

25. Carpenters, C. B., and Winn, H. J.   Hyperacute Rejection (Letter to Editor) *N. Engl. J. Med.* 280:47, 1969.

26. Ceppellini, R., Curtoni, E. S., Matting, P. L., Leighes, G., Visetti, M., and Colombi, A.   Survival of test skin graft in man. Effect of genetic relationship and of blood group incompatibility. *Ann. N.Y. Acad. Sci.* 129:421, 1966.

27. Cepellini, R.   Old and new facts and speculations about transplantation antigens of man. In B. Ames (ed.), *Progress in Immunology.* 1st International Congress of Immunology. New York and London: Academic Press, 1971, pp. 973–1025.

28. Chaplin, H., Jr.   Frozen red cell storage: Perspectives and potentials. In P. J. Schmidt (ed.), *Progress in Transfusion and Transplantation.* Proceedings of the 25th Annual Meeting of the American Association of Blood Banks and 13th Congress of the International Society of Blood Transfusion. Washington, D.C.: American Association of Blood Banks, 1972, pp. 329–342.

29. Clarke, C. A.   The prevention of Rh isoimmunization. *Hosp. Practice* 8:77, 1973.

30. Colombani, J., Colombani, M., and Dausset, J.   Cross-reactions in the HL–A system with special reference to DaG (cross-reacting group). In P. I. Terasaki (ed.), *Histocompatibility Testing 1970.* Baltimore: Williams & Wilkins, 1970, pp. 79–92.

31. Dammin, G. J.   The pathology of human renal transplantation. In F. T. Rapaport and J. Dausset (eds.), *Human Transplantation.* New York and London: Grune & Stratton, 1968, pp. 170–200.

32. Dausset, J., and Rapaport, F. T.   Blood group determinants of human histocompatibility. In F. T. Rapaport and J. Dausset (eds.), *Human Transplantation.* New York and London: Grune & Stratton, 1968, pp. 383–393.

33. Dausset, J., Walford, R. L., Colombani, J., Legrand, L., Feingold, N., Barge, A., and Rapaport, F. T.   The HL–A subloci and their importance in transplantation. *Transplant. Proc.* 1:331, 1969.

34. Dausset, J., and Hors, J.   Analysis of 221 renal transplants: Influence of cross-reactions between donors and recipient HL–A antigens. In F. T. Rapaport and J. Dausset (eds.), *Tissue Typing Today*. New York and London: Grune & Stratton, 1971, pp. 26–32.

35. Dausset, J.   Correlation between histocompatibility antigens and susceptibility to alleles. In R. S. Schwartz (ed.), *Progress in Clinical Imunology*. New York and London: Grune & Stratton, 1972, vol. 1, pp. 183–210.

36. Dausset, J.   Transplantation, clinical correlation with the HL–A system. In P. J. Schmidt (ed.), *Progress in Transfusion and Transplantation*. Proceedings of the 25th Annual Meeting of the American Association of Blood Banks and 13th Congress of the International Society of Blood Transfusion. Washington, D.C.: American Association of Blood Banks, 1972, pp. 257–271.

37. David, J. R.   Macrophage migration. *Fed. Proc.* 27:6, 1968.

38. David, J.   Lymphocyte mediators and cellular hypersensitivity. *N. Engl. J. Med.* 288:142, 1973.

39. Editorial.   Hyperacute rejection. *N. Engl. J. Med.* 279:657, 1968.

40. Falchuk, Z. M., Rogentine, G. N., and Strober, W.   Predominance of histocompatibility antigen HL–A8 in patients with gluten-sensitive enteropathy. *J. Clin. Invest.* 51:1602, 1972.

41. Festenstein, H., Oliver, R. T. D., and Saks, J. A.   A collaborative scheme for tissue typing and matching in renal transplantation: III. A preliminary assessment of the influence of histocompatibility matching grades on the outcome of renal transplantation. In F. T. Rapaport and J. Dausett (eds.), *Tissue Typing Today*. New York and London: Grune & Stratton, 1971, pp. 33–36.

42. Fischer, C. L., Daniels, J. C., Levin, W. C., Kimzey, S. L., Cobb, E. K., and Ritzmann, S. E.   Effects of the space flight environment on man's immune system: II. Lymphocyte counts and reactivity. *Aerosp. Med.* 43:1122, 1972.

43. Forbes, J. F., and Morris, P. J.   Leukocyte antigens in Hodgkin's disease. *Lancet* 2:849, 1970.

44. Freda, V. J.   The control of Rh disease. In R. A. Good and D. W. Fisher (eds.), *Immunobiology*. Stamford, Conn.: Sinauer Associates, 1971, pp. 266–273.

45. Fudenberg, H. H., Pink, J. R. L., Stites, D. P., and Wang, A. G.   *Basic Immunogenetics*. New York: Oxford University Press, 1972, p. 173.

46. Fulginiti, F. A., Hathaway, W. E., Pearlman, D. A., and Kempe, C.H.   Agammaglobulinemia and achondroplasia. *Br. Med. J.* 2:242, 1967.

47. Gewurz, H.   The immunologic role of complement. *Hosp. Practice* 2:45, 1967.

48. Gleason, R. E., and Murray, J. E.   Reports from Kidney-Transplant Registry. Analysis of variable in the function of human kidney transplants. I. Blood group compatibility in splenectomy. *Transplantation* 5:343, 1967.

49. Goldstein, I. M., Eyre, H. J., Terasaki, P. I., Henderson, E. S., and Graw, R. G., Jr.   Leukocyte transfusions: Role of leukocyte alloantibodies in determining transfusion response. *Transfusion* 11:19, 1971.

50. Good, R. A., Bigger, W. D., and Park, H. B.   Immunodeficiency diseases of man. In B. Amos (ed.), *Progress in Immunology*. 1st Inter-

national Congress of Immunology. New York and London: Academic Press, 1971, pp. 699–722.

51. Gordon, J. The mixed leukocyte culture reaction. *Med. Clin. North Am.* 56:337, 1972.

52. Gowans, J. L., and McGregor, D. D. The immunological activities of lymphocytes. *Prog. Allergy* 9:1, 1965.

53. Grumet, F. C., Conhell, A., Bodmer, J. G., Bodmer, W. F., and Mc-Devitt, H. O. Histocompatibility (HL–A) antigens associated with systemic lupus erythematosus. *N. Engl. J. Med.* 285:193, 1971.

54. Hathaway, W. E., Brangle, R. W., Nelson, T. L., and Roeckel, I. E. Aplastic anemia and alymphocytosis in an infant with hypogamma-globulinemia: Graft-versus-host reaction? *J. Pediatr.* 68:713, 1966.

55. Högman, C. F., and Lindbloom, J. B. The probability of donor-recipient histocompatibility in different HL–A-phenotype combinations. *Tissue Antigens* 1:197, 1971.

56. Högman, C., and Lindbloom, J. B. Transplantation—practical laboratory aspects. In P. J. Schmidt (ed.), *Progress in Transfusion and Transplantation*. Proceedings of the 25th Annual Meeting of the American Association of Blood Banks and 13th Congress of the International Society of Blood Transfusion. Washington, D.C.: American Association of Blood Banks, 1972, pp. 243–255.

57. Hong, R., Gatti, R. A., and Good, R. A. Hazards and potential benefits of blood transfusion in immunological deficiency. *Lancet* 2:388, 1968.

58. Hong, R., Kay, H. E. M., Cooper, M. D., Meuwissen, H., Allan, M. J. G., and Good, R. A. Immunological restitution in lymphopenic immunological deficiency syndrome. *Lancet* 1:503, 1968.

59. Hors, J., Fradelizi, D., Feingold, N., and Dausset, J. Critical evaluation of histocompatibility in 179 renal transplants. *Lancet* 1:609, 1971.

60. Huggins, C. E., Russel, P. S., Winn, H. J., Fuller, T. C., and Beck, C. H., Jr. Frozen blood in transplant recipients to avoid hepatitis and/or HL–A sensitization. *Transplant. Proc.* 4:574, 1972.

61. Hulme, B., and Pitcher, P. M. Rapid latex-screening test for detection of fibrin/fibrinogen degradation products in urine after renal transplantation. *Lancet* 1:6, 1973.

62. Hume, D. M., and Rapaport, F. T. Introduction. *Transplant. Proc.* 4:427, 1972.

63. Hunsicker, L. G., Wintroub, B. U., and Austen, K. F. Humoral amplification systems in inflammation. In F. H. Bach and R. A. Good (eds.), *Clinical Immunobiology*. New York and London: Academic Press, 1972, vol. 1, pp. 179–192.

64. Jacobs, J. C., Blanc, W. A., deCapoa, A., Heird, W. C., McGilvray, E., Miller, O. J., Morse, J. H., Rossen, R. D., Schullinger, J. N., and Walzer, R. A. Complement deficiency and chromosomal breaks in a case of Swiss-type agammaglobulinemia. *Lancet* 1:499, 1968.

65. Jersild, C., Svejgaard, A., and Fog, T. HL–A antigens and multiple sclerosis. *Lancet* 1:1240, 1972.

66. Johnson, A. H., Butler, W. T., Rossen, R. D., and Mittal, K. K. Lymphocytotoxic antibody response to cardiac allotransplantation in man: II. Characterization of antigenetic specificities and immunoglobulin class. *J. Immunol.* 105:1432, 1970.

67. Kissmeyer-Nielsen, F., Olsen, S., Petersen, V. P., and Fjeldborg, O.

Hyperacute rejection of kidney allografts associated with preexisting humoral antibodies against donor cells. *Lancet* 2:662, 1966.

68. Kissmeyer-Nielsen, F., and Thorsby, E.   Human transplantation antigens. Appendix: Current methods in histocompatibility testing. *Transplant. Rev.* 4:1, 1970.

69. Kissmeyer-Nielsen, F., Staub Nielsen, L., Lindholm, A., Sandberg, L., Svejgaard, A., and Thorsby, E.   The HL–A system in relation to human transplantation. In P. I. Terasaki (ed.), *Histocompatibility Testing.* Copenhagen: Munksgaard, 1970, pp. 105–135.

70. Kissmeyer-Nielsen, F., Svejgaard, A., Fjelsborg, O., et al.   Scandiatransplant: Preliminary report of a kidney exchange program. In F. T. Rapaport and J. Dausset, *Tissue Typing Today.* New York and London: Grune & Stratton, 1971, pp. 41–51.

71. Kissmeyer-Nielsen, F., Andersen, H., Hauge, M., Kjerbye, K. E., Mogensen, B., and Svejgaard, A.   HL–A types in Danish Eskimos from Greenland. *Tissue Antigens* 1:74, 1971.

72. Kissmeyer-Nielsen, F., Lamm, L., Svejgaard, A., and Thorsby, E. White cell and platelet antigens. In P. J. Schmidt (ed.), *Progress in Transfusion and Transplantation.* Proceedings of the 25th Annual Meeting of the American Association of Blood Banks and 13th Congress of the International Society of Blood Transfusion. Washington, D.C.: American Association of Blood Banks, 1972, pp. 91–100.

73. Koscielak, J., Gardas, A., Gorniak, H., Pacuszko, T., and Piasek, A. Chemistry of the ABO antigens on human erythrocytes. In P. J. Schmidt (ed.), *Progress in Transfusion and Transplantation.* Proceedings of the 25th Annual Meeting of the American Association of Blood Banks and 13th Congress of the International Society of Blood Transfusion. Washington, D. C.: American Association of Blood Banks, 1972, pp. 149–166.

74. Lance, E. M.   Antilymphocyte serum: Mechanism of action. *Transplant. Proc.* 4:473, 1972.

75. Lang, J. M., Oberling, F., Tongio, M. M., Mayer, S., and Waitz, S. Mixed lymphocyte reaction as assay for immunological competence of lymphocytes from patients with Hodgkin's disease. *Lancet* 1:1261, 1972.

76. Lawrence, H. S., and Landy, M. (eds.)   *Mediators of Cellular Immunity.* New York and London: Academic Press, 1969.

77. Lee, H. M., Hume, D. M., Vredevoe, D. L., Mickey, M. R., and Terasaki, P. I.   Serotyping for homotransplantation: IX. Evaluation of leukocyte antigen matching with the clinical course and rejection types. *Transplantation* 5:1040, 1967.

78. Leibowitz, S., and Schwartz, R. S.   Malignancy as a complication of immunosuppressive therapy. In G. H. Stollerman (ed.), *Advances in Internal Medicine.* Chicago: Year Book, 1971, vol. 17, pp. 95–123.

79. Levey, R. H.   The problems and practice of bone marrow transplantation in man: The severe combined immunodeficiency syndrome as the ideal model. *Transplant. Proc.* 4:565, 1972.

80. Lieber, E., Hirschhorn, K., and Fudenberg, H. H.   Response of agammaglobulinaemic lymphocytes in mixed lymphocyte culture. *Clin. Exp. Immunol.* 4:83, 1969.

81. Lischner, H. W., Punnett, H. H., and DiGeorge, A. M.   Lymphocytes in congenital absence of the thymus. *Nature* 214:580, 1967.

82. Mackenzie, I. F. C., and Whittingham, S.   Deposits of immunoglobulin and fibrin in human allografted kidneys. *Lancet* 2:1313, 1968.
83. Marshall, W. C., Cope, W. A., Soothill, J. F., and Dudgeon, J. A.   In vitro lymphocyte response in some immunity deficiency diseases and in intrauterine virus infections. *Proc. R. Soc. Med.* 63:351, 1970.
84. McDevitt, H. O., and Bodmer, W. F.   Histocompatibility antigens, immune responsiveness and susceptibility to disease. *Am. J. Med.* 52:1, 1972.
85. McDevitt, H. O.   Genetic control of the antibody response. *Hosp. Practice.* 8:61, 1973.
86. Meuwissen, H. J., Stutman, O., and Good, R. A.   Functions of lymphocytes. *Semin. in Hematol.* 4:28, 1969.
87. Miggiano, V. C., Bernoco, D., Lightbody, J., Trinchieri, G., and Ceppellini, R.   Cell mediated lympholysis in vitro with normal lymphocytes as target: Specificity and cross-reactivity of the test. *Transplant. Proc.* 4:231, 1972.
88. Milgrom, F., Titrak, B. J., Kano, K., and Witebsky, E.   Humoral antibodies in renal homografts. *J.A.M.A.* 198:226, 1966.
89. Miller, M. E.   Thymic dysplasia ("Swiss agammaglobulinemia"): I. Graft versus host reaction following bone-marrow transfusion. *J. Pediatr.* 70:730, 1967.
90. Mollison, P. L.   Rh immunization and its suppression. In P. J. Schmidt (ed.), *Progress in Transfusion and Transplantation.* Proceedings of the 25th Annual Meeting of the American Association of Blood Banks and 13th Congress of the International Society of Blood Transfusion. Washington, D.C.: American Association of Blood Banks, 1972, pp. 119–133.
91. Morgan, W. T. J., and Watkins, W. M.   The detection of the blood group O and the relationship of the so-called O substance to the agglutinogens A and B. *Br. J. Exp. Pathol.* 29:159, 1948.
92. Morris, P. J., Williams, G. M., Hume, D. M., and Terasaki, P. I.   Serotyping for homotransplantation: XII. Occurrence of cytotoxic antibodies following kidney transplantation in man. *Transplantation* 6:392, 1968.
93. Morris, P. J., Ting, A., and Kincaid-Smith, P.   Leukocyte antigens in renal transplantation: X. A clinical and histological evaluation of matching for HL–A in cadaver renal allotransplantation. In P. I. Terasaki (ed.), *Histocompatibility Testing.* Copenhagen: Munksgaard, 1970, pp. 371–380.
94. Morris, P. J., and Ting, A.   Leukocyte antigens in renal transplantation: IX. Matching for the HL–A system and the early course of cadaveric renal grafts. *Med. J. Aust.* 14:517, 1970.
95. Morris, P. J.   Analysis of histocompatibility in cadaveric renal transplantation. In F. T. Rapaport and J. Dausset (eds.), *Tissue Typing Today.* New York and London: Grune & Stratton, 1971, pp. 52–57.
96. Murray, J. E., Birtch, A., and Wilson, R. E.   Thoracic duct drainage as an aid for immunosuppression in human renal transplantation. *Transplant. Proc.* 4:465, 1972.
97. Naito, S., Namerow, N., Mickey, M. R., and Terasaki, P. I.   Multiple sclerosis: Associated with HL–A 3. *Tissue Antigens* 2:1, 1972.
98. Ogden, D. A., Porter, K. A., Terasaki, P. I., Marchioro, T. L., Holmes, J. H., and Starzl, T. E.   Chronic renal homograft function: Correlation

with histology and lymphocyte antigen matching. *Am. J. Med.* 43:837, 1967.

99. Oliver, R. T. D., Sachs, J. A., Festenstein, H., Pegrum, G. D., and Moorhead, J. F.   Influence of HL–A matching, antigenic strength, and immune responsiveness on outcome of 349 cadaver renal grafts. *Lancet* 2:1381, 1972.

100. Opelz, G., and Terasaki, P. I.   Histocompatibility matching untilizing responsiveness as a new dimension. *Transplant. Proc.* 4:433, 1972.

101. Oppenheim, J. J., Barlow, M., Waldmann, T. A., and Block, J. B.   Impaired in vitro lymphocyte transformation in patients with ataxia-tele-angiectasia. *Br. Med. J.* 2:330, 1966.

102. Patel, R., Terasaki, P. I., and Mickey, M. R.   Serotyping for homo-transplantation: XVI. Analysis of kidney transplants from unrelated donors. *N. Engl. J. Med.* 279:501, 1968.

103. Patel, R., and Terasaki, P. I.   Significance of the positive cross-match test in kidney transplantation. *N. Engl. J. Med.* 280:735, 1969.

104. Patel, R., Mickey, M. R., and Terasaki, P. I.   Leucocyte antigens and disease: I. Association of HL–A2 and chronic glomerulonephritis. *Br. Med. J.* 2:424, 1969.

105. Patel, R., and Myrberg, S.   Value of prospective tissue typing in kidney transplantation between HL–A identical siblings. *Br. Med. J.* 4:709, 1970.

106. Patel, R., and Briggs, N. A.   Limitation of the lymphocyte cytotoxic cross-match test in recipients of kidney transplants having preformed antileukocyte antibodies. *N. Engl. J. Med.* 284:1016, 1971.

107. Patel, R., Habel, M. B., Wilson, R. E., Birtch, A. G., and Moore, F. D.   Histocompatibility (HL–A) antigens and cancer of the breast. *Am. J. Surg.* 124:31, 1972.

108. Pegrum, G. D., Balfom, I. C., Evans, C. A., and Middleton, V. L.   HL–A antigens on leukaemic cells. *Br. J. Haematol.* 19:493, 1970.

109. Penn, I., Hammond, W., Brettschneider, L., and Starzl, T. E.   Malignant lymphomas in transplantation patients. *Transplant. Proc.* 1:106, 1969.

110. Penn, I., and Starzl, T. E.   A summary of the status of De Novo cancer in transplant recipients. *Transplant. Proc.* 4:719, 1972.

111. Perkins, H. A., Kountz, S. L., Payne, R., and Belzer, F. O.   Achievements and limitations of histocompatibility testing for 10 HL–A factors in kidney transplantation. *Transplant. Proc.* 3:130, 1971.

112. Petrakis, N. L., and Politis, G.   Prolonged survival of viable, mitotically competent mononuclear leukocytes in stored whole blood. *N. Engl. J. Med.* 267:286, 1962.

113. Pierce, J. C., Cobb, G. W., and Hume, D. M.   Relevance of HL–A antigens to acute humoral rejection of multiple renal allotransplants. *N. Engl. J. Med.* 285:142, 1971.

114. Pierce, J. C., and Sloane, C. E.   Azathioprine and prednisone. *Transplant. Proc.* 4:457, 1972.

115. Porter, K. A.   Pathological changes in transplanted kidneys. In T. E. Starzl (ed.), *Experience in Renal Transplantation.* Philadelphia: Saunders, 1964.

116. *Questions and Answers about Blood and Blood Banking.* Chicago: American Association of Blood Banks, 1970, p. 5.

117. Reisfield, R. A., and Edidin, M. Histocompatibility antigens: Characterization. In B. Amos (ed.), *Progress in Immunology*. 1st International Congress of Immunology. New York and London: Academic Press, 1971, pp. 1373–1377.
118. Ritzmann, S. E., and Daniels, J. C. Immunology of transplantation. *Tex. Med.* 66:48, 1970.
119. Ritzmann, S. E., Daniels, J. C., Sakai, H., and Beathard, G. A. Abberrations of cellular and humoral immunity in burned patients. In Pan American Medical Association Section on Burns, *Immunological Response*. Nov. 20, 1972, in press.
120. Ritzmann, S. E. Unpublished data.
121. Ritzmann, S. E., Vyvial, T. M., Levin, W. C., and Daniels, J. C. *Tissue Antigens*—submitted for publication.
122. Roberts, J. A. F. Blood groups and susceptibility to disease: A review. *Br. J. Prev. Soc. Med.* 11:107, 1957.
123. Roitt, I. M. *Essential Immunology*. Oxford: Blackwell, 1971.
124. Russell, P. S., and Monaco, A. P. *The Biology of Tissue Transplantation*. Boston: Little, Brown, 1964.
125. Russell, P. S., Austen, K. F., Flax, M. H., and Winn, H. J. Immunopathology of renal transplantation. In P. A. Miescher and H. J. Müller-Eberhard (eds.), *Textbook of Immunopathology*. New York and London: Grune & Stratton, 1969, vol. 2, pp. 752–767.
126. Sakai, H., Groves, L., Townsend, C. M., Jr., and Ritzmann, S. E. Mixed lymphocyte cultures (MLC). In *Workshop Manual, Histocompatibility Assays*. Chicago: American Society of Clinical Pathologists, 1973, pp. 187–203.
127. Sakai, H., Sarles, H. E., Remmers, A. R., Jr., and Ritzmann, S. E. Early detection of human MLC reactions. *Clin. Res.* 21:587, 1973.
128. Sarles, H. E., Thomas, F. D., Remmers, A. R., Jr., Canales. C. O., Smith, G. H., and Beathard, G. A. Review of the actions and effects of immunosuppressive drugs. *Tex. Rep. Biol. Med.* 27:327, 1969.
129. Sarles, H. E., Remmers, A. R., Jr., Fish, J. C., Canales, C. O., Thomas, F. D., Tyson, K. R. T., Beathard, G. A., and Ritzmann, S. E. Depletion of lymphocytes for the protection of renal allografts. *Arch. Intern. Med.* 125:443, 1970.
130. Schwartz, R. S. Immunosuppressive drug therapy. In F. T. Rapaport and J. Dausset (eds.), *Human Transplantation*. New York and London: Grune & Stratton, 1968, pp. 440–471.
131. Simonsen, M. Graft versus host reactions. Their natural history, and applicability as tools of research. *Prog. Allergy* 6:349, 1962.
132. Simonsen, M. Strong transplantation antigens in man. *Lancet* 1:415, 1965.
133. Singal, D. P., Mickey, M. R., and Terasaki, P. I. Serotyping for homotransplantation: XXIII: Analysis of kidney transplants from parental versus sibling donors. *Transplantation* 7:246, 1969.
134. Starzl, T. E., Marchioro, T. L., Holmes, J. H., Hermann, G., Brittain, R. S., Stonington, O. H., Talmage, D. W., and Waddell, W. R. Renal homografts in patients with major donor-recipient blood group incompatibilities. *Surgery* 55:195, 1964.
135. Starzl, T. E., Penn, I., and Halgrimson, C. G. Immunosuppression and malignant neoplasms. *N. Engl. J. Med.* 283:934, 1970.

136. Starzl, T. E., Putnam, C. W., Halgrimson, C. G., Groth, C. G., Booth, A. S., Jr., and Penn, I.   Renal transplantation under cyclophosphamide. *Transplant. Proc.* 4:461, 1972.

137. Starzl, T. E., and Putnam, C. W.   Transplantation immunology. In F. H. Bach and R. A. Good (eds.), *Clinical Immunobiology*. New York and London: Academic Press, 1972, vol. 1, pp. 75–112.

138. Stewart, J. H., Sheil, A. G. R., Johnson, J. R., Wyatt, F. M., Sharp, A. M., and Johnston, J. M.   Successful renal allotransplantation in presence of lymphocytotoxic antibodies. *Lancet* 1:176, 1969.

139. Stickel, D. L., Seigler, H. F., Amos, D. B., Ward, F. E., Price, A. R., and Anderson, E. E.   Immunogenetics of consanguinous allografts in man: II. Correlation of renal allografting with HL–A genotyping. *Ann. Surg.* 172:160, 1970.

140. Stiehm, E. R., Lawlor, G. J., Kaplan, M. S., Greenwald, H. L., Neerhout, R. C., Sengar, D. P. S., and Terasaki, P. I.   Immunologic reconstitution in severe combined immunodeficiency without bone-marrow chromosomal chimerism. *N. Engl. J. Med.* 286:797, 1972.

141. Sturgeon, P.   Erythrocyte antigens and antibodies. In W. J. Williams, E. Beutler, A. J. Erslev, and R. W. Rundles (eds.), *Hematology*. New York: McGraw-Hill, 1972, pp. 1266–1283.

142. Szulman, S. E.   The biological distribution of blood group substances A and B in man. *J. Exp. Med.* 111:785, 1960.

143. Szulman, A. E.   Chemistry, distribution, and function of blood group substances. In A. D. DeGraff and W. C. Creger (eds.), *Annual Review of Medicine*. Palo Alto: Annual Review, 1966, vol. 17, pp. 307–322.

144. Tanigeki, N., Miyakawa, Y., Yagi, Y., and Pressman, D.   HL–A antigens from hematopoietic cell lines: Molecular size and electrophoretic mobility. *J. Immunol.* 107:402, 1971.

145. Tapai, H. R., Holley, K. E., Woods, J. E., and Johnson, W. J.   Causes of death after renal transplantation. *Arch. Intern. Med.* 131:204, 1973.

146. Terasaki, P. I., Trasher, D. L., and Hauber, T. H.   Serotyping for homotransplantation: XIII. Immediate kidney transplant rejection and associated preformed antibodies. In P. I. Terasaki, (ed.), *Advances in Transplantation*. Copenhagen: Munksgaard, 1968, pp. 225–229.

147. Terasaki, P. I., Mottironi, V. D., and Barnett, E. V.   Cytotoxins in disease. Autocytotoxin in lupus. *N. Engl. J. Med.* 283:724, 1970.

148. Terasaki, P. I., Kreisler, M., and Mickey, R. M.   Presensitization and kidney transplant failures. *Postgrad. Med.* 47:89, 1971.

149. Terasaki, P. I., Mickey, M. R., Yamezaki, J. N., and Vrederoe, D.   Maternal-fetal incompatibility: I. Incidence of HL–A antibodies and possible association with congenital anomalies. *Transplantation* 9:538, 1970.

150. Terasaki, P. I., Miyajim, T., Sengar, D. P. S., and Stiehm, E. R.   Extraneous lymphocytic HL–A antigens in severe combined immunodeficiency disease. *Transplantation* 13:250, 1972.

151. Ting, A., Wee, G. B., Simons, M. J., and Morris, P. J.   The distribution of HL–A leukocyte antigens in Singapore Chinese, Malays and Indians. *Tissue Antigens* 1:258, 1971.

152. Tovey, G.   National and international cooperation in transplantation. In P. J. Schmidt (ed.), *Progress in Transfusion and Transplantation*.

Proceedings of the 25th Annual Meeting of the American Association of Blood Banks and 13th Congress of the International Society of Blood Transfusion. Washington, D.C.: American Association of Blood Banks, 1972, pp. 273–284.

153. Townsend, C. M., Jr., Sakai, H., Ritzmann, S. E., and Fish, J. C. Lymphocyte reactivity in patients with regional enteritis. *Surg. Forum* 23:394, 1972.

154. Townsend, C. M., Jr., Sakai, H., Fish, J. C., and Ritzmann, S. E. T-cell functions in patients with inflammatory bowel disease. *Clin. Res.* 21:97, 1973.

155. Townsend, C. M., Jr., Sakai, H., Fish, J. C., and Ritzmann, S. E. Disparity of the T-cell functions in patients with regional enteritis. *J. Reticuloendothel. Soc.* 13:344, 1973.

156. Van Hooff, J. P., Van der Steen, G. J., Schippers, H. M. A., and Van Rood, J. J. Efficacy of HL–A matching in eurotransplant. *Lancet* 2:1385, 1972.

157. Van Rood, J. J., Von Leeuwen, A., and Bruning, J. W. The relevance of leukocyte antigens for allogeneic renal transplantation. *J. Clin. Pathol.* 20:504, 1967.

158. Van Rood, J. J., and Earnisse, J. G. The detection of transplantation antigens in leukocytes. *Semin. Hematol.* 5:187, 1968.

159. Van Rood, J. J. Tissue typing and organ transplantation. *Lancet* 1:1142, 1969.

160. Van Rood, J. J., Van Leeuwen, A., Freudenberg, J., and Rubinstein, P. Prospects in host-donor matching. *Transplant. Proc.* 3:1042, 1971.

161. Van Rood, J. J., Van Leeuwen, A., Freudenberg, J., and Rubinstein, P. Prospects in host-donor matching. In F. T. Rapaport and J. Dausset (eds.), *Tissue Typing Today*. New York and London: Grune & Stratton, 1971, pp. 64–72.

162. Van Rood, J. J. The (relative) importance of HL–A matching in kidney transplantation. In B. Amos (ed.), *Progress in Immunology*. 1st International Congress of Immunology. New York and London: Academic Press, 1971, pp. 1027–1043.

163. Van Rood, J. J. Transplantation, a serological introduction. In P. J. Schmidt, *Progress in Transfusion and Transplantation*. Proceedings of the 25th Annual Meeting of the American Association of Blood Banks and 13th Congress of the International Society of Blood Transfusion. Washington, D.C.: American Association of Blood Banks, 1972, pp. 231–242.

164. Villari, P. The history of Girolomo Savanarola and his times. Cited in R. A. Kilduffe and M. DeBakey, *The Blood Bank and the Technique and Therapeutics of Transfusion*. St. Louis: Mosby, 1942, pp. 17–18.

165. Vyvial, T. M., Remmers, A. R., Jr., Sarles, H. E., Fish, J. C., Lindley, J. D., Beathard, G. A., and Ritzmann, S. E. Specificity of cytotoxic antibodies. Assay for anti-I, anti-P+P_1 and heterophile antibody activity. *Transplantation* 10:559, 1970.

166. Walford, R. L., Gallager, R., and Sjaarda, J. R. Serologic typing of human lymphocytes with immune serum obtained after homografting. *Science* 144:868, 1964.

167. Walford, R. L. Production and analysis of HL–A typing serums. A

seminar on histocompatibility testing. Annual Meeting of the American Association of Blood Banks, San Francisco: 1970, pp. 37–44.

168. Walford, R. L., Finkelstein, S., Neerhout, R., Konrad, P., and Shanbrom, E. Acute childhood leukaemia in relation to the HL–A human transplantation genes. *Nature* 225:461, 1970.

169. Ward, F. A. *A Primer of Immunology*. New York and London: Appleton, 1970, pp. 1–130.

170. Watkins, W. M. Blood group substance. *Science* 152:172, 1966.

171. Wiener, A. S. *Blood Groups and Transfusion*. Springfield, Ill.: Thomas, 1943, reprinted. New York: Hafner, 3rd ed., p. 438.

172. Williams, G. M., Hume, D. M., Hudson, R. P., Jr., Morris, P. J., Kano, K., and Milgrom, F. "Hyperacute" renal-homograft rejection in man. *N. Engl. J. Med.* 279:611, 1968.

173. Wintrobe, M. M. Blood groups and blood transfusion. In M. M. Wintrobe (ed), *Clinical Hematology*. Philadelphia: Lea & Febriger, 1967, 6th ed., pp. 367–409.

174. Wolf, J. S. Extracorporeal irradiation of blood as an immunosuppressive agent. *Transplant. Proc.* 4:469, 1972.

175. Wonham, V. A., Winn, H. J., and Russell, P. S. Serotyping and genetic analysis in the selection of related renal allograft donors. *N. Engl. J. Med.* 284:509, 1971.

176. Workshop "Blood Group Antigens." Chairmen: E. A. Kabat and W. M. Watkins. In B. Amos (ed.), *Progress in Immunology*. 1st International Congress of Immunology. New York and London: Academic Press, 1971, pp. 1169–1173.

177. Yamada, T., and Kay, J. H. Kidney homotransplantation with special reference to cytotoxic antibody response. *Surgery* 63:637, 1968.

178. Yankee, R. A., Grumet, F. C., and Rogentine, G. N. Platelet transfusion therapy. The selection of compatible platelet donors for refractory patients by lymphocyte HL–A typing, *N. Engl. J. Med.* 281:2308, 1969.

179. Yust, I., Schwartz, J., and Dreyfuss, F. A cytotoxic serum factor in polyarteritis nodosa and related conditions. *Am. J. Med.* 48:472, 1970.

180. Zervas, J. D., Delamore, I. W., and Israels, M. C. G. Leukocyte phenotypes in Hodgkin's disease. *Lancet* 2:634, 1970.

181. Zmijewsky, C. M., and Fletcher, J. L. Preoperative assessment of histocompatibility. *Arch. Intern. Med.* 123:524, 1969.

182. Zmijewsky, C. M. *Immunohematology*. New York: Appleton, 1972, 2nd ed., pp. 214–274.

18

Tissue Typing Techniques in the Clinical Laboratory

Stephan E. Ritzmann, Theona M. Vyvial,
Hideto Sakai, and Jerry C. Daniels

E valuation of histocompatibility for allotransplantation includes assays for the ABO blood group system, HL–A tissue antigens, reactivity, and preformed cytotoxic antibodies (see Chapter 17). Therefore, the methodology for these assays will be described.

The ABO System

Cell Preparation
In connection with histocompatibility assays for organ allotransplantation, venous blood is used for the various aspects of ABO blood group typing and cross matching (Fig. 18-1).

ABO Typing
The principle of ABO blood group typing is simple [22]. Two separate mixtures of the blood being tested are prepared, either in test tubes or on open slides, with two different testing sera called anti-A and anti-B, respectively. These sera are added to aliquots of an individual's blood and examined for the presence or absence of clumping (agglutination) of the red cells (Fig. 18-2) [13].

Blood types may be identified by 4 possible combinations which determine whether a person's blood is type A, B, AB, or O. These letters correspond to the type of antigenic substance that is an inherited characteristic of the red blood cell.

A. Type A blood has A substance on the red blood cells, and anti-B antibodies in the plasma.

B. Type B blood has B substance on the red cells, and anti-A antibodies in the plasma.

C. Type AB blood has both A and B substances on the red cells, but neither anti-A nor anti-B antibodies in the plasma.

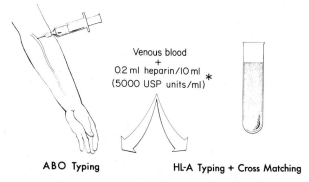

Figure 18-1
Preparation of venous blood used for both ABO typing and cross-matching, and HL–A typing and cross-matching.

D. Type O blood has neither A nor B substance on the red cells, but both anti-A and anti-B antibodies in the plasma.

Blood groups are determined as follows (see Fig. 18-2): On the left side of a glass slide, a drop of serum containing anti-A substance is placed. On the right, a drop of serum containing anti-B substance is placed. A drop of a person's blood being typed is then added to each drop of antiserum and mixed. After rotation or tilting of the slide, observations are made for one of four possibilities visible to the unaided eye.

A. If the anti-A serum alone causes the red cells to clump (agglutinate), the blood is type A.

B. If the anti-B serum alone causes the red cells to clump (agglutinate), the blood is type B.

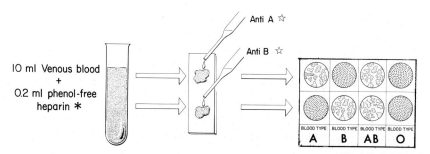

Figure 18-2
ABO typing: How blood types are determined [13, 21]. See text for detailed description.
☆ Anti-A, Anti-B blood grouping serum: Dade.
* Heparin: Riker.

C. If both anti-A and anti-B sera cause the red cells to clump (agglutinate), the blood is type AB.
D. If neither anti-A nor anti-B sera cause the red cells to clump (agglutinate), the blood is type O.

Cross-Matching
To assure minimal risk of incompatibility, cross-matching of the red
cells is performed. There are two types of cross-matches: (a) the *major
cross-match,* or the incubation of the prospective donor's red cells with
the recipient's serum; and (b) the *minor cross-match,* or the incubation
of the recipient's red cells with the prospective donor's serum. In each
case, the cell suspensions are incubated, centrifuged, and examined for
antibody reactions (agglutination).

Coombs' Test
The final step of red blood cell compatibility testing is carried out: the
indirect antiglobulin or indirect Coombs' test (see Fig. 18-3). The cell

Table 18-1. Blood Group Antibodies—Characteristics.

Functional Denomination	Definition	Immunoglobulin Class
1. Naturally occurring antibodies	Present without any known antigenic stimulants (e.g., anti-A, B, I)	IgM
2. Immune antibodies	Formed as a result of exposure to foreign antigens (e.g., transfusion, pregnancy)	IgG
3. Complete antibodies	Agglutinate saline-suspended red cells (e.g., anti-A, B, H, I)	IgM
4. Incomplete antibodies	Do not agglutinate saline-suspended red cells	IgG
5. Cold antibodies	React maximally with red cells at 4° C	IgM
6. Warm antibodies	React maximally with red cells at 37° C	IgG
7. Blocking antibodies	Thought to block the reaction with red cells	IgG
8. Saline antibodies	See 3	IgM
9. Coombs' antibodies	Agglutinate red cells in the presence of Coombs' serum, see 2	IgG

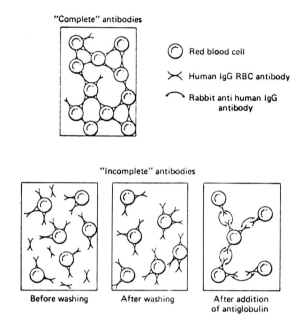

"Complete" antibodies

◯ Red blood cell

✕ Human IgG RBC antibody

⌒ Rabbit anti human IgG antibody

"Incomplete" antibodies

Before washing   After washing   After addition of antiglobulin

Figure 18-3

"Complete" and "incomplete" antibodies. Reaction of complete antibodies: No Coombs' test needed. Reaction of incomplete antibodies: Coombs' test needed to "enlarge" the IgG–anti-red cell antibody to bridge the gap between two adjacent cells leading to agglutination. (The so-called *non-γ type of Coombs' test* is based on the identical principle, with the substitution of antibody to human complement components for the anti-human IgG antibody as the bridging antibody. This test may be positive in patients whose red cells carry such complement components as a reflector of immune sensitization.) Indirect Coombs' test: Detects incomplete antibodies in the serum. Direct Coombs' test: Detects incomplete antibodies on red cells. (With permission from Fudenberg, Pink, Stites, and Wang, *Basic Immunogenetics,* Oxford University Press [5]).

suspensions are washed in saline solution, Coombs' serum (antiglobulin serum) is added, and the suspensions are then centrifuged and examined for agglutination. No reaction confirms a negative cross-match test. This approach detects errors in ABO typing, irregular antibodies in the recipient's serum that are directed against the donor's red cells, and in the case of the minor cross-match, donor antibodies directed against the recipient's red cells.

Blood Group Antibodies

Blood group antibodies belong usually to the IgM or IgG classes. They are further distinguished by their functional characteristics (Table

18-1). Complete antibodies (usually identical with IgM class antibodies; synonyms: naturally occurring antibodies, cold antibodies, saline antibodies) agglutinate red blood cells in saline suspensions. In contrast, the incomplete antibodies (usually identical with IgG class antibodies; synonyms: immune antibodies, warm antibodies, blocking antibodies, Coombs' antibodies), do not directly agglutinate saline-suspended red cells. These IgG antibodies are not large enough to bridge the gap between adjacent red cells, in contrast to the larger complete IgM molecules. The red cells can be brought close enough together to allow IgG molecules to agglutinate by altering the electrical forces which repel two cells (zeta potential). This can be done by adding bovine albumin, or enzymes such as trypsin. Another way of detecting IgG incomplete antibodies is by means of the antiglobulin (Coombs') test (see Fig. 18-3).

Incomplete antibodies usually produce no agglutination when blood group antibodies are added to red cells. These antibodies are detected by subsequent washing of the coated red blood cells to remove all extraneous proteins, followed by the addition of a rabbit antiserum to human globulin (Coombs' serum). The antiglobulin reacts with the incomplete antibodies on the red cells and causes agglutination.

Application to Allotransplantation
See Chapter 17, Immunologic Donor Selection.

HL–A System

A variety of techniques is available for the detection of HL–A antigens and the assay for anti-HL–A (cytotoxic) antibodies [1, 8, 17]. In general, these are the agglutination and cytotoxicity techniques [7, 9, 20]. The following procedure is most widely used in the United States (Fig. 18-4).

Microdroplet Lymphocyte Cytotoxicity One-Stage Method of Terasaki [17, 18]: Lymphocyte Preparation

MATERIALS AND REAGENTS
A. Phenol free heparin (Riker)
B. Heparinized blood (0.2 ml phenol free heparin + 10 ml venous blood)
C. Fisher Centrifuge Model No. 59 (Fisher)
D. Fisher centrifuge tubes (Fisher)
E. Anti-A, Anti-B blood grouping sera (Dade)
F. Anti-H (*Ulex europaeus* seeds) (Schumacher)
G. Ficoll (Pharmacia)
H. Isopaque (75% metrizoat) (Nyegaard)
 I. Beckman Spinco Microfuge Model No. 152 (Beckman)
 J. Beckman Centrifuge Microtest Tube (Beckman)

K. Hank's balanced salt solution (Grand Island)
L. McCoy's 5a medium with 30% fetal calf serum (Grand Island)
M. Microdroplet typing trays (Falcon Microtest Tissue Culture Plate No. 3034)
N. Hamilton Syringe No. 705, Cat. 83726 (50 μl with PB 600 repeating dispenser) (Hamilton)
O. Hamilton Syringe No. 725, Cat. 83725 (250 μl with PB 600 repeating dispenser)
P. Hamilton Syringe No. 1001 with PB 600 repeating dispenser (Hamilton)
Q. Multiple needle dispenser (6 20-gauge needles embedded in plastic) (Aoki)
R. Hamilton Syringe No. 1002 with PB 600 repeating dispenser and multiple needle dispenser)
S. Microcover slide: 50 × 75 mm (Clay Adams)
T. Nikon Model M Inverted Microscope (Dolan)
U. Pasteur pipette

USING FRESHLY DRAWN BLOOD (Fig. 18-4a) [21]
1. Place 2 ml of heparinized blood into 2-ml centrifuge tubes.
2. Centrifuge for 2 min at 3,500 g.
3. Remove the buffy coat and place in a dispo beaker containing 0.3 ml of anti-A, B, or H, depending on ABO blood type.
4. Agglutinate red blood cells by mixing on rotator for 5 min.
5. Place the suspension in a Fisher tube and spin for 3 sec at 1,000 g to remove the agglutinated red cells.
6. Layer the supernatant onto 0.3 ml Ficoll-Isopaque mixture in a Fisher tube. Centrifuge for 3 min at 2,000 g.
7. Remove the hazy white interface and place in a Beckman centrifuge tube. Centrifuge for 10 sec at full speed (controlled by a transformer, approximately 1,000 g) in a Beckman Microfuge.
8. Discard the supernatant and suspend the lymphocytes in Hank's BSS, mixing well with a Pasteur pipette.
9. Centrifuge for 10 sec at full speed in a Beckman Microfuge. Discard the supernatant and resuspend the lymphocytes in 0.4 ml McCoy's 5a medium with 30% fetal calf serum.
10. Centrifuge for 3 sec at $\frac{1}{3}$ speed (approximately 3,500 g in Beckman Microfuge) to remove large clumps and debris. Transfer upper $\frac{3}{4}$ to a new Beckman tube and adjust cell count to $1 - 2 \times 10^3/$ mm^3 using phase contrast microscopy.

BLOOD MAILED INTO THE LABORATORY (utilizing Terasaki Mailing Bags and Supplies) (Life Instrumentation) [21]
1. Place the blood-filled cotton pad into a 50 ml syringe and add 8 ml of normal saline solution; squeeze into a 20 ml centrifuge tube.
2. Centrifuge 10 min at 500 g in a clinical centrifuge.

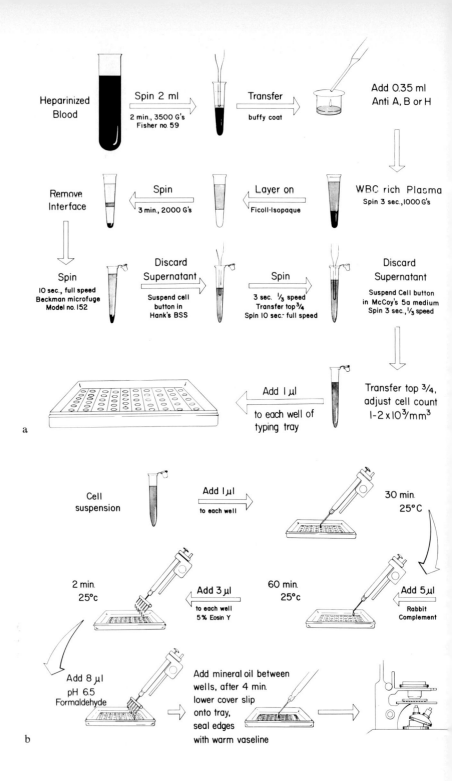

a

b

3. Transfer the buffy coat to a Fisher tube and spin 2 min at 3,500 g (this step concentrates the lymphocytes).
4. Remove the buffy coat and agglutinate the red blood cells as described in the previous procedure.
5. Remove the agglutinated red cells by spinning for 3 sec at 1,000 g in Fisher centrifuge.
6. Transfer the supernatant to a Beckman tube and spin for 10 sec at full speed to agglutinate any remaining red cells.
7. Discard the supernatant and gently resuspend the cells in Hank's BSS with a Pasteur pipette; this separates the lymphocytes from the clumped red cells.
8. Spin 3 sec at ⅓ speed to remove residual red cell clumps, transfer the lymphocyte-rich supernatant to a new Beckman tube and spin for 10 sec at full speed (this washes out the red cell-agglutinating antiserum).
9. Discard the supernatant and resuspend the button in 0.4 ml McCoy's 5a medium. Centrifuge for 3 sec at ⅓ speed to remove debris.
10. Transfer supernatant to another Beckman tube, adjust cell count to $1–2 \times 10^3/mm^3$ using phase contrast microscopy.

HL–A Typing and Cross-Matching for Cytotoxic Antibodies

MATERIALS AND REAGENTS
A. Typing tray (NIH) [21]
B. Freezer to $-70°$ C
C. 50 μl multiple repeating dispenser
D. Cell suspension
E. Incubator at $25°$ C
F. Rabbit complement stored in liquid nitrogen
G. 5% aqueous Eosin Y
H. 1,000 μl syringe fitted with multiple needle dispenser
I. Formaldehyde (pH 6.5–7.0)
J. 2,500 μl syringe fitted with multiple needle dispenser
K. Heavy mineral oil
L. 50×75 mm glass slide
M. Heated vaseline (to seal tray)

HL–A PROCEDURE FOR TYPING (Fig. 18-4B)
1. Remove typing trays from $-70°$ C and thaw just before use.
2. Thoroughly mix the cell preparation and, with a 50 μl multiple repeating dispenser, add 0.001 ml cell suspension to each well, being careful not to touch the antisera with the needle.

Figure 18-4
HL–A typing and cross-matching. (a) Blood and cell preparation; (b) procedures.

3. Ascertain that all cells and antisera are mixed, and incubate for 30 min at 25° C.
4. Add 0.005 ml rabbit complement (stored in liquid nitrogen) to each well with a 250 µl multiple repeating dispenser, and incubate for 60 min at 25° C.
5. Add 0.003 ml of 5% aqueous Eosin Y to each well with a 1,000 µl syringe fitted with a multiple needle dispenser.
6. After 2 min gently add 0.008 ml formaldehyde (pH 6.5–7.0) to each well, using a 2,500 µl syringe fitted with a multiple needle dispenser.
7. After 4 min add heavy mineral oil between the wells and lower a 50 × 75 mm glass slide onto the wells, seal with heated petroleum jelly to prevent evaporation and siphoning off of fluid from individual wells.

PROCEDURE FOR CROSS-MATCH TESTS FOR CYTOTOXIC ANTIBODIES
   Standard technique [21]
1. Prepare lymphocyte suspension as previously described.
2. Collect fresh serum samples from prospective recipients and dilute 1:2, 1:4.
3. Prepare recipient serum spectrum as follows (by this method one recipient can be tested in a row of 6 wells): 1 µl 1:4 dilution of patient's serum; 1 µl 1:2 dilution of patients' serum; 1 µl of patient's whole serum; 3 parts of whole serum (3 µl) (i.e., 3:1); 6 parts patient's serum (i.e., 6:1); and 9 parts of patient's serum (i.e., 9:1).
4. Add lymphocytes to wells as described before.
5. After 30 min at 25° C add rabbit complement.
6. After 60 min at 25° C add Eosin Y and formaldehyde.
7. Seal trays and interpret results as described below.

Double time procedure (to evoke increased sensitivity of the test)
1. Prepare lymphocytes and serum spectrum as described in the previous section.
2. Add lymphocytes to tray and incubate for 60 min at 25° C.
3. Add rabbit complement and incubate for 120 min.
4. Add Eosin Y and formaldehyde and seal as described.
5. Interpret results as described below [21].

"Contamination" by Blood Transfusion
"Antigenic contamination" by blood transfusion poses a major obstacle in evaluating the effects of various blood group and HL–A antigens in renal allotransplanted patients. The theoretical contamination of the recipient's leukocytes with leukocytes from a single unit of blood is shown in Table 18-2.

This "contamination" of blood by HL–A-bearing lymphocytes, granulocytes, and platelets poses additional problems in the prospective allograft recipients. The required hemodialysis and blood transfusions often result in presensitization of transplant recipients by the formation of cytotoxic antibodies, with the attendant danger of hyperacute rejection of allografts. Van Rood [19] refers to this dilemma: "It is evident that as long as we are not better informed on the immune potential of our patients, giving blood transfusions and hoping for the best is playing Russian roulette with the prognosis of the graft at stake." Clearly, HL–A typing of blood for such patients ought to be performed. It is imperative that the blood transfusions are obtained from donors who are either HL–A identical or compatible. Using a blood donor pool of 1685 Dutch individuals, an average of 8.4 HL–A identical donors and patients was found [19].

Interpretation of Results
The grading of the results of the cytotoxicity assay is based upon the degree of cell death in the lymphocytotoxicity tests both for HL–A typing and for cytotoxic antibodies. Examples of these reaction grades are shown in Fig. 18-5.

There are several modes of expressing the results of HL–A typing, including the A to F classification of Terasaki et al. [10], net histo-compatibility ratio of Rapaport and Dausset [14], and the use of re-sponsiveness [11]. The A–E classification of Terasaki is based upon estimation of the number of mismatched HL–A antigens (see Fig. 17-4).

Application to Allotransplantation
See Chapter 17, Immunologic Donor Selection.

Mixed Lymphocyte Cultures (MLC)

MATERIALS AND REAGENTS
A. Heparin (Riker)
B. 6% Gentran 75 (Dextran 75) in 0.9% NaCl (Travenol)
C. Ficoll (Pharmacia)

Table 18-2. Theoretical Contamination of Patient's WBC with Leukocytes from a Single Unit of Blood.

Blood volume	6,000 ml
WBC	7,000/mm^3
Polymorphonuclear granulocytes	50%
Lymphocytes	30%
Transfusion volume	500 ml
% contamination	8.3% granulocytes with granulocytes
	13.9% lymphocytes with granulocytes
	5% granulocytes with lymphocytes

SOURCE: C. M. Zmijewsky, *Immunohematology* (2d ed.), New York: Appleton, 1972.

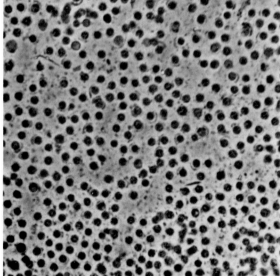

a

b

Figure 18-5
HL–A Reactions. (a) Negative reaction: viability is same as in controls. (b)
Positive reaction: viability is clearly different from that of controls (10–90%
cell death).

D. Hypaque, Sodium 50% (W/V) (Winthrop)
E. Working Ficoll solution: Solution A: 9.54 gm Ficoll + 106 ml distilled water. Solution B: 50 ml Hypaque + 23.5 ml distilled water. Mix 106 ml solution A + 44 ml solution B; sterilize by autoclaving.
F. International Centrifuge Model HN–S (Scientific Products)
G. Medium 199 (1 X with Hank's Salts and L-glutamine) (Grand Island)
H. Human AB serum: Sterile, decomplemented, stored at −20° C
 I. Owen Oval Prescription Bottle (Jefferson)
 J. Mitomycin C, 2 mg/ampule (Nutritional Biochemicals)
K. H^3-Thymidine, 6.0 c/m mole (Schwarz-Mann)
L. Thymidine (Sigma)
M. Trichloracetic Acid (Curtin)
N. Hydroxide of hyamine (Packard)
O. Diatol Scintillation Cocktail: POPOP 150 mg (Scintillation Grade, Packard)
P. PPO (Scintillation Grade, Packard)—5 gm
Q. 1,4 Dioxane (Spectroquality, Curtin)—500 ml
R. Naphthalene (Curtin)—100 ml
S. Methanol (Spectroquality, Curtin)—300 ml
T. Toluene (Spectroquality, Curtin)—500 ml
U. Liquid scintillation counter (Packard, Nuclear Chicago, or Beckman)
V. Incubator at 37° C; at 5% CO_2 atmosphere

PROCEDURE

Culture preparation [4, 12, 16].   Strict sterile technique is required throughout preparation and culture procedures.

1. Obtain 30 ml venous blood and mix with 0.5 ml phenol free heparin from the following: potential donor, recipient, and two healthy, unrelated persons (controls).
2. Add 3 ml 6% Dextran to each sample, mix, and sediment red cells for 40 min at 37° C.
3. Layer the leukocyte-rich supernatant onto 3 ml working Ficoll solution, the final supernatant-to-Ficoll ratio should be 4:1. Centrifuge for 30 min at 1,000 g.
4. Remove the interface (91–96% lymphocytes) and mix with 5–10 ml Medium 199 and centrifuge for 10 min at 1,000 g.
5. Decant the supernatant and resuspend the cell button in 2 ml 10% human AB serum in Medium 199.
6. Calculate the amount of suspension needed to provide each of the 23 cultures with 0.75×10^6 responding cells (see Table 18-3 for cell combinations).
7. After removal of the necessary cell suspension from step 6, restore the responding cell suspension to 2 ml with Medium 199. Recon-

Table 18-3. Cell Combinations for MLC.

Cell	Response	Location
R.Dm R.Dm' R.Dm"	MLC response	Patient
D.Rm D.Rm' D.Rm"	MLC stimulation	Patient
R.Am R.Am' R.Am"	Positive control	Patient
R.Rm R.Rm' D.Dm D.Dm'	Negative control	Patient and donor
A.Bm A.Bm' A.Bm" B.Am B.Am' B.Am"	Positive controls	Normal adults (controls)
A.Am A.Am' B.Bm B.Bm'	Negative controls	Normal adults (controls)

R	= Recipient's responding cells	B	= Control B's responding cells
Rm*	= Recipient's stimulating cells	Bm*	= Control B's stimulating cells
D	= Donor's responding cells	m*	= Mitomycin C-treated stimulating cells
Dm*	= Donor's stimulating cells	m'	= duplicate cultures
A	= Control A's responding cells	m"	= triplicate cultures
Am*	= Control A's stimulating cells		

stitute 2 mg mitomycin C with 2 ml Medium 199, prepare a 1:4 dilution of the mitomycin C using Medium 199 as a diluent.

8. Add 0.20 ml diluted mitomycin C to the cell suspension, incubate at 37° C for 20 min. Wash the treated cells twice with 5 ml Medium 199, centrifuge at 200 g for 6 min for each wash.

9. Following the last wash, suspend the cells in 2 ml Medium 199 with 10% AB serum. Calculate the amount of suspension needed to provide each of the cultures with 1.25×10^6 stimulating cells.

10. Add the amount of suspension calculated in step 9 to the cultures, bring the total volume of each culture combination to 2.5 ml using Medium 199 with AB serum, and incubate in a 5% CO_2 atmosphere for 7 days.

HARVESTING PROCEDURE
1. On day 7, sterility of the cultures is documented by blood agar plates, the media color is noted (see Sources of Error) and 2 μc H^3-thymidine are added to each culture. The cultures are reincubated for 5 hours, then each is transferred to an appropriately labeled centrifuge tube.
2. The harvesting procedure consists of a series of washes at 200 g for 6 min each:
   a. One wash with 10 ml saline solution containing 100 mg/liter thymidine
   b. Repeat with 5 ml saline solution/thymidine.
   c. Two washes with 5% trichloroacetic acid (TCA). NOTE: Completely resuspend button with a wooden stick after each TCA wash.
   d. One wash with methanol.
3. Add 0.5 ml hydroxide of hyamine and let stand at room temperature for 20 min.
4. Dilute each culture into scintillation vials with 15 ml Diatol.
5. Cap the vials tightly and place in scintillation counter. Results are reported in DPM/culture (Disintegrations/minute/culture; DPM = counts/minute $\div$ counting efficiency of H^3).

COUNTING AND CALCULATION PROCEDURE.   A sample scintillation counter print-out for a positive MLC culture is presented:

E. S. Ratio	Sample No.	Time (min)	Gross Count	Count/Min
0.4608	116	10.00	80543	8054.3

Efficiency of H^3 is obtained from the standard quench curve by using the E.S. Ratio (External Standard Ratio).

$$\frac{CPM}{\text{Efficiency of } H^3} = \frac{8054.3}{0.2247} = 35,843 = DPM/culture$$

SOURCES OF ERROR
A. Color changes of the media indicate pH changes or bacterial contamination. An alkaline pH of the media (purple color) may result in depressed MLC response; results from such cultures cannot be utilized.
B. Contamination is indicated by yellow media and bacterial growth on blood agar plates. This may cause spuriously positive counts; results from such cultures cannot be accepted.
C. AB serum including cytotoxic antibodies and/or immunosuppressive agents may depress the MLC activity.
D. Red cell fragments in the interface may cause a high degree of quenching in the scintillation counter.
E. Contamination by polymorphonuclear leukocytes may cause erroneously low results.

Table 18-4. Examples of Negative and Positive MLC Results.

Lymphocyte Combinations	HL–A Matching Grades	MLC Response of Recipient
Recipient A vs. potential donor for A	A (HL–A identity)	484 DPM/culture
Recipient B vs. potential donor for B	C (one HL–A antigen mismatch)	48,343 DPM/culture

F. Careless washing procedures during the culture harvest may result in low radioactivity counting.
G. Inaccurate cell counting or calculations lead to erroneous results.
H. The multitude of technical steps involved in this procedure invites errors (e.g., adding inappropriate reagents or cells), so that alert caution is required throughout the procedure.

INTERPRETATION OF RESULTS.   Normal mean values and 90th percentile normal ranges, obtained from 72 healthy adults, have been found to be as follows:
    Normal mean values: 47,332 DPM/culture; and
    90th percentile normal range: 14,862–96,796 DPM/culture
A. MLC values in the positive range (within the normal range obtained from unrelated pairs) reflect histoincompatibility (Table 18-4, bottom). Abnormally high DNA synthesis rates in "negative control" cultures (MLC of autologous cells) may be observed in patients with certain infectious diseases, as well as in contaminated cultures.
B. Decreased MLC values (below the normal range) reflect either (a) high degree of histocompatibility (Table 18-4, top) or (b) lack of immunocompetent lymphocytes. Technical reasons for low MLC values can be excluded by the strong MLC response obtained from simultaneous MLC with lymphocytes from two unrelated healthy adults (stimulatory controls).

APPLICATION TO CLINICAL ALLOTRANSPLANTATION.   See Chapter 17, Immunologic Donor Selection, MLC.

APPENDIX
    Micromethod of MLC.   Recently, Hartman et al. [6] introduced a micromethod of MLC. The advantage of this technique is the economic use of lymphocytes and supplies. Lymphocytes are cultured in 0.2 ml of medium, in small wells of plastic trays. The culture conditions are essentially the same as those described for the standard MLC procedure. At 96 hours of culture, 2 μc of H^3-thymidine are added to the wells, and

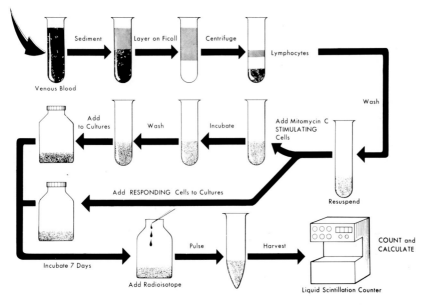

Figure 18-6
MLC procedures. (From Sakai, Groves, Townsend, and Ritzmann [16].)

then the whole culture is incubated for an additional 20 hour period. At the end of the harvesting, individual cultures are aspirated and washed by a semiautomatic cell aspirator (Hiller; Microbiological Associates). Radioactivity in the cells, which are trapped on small glass filters, is then determined by liquid scintillation spectrophotometry. The results are expressed as DPM/culture.

Rapid MLC.   The standard MLC test requires 4 to 7 days [2, 3], which renders this test impractical for immunologic selection of cadaveric donors for organ allotransplantation. A technique has recently been developed [15] which allows the detection of MLC reaction within 24 hours of culture. Peripheral blood lymphocytes are obtained by Ficoll density gradient centrifugation [12]. One $\times$ 10^6 responding cells are cultured with 1×10^6 mitomycin C-treated autologous cells [2] or allogeneic stimulating cells in 2.5 ml of 10% homologous AB serum in TC–199 with HEPES buffer (Gibco), in 5% CO_2–air at 37° C. At 18.5 hours of culture, the MLC is washed with, and resuspended in 1.0 ml of leucine free MEM (Gibco). The cell suspensions are then pulsed with 2 μc of H^3-leucine (51 C/mM, Schwarz-Mann) in 5% CO_2–air at 37° C for 5 hours. The cells are washed 3 times with saline solution containing 1 mg/ml of nonradiolabeled L-leucine. The radioactivity is determined by liquid scintillation spectrophotometry, the results are expressed as DPM/culture, and a stimulation index is calculated.

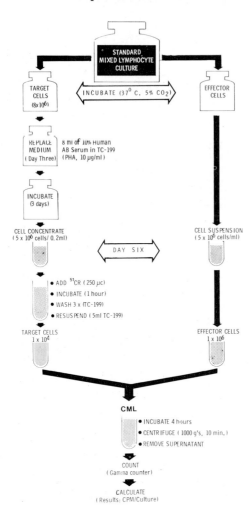

Figure 18-7
CML procedure. (From Sakai, Groves, Townsend, and Ritzmann [16].)

Cell-mediated lymphocytolysis (CML). MLC cultures are prepared as depicted in Fig. 18-6. Simultaneously, the lymphocytes used as stimulating cells in these MLC are cultured separately to be used as target cells (Fig. 18-7). After 3 days of culture, these target cells are washed and resuspended in fresh medium with phytohemagglutinin (PHA). PHA increases the sensitivity of the test system. At the end of the sixth day, these PHA-treated target cells are labeled with Cr^{51} and added to the MLC, which has been prepared simultaneously. The optimal ratio of the target cells and the effector cells in CML is about 1:100. The cell mixtures are incubated for 4 hours and then centrifuged. The radioactivity released from the target cells, determined in a γ-ray counter, reflects the degree of the cell-mediated lymphocytolysis of the target cells [24].

References

1. Ahrous, S.   Cytotoxic HL–A antibodies, methodological considerations. *Scand. J. Haematol.* 7:498, 1970.
2. Bach, F. H., and Voynow, N. K.   One-way stimulation in mixed leukocyte cultures. *Science* 153:545, 1966.
3. Bach, J. F., Debray-Sachs, M., Crosnier, J., Kreis, H., and Dormont, J. Correlation between mixed lymphocyte culture performed before renal transplantation and kidney function. *Clin. Exp. Immunol.* 6:821, 1970.
4. Cutts, J.   *Cell Separation—Methods in Hematology.* New York: Academic Press, 1970, pp. 49–54, 125–126.
5. Fudenberg, H. H., Pink, J. R. L., Stites, D. P., and Wang, A. C.   *Basic Immunogenetics.* New York: Oxford University Press, 1972, pp. 1–214.
6. Hartman, R. J., Segall, M., Bach, M. L., and Bach, F. H.   Histocompatibility matching: VI. Miniaturization of the mixed leukocyte culture tests: A preliminary report. *Transplantation* 11:268, 1971.
7. Högman, C., and Lindbloom, J. B.   Transplantation—practical laboratory aspects. In P. J. Schmidt (ed.), *Progress in Transfusion and Transplantation.* Proceedings of the 25th Annual Meeting of the American Association of Blood Banks and 13th Congress of the International Society of Blood Transfusion. Washington, D.C.: American Association of Blood Banks, 1972, pp. 243–255.
8. Kissmeyer-Nielsen, F., Lamm, L., Svejgaard, A., and Thorsby, E. White cell and platelet antigens. In P. J. Schmidt (ed.) *Progress in Transfusion and Transplantation.* Proceedings of the 25th Annual Meeting of the American Association of Blood Banks and 13th Congress of the International Society of Blood Transfusion. Washington, D.C.: American Association of Blood Banks, 1972, pp. 91–100.
9. Kissmeyer-Nielsen, F., and Van Rood, J. J.   Micro-agglutination test. In J. G. Ray, R. C. Scott, D. B. Hare, C. E. Harris, and D. E. Kayhoe (eds.), *Manual of Tissue Typing Techniques.* Bethesda, Md.: Transplantation and Immunology Branch, National Institute of Allergy and Infectious Diseases, National Institutes of Health, 1972.
10. Lee, H. M., Hume, D. M., Vredevoe, D. L., Mickey, M. R., and Terasaki, P. I.   Serotyping for homotransplantation: IX. Evaluation of leukocyte antigen matching with the clinical course and rejection types. *Transplantation* 5:1040, 1967.
11. Opelz, G., and Terasaki, P. I.   Histocompatibility matching utilizing responsiveness as a new dimension. *Transplant. Proc.* 4:433, 1972.
12. Parker, K. L., Schreinemachers, D. M., and Meuwissen, H. J.   Lymphocyte recovery, purification, and stimulation. *Transplantation* 14:135, 1972.
13. *Questions and Answers about Blood and Blood Banking.* Chicago: American Association of Blood Banks, 1970, p. 5.
14. Rapaport, F. T., and Dausset, J.   Ranks of donor-recipient histocompatibility for human transplantation. *Science* 167:1260, 1970.
15. Sakai, H., Sarles, H. E., Remmers, A. R., Jr., and Ritzmann, S. E. Early detection of human MLC reactions. *Clin. Res.* 21:587, 1973.

16. Sakai, H., Groves, L., Townsend, C. M., Jr., and Ritzmann, S. E.   Mixed lymphocyte cultures (MLC). In *ASCP Workshop Manual, Histocompatibility Assays*. Chicago: American Society of Clinical Pathologists, 1973, pp. 187–203.
17. Terasaki, P. I., and McClelland, J. B.   Microdroplet assay of human serum cytotoxins. *Nature* 204:998, 1964.
18. Terasaki, P. I.   Microdroplet lymphocyte cytotoxicity test. In A. L. Brand and J. G. Ray (eds.), *Manual of Tissue Typing Techniques*. Bethesda, Md.: Transplantation and Immunology Branch, National Institute of Allergy and Infectious Diseases, National Institutes of Health, 1970, pp. 42–45.
19. Van Rood, J. J.   The (relative) importance of HL–A matching in kidney transplantation. In B. Amos (ed.), *Progress in Immunology*. 1st International Congress of Immunology. New York and London: Academic Press, 1971, pp. 1027–1043.
20. Van Rood, J. J.   Transplantation, a serological introduction. In P. J. Schmidt (ed.), *Progress in Transfusion and Transplantation*. Proceedings of the 25th Annual Meeting of the American Association of Blood Banks and 13th Congress of the International Society of Blood Transfusion. Washington, D.C.: American Association of Blood Banks, 1972, pp. 231–242.
21. Vyvial, T. M., Kiamar, M. S., Townsend, C. M., Jr., and Ritzmann, S. E.   B. ABO system, Inc. In *ASCP Workshop Manual, Histocompatibility Assays*. Chicago: American Society of Clinical Pathologists, 1973, pp. 135–149.
22. Wiener, A. S.   *Blood Groups and Transfusion*. Springfield, Ill.: Thomas, 1943, 3rd ed., reprinted New York: Hafner, 1962, p. 438.
23. Zmijewsky, C. M.   *Immunohematology*. New York: Appleton, 1972, 2nd ed., pp. 214–274.
24. Miggiana, V. C., Bernoco, D., Lightbody, J., Trinchieri, G., and Ceppellini, R.   Cell mediated lympholysis in vitro with normal lymphocytes as target: Specificity and crossreactivity of the test. *Transpl. Proc.* 4:231–239, 1972.

19

Laboratory Tests for the Diagnosis and Evaluation of Human Tumors

M ajor advances have been made in the field of tumor immunology, and several excellent reviews on various aspects of tumor
immunology have been written [25, 52, 87, 88, 91, 102, 118,
124, 139, 162, 163, 164, 165]. The most significant advances have been
made in the development of sensitive in vitro assay procedures. At the
present time, most of the procedures are employed as basic and clinical
research tools. However, one can anticipate that some of the methods will
become routine procedures in a hospital clinical laboratory for (a) the
diagnosis of human tumors, (b) the evaluation of the immune status of
the patient, and (c) the selection and monitoring of therapy. In this
chapter an attempt will be made to cover certain aspects of human tumor
immunology briefly, but with emphasis on methods and topics of general
interest to clinical laboratory workers.

Hypotheses as to the Nature of Malignancy

Cancer may be a nonspecific reaction of the host to a large variety of
factors similar to the inflammatory response, or a disease with a common
mechanism which is triggered off and influenced by a wide variety of
factors such as viruses, genes, and chemical and physical agents. The
factor involved in a particular tumor may be single or multiple.

Immunologic Aspects in the Theory of Cancer

Any mechanism which would result in the aberration or imbalance of
the immune surveillance mechanism of the host immune system is related
to the development of neoplasms. In the immunologic theory of cancer
forwarded by Green in 1954 [72], tumor cells become malignant because they have lost tissue specific antigens and are no longer subject to
tissue homeostatic control mechanisms. Autoimmune disease may predispose to malignancy [73]. Goudie [70] has suggested that the association of malignant changes with organ specific autoimmune disease

527

possibly results from the autoimmune selection of tumor cells. The auto-immune attack of the tissue specific site would lead to a loss of a component characteristic of the tissue which is involved in the homeostatic control mechanisms. The mechanism of action of autoantibody in the induction of malignancy is consistent with Green's hypothesis of the immunologic theory of cancer.

Chemical Carcinogens

Chemical carcinogens form strong attachments to cellular macromolecules of DNA, RNA, and protein [154]. With the same chemical carcinogen, each new tumor has unique properties of its own unique antigenic specificity, regardless of the similar morphologic appearance, in contrast to the virus-induced tumor. Tumors induced by the same virus in different species display identical tumor antigens specific for the inducer virus, whereas several tumors of one host induced by the same chemical carcinogens may show individually specific neoantigens [73, 101, 175]. Absence of immunologic cross-reactivity in certain antigens by methylcholanthrene-induced and dimethylaminoazobenzene-induced tumors has been demonstrated. The neoantigens in chemically induced tumors are best demonstrated by in vitro serologic techniques such as immunodiffusion and immunofluorescence.

Viruses

The widespread presence of oncogenic RNA viruses in mammalian cells leads to the recent hypothesis that viruses are the causative agents of most naturally occurring cancer in man [2, 133, 186]. Depending on the host genome and environmental factors, the latent viral genome may code from virus replication or may effect malignant transformation of host cells. One theory proposes that certain viruses, such as those of the highly oncogenic Papova group, become activated upon additional infection with a syncitium-inducing paramyxovirus. This phenomenon is observed in sclerosing panencephalitis following measles, in multifocal leukoencephalopathy-associated measles, and in multifocal leukoencephalopathy associated with Hodgkin's disease.

In humans, one tumor associated virus is the Epstein virus, which is a herpes virus associated with Burkitt's lymphoma and infectious mononucleosis [133]. Best candidates for the induction of natural tumors are those related to the RNA-containing leukomogenic and tumor-inducing viruses, since they are ubiquitous and spread vertically and may exist within the host cell. The viral genome may be suppressed by the genome of the host cell; however, upon injury such as exposure to radiation, chemicals, or other viruses, suppression of the viral genome of the host may be abolished. The unmasking of the viral genome initiates reproduction of the RNA and coating for synthesis of viral proteins. The genome may consist of two major parts, one part for coating for the resynthesis of viral particles and components, and the other part carrying information for malignant transformation of the host cell. Defective viral particles may replicate in the host without causing malignant transformation, but immunosuppression or autoimmune reaction may result in the virus carrier host. Such tumor cells carrying defective virus possess tumor-associated transplantation antigen.

Physical Agents

The carcinogenic effect of ionizing radiation is well known. However, the exact pathogenesis of radiation carcinogenesis is not always known. In animals, radiation and chemicals may activate latent oncogenic viruses and cause immunosuppression which can contribute to the neoplastic alteration.

Genetic Factors

The genetic factors are important in several human tumors. Retinoblastoma is an example which follows an autosomal dominant inheritance [122]. Chromosomal defects have been found in chronic granulocytic leukemia [137], chronic lymphocytic leukemia [74], Waldenström's macroglobulinemia [32], and Burkitt's lymphoma [104].

Antigenic and Surface Membrane Modification of Tumors

Antigens which are present in tumor cells but absent in normal cells have been called tumor specific antigens. Antigens able to induce an immune response or resistance to tumor growth in the autochthonous host have been called tumor specific transplantation antigens [91]. However, the presence of many of these antigens in normal tissue depends upon the age and types of normal cells examined. Many embryonic antigens have been discovered in certain fetal and tumor tissues and are undetectable in normal adult tissue. Thus, some antigens may be phase specific rather than tumor specific [7].

Thus, the term *tumor-associated antigen* is a more appropriate term, for the antigen associated with the tumor can be qualitatively, quantitatively, or temporally different from normal cells [91]. Similarly, the term *tumor-associated transplantation antigen* should be used. The tumor cells when compared to their normal counterparts may show

A. Deletion of normal surface cell antigens
B. Formation of tumor-associated transplantation antigens (TATA)
C. Retrogressive dedifferentiation with formation of fetal antigens
D. Membrane alteration with changes in composition and immunochemical reactivity

Deletion of Normal Surface Cell Antigens

Deletion and loss of cellular antigens have been noted in many human tumors [73]. Many of the human epithelial cancers show an early loss of the blood group antigens A, B, and H. Davidsohn and co-workers [29, 31, 105] have tested for the presence of A, B, and H antigens in human cancer and used the procedure for the early immunologic diagnosis of carcinoma. The cell surface structure may combine with a carcinogen and act as neoantigens, leading to antibody production, and the autoantibody would result in deletion of the surface antigen [73].

Tumor-Associated Transplantation Antigen (TATA)
The TATA are under genetic control and are transmitted from each generation of cells to the next. Tumors which are induced by chemical carcinogens or by physical agents such as radiation are unique in that each tumor has its own antigenic specificity. Tumor specific antigens induced by viruses show similar antigenic specificity, since each tumor induced by a single virus contains the same tumor specific antigens on the surface.

DNA tumor viruses form viral coantigens which are less readily detected on the surface of the tumor cells, whereas the RNA viruses are demonstrable on both the membrane and the cytoplasm. On the membrane the RNA viruses form buds. A unique aspect of the RNA viruses is a coantigen which is a RNA dependent RNA polymerase called *reverse transcriptase* [2]. Most of the evidence on virus-induced antigens is confined to the animal system; however, there is evidence available that Burkitt's lymphoma, melanomas, neuroblastoma of infancy, osteogenic sarcoma, bladder tumors, and Hodgkin's disease may be possibly virus induced [2, 25, 133].

Embryonic or Fetal Antigens in Human Cancer
Postulated during the events of carcinogenesis is a depressive dedifferentiation or retrodifferentiation which leads to increased expression of the genetic information which is normally repressed in the mature cell. This leads to formation of fetal or embryonic components of the cell. There has been increasing evidence that in normal individuals there is formation of small amounts of fetal antigens with formation of tumor. There is a reversion of the cell to the embryonic form, and the fetal antigens are formed in increasing amounts and released into the circulation. Therefore, the measurement of fetal antigens and a quantitative factor in large amounts are practically diagnostic of some form of tumor; however, extremely small amounts may be found in normal individuals and in other benign conditions. Some of the fetal antigens which have been found in human tumor are as follows:

A. Carcinoembryonic antigens of the gastrointestinal tract [62, 63]
B. α_1-fetoprotein antigen produced in liver and hepatomas [1, 5]
C. α_2-H ferroprotein, which is found in sera of children with tumor [14]
D. Regan alkaline phosphatase (placental alkaline phosphatase) [53, 54, 55, 134]
E. Fetal sulfoglycoprotein antigen [75, 76, 77]
F. γ-fetoprotein (heterophile fetal antigen) [34, 35]

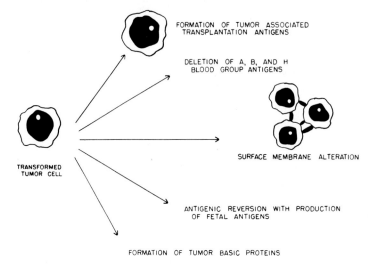

Figure 19-1
Antigen and surface membrane modifications in human tumors.

Membrane Alterations of Tumor Cells

The tumor cell membrane has been altered, and the many properties which make it different from normal membranes are not confined only to a loss in acquisition of antigens. There is a change in distribution of the density of normal membrane macromolecules which may be demonstrated by differences in the interaction of normal and transformed cells with carbohydrate-containing proteins such as concanavalin A, wheat germ agglutinin, and soy bean agglutinin [135, 136, 157]. Transformed cells are more susceptible to agglutination than normal cells by the plant agglutinins such as concanavalin A and wheat germ agglutinins. Also, transformed tumor cells may show little or no tendency to aggregate after exposure of cell membrane to trypsin digestion, whereas normal cells tend to adhere and aggregate when treated with trypsin [33].

It is also known that lipids are extensively changed in the tumor cell membranes, affecting the distribution of other antigens [155]. The substances combine with membrane sites which are more accessible in the tumor cells than in normal cells, and the position and binding density of the binding sites are altered in the course of the malignant transformation (Fig. 19-1).

General Laboratory Tests for the Detection of Tumor-Associated Antigens and Humoral Antibodies

The basic principle to measure circulating antibodies to tumor cells is to measure the interaction of serum immunoglobulins with the patient's tumor or a specific component. Different tests can be employed to detect tumor antigens. Circulating antigens can be detected by standard immunochemical techniques such as (a) double diffusion, (b) electro-immunodiffusion, and (c) radioimmunoassay. Antigens which are found in tumor tissue and not released in appreciable quantities in the serum can be detected by the (a) cytotoxic test, (b) colony inhibition test, (c) immunofluorescence test, and (d) electron microscopy.

Cytotoxic Test

In this test, tumor cells must be obtained in a viable state. The antibodies will react with the surface of the tumor cells in the presence of complement and cause lysis [9]. The cytotoxic reaction can be measured by the ability of the viable cells to prevent certain vital dyes such as trypan blue or eosin from entering the cytoplasm [156]. Also, the cells may be labeled with radioactive chromium and the release of radioactive chromium following a cytotoxic reaction may be measured [13, 17].

Circulating cytotoxic antibodies to human melanoma have been studied by the cytotoxic method. Cell suspensions are made from freshly removed tumor and cultured and grown on coverslips [119]. The viable cells will adhere to coverslips; and the addition of serum containing cytotoxic antibody, will cause the cells to round up and fall away from the coverslip [118]. The degree of cytotoxicity is measured by comparison of the test serum with controls.

A microplate method requiring small numbers of tumor cells has been used to measure cytotoxicity. The plastic plate contains small wells in which the tumor cells are seeded; then serum dilutions containing cytotoxic antibody and complement are added to the wells. After incubation and washing of plates, the viable cells remain attached while the dead cells are washed away. The adherent cells may be stained with trypan blue or examined with a phase contrast microscope [119].

Inhibition of Tumor Cell Growth or Colony Formation

Many human tumors can be grown in tissue culture and have the ability to form colonies [79, 80, 81, 85, 86]. The effect of adding antibody-containing sera to the cultures can be measured. The system has been used to measure cytotoxic antibodies [85], cell-mediated immune response [80, 81], and also to demonstrate blocking or enhancing antibodies [86].

Immunofluorescence Tests

The immunofluorescence method has been used in the detection of the presence of tumor antibodies and antigens in a wide variety of tumors [69, 118]. The tumor cells can be frozen and fixed on slides before appropriate antisera are added. In many cases, viable tumor cell suspensions are used to react surface membrane antigens with the antibody.

Usually an indirect fluorescence method is employed to detect the primary tumor antigen and antibody reaction. However, a direct method is often employed for the detection and localization studies of specific tumor antigens.

Electron Microscopy

The electron microscope is an excellent tool to localize the site of tumor antigen-antibody reactions on the cell surface or cytoplasm [8]. The ferritin-labeled or enzyme-labeled antibody method may be employed.

Tests for the Evaluation of Cell-Mediated Immune Reactions to Tumors

The T-lymphocytes play a part in cellular immunity to cancer. The lymphocytes have specific receptors which interact with the tumor antigen and which can be directly and indirectly involved in the destruction of target cells bearing the tumor antigen. The target cell can be directly destroyed by immediate contact with a sensitized lymphocyte bearing the specific receptor [178]. The sensitized lymphocyte in turn can interact with the surface-bound or free antigen, and it is stimulated to proliferate and produce a number of highly potent soluble factors [111, 143]. The soluble factors have certain biologic and chemical properties, and similar factors can be released from lymphocytes regardless of the specificity of the immunologic reaction. The soluble factors include (a) migration inhibitory factor, which prevents macrophages from migrating; (b) lymphotoxin, a cytotoxic factor; (c) blastogenic factor, which causes transformation of sensitized lymphocytes; (d) chemotactic factors, which attract neutrophils, eosinophils, and macrophages; (e) skin reactive factor, which can produce an inflammatory reaction similar to the delayed hypersensitivity type in the skin of guinea pigs; and (f) interferon, which helps the host cells to become resistant to virus infection.

There are two other soluble factors which are produced by lymph nodes, but their production is not contingent upon specific antigen stimulation. These factors are (a) lymph node permeability factor, which increases local vascular permeability [183], and (b) the transfer factor [112, 113], which has immunologic specificity. The transfer factor is a dialyzable substance from lymphocytes which is most likely a polynucleotide. The administration of the transfer factor can confer on nonimmune recipients the ability to demonstrate specific cellular immune reactions to the specific antigens to which the donor has been sensitized. The transfer factor confers on the nonsensitive human recipient and his lymphocytes the cellular immunologic memory mechanisms found in the donor. The transfer factor isolated from selected donors can be used to treat immune deficiency diseases, cases of disseminated intracellular infections, and cancer patients [112, 113].

Delayed Skin Reactions

Delayed hypersensitivity reactions to intradermal inoculation of autologous tumor antigens have been demonstrated for a number of human tumors including malignant melanoma, Burkitt's lymphoma, acute leukemia, fibrosarcoma, and carcinoma of the breast, colon, lung, stomach, and ovary [38, 95, 166].

It is difficult to evaluate positive skin test reactions because of the complexity of the tumor antigens, and because of problems of relating to an adequate number of control patients. Oren and Herberman [142] studied delayed cutaneous hypersensitivity reactions to membrane extracts of human tumor cells. They observed that positive reactions were seen in 50% of the nonanergic cancer patients; the incidence of positive reactions in normals was less than 10%. Also, they observed that the protein concentration of the tumor antigen used in the test was important, since high protein concentrations of test antigen may elicit positive reactions in both the patients and the normal controls. In a study of immune reactivity of leukemic patients to autologous blast cells, Leventhal et al. [116] observed that positive skin tests tended to correlate inversely with the activity of the disease. The patients usually showed positive skin tests during remission which may become negative during relapse. One can conclude that immune reactivity of patients to their own leukemic cells does exist and can be used to monitor therapy. The leukemic patients were also studied with the mixed leukocyte culture test and lymphocyte cytotoxicity test, and these tests did not appear to correlate with one another [116].

The cellular immune mechanisms in a particular patient to specific tumors can be evaluated in the laboratory by various in vitro tests.

Lymphocyte Transformation Tests

The transformation of lymphocytes in vitro by antigens has been applied to the study of glioblastoma, leukemia, and breast cancer as well as to many other tumors [139].

Colony Inhibition Test

In this method the ability of tumor cells to divide and form colonies is measured under various conditions. Sensitized lymphocytes will inhibit colony formation. The method has been used extensively to detect tumor specific cellular immunity [80, 82, 85].

Cytotoxic Plaque Assay Tests

In this method, when immune lymphocytes are placed on a sheet of tissue culture tumor cells, a plaque is formed [71, 82]. The sensitized lymphocytes will cause focal destruction of tumor cells at the point of application. The procedure has been used to study cellular immunity to postnasal carcinoma [22].

Inhibition of Migration of Macrophages
When sensitized lymphocytes are exposed to tumor antigens a migration inhibitory factor is produced. This test has been used to detect cellular immunity in cases of breast cancer and can be used to study a wide variety of tumors [25, 139].

Antigens Associated with Human Cancer

Epstein-Barr Virus (EBV)-Related Antigens
The EBV-related antigens may be found in cultured lymphoblastoid tumor cells. Antibodies to EBV antigens were observed in high titers, too, in patients with Burkitt's lymphoma, nasopharyngeal carcinoma, infectious mononucleosis, sarcoidosis, and Crohn's disease [89, 90, 92, 96, 103, 133]. The demonstration of antibody to EB virus may have limited diagnostic usefulness since 70–85% of normal adults have antibodies against the Epstein-Barr virus. The detection of virus antibody will have little diagnostic value except in terms of fluctuation in titers of the virus antibody.

Sarcoma Antigens
The sarcoma (S) antigens have been noted in cultured cells of human sarcomas. Similar to EBV antigens, antibodies to human sarcoma antigens are found commonly in the human population [57, 130, 131, 184]. Patients with sarcomas and persons in close contact show high titers of antibody to certain of the sarcoma (S) antigens.

Malignant Melanoma Antigens
Two classes of melanoma antigens have been demonstrated with human serum [97, 119, 131, 137]. The first is a common intracellular antigen found in all malignant melanomas, and the second is a cell surface antigen which is specific for each individual tumor. High titers of antibody to intracellular melanoma antigen are found in patients with malignant melanoma, whereas the cell surface antibodies are seen only in the serum of patients from whom the melanoma cells are taken [117].

Tumor-Associated Antigen in Hodgkin's Disease
Order and co-workers [141] have shown by an indirect immunofluorescence method that a tumor-associated antigen may be seen in tumor tissue from cases of Hodgkin's disease. This would correlate with the observation that the presence of many lymphocytes in the tissue of cases of Hodgkin's indicates a more favorable prognosis [6].

*Antigens Specific for Human Lymphocytic and
Myeloid Leukemia*
Metzgar and co-workers [126] have shown that antigens specific for lymphocytic and myeloid leukemic cells are present. Antisera were pro-

duced in monkeys following the injection of human leukemic cells. The monkey antisera are type specific and can detect antigens that distinguish chronic lymphocytic leukemia or acute lymphocytic leukemia from acute and chronic myelogenous leukemia. The antigens detected on the leukemic cells are lost by digestion with trypsin or neuraminidase.

Cytolipin H and T-Globulin
Tal and co-workers [170, 171, 172] have presented evidence of a T-globulin in the serum of cancer patients and pregnant women at delivery. The T-globulin apparently is not detected in the serum of patients with other diseases or in normal individuals. The T-globulin is capable of combining with a lipid, ceramide-lactoside (cytolipin H) which is found in high concentration in the membrane of tumor cells and in trophoblastic tissue. The hypothesis is that the cytolipid H cancer antigen complex will stimulate the appearance of a specific anticeramide-lactoside globulin in the serum of cancer patients [171]. Since the ceramide-lactoside hapten of the tumor cell antigen is not soluble in aqueous media, a simple direct serologic test with serum T-globulin is not available. Tal and Halperin [172] made antisera to T-globulin in rabbits and detected T-globulin in cancer patients by an immunoelectrophoretic technique in which the globulin fraction of the patient reacted with rabbit antisera. The presence of T-globulin and the value and significance of the test still remain to be confirmed.

Basic Protein Antigens in Human Cancer
Field and Caspary [21, 41] noted that the lymphocytes of cancer patients with an early malignant tumor are sensitized to basic proteins of cancer and nervous tissue. The patients show a much greater sensitivity to basic proteins extracted from cancer as compared to basic proteins derived from the brain and central nervous system. On the basis of their fundamental observations, Field and Caspary have developed a macrophage electrophoretic migration (MEM) test for malignant disease. The nature of cellular sensitivity to basic proteins and the MEM test are discussed in greater detail below.

Tests for Embryonic or Fetal Antigens and Their Significance in Human Cancers
These antigens may be active during fetal life, not expressed during adult life, and reactivated in tumor and disease states by a mechanism of depressive dedifferentiation [7, 67, 175].

Carcinoembryonic Antigen (CEA)
Carcinoembryonic antigen (CEA) was first discovered by Gold and Freedman in 1965 [62, 63]. The CEA antigen was found to be present in adenocarcinomas of the gastrointestinal tract and embryonic and

fetal digestive systems during the first two trimesters [62, 63, 67]. The CEA is found on the surface of the cells by fluorescence microscopy [65, 180] and is found in the glycocalyx of intestinal cells [66, 180].

Excellent preparations of CEA have been isolated from tumors of the digestive tract [26, 107] and found in two molecular sizes of 6.8 S and 10.1 S. The 6.8 S molecular size is the one usually present in the various tumors [26]. Preliminary studies of CEA indicated it was a glycoprotein [108]. Amino acid sequence studies of CEA preparations from two different tumors suggest that the polypeptide chains are identical [173]. However, the material carrying the CEA activity may or may not be identical with the protein [173]. A heterosaccharide grouping with a high content of N-acetyl-glucosamine may be the major immunologic determinant of CEA [12]. The CEA preparations have been found to cross-react with a glycoprotein of normal tissue [123, 181] and the fetal sulfoglycoprotein antigen of cancerous gastric juice [77].

HUMAN ANTI-CEA ANTIBODIES.   There has been some controversy as to the existence and nature of anti-CEA antibodies in human patients. In 1967, with the use of a bis-diazotized benzidine hemagglutination technique, Gold [64] demonstrated IgM anti-CEA antibodies in 70% of 30 patients with nonmetastatic digestive system cancers, and in approximately 70% of 18 women in all trimesters of pregnancy. Burtin and co-workers showed that circulating antibodies in patients with colon-rectal cancer could be absorbed out by preparations of normal bowel tissue [27, 179]. Other investigators could not demonstrate circulating antibodies to CEA in patients with gastrointestinal malignancies with a sensitive radioimmunoassay method [27, 121]. Gold and co-workers [61] demonstrated that anti-CEA antibodies were present in patients with digestive and nondigestive system cancers and in pregnant women by use of a radioimmunoelectrophoresis method. Further, there was a degree of cross-reactivity among CEA, blood group A substance, and anti-A antibodies combined with CEA [61]. The addition of blood group A substance fails to alter the binding of anti-CEA antisera to ^{125}I-CEA. This differentiates the "A-like" site of the CEA from the major antigenic site. The human anti-CEA antibodies do not appear to play any significant role in the protection of the host against the tumor.

There is some evidence that the immune response to CEA in the adult host is not significant. The in vitro tests of the lymphocytes from patients with gastrointestinal cancer in the presence of CEA failed to demonstrate transformation and increased tritiated thymidine incorporation [115]. With the use of the colony inhibition assay, Hellström et al. [84] have demonstrated cellular sensitivity of the lymphocytes of patients with gastrointestinal cancer against human colonic carcinoma.

Skin reactions of the delayed hypersensitivity type were observed in 17 of 19 patients with carcinoma of the colon and rectum when soluble membrane fractions of autologous tumor cells were used as antigens

[93]. Further studies of the soluble fractions of human intestinal tumors showed that the skin reactive intestinal cancer antigen was separate and distinct from CEA [94].

LOCALIZATION OF CEA BY IMMUNOFLUORESCENCE IN NORMAL AND TUMOR TISSUE.   The CEA antigen was noted to be on the surface and glycocalyx of intestinal tumors, fetal cells [180], and colonic cells of normal children [16]. Burtin and co-workers [15] studied intestinal polyps of various histologic types by immunofluorescence. They detected CEA reactive antigen in normal intestinal mucosa as well as in all intestinal polyps independent of their state of differentiation. The CEA appeared more abundant in differentiated polyps than in the undifferentiated polyps. The localization of CEA in normal tissue may be explained by the presence of normal glycoproteins which can cross-react with CEA [123, 181].

ASSAY FOR CEA IN CIRCULATION.   A hemagglutination inhibition test has been reported for CEA [109]. The preliminary result showed that all 33 patients with endodermally derived carcinoma gave positive results. Also, positive results were seen in some controls and in 60% of patients with rectal polyps, chronic ulcerative colitis, and cirrhosis.
    Thompson and co-workers developed a radioimmunoassay for CEA [174]. Briefly, the method involves the following:
1. Glycoproteins are extracted from the serum with perchloric acid. The material is dialyzed, lyophilized, and converted to a powdered extract.
2. The powdered extract is added to a known anti-CEA and radiolabeled CEA system.
3. The unknown CEA in the perchloric acid extract is quantitated by the inhibition radioimmunoassay procedure.
4. The bound and unbound CEA antigen are separated by coprecipitation of antibody-bound CEA with 50% ammonium sulfate.
The method can detect a level of 2.5 ng CEA/ml; circulating CEA up to 320 ng/ml may be seen in patients with adenocarcinoma of the colon and rectum [68, 174]. Preoperative levels of serum CEA in cases of colon or rectal cancer may range from 5 to 160 ng/ml.
    Several investigators [23, 120] used a CEA radioimmunoassay which detects an antigenic site on CEA exposed at low ionic strength. Since CEA was found in the serum of both endodermal and ectodermal tumors, they postulated an antigenic site on CEA common to several types of tumors [120]. This assay requires a perchloric acid extraction of plasma, and zirconyl phosphate gel is used to separate antibody-bound CEA from unbound CEA in the radioimmunoassay procedure.
    A radioimmunoassay more conveniently adaptable to screening in the clinical laboratory has been developed by Egan and co-workers [36, 37] and is described in detail in Chapter 20. The radioimmuno-

assay utilizes a double antibody method for the separation of bound and unbound CEA. The assay may be performed on a direct 0.2 ml serum sample, avoiding time-consuming extraction and concentration procedures. Lawrence et al. [78, 110] used a modified procedure described by Egan et al. [36, 37] and compared it to the procedure of LoGerfo et al. [120]. Lawrence et al. [110] noted that the upper limit of normal, 2.5 ng CEA/ml, by the method of LoGerfo et al. [120], was 12.5 ng CEA/ml plasma [110], and values of 9 ng and 24 ng/ml of Lo Gerfo corresponded to volumes of 20 and 40 ng/ml. By the use of a sensitive radioimmunoassay procedure, Chu et al. [24] demonstrated CEA in normal human plasma. The level of plasma CEA in so-called normal individuals is believed to be 2.5 ng/ml [120, 150]. In an extensive study by Reynoso et al. [150], elevated CEA levels were noted in 39 of 48 patients with gastrointestinal cancers and 90 of 281 of non-endodermally derived tumors. Other investigators have reported CEA levels in a wide variety of diseases other than malignancy, such as severe alcoholic cirrhosis, uremia, and benign inflammatory conditions of the bowel [110, 114, 185].

It is obvious that much work remains to be done as to the exact nature and chemical structure of CEA in normal and tumor tissue, as well as to the properties of CEA bound in tissue and released into the circulation in different diseases. The CEA assay procedure is limited as a diagnostic tool today, although it is of value as a presumptive diagnostic test. The CEA assay procedure will not screen all patients with cancer, and a positive result is seen in many nonneoplastic diseases. In its present form, the major value of CEA assay is that it may be used to monitor known cancer patients on therapy. The test can be used to detect recurrences of tumor, for reappearance of CEA will indicate renewed activity of tumor. Serial assays of CEA along with the quantitative levels may be helpful to differentiate cancer of the bowel from benign inflammatory conditions. Patients with inflammatory disease of the bowel may have a transient CEA level elevation which disappears with remission [129, 151].

α_1-Fetoprotein (AFP)

Normally, α_1-fetoprotein (AFP) is synthesized in the fetus of 14–40 weeks and the level of AFP declines rapidly after 2 weeks of age [99, 160]. The AFP is produced by embryonic liver and yolk sac tissues. The AFP has been found in the serum of adults associated primarily with hepatocellular cancer of the liver and embryonic tumors of the ovary and testes [1, 5, 148, 159, 161]. Immunofluorescence studies have shown that α-fetoprotein is present in human fetal liver and hepatoma tissue [146]. More recently, serum AFP has been detected in cases of gastric carcinoma and prostatic carcinoma [4, 106, 125], viral hepatitis [160], and cirrhosis [149]. Thus, it appears that the relative specificity of AFP for hepatomas and embryonal carcinomas is a quantitative phenomenon. Of 380 patients with the diagnosis of hepatoma, 159 or 68% were positive when tested for serum AFP [167]. Of 355 patients with a neoplasm of other than primary hepatoma, only 3.1% were positive for AFP, and each of these patients had a teratoblastoma [167].

The diagnostic usefulness of AFP detection in serum for the confirmation of a diagnosis of primary liver cancer is well documented [148, 159, 161]. Most commonly, agar gel double diffusion methods are used, and the sensitivity of the test is approximately 0.3 mg AFP/100 ml [147, 149]. Such levels of AFP are almost always associated with liver or embryonic tumors.

METHODS FOR THE DETECTION OF α_1- FETOPROTEIN

A. Agar gel double diffusion. This method is very insensitive, but a positive test is almost diagnostic since the sensitivity of the test is 0.3 mg AFP/100 ml [147, 149].

B. Rivanol precipitation combined with double diffusion agar gel. In this procedure, α_1-fetoprotein is precipitated with Rivanol (2 ethoxy-6,9,diaminoacridine lactate) before a double diffusion test is carried out. The sensitivity of the test is such that it can detect approximately 1.5 to 3.0 μg per ml of AFP [127]. The procedure can be briefly outlined as follows:

   1. Two ml 0.4% aqueous solution of Rivanol (Calbiochem) are added to 1 ml serum and then mixed to precipitate. The suspension is left at room temperature for 2 hours and then centrifuged.

   2. The precipitate is redissolved in 0.1 ml 2% sodium chloride in phosphate buffer (pH 7.4, ionic strength 0.17) and kept overnight at 4° C.

   3. The extract is then reacted against anti-AFP antisera in an agar gel double diffusion test.

   A positive test for AFP can then be quantitated by electroimmunodiffusion [158].

C. Cross-electrophoresis. Counter-electrophoresis may be used and is much more sensitive than a double diffusion method [13, 11, 56]. Smith utilized a sandwich cross-electrophoresis method and was able to detect AFP in cases of acute viral hepatitis [160]. In the latter method:

   1. The serum containing unknown AFP is placed in the well near the cathode. Rabbit anti-AFP is placed in the opposite well near the anode.

   2. The plate is then subjected to electrophoresis for 1 hour. The wells are cleared and sheep anti-rabbit IgG is placed in the anodal well. This step is not necessary if a clear precipitin line is observed.

   3. Electrophoresis is again carried out for 45 min and precipitin bands may be seen after 2 to 3 hours' incubation at room temperature. The procedure is sensitive for AFP concentrations of 0.5 μg/ml or less [160].

D. Electroimmunodiffusion. This technique, a rapid method to measure serum AFP levels, can detect levels at or above 0.35 μg/ml. The procedure has the advantage in that AFP can be quantitated [158].
E. Radioimmunoassay of AFP. With a sensitive immunoassay procedure, AFP may be detected in apparently normal individuals [147, 149, 152]. Levels to the order of 25 ng/ml of AFP have been found in normal persons [153]. AFP levels in the sera of pregnant women at different stages of gestation may range from 100 to 800 ng/ml and are presumed to be of fetal origin [149].

The tests for AFP in serum must be interpreted in light of the method of assay used, and must be correlated with the clinical history and physical findings in a particular patient.

α_2-H Ferroprotein

The α_2-H globulin is protein formed in the liver and found in fetal organs and serum. By conventional serologic methods, the protein has not been detected in normal children beyond the age of 2 months. With the use of a radioimmunodiffusion method, the protein was detected in the sera of 81% of 334 children with malignant tumors [14]. The tumors noted to be associated with α_2-H ferroprotein are nephroblastoma, neuroblastoma, hepatoma, teratoma, lymphomas, osteogenic sarcoma, and brain tumors. On the other hand, 8% of 122 children with noncancerous diseases had positive results [14].

Regan Alkaline Phosphatase

An isoenzyme of alkaline phosphatase normally absent from adult tissue has been found in the serum of 12% of cancer patients [53, 54, 55, 134]. The isoenzyme was named for the patient in whom it was first discovered (Regan) and is biochemically and immunologically similar to placental alkaline phosphatase. It is identical to placental alkaline phosphatase with respect to L-phenylalanine sensitivity, heat stability at 65° C. The Regan enzyme is probably a product of the tumor, and minute amounts of enzyme may be present in the sera of cancer patients. The Regan isoenzyme is not organ specific and has been observed in many cancer patients with a wide variety of cellular types including lung, ovary, testicle, liver, colon, uterus, and lymphomas [98, 134, 168, 182].

Usategui-Gomez and associates [177] have developed an assay to quantitate extremely small amounts of Regan alkaline phosphatase. An antibody is produced to the Regan isoenzyme and polymerized into a solid immunoadsorbent pellet with ethylchloroformate [10]. The immunoadsorbent allows concentration of the Regan isoenzyme 10 to 20 fold by reaction with the antibody. The pellet is then assayed for enzymatic activity, since the antibody complex with enzyme does not interfere with the enzyme activity. With the sensitive assay, the Regan isoenzyme has been noted in normal individuals. The average value obtained in normal sera was 0.29 ± 0.21 IU/liter. Cancer patients with abnormal levels contain 5 to 300 times the average normal value [176]. Thus, the Regan alkaline phosphatase may be another fetal antigen which may be found in significant amounts in fetal, embryonic, or tumor tissue.

Fetal Sulfoglycoprotein

Fetal sulfoglycoprotein (FSA) can be found in the gastric juice from 0 to 6.67% of a normal population between 45 to 65 years of age [75, 76]. However, the antigen is usually lacking in younger adults. FSA appears to share with CEA a common antigenic determinant which is not the colon cancer specific determinant of the CEA molecule [77]. FSA in gastric secretion was found to precede the development of definite cancer cells, and a relationship of FSA to carcinogenesis was suggested. The detection of FSA in the young adult population may be helpful in suspected cases of stomach cancer.

γ Fetoprotein (γFP)

A fetal protein distinct from α_1 fetal protein and CEA has been found associated with human neoplasms and some tissues of the normal fetus [34, 35]. γFP was present in 75% of a wide variety of benign and malignant human tumors, the serum of 11% (23 of 210) of patients and 2 of 101 specimens of nonneoplastic diseased tissue. The antigen was not detected by immunodiffusion tests in normal human tissue or in adult human serum. γFP does not show species specificity, for it is observed in the sera of 4 of 6 other mammalian species, but no tumors of the animals were γFP positive [34, 35]. The original serum detecting γFP was obtained from a 49-year-old female patient with localized medullary carcinoma of the breast.

Tests for Deletion of A, B, and H Tissue Isoantigens

Davidsohn and co-workers [29, 30, 31, 105] have developed a technique valuable in the early diagnosis of carcinoma. Tissues which normally contain A, B, and H blood antigen will demonstrate a deletion or absence of the antigens with carcinomatous change. Although there are several technical problems, the tests for deletion of A, B, and H antigen may be done with tissue frozen sections and paraffin sections of formalin-fixed tissues [31, 100]. The procedures used for the deletion of A, B, and H isoantigens in tissues are:
1. Immunofluorescence [29]
2. Modified Coombs' mixed cell agglutination reaction (MCAR) [39] or the specific red cell adherence (SRCA) test [105]

Many tissues normally contain the A, B, H blood group isoantigens. Since blood vessel endothelial cells also contain the antigens, a tissue with tumor will contain blood vessels which provide a positive control on the same section.

There have been some conflicting reports on the presence of A, B, and H antigens in human cancers when studied by immunofluorescence methods [39, 59, 60]. Davidsohn and co-workers [29] used immunofluorescence methods and studied formalin-fixed normal tissues, benign neoplasms, and carcinomas of the gastrointestinal tract. They observed that the antigens A, B, and H were present in normal tissue epithelial cells and in benign neoplasms, and were absent in 28 of 45 or 62% of carcinomas of the stomach [29].

The specific red cell adherence test (SRCA) is a "sandwich" type of reaction in which anti-A, anti-B or the lectin *Ulex europeus* reacts with tissue A, B, or H antigens, respectively, and the second step includes the overlaying of specific indicator erythrocytes. Human anti-A or anti-B antiserum with a titer of 1:500 is used for the detection of A and B, and extracts of *Ulex europeus* with titers from 500 to 1,000 are used for the detection of H antigen in group 0 patients. Apparently, none of the commercially available extracts of *Ulex europeus* can be used; a special preparation of *Ulex europeus* is needed. The method appears very promising. It is advisable to obtain some instruction from Davidsohn and his group when the procedure is instituted in the hospital laboratory.

Test for Lymphocyte Sensitization to Basic Proteins in Cancer Patients

Field and Caspary [41] first noted that blood lymphocytes of patients with an early malignant neoplasm are sensitized to basic proteins derived from the central and peripheral nervous systems [19] and malignant tumors [21]. The sensitization to basic proteins does not occur with benign neoplasms and has the following characteristics:
1. It is independent of the type of malignant neoplasm.
2. It is long lasting and does not disappear after removal of the neoplasm; it is known to be present 24 years after carcinoma of the tongue [48].
3. It is independent of tumor involvement of the nervous system.

The proteins to which sensitization occurs in cancer patients are the encephalitogenic factor (EF), which is a basic protein of histone-like character derived from the human brain [19], and a basic protein derived from human sciatic nerve. Further studies have shown that basic protein can be extracted from tumor tissue and will be a more effective antigen than the brain basic protein in the macrophage electrophoretic migration (MEM) test for malignant disease [21]. The basic proteins from the brain and from tumors have some degree of cross-reactivity. Cancer basic proteins are at least 10,000 times more antigenically active than EF on a molecular basis. It is estimated that cancer antigens from 1,000 malignant cells may initiate lymphocyte sensitization and result in a positive MEM test [48]. Carnegie [18] had suggested that EF may be a receptor for serotonin (5-hydroxytryptamine). With this postulate, experiments were conducted, and indeed serotonin was shown to block the interaction of EF and sensitized lymphocytes in cancer. Serotonin is much more effective in blocking EF than basic proteins extracted from cancer tissues. There is evidence that EF shares antigenic determinants with the purified protein derivative PPD of *Mycobacterium tuberculosis,* and with basic proteins extracted from cancer [40, 48].

Macrophage Electrophoretic Migration (MEM) Test [41, 144]

PREPARATION
1. Venous blood is drawn from patients with a heparinized syringe. The lymphocytes are isolated by various means to have minimal contamination with red cells, macrophages, and neutrophils [41, 43, 143, 144].
2. The isolated lymphocytes are washed and resuspended in Medium 199 and adjusted to a concentration of 10^6 cells/ml.
3. The encephalitogenic factor (EF) is prepared from a human brain, according to the method of Caspary and Field [19, 21]; 1.0 mg of EF is dissolved in Medium 199, so that the final concentration is 100 μg/0.1 ml.
4. Macrophages are prepared from peritoneal exudate of 400 to 600 gm Hartley albino guinea pigs 4 to 10 days after the injection of 20 ml sterile liquid paraffin into the peritoneum. The cells are washed and resuspended in Medium 199 to a concentration of 10^7 cells/ml and then irradiated with a dose of 200 rad.

PROCEDURE
1. 1.5 Medium 199, 0.1 ml antigen, 0.5 ml lymphocyte preparation, and 1 ml macrophage suspension are incubated at room temperature for 90 min.
2. A duplicate suspension without antigen is prepared as a control for each sample.
3. The electrophoretic mobility of the macrophages is measured in a Zeiss cytopherometer.

If the time of macrophage migration in the presence of human lymphocytes without antigen is t_c or control time, and if t_e = time of migration in the presence of lymphocytes together with antigen, then

$$\frac{t_e - t_c}{t_c} \times 100$$

represents the percentage slowing of macrophages induced by the antigen. The percentage slowing of macrophages in normal patients is 0.9–3.6%. Patients with neoplastic disease showed a percentage slowing of macrophages of 8.2–29.9% [41].

Pritchard and co-workers [144] have made several improvements on the MEM test, increasing its sensitivity. In their new method, which they call the modified MEM or Mod-MEM test, the main points of their test are as follows:

1. The human lymphocytes are first isolated and incubated with EF antigen to release the soluble macrophage inhibitory factor (MIF), which is then separated from the cells by centrifugation.
2. The MIF is added as a cell free supernatant to a suspension of irradiated guinea pig macrophages for a second period of incubation.
3. The migration rate of the macrophages is then measured in a Zeiss cytopherometer. With this procedure, the two different populations from human and guinea pig are kept apart and a possible mixed interaction does not occur.

With the use of the MOD-MEM procedure, Pritchard et al. [144] have found that the percentage slowing of macrophages over the control in cancer patients jumped to a new range of 22.6–40% without affecting the corresponding low values from "normal patients."

The MEM technique has been used to study the length of time a cancer may be present in the quiescent phase. Field and Caspary [44] observed that lymphocyte sensitization possessed by the mother is passed on to the child. Apparently, intact lymphocytes or information-carrying materials from maternal lymphocytes pass to the offspring. If the mother has had a cancer and carries sensitization to cancer basic proteins, the newborn child will also show evidence of sensitization which may be detectable up to 12 years [48]. By the study of a family to which children were born before the mother developed clinical evidence of cancer, one can estimate the latent period. In cases of cancer of the breast, there is evidence that tumor was present for at least 7 years before it was detected clinically.

INTERPRETATION.   Difficulties in the interpretation of the MEM test are as follows:
A. Patients with cancer may show a positive test as long as 24 years after removal of the tumor [48].
B. Positive tests are also seen in (a) offspring of mothers who have had cancer [41]; (b) patients with demyelinizing neurologic diseases, such as multiple sclerosis [139]; (c) patients with intrinsic asthma [49]; (d) patients exposed to influenza virus [50]. Guinea pigs used as a source of macrophages if exposed to influenza should not be used for the tests; and (e) active pulmonary tuberculosis, as basic protein and tubercle bacillus, may share antigenic determinants [40, 45, 48].
C. The test may be positive in patients with latent cancer and appears as false positives.

D. False negative reactions may be seen in patients whose lymphocytes do not respond to antigens such as PPD and thyroglobulin.
E. Advanced cancers tend to show low results which may be due to reduced numbers of sensitized lymphocytes [51]. In the serum of cancer patients, there is a lymphocyte response-depressing factor whose levels rise in advanced cancer [46, 47, 51]. However, the decreased lymphocyte sensitization in advanced cancers is not directly due to serum depressive factor.

The test does not appear to demonstrate overlapping values between the so-called normal and cancer patients, and it has advantages over previous tests for the detection of cancer. The MEM test for sensitivity to cancer basic proteins will have limited value as a screening procedure for cancer. It may be used in selected cases of patients who display specific localizing signs or symptoms, such as noted in cancers of the cervix and breast. It may be of value to follow patients who are exposed to environmental carcinogens, such as rubber, dye, and asbestos workers [48].

Cell Inhibition

Quantitative Lymphocyte-Tumor Cell Inhibition Assay
(Method of S. Deodhar and B. Barna, Division of Immunology, Cleveland Clinic, Cleveland, Ohio. Modified from method of Hellström and Hellström [85])

The cell inhibition test provides a means of quantitating the extent of target cell destruction by lymphocytes. In addition, the capacity of the patient's serum to block this lymphocyte-mediated destruction can also be measured. The assay requires a preparation of tumor cells grown in vitro from the original tissue explant, lymphocytes obtained from heparinized blood, and serum. All the following procedures require aseptic techniques, materials, and reagents.

MATERIALS AND REAGENTS
A. Tissue collected at surgery in a sterile petri dish
B. Heparinized blood from patient for isolation of lymphocytes (15–20 ml)
C. Clotted blood (10 ml) for patient's serum sample
D. Heparin 1,000 units/ml (Lipo-hepin, Riker Lab)
E. Waymouth medium (Gibco No. 122)
F. Fetal calf serum, heat inactivated (Gibco No. 614H)
G. l-Glutamine (Gibco No. 503)
H. Penicillin-streptomycin solution (Gibco No. 514)
I. Nonessential amino acids, 100 X solution (Gibco No. 114)—1%
J. Sodium pyruvate, 100 mM solution (Gibco No. 136)—1%

K. Hepes buffer solution (N-2-hydroxyethylpiperazine-N'-2-ethane-sulfonic acid) (MW 238.3 gm) (Calbiochem)—see below for prep-aration of 1% solution
L. Mycostatin, 100 X solution (Gibco No. 532)
M. Trypsin, 2.5% stock solution (Gibco No. 509)
N. Hanks' balanced salt solution (Gibco No. 402)
O. Hanks' balanced salt solution, calcium and magnesium free (Gibco No. 417)
P. Trypan blue, 1% in 0.5% chlorobutanol in H_2O (Medical Chem-icals)
Q. Collagenase (Nutritional Biochemicals)
R. Phosphate-buffered saline solution
S. 10% Formalin
T. Crystal violet, 0.1% filtered (Fisher)
U. Distilled water
V. Normal saline solution
W. Methanol
X. May-Grünwald and Giemsa stains

PREPARATION OF HEPES BUFFER FOR USE AS A 1% SOLUTION.
Stock solution = 1 Molar. To prepare 100 ml:
1. Dissolve 23.83 gm in 50 ml double-distilled H_2O with mixing.
2. Titrate with approximately 13 ml 5 N NaOH to pH 8.1.
3. Bring to 100 ml in volumetric flask.
4. Sterilize by millipore filtration.

EQUIPMENT
A. 250 ml tissue culture flasks (Falcon)
B. Incubator at 37° C in 5% CO_2
C. Trypsinizing flask (Bellco)
D. Inverted microscope
E. Centrifuge
F. Incubator at 37° C
G. Hemocytometer
H. Digestion flask
I. Mixer
J. Erlenmeyer flask
K. Magnetic stirrer
L. Sterile gauze
M. Pipette
N. Heparinized plastic syringe
O. Pasteur pipette
P. Sterile applicator swabs
Q. Microtest plates, 96 well (Falcon No. 3040)
R. Microtest plate lids (Falcon)
S. Leighton tubes and coverslips (Bellco)
T. Sterile forceps

PREPARATION OF TARGET CELLS

1. Tissue is collected at surgery in a sterile petri dish. A section of the sample is processed for histologic examination to confirm the presence of malignant cells.

2. Soft tumors (melanomas) are finely minced in complete Waymouth's medium (Waymouth's medium supplemented with 30% fetal calf serum; 292 mcg/ml. 1-glutamine; 100 units/ml penicillin; 100 mcg/ml streptomycin; 1% of a 100 x solution of nonessential amino acids; 1% of a 100 mM solution of sodium pyruvate; 1% Hepes buffer; and 1% of a 100 x solution of mycostatin). The mince is transferred to 250 ml plastic flasks, each with 15 ml medium, and incubated at 37° C under 5% CO_2 until a cell monolayer has been established (from 3 to 21 days, depending on sample). Growth is checked daily by means of an inverted microscope. Flasks should receive 15 ml fresh medium at 72 hours. The old medium may be centrifuged and the pellet and large pieces transferred to another flask with 15 ml fresh medium.

3. For testing, the monolayer is trypsinized (0.25% trypsin in Hanks' balanced salt solution, calcium and magnesium free) as follows:
   a. Pour off medium from 250 ml flask.
   b. Rinse out flask with 3 ml trypsin solution.
   c. Add 5 ml trypsin solution which has been warmed to 37° C.
   d. Let flask stand at room temperature for 5 to 10 min. Cells should begin to detach from flask wall. Shake flask gently to remove monolayer, which should "peel" off.
   e. Pour off trypsin. Add 5 ml complete Waymouth's medium to rinse flask. Pool with trypsin. Centrifuge.
   The cells are resuspended in complete Waymouth's medium, counted in a hemocytometer, and viability determined with 1% trypan blue. Cells for testing are diluted to 1,000 cells per ml in complete Waymouth's medium for use in cell inhibition test described below.

4. Hard tumors (breast carcinomas) are minced and the pieces placed in a digestion flask with 25 ml 0.25% trypsin, 1 mg/ml collagenase, 100 units/ml penicillin, and 100 mcg/ml streptomycin in Hanks' balanced salt solution, calcium and magnesium free. Digestion is maintained on a mixer for 3–4 hours or until a cell suspension has been obtained. Trypsin solution is poured off every hour and centrifuged to collect free cells. Fresh trypsin is added to flask after each pour-off. Cell pellets should be immediately washed with complete Waymouth's medium and resuspended in medium. Viability is determined with trypan blue and the cells counted. Flasks may be seeded at this time (2×10^6 cells per flask) or the cells may be diluted to 1,000 per ml for use directly in the cell inhibition test.

OUTLINE OF STEPS IN THE PREPARATION OF TISSUE CULTURE OF TUMORS
FOR IN VITRO TESTING

1. Obtain tumor tissue and place immediately in a container with Hanks' BSS, calcium and magnesium free.
2. Mince tissue into 1 mm fragments with scissors.
3. Transfer fragments to erlenmeyer flask with trypsin solution. Mix with magnetic stirrer.
4. When trypsinization is completed, strain suspension through gauze into a centrifuge tube and centrifuge at 500–900 rpm for 5 to 10 min.
5. Pour off supernatant from packed cells and add a measured amount of complete Waymouth's medium. Resuspend cells by vigorous pipetting.
6. Perform a viable cell count using trypan blue stain and a hemocytometer:
   a. Take a 1 ml sample of suspension for counting.
   b. Dilute 1 ml suspension with 1 ml trypan blue to obtain a 1:2 dilution.
   c. Aspirate several times to mix thoroughly and break up cell clumps.
   d. Charge counting chambers of hemocytometer without flooding and count the unstained cells in 10 squares (5 squares in each chamber).
   e. Calculate concentration of cells per milliliter.
      Example: Total cells counted = 100
      Multiply by dilution factor $\times$ 2 = 200
      Add 3 zeroes = 200,000 cells/ml
7. The volume of the cell suspension is adjusted with complete Waymouth's medium to obtain the desired cell concentration.
8. The cells may be used for cell inhibition or for seeding flasks.
9. The tumor cells are cultured in flasks, and when a monolayer is established, cells are removed by trypsinization. First the medium is poured out, 3 ml 0.25% trypsin is added, swirled briefly, and poured out.
10. Then 5 ml trypsin is added. The flask is allowed to stand at room temperature for 5–10 min, until cells begin to detach. The suspension is transferred to a centrifuge tube, mixed with medium, spun, and the supernatant decanted. Cells are resuspended in fresh medium, counted, and viability determined. The suspension is then adjusted to the desired concentration and can be used for testing.

PREPARATION OF LYMPHOCYTES

1. Draw 15–20 ml blood into a heparinized plastic syringe (Lipo-hepin, Riker Lab, 1,000 units/ml) containing 100–200 units heparin.
2. Proceed with removal of plasma and filtration as in steps 4 through

16 of the method for Lymphocyte Transformation with Phytohemag-glutinin (Chapter 3).

3. The final cell suspension is adjusted to a concentration of 1 million lymphocytes/ml in complete Waymouth's medium and is ready for use in the cell inhibition test described below.

PREPARATION OF SERUM

1. Draw 10 ml clotted blood. Centrifuge and remove serum with a Pasteur pipette.
2. Inactivate 56° C for 30 min. Serum is ready for testing in the cell inhibition test.

CELL INHIBITION TEST

1. Target cell concentration is adjusted to give 1,000 viable cells per milliliter of complete Waymouth's medium, and 0.2 ml of the suspension is added to each well of a Falcon microtest plate. NOTE: Although 200 cells are added per well, only 50 to 100 cells may actually appear on the final stained test plate because of the low plating efficiency demonstrated by most human tumors. If human fibroblasts are used as the target cell, add only 50 cells in 0.2 ml per well.
2. Incubate test plate with an unsealed plastic lid at 37° C under 5% CO_2 overnight (or 16 to 24 hours).
3. The following day, invert the plate and shake out the medium; the cells will adhere to the plate. Sterile applicator swabs may be used to dry spills on the rims of the test plate.
4. A protocol similar to that shown in Fig. 19-2 should be prepared. Allow 5 to 10 replicate wells for each variation tested.
5. Add 0.1 ml inactivated serum to a series of test wells. Add 0.1 ml complete Waymouth's medium to all other wells. Incubate 45 min (preferably on a rocker platform) at 37° C. NOTE: This step is necessary for determination of serum blocking activity only. If patient's serum is not available, omit this step.
6. Shake out the serum and medium as before.
7. Add 1×10^5 lymphocytes in 0.1 ml medium to a series of wells. Allow one row of lymphocytes on untreated target cells and one row of lymphocytes on the serum-treated target cells prepared in step 5. Add 0.1 ml complete Waymouth's medium to all other wells.
8. Incubate 45 min at 37° C as above.
9. Add 0.1 complete Waymouth's medium to all wells.
10. Incubate at 37° C under 5% CO_2 for 72 hours.
11. Shake out medium and gently flood plate with phosphate-buffered saline solution (PBS). Shake out PBS.
12. Add 10% formalin in PBS to all wells for a minimum of 20 min.
13. Shake out fixative and stain with 0.1% filtered crystal violet for 20 min.

Lymphocyte — Tumor Cell Interaction Form for Recording
Cell Inhibition Assay Results

Expt. # _____ Date _____

(Cell Counts/Well Recorded Here)

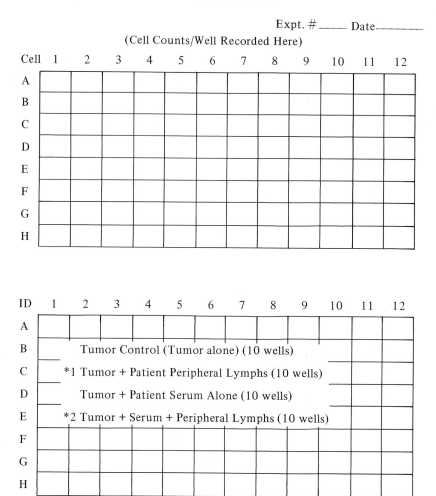

Figure 19-2
Sample assay protocol using diagrammatic representation of falcon no. 3040 microtest plate. *1 tumor: purpose: test capacity of lymphocytes to kill target cells. Results = % cell inhibition. *2 tumor: purpose: test capacity of serum to block lymphocyte killing of target cells. Results = % blocking activity.

Name _____ Clinic No. _____ Date_____

   I. Tumor Specimens   (1)

        Received _____   Received _____

        Path. Report _____   Path. Report _____

        * Culture Report _____   * Culture Report _____

  II. Lymphocyte Specimens (1)

        Received _____ Tested _____ Received _____ Tested _____

        Tumor Donor _____   Tumor Donor _____

        * Culture Report _____   * Culture Report _____

 III. Serum Specimens

        Received _____ Tested _____ Received _____ Tested _____

        Tumor Donor _____   Tumor Donor _____

        * Culture Report _____   * Culture Report _____

        * Blocking Antibody _____   * Blocking Antibody _____

 IV. MIF Test—Dated Tested _____

        Source—Tumor Homogenate _____

        * Result _____

  V. Lymphocyte Transformation Test—Date Tested _____

        Source—Tumor Homogenate _____

        * Result   (No)   (Questionable)   (Significant)

        Blast Cell Formation   (   ) % with Tumor
                                (   ) % with Control

                 Signed _____

Figure 19-3
In vitro cancer immunology studies: clinical report form.

14. Rinse plate with tap water and dry, inverted, at room temperature.
15. Microscopically count all remaining target cells in each well, and obtain a mean for each test series.
16. Calculate results as follows:

% cell inhibition

$$= \frac{\text{average (tumor control) wells} - \text{average (tumor + lymph) wells}}{\text{average (tumor control) wells}} \times 100$$

% blocking activity

$$= \frac{\text{average (tumor + lymph + serum)} - \text{average (tumor + lymph)}}{\text{average (tumor + lymph)}} \times 100$$

COVERSLIP TECHNIQUE FOR VISUALIZATION OF TARGET CELLS.   This is a simple method of obtaining permanent slides of in vitro target cell growth.

1. Leighton tubes and coverslips are soaked in Hanks' balanced salt solution (GIBCO, Cat. No. 402) overnight, rinsed with distilled water, dried, and sterilized.
2. Drop coverslip into Leighton tube with sterile forceps.
3. Add 2–3 × 10^5 target cells in 2 ml complete Waymouth's medium.
4. Incubate at 37° C for 48 hours.
5. Pour off medium. Gently add 2 ml normal saline solution down side of tube to wash coverslip.
6. Pour off saline solution. Add 2 ml methanol and fix for a minimum of 30 min.
7. Stain with May-Grünwald and Giemsa stains as given in Methods for Lymphocyte Transformation with Phytohemagglutinin in Chapter 3.

REPORT FORM.   Fig. 19-3 demonstrates the manner in which cell inhibition tests as well as other assays for cellular immunity are reported for cancer patients involved in special studies of the Cleveland Clinic.

References

1. Abelev, G. I.   Production of embryonal serum α globulin by hepatomas: Review of experimental and clinical data. *Cancer Res.* 28:1344, 1968.
2. Allen, D. W., and Cole, P.   Viruses and human cancer. *N. Engl. J. Med.* 286:70, 1972.
3. Alpert, E., Hershberg, R., Schur, P. H., and Isselbacher, K. J.   Alpha fetoprotein in human hepatomas: Improved detection in serum and quantitative studies using a new sensitive technique. *Gastroenterology* 61:137, 1971.
4. Alpert, E., Pinn, V. W., and Isselbacher, K. J.   Alpha-fetoprotein in a patient with gastric carcinoma metastatic to the liver. *N. Engl. J. Med.* 285:1058, 1971.

5. Alpert, M. E., Uriel, J., and De Nechaud, B.   Alpha₁ fetoglobulin in the diagnosis of human hepatoma. *N. Engl. J. Med.* 278:984, 1968.

6. Anderson, A. P., Brincker, H., and Lass, F.   Prognosis in Hodgkin's disease with special reference to histologic type: Results of treatment predominantly by cyto-status. *Acta Radiol.* (Stockh.) 9:81, 1970.

7. Anderson, N. G., and Coggins, J. H., Jr.   *Proceedings of the First Conference and Workshop in Embryonic and Fetal Antigens in Cancer* at Oak Ridge National Laboratory, Oak Ridge, Tenn. Springfield, Va.: National Technology Information Service, May, 1971.

8. Andres, G. A., Hsu, K. C., and Seegal, B. C.   Immunoferritin technique for the identification of antigens by electron microscopy. In D. M. Weir (ed.), *Handbook of Experimental Immunology.* Oxford: Blackwell, 1967.

9. Arpels, C., and Southam, C. M.   Cytotoxicity of sera from healthy persons and cancer patients. *Int. J. Cancer* 4:548, 1969.

10. Avrameas, S., and Ternynck, T.   Biologically active water insoluble protein polymers. *J. Biol. Chem.* 242:1651, 1967.

11. Ballas, M.   Yolk sac carcinoma of the ovary with alpha-fetoprotein in serum and ascitic fluid demonstrated by immunoosmophoresis. *Am. J. Clin. Pathol.* 57:511, 1972.

12. Banjo, C., Gold, P., Freedman, S. O., and Krupey, J.   Immunologically active heterosaccharides of carcinoembryonic antigen of human digestive system. *Nature [New Biol.]* 238:183, 1972.

13. Brunner, K. T., Mauel, J., Cerottini, J. C., and Chapius, B.   Quantitative assay of the lytic action of immune lymphoid cells on Cr⁵¹ labeled allogenic target cells in vitro. Inhibition by isoantibody and by drugs. *Immunology* 14:181, 1968.

14. Buffe, D., Rimbaut, C., Lemerle, J., Schweisguth, O., and Burtin, P.   Presence d'une ferroproteine d'origine tissulaire l'α_2 H dans le serum des enfants porteurs de tumeurs. *Int. J. Cancer* 5:85, 1970.

15. Burtin, P., Martin, E., Sabine, M. C., and Von Kleist, S.   Immunological study of polyps of the colon. *J. Natl. Cancer Inst.* 48:25, 1972.

16. Burtin, P., Sabine, M. C., and Chavonel, G.   Presence of carcinoembryonic antigen in children's colonic mucosa. *Int. J. Cancer* 10:72, 1972.

17. Canty, T. G., and Wunderlich, J. R.   Quantitative in vitro assay of cytotoxic cellular immunity. *J. Nat. Cancer Inst.* 45:761, 1970.

18. Carnegie, P. R.   Properties, structure and possible neuroreceptor role of the encephalitogenic protein of human brain. *Nature* 229:25, 1971.

19. Caspary, E. A., and Field, E. J.   An encephalitogenic protein of human origin: Some chemical and biological properties. *Ann. N.Y. Acad. Sci.* 122:182, 1965.

20. Caspary, E. A.   Lymphocyte-antigen interaction in electrophoretic mobility test for cellular sensitization. *Nature [New Biol.]* 231:24, 1971.

21. Caspary, E. A., and Field, E. J.   Specific lymphocyte sensitization in cancer: Is there a common antigen in human malignant neoplasia? *Br. Med. J.* 2:613, 1971.

22. Chu, E., Stjernsuard, J., Clifford, P., and Klein, G.   Reactivity of human lymphocytes against autochthonous and allogeneic normal and tumor cells in vitro. *J. Nat. Cancer Inst.* 39:595, 1967.

23. Chu, T. M., and Reynoso, G.   Evaluation of a new radioimmunoassay method for carcinoembryonic antigen in plasma with use of zirconyl phosphate gel. *Clin. Chem.* 18:918, 1972.
24. Chu, T. M., Hansen, H. J., and Reynoso, G.   Demonstration of carcinoembryonic antigen in normal human plasma. *Nature* (Lond.) 238:152, 1972.
25. Cinader, B.   The future of tumor immunology. *Med. Clin. North Am.* 56:801, 1972.
26. Coligan, J. E., Lautenschleger, J. T., Egan, M. L., and Todd, C. W.   Isolation and characterization of carcinoembryonic antigen. *Immunochemistry* 9:377, 1972.
27. Collatz, E., Von Kleist, S., and Burtin, P.   Further investigations of circulating antibodies in colon cancer patients: On the autoantigenicity of the carcinoembryonic antigen. *Int. J. Cancer* 8:298, 1971.
28. Coombs, R. R. A., Bedford, D., and Rouillard, I. M.   A and B blood group antigens on human epidermal cell demonstrated by mixed agglutination. *Lancet* 1:461, 1956.
29. Davidsohn, I., Kovarik, S., and Lee, C. L.   A, B, and O substances in gastrointestinal carcinoma. *Arch. Pathol.* 81:381, 1966.
30. Davidsohn, I., Ni, L. Y., and Stejskal, R.   Tissue isoantigens A, B, and H in carcinoma of the stomach. *Arch. Pathol.* 92:456, 1971.
31. Davidsohn, I.   Early immunologic diagnosis and prognosis of carcinoma. *Am. J. Clin. Pathol.* 57:715, 1972.
32. DeGrouchy, J., and DeNava, C.   A chromosomal theory of carcinogenesis. *Ann. Intern. Med.* 68:381, 1968.
33. Edwards, J. G., Campbell, J. A., and Williams, J. F.   Transformation by polyoma virus affects adhesion of fibroblasts. *Nature [New Biol.]* 231:147, 1971.
34. Edynak, E. M., Old, L. J., Vrana, M., and Lardis, M.   A fetal antigen in human tumors detected by an antibody in the serum of cancer patients [abstract]. *Proc. Am. Assoc. Can. Res.* 11:22, 1970.
35. Edynak, E. M., Old, L. J., Vrana, M., and Lardis, M. P.   A fetal antigen associated with human neoplasia. *N. Engl. J. Med.* 286:1178, 1972.
36. Egan, M. L., Lautenschleger, J. T., Coligan, J. E., and Todd, C. W.   Radioimmune assay of carcinoembryonic antigen. *Immunochemistry* 9:289, 1972.
37. Egan, M., Coligan, J. E., Lautenschleger, J. T., and Todd, C. W.   A test for the carcinoembryonic antigen in serum. In press.
38. Eilber, F. R., and Morton, D. L.   Immunologic studies of human sarcomas: Additional evidence suggesting an associated sarcoma virus. *Cancer* 26:588, 1970.
39. Eklund, A. E., Gullbring, B., and Lagerlof, B.   Blood group specific substances in human gastric carcinoma: A study using the fluorescent antibody technique. *Acta Pathol. Microbiol. Scand.* 59:447, 1963.
40. Field, E. J., Caspary, E. A., and Ball, E. J.   Some biological properties of a highly active encephalitogenic factor isolated from human brain. *Lancet* 2:11, 1963.
41. Field, E. J., and Caspary, E. A.   Lymphocyte sensitization: An in vitro test for cancer? *Lancet* 2:1337, 1970.
42. Field, E. J., Caspary, E. A., and Carnegie, P. R.   Lymphocyte sensitization to basic protein of brain in malignant neoplasia: Experiments with serotonin and related compounds. *Nature* (Lond.) 233:284, 1971.

43. Field, E. J., and Caspary, E. A.   Demonstration of sensitized lymphocytes in blood. *J. Clin. Pathol.* 24:179, 1971.
44. Field, E. J., and Caspary, E. A.   Is maternal lymphocyte sensitization
passed to the child? *Lancet* 2:337, 1971.
45. Field, E. J., and Caspary, E. A.   Lymphocyte sensitization in cancer.
Lancet 1:189, 1971.
46. Field, E. J., and Caspary, E. A.   Inhibition of lymphocyte response
by serum. *Lancet* 2:95, 1971.
47. Field, E. J., and Caspary, E. A.   Lymphocyte reactivity in cancer.
Lancet 2:877, 1971.
48. Field, E. J., Caspary, E. A., and Shepherd, R. T. H.   Immunodiagnosis
of cancer. *Br. Med. J.* 3:641, 1972.
49. Field, E. J., and Caspary, E. A.   M.E.M. Test for malignant disease.
Lancet 2:826, 1972.
50. Field, E. J., and Caspary, E. A.   "Spontaneous" lymphocyte reactivity
in the presence of virus infection. *Lancet* 1:963, 1972.
51. Field, E. J., and Caspary, E. A.   Lymphocyte sensitization in advanced malignant disease: A study of serum lymphocyte depressive
factor. *Br. J. Cancer* 26:164, 1972.
52. Fisher, B.   The present status of tumor immunology. *Adv. Surg.* 5:189,
1971.
53. Fishman, W. H., Inglis, N. R., Green, S., Anstiss, C. L., and Gosh, M. K.
Immunology and biochemistry of Regan isoenzyme of alkaline phosphatase in human cancer. *Nature* 219:697, 1968.
54. Fishman, W. H.   Immunologic and biochemical approaches to alkaline
phosphatase isoenzyme analysis: The Regan isoenzyme. *Ann. N.Y.
Acad. Sci.* 166:745, 1969.
55. Fishman, W. H., Inglis, N. R., and Green, S.   Regan isoenzyme: A
carcinoplacental antigen. *Cancer Res.* 31:1054, 1971.
56. Franco, J., Coppler, M., and Kovaleski, B.   Crossover electrophoresis
for the detection of serum alpha$_1$-fetal protein. *Am. J. Clin. Path.*
57:267, 1972.
57. Giraldo, G., Beth, E., Hirshaut, Y., Aoki, T., Old, L. J., Boyse, E. A.,
and Chopra, H. C.   Human sarcoma in culture. Foci of altered cells
and a common antigen: Induction of foci and antigen in human fibro-
blast cultures by filtrates. *J. Exp. Med.* 133:454, 1971.
58. Gitlin, D., and Boesman, M.   Sites of serum α-fetoprotein synthesis in
the human and in the rat. *J. Clin. Invest.* 46:1010, 1967.
59. Glynn, L. E., Holborow, E. J., and Johnson, G. D.   The distribution
of blood group substance in human gastric and duodenal mucosa. *Lancet*
2:1083, 1957.
60. Glynn, L. E., and Holborow, E. J.   Distribution of blood group substances in human tissues. *Br. Med. Bull.* 15:150, 1959.
61. Gold, J. M., Freedman, S. O., and Gold, P.   Human anti-CEA antibodies detected by radioimmunoelectrophoresis. *Nature* [*New Biol.*]
239:60, 1972.
62. Gold, P., and Freedman, S. O.   Demonstration of tumor specific antigens in human colonic carcinomata by immunological tolerance and
absorption techniques. *J. Exp. Med.* 121:439, 1965.
63. Gold, P., and Freedman, S. O.   Specific carcinoembryonic antigens of

the human digestive system. *J. Exp. Med.* 122:467, 1965.

64. Gold, P.   Circulating antibodies against carcinoembryonic antigens of the human digestive system. *Cancer* 20:1663, 1967.

65. Gold, P., Gold, M., and Freedman, S. O.   Cellular location of carcino-embryonic antigens of the human digestive system. *Cancer Res.* 28:1331, 1968.

66. Gold, P., Krupey, J., and Ansari, H.   Position of the carcinoembryonic antigen of the human digestive system in ultrastructure of the tumor cell surface. *J. Natl. Cancer Inst.* 45:219, 1970.

67. Gold, P.   Antigenic reversion in human cancer. *Ann. Rev. Med.* 22:85, 1971.

68. Gold, P.   Tumor specific antigen in GI cancer. *Hosp. Practice* 7:85, 1972.

69. Goldstein, G.   Immunofluorescent detection of human antibodies re-active with tumor. *Ann. N.Y. Acad. Sci.* 177:279, 1971.

70. Goudie, R. B.   Autoimmune selection of carcinoma cells in man. *Nature* 197:1020, 1963.

71. Granger, G. A., and Weiser, R. S.   Homograft target cells: Specific destruction in vitro by contact interaction with immune macrophages. *Science* 145:1427, 1964.

72. Green, H. N.   An immunological concept of cancer. *Br. Med. J.* 2:1374, 1954.

73. Green, H. N., Anthony, H. M., Baldwin, R. W., and Westrop, J. W. *An Immunological Approach to Cancer.* London: Butterworths, 1967.

74. Gunz, F. W., Fitzgerald, P. H., and Adams, A.   An abnormal chromo-some in chronic lymphocytic leukemia. *Br. Med. J.* 2:1097, 1962.

75. Häkkinen, I. P. T., Korhoren, L. K., and Saxé, L.   The time of appear-ance and distribution of sulphoglycoprotein antigens in the human fetal alimentary canal. *Int. J. Cancer* 3:582, 1968.

76. Häkkinen, I. P. T., and Viikari, S.   Occurrence of fetal sulfoglycopro-tein antigen in the gastric juice of patients with gastric disease. *Ann. Surg.* 169:277, 1969.

77. Häkkinen, I. P. T.   Immunological relationships of the carcinoem-bryonic antigen and the fetal sulfoglycoprotein antigen. *Immunochem-istry* 9:1115, 1972.

78. Hall, R. R., Lawrence, D. J. R., Darcy, D., Stevens, V., James, R., Roberts, S., and Neville, A. M.   Carcinoembryonic antigen in the urine of patients with urothelial carcinoma. *Br. Med. J.* 2:609, 1972.

79. Hellström, I., and Sjögren, H. O.   Demonstration of H-2 isoantigens and polyoma specific tumor antigens by measuring colony formation in vitro. *Exp. Cell Res.* 40:212, 1965.

80. Hellström, I.   A colony inhibition (CI) technique for demonstration of tumor cell destruction by lymphoid cells in vitro. *Int. J. Cancer* 2:65, 1967.

81. Hellström, I., Hellström, K. E., and Pierce, G. E.   In vitro studies of immune reactions against autochthonous and syngeneic mouse tumors induced by methylcholanthrene and plastic discs. *Int. J. Cancer* 3:467, 1968.

82. Hellström, I., Hellström, K. E., Pierce, G. E., and Bill, A. H.   Demon-stration of cell bound and humoral immunity against neuroblastoma cells. *Proc. Natl. Acad. Sci. U.S.A.* 60:1231, 1968.

83. Hellström, I., Pierce, G. E., and Hellström, K. E.   Human tumor specific antigens. *Surgery* 65:984, 1964.
84. Hellström, I., Hellström, K. E., and Shepard, T. H.   Cell mediated immunity against antigens common to human colonic carcinomas and fetal gut epithelium. *Int. J. Cancer* 6:346, 1970.
85. Hellström, I., and Hellström, K. E.   Colony inhibition and cytotoxic assays. In B. R. Bloom and P. R. Glade (eds.), *In Vitro Methods in Cell Mediated Immunity* New York: Academic Press, 1971.
86. Hellström, I., Sjögren, H. O., Warner, G., and Hellström, K. E.   Blocking of cell-mediated tumor immunity by sera from patients with growing neoplasms. *Int. J. Cancer* 7:226, 1971.
87. Hellström, K. E., and Hellström, I.   Cellular immunity against tumor antigens. *Adv. Cancer Res.* 12:167, 1969.
88. Hellström, K. E., and Hellström, I.   Immunological enhancement as studied by cell culture techniques. *Ann. Rev. Microbiol.* 24:373, 1970.
89. Henle, G., and Henle, W.   Immunofluorescence in cells derived from Burkitt's lymphoma. *J. Bacteriol.* 91:1248, 1966.
90. Henle, G., Henle, W., and Diehl, V.   Relation of Burkitt's tumor-associated herpes-type virus to infectious mononucleosis. *Proc. Natl. Acad. Sci. U.S.A.* 59:94, 1968.
91. Herberman, R.   Immunological reactions of experimental animals to tumor associated cell surface antigens. *Pathobiology Annual,* 1972.
92. Hirshaut, Y., Glade, P., Vieira, L. O. B. D., Ainbender, E., Dvorak, B., and Siltzbach, L.   Sarcoidosis, another disease associated with serologic evidence for herpes-like virus infection. *N. Engl. J. Med.* 283:502, 1970.
93. Hollinshead, A., Glew, D., Bunnay, B., Gold, P., and Herberman, R.   Skin reactive soluble antigen from intestinal cancer cell membranes and relationship to carcinoembryonic antigens. *Lancet* 1:1191, 1970.
94. Hollinshead, A. C., McWright, C. G., Alford, T. C., Glew, D. H., Gold, P., and Herberman, R. B.   Separation of skin reactive intestinal cancer antigen from the carcinoembryonic antigen of Gold. *Science* 177:887, 1972.
95. Hughes, I. F., and Lytton, B.   Antigenic properties of human tumors: Delayed cutaneous hypersensitivity reactions. *Br. Med. J.* 1:209, 1964.
96. Järnerot, G., and Lantorp, K.   Antibodies to EB virus in cases of Crohn's disease. *N. Engl. J. Med.* 286:1215, 1972.
97. Jehn, U. W., Nathanson, L., Schwartz, R. S., and Skinner, M.   In vitro lymphocyte stimulation by a soluble antigen from malignant melanoma. *N. Engl. J. Med.* 283:329, 1970.
98. Kang, K. Y., Higashino, K., Hashinotsume, M., Takahashi, Y., Aoki, T., Tsubura, E., and Yamamura, Y.   Production of placental type alkaline phosphatase isoenzyme by lung cancer tissue. *Gann* 63:217, 1972.
99. Kang, K. Y., Higashino, K., Takahashi, Y., Hashinotsume, M., and Yamamura, W.   α fetoprotein in ill infants. *N. Engl. J. Med.* 287:48, 1972.
100. Kent, S. P.   The demonstration and distribution of water soluble blood group O (H) antigen in tissue sections using a fluorescein labelled extract of *Ulex europeus* seed. *J. Histochem. Cytochem.* 12:591, 1964.
101. Klein, G.   Tumor antigens. *Ann. Rev. Microbiol.* 20:723, 1966.

102. Klein, G. Experimental studies in tumor immunology. *Fed. Proc.* 28:1739, 1969.
103. Klein, G., Geering, G., Old, L. J., Henle, G., Henle, W., and Clifford, P. Comparison of the anti EBV titer and the EBV associated membrane reactive and precipitating antibody levels in the sera of Burkitt lymphoma and nasopharyngeal carcinoma patients and controls. *Int. J. Cancer* 5:185, 1970.
104. Kohn, G., Mellman, W. J., Moorhead, P. S., Loftus, J., and Henle, G. Involvement of C-group chromosomes in five Burkitt lymphoma cell lines. *J. Nat. Cancer Inst.* 38:209, 1967.
105. Kovarik, S., Davidsohn, I., and Stejskal, R. ABO antigens in cancer. Detection with the mixed cell agglutination reaction. *Arch. Pathol.* 86:12, 1968.
106. Kozower, M., Fawaz, K. A., Miller, H. M., and Kaplan, M. M. Positive alpha-fetoglobulin in a case of gastric carcinoma. *N. Engl. J. Med.* 285:1059, 1971.
107. Krupey, J., Wilson, T., Freedman, S. O., and Gold, P. The preparation of purified carcinoembryonic antigen of the human digestive system from large quantities of tumor tissue. *Immunochemistry* 9:617, 1972.
108. Krupey, J., Gold, P., and Freedman, S. O. Physicochemical studies of the carcinoembryonic antigens of the human digestive system. *J. Exp. Med.* 128:387, 1968.
109. Lange, R. D., Chernoff, A., and Collman, R. I. Experience with a hemagglutination inhibition test for carcinoembryonic antigen. Preliminary report. In M. G. Anderson and J. H. Coggin (eds.), *Proceedings of the 1st Conference and Workshop on Embryonic and Fetal Antigens in Cancer.* Springfield, Va.: Oak Ridge National Laboratory, National Technical Information Service, 1971.
110. Lawrence, D. J. R., Stevens, V., Bettelheim, R., Darcy, D., Leese, C., Turberville, C., Alexander, P., Johns, E. W., and Neville, A. M. Role of plasma carcinoembryonic antigen in diagnosis of gastrointestinal, mammary, and bronchial carcinoma. *Br. Med. J.* 2:605, 1972.
111. Lawrence, H. S., and Landy, M. *Mediators of Cellular Immunity.* New York: Academic Press, 1969.
112. Lawrence, H. S. Transfer factor. *Adv. Immunol.* 11:195, 1969.
113. Lawrence, H. S. Transfer factor and cellular immune deficiency disease. *N. Engl. J. Med.* 283:411, 1970.
114. LeBel, J. S., Deodhar, S. D., and Brown, C. H. Evaluation of a radioimmunoassay for carcinoembryonic antigen of the human digestive system. *Clev. Clin. Q.* 39:25, 1972.
115. Letjtenji, M. C., Freedman, S. O., and Gold, P. Response of lymphocytes from patients with gastrointestinal cancer to the carcinoembryonic antigen of the human digestive system. *Cancer* 28:115, 1971.
116. Leventhal, B. G., Halterman, R. H., Rosenberg, E. B., and Herberman, R. B. Immune reactivity of leukemic patients to autologous blast cells. *Cancer Res.* 32:1820, 1972.
117. Lewis, M. G., and Phillips, T. M. The specificity of surface membrane immunofluorescence in human malignant melanoma. *Int. J. Cancer* 10:105, 1972.

118. Lewis, M. G.   Circulating humoral antibodies in cancer. *Med. Clin. North Am.* 56:481, 1972.
119. Lewis, M. G., Ikonopisov, R. L., Nairn, R. C., Phillips, T. M., Hamilton-Fairley, G., Bodenham, D. C., and Alexander, P.   Tumor specific antibodies in human malignant melanoma and their relationship to the extent of the disease. *Br. Med. J.* 3:547, 1969.
120. LoGerfo, P., Krupey, J., and Hansen, H. J.   Demonstration of an antigen common to several varieties of neoplasia. *N. Engl. J. Med.* 285:138, 1971.
121. LoGerfo, P., Herter, F. P., and Bennett, S. J.   Absence of circulating antibodies to carcinoembryonic antigen in patients with gastrointestinal malignancies. *Int. J. Cancer* 9:344, 1972.
122. Lynch, H. T.   Genetic factors in carcinoma. *Med. Clin. North Am.* 53:923, 1969.
123. Mach, J. P., and Pusztaszeri, G.   Carcinoembryonic antigen (CEA): Demonstration of a partial identity between CEA and a normal glycoprotein. *Immunochemistry* 9:1031, 1972.
124. Malmgren, R. A., and Morton, D. L.   Viral and immunologic studies of human neoplasms. *Pathobiology Annual* 1:63, 1971.
125. Mehlman, D. J., Buckley, B. H., and Wiernik, P. H.   Serum alpha$_1$-fetoprotein with gastric and prostatic carcinoma. *N. Engl. J. Med.* 285:1060, 1971.
126. Metzgar, R. S., Mohanakumar, T., and Miller, D. S.   Antigens specific for human lymphocytic and myeloid leukemic cells: Detection by non-human private antiserums. *Science* 178:986, 1972.
127. Mody, M. J., Vogel, C. L., Patel, I. R., and McIntire, K. R.   Rivanol precipitation technique for the detection of alpha-fetoprotein. *J. Lab. Clin. Med.* 80:125, 1972.
128. Moore, T. L., Kupchik, H. Z., Marcon, N., and Zamcheck, M.   Carcinoembryonic antigen assay in cancer of the colon and pancreas and other digestive tract disorders. *Am. J. Dig. Dis.* 16:1, 1971.
129. Moore, T. L., Kantrowitz, P. A., and Zamcheck, N.   Carcinoembryonic antigen (CEA) in inflammatory bowel disease. *J.A.M.A.* 222:944, 1972.
130. Morton, D. C., Malgren, R. A., Hall, W. T., and Schidlovsky, G.   Immunologic and virus studies with human sarcoma. *Surgery* 66:152, 1969.
131. Morton, D. L., Holmes, E. C., Eilber, F. R., and Wood, W. C.   Immunological aspects of neoplasia: A rational basis for immunotherapy. *Ann. Intern. Med.* 74:587, 1971.
132. Muna, N. M., Marcus, S., and Smart, C.   Detection by immunofluorescence of antibodies specific for human malignant melanoma cells. *Cancer* 28:88, 1969.
133. Nakahara, W., Nishioka, K., Hiroyama, T., and Ito, Y.   *Recent Advances in Human Tumor Virology and Immunology.* Baltimore: University Park Press, 1971.
134. Nathanson, L., and Fishman, W. H.   New observations on the Regan isoenzyme of alkaline phosphatase in cancer patients. *Cancer* 27:1388, 1971.
135. Nicolson, G. L.   Difference in topology of normal and tumor cell membranes shown by different distribution of ferritin conjugated concanavalin A. *Nature [New Biol.]* 233:244, 1971.

136. Nicolson, G. L.   Topography of membrane concanavalin A sites modified by proteolysis. *Nature [New Biol.]* 239:193, 1972.
137. Nowell, P. C., and Hungerford, D. A.   A minute chromosome in human chronic granulocytic leukemia. *Science* 132:1497, 1960.
138. Oettgen, H. R., Aoki, T., Old, L. J., Boyse, E. A., DeHarven, E., and Mills, G.   Suspension culture of a pigment producing cell line derived from a human malignant melanoma. *J. Natl. Cancer Inst.* 41:827, 1968.
139. Oettgen, H. F., Old, L. J., and Boyse, E. A.   Human tumor immunology. *Med. Clin. North Am.* 55:761, 1971.
140. Old, L. J., Boyse, E. A., Oettgen, H. F., DeHarven, E., Geering, G., Williamson, B., and Clifford, P.   Precipitating antibody in human serum to an antigen present in culture of Burkitt's lymphoma cells. *Proc. Nat. Acad. Sci. U.S.A.* 56:1699, 1966.
141. Order, S. E., Porter, M., and Hellman, S.   Hodgkin's disease: Evidence for a tumor associated antigen. *N. Engl. J. Med.* 285:471, 1971.
142. Oren, M. E., and Herberman, R. B.   Delayed cutaneous hypersensitivity reactions to membrane extracts of human tumor cells. *Clin. Exp. Immunol.* 9:45, 1971.
143. Pick, E., and Turk, J. L.   Review: The biological activities of soluble lymphocyte products. *Clin. Exp. Immunol.* 10:1, 1972.
144. Pritchard, J. A. V., Moore, J. L., Sutherland, W. H., and Joslin, C. A. F.   Immunodiagnosis of cancer. *Br. Med. J.* 3:823, 1972.
145. Pritchard, J. A. V., Moore, J. L., Sutherland, W. H., and Joslin, C. A. F.   Macrophage electrophoretic mobility (M.E.M.) test for malignant disease: An independent confirmation. *Lancet* 3:627, 1972.
146. Purtilo, D. T., and Yunis, E. J.   α-fetoprotein: Its immunofluorescent localization in human fetal liver and hepatoma. *Lab. Invest.* 25:291, 1971.
147. Purves, L. R., MacNab, M., and Bersohn, I.   Serum alpha-fetoprotein: I. Immunodiffusion and immunoassay results in cases of primary cancer of the liver. *S. Afr. Med. J.* 42:1138, 1968.
148. Purves, L. R., Bersohn, I., and Geddes, E. W.   Serum alpha-fetoprotein and primary cancer of the liver in man. *Cancer* 25:1261, 1970.
149. Purves, L. R., and Geddes, E. W.   A more sensitive test for alpha-fetoprotein. *Lancet* 1:47, 1972.
150. Reynoso, G., Chu, T. M., Holyoke, D., Cohen, E., Nemoto, T., Wang, J. J., Chuang, J., Guinan, P., and Murphy, G. P.   Carcinoembryonic antigen in patients with different cancers. *J.A.M.A.* 220:361, 1972.
151. Rule, A. H., Straus, E., VandeVoorde, J., and Janowitz, H. D.   Tumor associated (CEA reacting) antigen in patients with inflammatory bowel disease. *N. Engl. J. Med.* 287:24, 1972.
152. Ruoslahti, E., and Seppala, M.   Studies of carcino-fetal proteins: III. Development of a radioimmunoassay for alpha-fetoprotein. Demonstration of alpha fetoprotein in serum of healthy human adults. *Int. J. Cancer.* 8:374, 1971.
153. Ruoslahti, E., and Seppala, M.   Normal and increased alpha-fetoprotein in neoplastic and in nonneoplastic liver disease. *Lancet* 2:278, 1972.
154. Ryser, H. J. P.   Chemical carcinogenesis. *N. Engl. J. Med.* 285:721, 1971.
155. Sanders, F. K.   Problems in the study of oncogenic   in vitro. *Med. Clin. North America* 55:653, 1971.

156. Schrèck, R.   Use of eosin dye to distinguish live and dead cells. *Am. J. Cancer* 28:389, 1936.
157. Sharon, N., and Lis, H.   Lectins: Cell agglutinating and sugar specific proteins. *Science* 177:949, 1972.
158. Sizaret, P. P., McIntire, K. R., and Princler, G. L.   Quantitation of human α-fetoprotein by electroimmunodiffusion. *Cancer Res.* 31:1899, 1971.
159. Smith, J. B.   Alpha-fetoprotein: Occurrence in certain malignant diseases and review of clinical applications. *Med. Clin. North Am.* 54·797, 1970.
160. Smith, J. B.   Occurrence of alpha-fetoprotein in acute viral hepatitis. *Int. J. Cancer* 8:421, 1971.
161. Smith, J. B., and O'Neill, R. T.   Alpha-fetoprotein: Occurrence in germinal cell and liver malignancies. *Am. J. Med.* 51:767, 1971.
162. Smith, R. T.   Tumor specific immune mechanisms. *N. Engl. J. Med.* 278:1207, 1968.
163. Smith, R. T., and Landy, M. *Immune Surveillance.* New York: Academic Press, 1970.
164. Smith, R. T.   Possibilities and problems of immunologic intervention in cancer. *N. Engl. J. Med.* 287:439, 1972.
165. Southam, C. M.   Cancer specific antigens in man. In M. Samter (ed.), *Immunological Diseases.* Boston: Little, Brown, 1971, 2nd ed., vol. 1, p. 743.
166. Stewart, T. H. M.   The presence of delayed hypersensitivity reactions in patients toward cellular extracts of their malignant tumors. *Cancer* 23:1368, 1969.
167. Stillman, A., and Zamcheck, M.   Recent advances in immunological diagnosis of digestive tract cancer. *Am. J. Dig. Dis.* 15:1003, 1970.
168. Stolbach, L. L., Krant, M. J., and Fishman, W. H.   Ectopic production of an alkaline phosphatase isoenzyme in patients with cancer. *N. Engl. J. Med.* 281:757, 1969.
169. Takasugi, M., and Klein, E.   A microassay for cell-mediated immunity. *Transplantation* 9:219, 1970.
170. Tal, C., Dishon, T., and Gross, J.   The agglutination of tumor cells in vitro by sera from tumor patients and pregnant women. *Br. J. Cancer* 18:111, 1964.
171. Tal, C.   The nature of cell membrane receptor for the agglutination factor present in the sera of tumor patients and pregnant women. *Proc. Nat. Acad. Sci. U.S.A.* 54:1318, 1965.
172. Tal, C., and Halperin, M.   Presence of serologically distinct protein in serum of cancer patients and pregnant women. An attempt to develop a diagnostic cancer test. *Isr. J. Med. Sci.* 6:708, 1970.
173. Terry, W. D., Henkart, P. A., Coligan, J. T., and Todd, C. W.   Structural studies of the major glycoprotein in preparations with carcinoembryonic antigen activity. *J. Exp. Med.* 136:200, 1972.
174. Thompson, D. M. P., Krupey, J., Freedman, S. O., and Gold, P.   The radioimmunoassay of circulating carcinoembryonic antigen of the human digestive tract. *Proc. Nat. Acad. Sci. U.S.A.* 64:161, 1969.
175. Ting, C. C., Lavrin, D. H., Shiu, G., and Herberman, R. B.   Expression of fetal antigen in tumor cells. *Proc. Nat. Acad. Sci. U.S.A.* 69:1664, 1972.

176. Usategui-Gomez, M., Yeager, F., and Fernandez de Castro, F.   Unpublished data, personal communication, 1973.
177. Usategui-Gomez, M., Yeager, F., and Fernandez de Castro, F.   A sensitive immunochemical method for the determination of Regan isoenzyme in serum. *Cancer Res.* 33:1574, 1973.
178. Valentine, F. T., and Lawrence, H. S.   Cell mediated immunity. *Adv. Intern. Med.* 17:51, 1971.
179. Von Kleist, S., and Burtin, P.   On the specificity of autoantibodies present in colon cancer patients. *Immunology* 10:507, 1966.
180. Von Kleist, S., and Burtin, P.   Localization cellulaire d'une antigene embryonnaire de tumeurs coliques humaines. *Int. J. Cancer* 4:874, 1969.
181. Von Kleist, S., Chavenel, G., and Burtin, P.   Identification of an antigen from normal human tissue that cross reacts with the carcinoembryonic antigen. *Proc. Nat. Acad. Sci. U.S.A.* 69:2492, 1972.
182. Warnock, M. L., and Reisman, R.   Variant alkaline phosphatase in human hepatocellular cancers. *Clin. Chim. Acta* 24:5, 1969.
183. Willoughby, D. A., Boughton, B., and Schild, H. O.   A factor capable of increasing vascular permeability present in lymph node cells. A possible mediator of the delayed reaction. *Immunology* 6:484, 1963.
184. Wood, W. C., and Morton, D. L.   Host response to a common cell surface antigen in human sarcoma. *N. Engl. J. Med.* 284:569, 1971.
185. Zamcheck, N., Moore, T. C., Dhar, P., and Kupchick, H.   Immunologic diagnosis and prognosis of human digestive tract cancer: Carcinoembryonic antigens. *N. Engl. J. Med.* 286:83, 1972.
186. Zilber, L. A., and Abelev, G. T.   *The Virology and Immunology of Cancer.* New York: Pergamon Press, 1968.

20

Carcinoembryonic Antigen

Marianne L. Egan

The carcinoembryonic antigen (CEA) is a glycoprotein present in adenocarcinomas of the entodermally derived digestive tract epithelium and in fetal intestine. It was originally described by Gold and Freedman in 1965 [18–20]. When this antigen was also detected in the blood of patients with adenocarcinoma [48], its potential as a diagnostic test for cancer was immediately recognized. Several methods of radioimmunoassay for CEA have been developed. These include the ammonium sulfate precipitation method [48], the zirconyl phosphate method [29], and the double antibody method [13].

Numerous laboratories in several countries are engaged in studies to determine whether the serum level of CEA will be an aid in the diagnosis and prognosis of cancer. In spite of findings that the antigen may have a wider distribution than originally reported, there seems to be a general concensus that CEA levels are helpful as a prognostic tool once a tumor has been surgically removed [27, 30, 40, 42, 52]. However, much additional research and a more detailed knowledge of the structure of CEA are necessary to determine whether CEA will be the basis of a reliable test for the diagnosis and detection of cancer.

Distribution of CEA in Adenocarcinomas of the Digestive Tract and in Other Tumors

Colonic adenocarcinoma was recognized by Gold and Freedman as material especially suitable for the isolation of a human tumor specific antigen [18, 19]. Since these adenocarcinomas usually do not penetrate very far and at surgery a considerable amount of normal tissue is removed along with the primary tumor, it was possible to overcome one of the major criticisms of previously reported cancer specific antigens, namely, these antigens were due not to a unique antigen present in tumors but rather to antigens unique for a given individual from which the tumor had been isolated. By first tolerizing rabbits with normal human

564

colon and then injecting tumor tissue from the same donor as the normal tissue, Gold and Freedman were able to obtain specific anticolonic adenocarcinoma antiserum [19].

The first report of CEA levels in colonic adenocarcinoma patients indicated that 97% of all patients with colonic adenocarcinoma had serum levels greater than 2.5 ng/ml, and that a normal population had no detectable CEA. Tumors other than colonic adenocarcinomas were negative [48]. Subsequent reports from other laboratories indicated that the number of adenocarcinoma patients with positive CEA serum assays greater than 2.5 ng/ml ranged from 64 to 97% [27–30, 36, 42, 48]. There is general agreement that the degree of metastatic spread of a tumor will influence the CEA serum values [27, 40]. The correspondence of degree of differentiation and amount of CEA in tumor tissue has been demonstrated by indirect immunofluorescence studies [12]. However, there seems to be no correlation between the degree of differentiation and serum CEA levels [27].

It now appears that the CEA has a wider distribution than initially described. Material reactive in CEA assays has been found in the serum of patients with breast, genitourinary tract, and respiratory tract adenocarcinoma; osteogenic sarcoma; neuroblastoma; leukemia; and Hodgkin's disease [8, 27–29, 35, 40, 42, 43]. A positive serum result is based on inhibition of binding of a radiotagged antigen with antibody. Since similar substances will also inhibit in a radioimmune assay, positive tests with these other tumors do not necessarily indicate the presence of CEA. Final proof that these tumors contain a molecule identical to the CEA of colonic adenocarcinoma will rest on the isolation and chemical characterization of these molecules.

Possible Presence of CEA in Normal and Diseased Tissue

Opinions have differed on whether or not, or to what extent, CEA is present in normal tissue [4, 6, 7, 26, 31–35]. This question is of obvious practical importance when using a serum CEA assay for the early detection of cancer. A substance with CEA activity extracted from pooled normal serum is soluble in perchloric acid and elutes from a Sephadex G-200 (Pharmacia) column in the same position as CEA [7, 26]. A substance has been extracted from normal liver which is immunologically similar to CEA when tested by radioimmunoassay, Ouchterlony double diffusion, immunoprecipitation inhibition, and immunoelectrophoresis [26]. Whether or not this substance with antigenic components similar to CEA is in fact CEA remains to be determined by chemical characterization.

The serum or tissue extract of patients with alcoholic cirrhosis, ulcerative colitis, inflammatory bowel disease, inflammatory chest disease, renal failure, and benign polyps is positive in a CEA assay [5, 8, 26–28,

35–38, 40, 46]. The CEA assay levels in these diseases are generally lower than in patients with metastatic colonic adenocarcinoma. Again, more detailed information on the structure of these molecules is necessary to determine whether they are identical to CEA or merely cross-reactive in a radioimmune assay.

Distribution of CEA in Urine, Feces, Saliva, and Meconium
Material reactive in a CEA radioimmune assay is present in the urine of patients with urinary tract adenocarcinoma. Lower values are present in the urine of healthy control subjects [23].

CEA or a molecule similar to CEA has been extracted from the feces of patients with gastrointestinal cancers and from the feces of healthy individuals [17]. A substance which inhibits in the radioimmune assay of CEA has also been found in meconium [21] and in saliva of patients with cystic fibrosis and asthma [1].

Chemical Studies on the Structure of CEA

Most of the studies describing the presence of CEA in the serum of cancer patients, patients with nonmalignant disease, and healthy controls were concerned with the measurement of CEA by immunologic methods. Although antibodies have the greatest affinity for their respective antigens they will also react with substances similar to the stimulating antigen, although with lower affinity. Thus, a substance which triggers the CEA assay is not necessarily CEA.[1] The only definitive proof that the molecule isolated from hepatic metastases of colonic adenocarcinoma is identical to a molecule present in normal liver and in an alcoholic cirrhotic liver is chemical characterization of these molecules [10].

CEA is a glycoprotein soluble in 1 M perchloric acid [18]. It has a β electrophoretic mobility and a sedimentation coefficient of 7–8 S [9, 25, 49]. It is possible to extract CEA from other tissue components by homogenization of tumor tissue in deionized water, followed by perchloric acid to precipitate the proteins [9, 18, 51]. It may also be obtained by extraction with butanol [32] or lithium diiodosalicylate [45] followed by partition in a phenol-water system and ethanol extraction of the glycoprotein fraction.

The amount of carbohydrate of individual preparations of CEA varies between 50% and 75% [11, 25, 47]. CEA is electrophoretically heterogeneous in isoelectric focusing [11, 50]. This heterogenity is due in part, but not entirely, to the sialic acid residues. Removal of the sialic acid does not affect the behavior of the molecule in a radioimmune assay [11].

---

[1] It is not even necessarily a substance reacting with the antibody against CEA. See [41] for a reference describing a case in which an enzyme which hydrolyzed the radiotagged antigen mimicked the antigen itself in the assay.

Although some investigators have found blood group A activity in several preparations of CEA, only trace amounts of N-acetylgalactosamine, the sugar responsible for blood group A immunologic activity, have been reported in some preparations of CEA [11]. Others have found no N-acetylgalactosamine [2]. The major sugars present are L-fucose, D-mannose, D-galactose, N-acetylglucosamine, and sialic acid [2, 24, 25].

The amino acid compositions of different CEA preparations are very similar [25, 47]. CEA preparations from five different tumors had identical N-terminal amino acid sequences [47, and unpublished observations]. The investigators were able to sequence 20 residues.

An antigenic determinant has been isolated by controlled acid hydrolysis and paper chromatography of the CEA fragments [2]. The fragment with the most immunologic activity contained mannose and N-acetylglucosamine. No detectable amino acids were present in the immunologically active fragment.

The Triple Isotope Double Antibody Assay for CEA

Studies on the chemical structure of CEA require the isolation of large quantities of CEA. Because of the necessity to analyze a great many Sepharose and Sephadex column fractions for CEA activity, a radioimmune assay for CEA has been devised which is simple and rapid, and which can be performed from start to finish in the same tube [13–16]. Since it is done in microtest tubes, a large number of assays may be conveniently handled at one time. A general outline of the procedure is given in Fig. 20-1.

Figure 20-1
General protocol for the radioimmune assay of CEA by the double antibody triple isotope technique. The radioactive cocktail is incubated with the sample to be assayed and anti-CEA for 2 hours at 37° C. Horse anti-goat IgG is added and the incubation continued for 1 hour at 37° C and 15 min at −4° C.

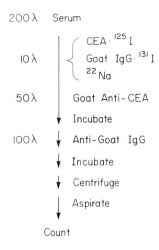

Double Antibody

This assay is based on a technique originally described by Morgan and Lazarow [39] and later developed by Berson and Yalow as a practical routine laboratory technique for the measurement of insulin [3]. In a radioimmune assay small amounts (nanograms, 10^{-9} gm, to picograms, 10^{-12} gm) of radiotagged antigen are mixed with a correspondingly small amount of antibody. The antigen and antibody combine but do not precipitate since they are present in low concentrations. In a double antibody radioimmune assay, precipitation of the antigen-antibody complex is effected by the addition of a second antibody directed against the immunoglobulins of the species making the first antibody.[2] For example, for the radioimmune assay of CEA we use anti-CEA antibody made in a goat. This antibody is diluted with normal goat serum to achieve an optimal concentration of both specific anti-CEA antibody and other immunoglobulins. An amount of horse anti-goat IgG sufficient to precipitate all the goat immunoglobulin is added. Thus, radiotagged CEA bound to specific antibody is precipitated along with all the other immunoglobulin present. The amount of antigen not bound by antibody may be measured by counting the radioactivity in a portion of the supernate or by counting the precipitate and subtracting these counts from the total counts in the system.

The principle of radioimmune assay is based on competition between radiotagged (hot) antigen and nontagged (cold) antigen for a limited number of antibody-combining sites. Usually the initial concentrations of reactants are adjusted so that 30–50% of the radiotagged antigen is bound. Increasing amounts of nonradiotagged antigen are added to a series of tubes containing a constant amount of antibody and radiotagged antigen. The competition of the hot and cold antigen for the antibody sites is measured by a decrease in the counts in the precipitate. A standard curve may be constructed in which the amount of cold antigen added is plotted versus the percent inhibition of counts obtained in the precipitate (Fig. 20-2).

There are many ways of statistically analyzing the data from a radioimmune assay. A detailed description of these methods will be found in [44]. One method is to plot the data as shown in Fig. 20-2 and use the approximately linear portion of the plot to determine the concentration of CEA in unknown samples.

Triple Isotope

The double antibody technique as originally described employed one isotope. The assay has been modified by incorporating two additional isotopes. Although at first glance these additional isotopes appear to

---

[2] In this discussion the term *antibody* is used to describe a molecule reacting against a specific antigen in question, and the term *immunoglobulin* is used to refer to all antibodies in general. IgG refers to a specific class of immunoglobulins.

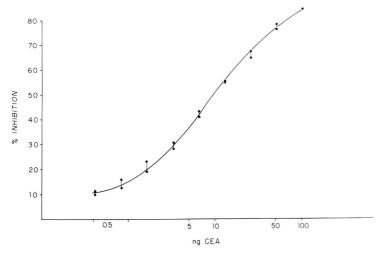

Figure 20-2
Standard inhibition curve obtained by the addition of unlabeled CEA to a constant amount (0.5 ng) of CEA · ^{125}I. The anti-CEA was diluted 1:1600.

complicate the assay, they actually serve to streamline it and to provide controls for the most likely sources of error when large numbers of unrelated samples are assayed.

^{22}Na is included as a volume marker [23]. This eliminates the necessity of removing a precise amount of supernate or washing the precipitate at the completion of the assay. A detailed explanation of the use of ^{22}Na as a volume marker in the CEA assay will be found in [13] and [14]. Briefly, since all the ^{22}Na is in the supernate, the following relationship holds:

$$\frac{^{22}\text{Na discarded}}{^{22}\text{Na total}} = \frac{^{125}\text{I discarded}}{^{125}\text{I total in supernate}}$$

The equation can be solved for ^{125}I in the supernate, and the results subtracted from the ^{125}I total to obtain the ^{125}I in the precipitate. The use of the ^{22}Na as a volume marker eliminates a time-consuming step necessary at the completion of a radioimmune assay—either washing the precipitate or removing an exact amount of supernate. When large numbers of assays are processed each day the time saved by the use of ^{22}Na as a volume marker becomes very significant. Since it is not necessary to disturb the precipitate, losses inadvertently incurred in the washing step are eliminated.

Goat IgG tagged with ^{131}I is added in trace quantities to each tube to check for completeness of precipitation of all the goat IgG. The conditions of the assay are adjusted so that all the goat IgG · ^{131}I should be precipitated. If there is less than 100% in the precipitate, either the antigen or antibody solutions were not added correctly, for some reason something interfered with the precipitation step, or the precipitate was inadvertently removed in the aspiration step.

Automatic Processing of Radioimmune Assay Data
In addition to the calculations involving the supernate when ^{22}Na is used as a volume marker, it is necessary to correct the ^{125}I counts for overlap from the higher energy isotopes, ^{131}I and ^{22}Na, and the ^{131}I counts for overlap from the ^{22}Na to obtain the ^{131}I and ^{125}I in the precipitate. From these latter values the percent precipitation of these two isotopes can be obtained. Processing all this data is not complicated, but it involves numerous repetitive corrections of counts and calculations of percent bound, percent precipitation, and percent inhibition. To facilitate these calculations, a program has been written for the Wang 700 Programable Calculator which will analyze the results from each assay tube and print out the results of the calculations, including a value for CEA expressed as total nanograms in the sample [15]. Radioactivity counts are registered on punched tape by a teletype connected to a Nuclear Chicago Gamma Scintillation Spectrometer equipped with a 512 channel spectrum analyzer and a multiple region of interest accessory. The data are fed into the Wang through a Wang 703 Paper Tape Editor. The results are printed out on a Wang 701 Output Writer. A copy of this program is available on request to the author.

The program is written in 5 parts. In the first part, 3 tubes containing either ^{125}I, ^{131}I, or ^{22}Na are counted. ^{125}I is counted from 10 to 70 kev, ^{131}I from 320 to 400 kev, and ^{22}Na from 470 to 550 kev. The required values for the percent overlap are calculated by the Wang 700 and stored for correcting the counts in each assay tube (Fig. 20-3).

Determination of ^{125}I, ^{131}I, and ^{22}Na Overlap

	Sample No.	Counts x 1/1000 Channel		
		1	2	3
^{125}I	101	5.334	.045	.164
^{131}I	102	5.927	26.334	.337
^{22}Na	103	6.920	3.689	31.675
^{131}I	Ratio ½	.225	Stored in Reg 3	
^{22}Na	Ratio ⅔	.116	Stored in Reg 1	
	Ratio ⅓	.218	Stored in Reg 2	

Figure 20-3
Part 1 of the program. The percent overlap is calculated.

Standardization

---

ng CEA $= Kf(x)$ $K = .483$ ng CEA/unit Reg 4

^{125}I $=$ Ch 1 $-$ Ch 3 $\times$ Reg 2 $-$ (Ch 2 $-$ Ch 3 $\times$ Reg 1) Reg 3

^{131}I $=$ Ch 2 $-$ Ch 3 $\times$ Reg 1

^{22}Na $=$ Ch 3

^{22}Na Ch 2/Ch 3 $= .116$ Reg 1

Ch 1/Ch 3 $= .218$ Reg 2

^{131}I Ch 1/Ch 2 $= .225$ Reg 3

All counts $\div$ 1000

$$\% \; ^{131}I = \frac{100 \, [1 - (\text{Reg } 5 - \; ^{131}I) \; \text{Reg } 6]}{(\text{Reg } 6 - \; ^{22}\text{Na}) \; \text{Reg } 5}$$

$$^{125}I \; \text{pptd} = \frac{\text{Reg } 7 - (\text{Reg } 7 - \; ^{125}I) \; \text{Reg } 6}{(\text{Reg } 6 - \; ^{22}\text{Na})}$$

$$\% \; \text{Pptd} = \frac{100 \times \; ^{125}I \; \text{pptd}}{\text{Reg } 7}$$

$$\% \; \text{Inhib} = \frac{100 \, (1 - \; ^{125}I \; \text{pptd})}{\text{Reg } 8}$$

Figure 20-4
Part 2 of the program. The calculations used to compute nanograms of CEA are printed out.

Part 2 prints out the K value described below and the calculations performed in the following three parts of the program, and sets the heading for the third part (Fig. 20-4).

The standard curve is calculated in program part 3 (Fig. 20-5). The data from tubes 4 to 14 are used to calculate this curve. Tube 4 contains 10λ of the cocktail (CEA · ^{125}I, 0.5 ng; goat IgG · ^{131}I, 1 μg; and ^{22}Na, 40,000 cpm), which has also been pipetted into each of the other assay tubes.[3] The counts in this tube are used to determine the number of counts originally present in each assay tube. Tube 5 includes radioactive cocktail and an amount of anti-CEA which will bind approximately 40% of the CEA · ^{125}I. All other tubes in the assay will be compared to this tube to determine if inhibition of binding has occurred. Tubes 6–14 include, in addition to the cocktail and antibody, doubling concentrations of unlabeled CEA, usually from 0.5 to 128 ng. Since the amount of cold CEA used in each assay may vary, the nanograms of CEA are expressed as units. These units are then converted to actual

---

[3] It is convenient to use a Micromedic Automatic Pipettor 25000 for the addition of cocktail to the tubes [15]. This ensures reproducible pipetting of the radioactive cocktail.

Units	Sample No.	Ch 1	Ch 2	Ch 3	^{131}I	% ^{131}I	^{22}Na	^{125}I	^{125}I Pptd	% Pptd	% Inhib	Reg
Blank	4	37.692	63.465	42.542	58.484 Reg 5	—	42.542 Reg 6	14.471 Reg 7	—	—	—	—
0	5	22.357	58.868	5.143		99.5	5.143	7.483	6.522 Reg 8	100	.0	1–06
1	6	21.366	58.425	4.577	57.889	98.8	4.577	6.707	5.771	39.8	11.5	1–07
2	7	20.737	57.389	5.424	56.754	96.6	5.424	6.157	4.942	34.1	24.2	1–08
4	8	20.707	58.421	5.236	57.808	98.6	5.236	5.921	4.721	32.6	27.6	1–09
8	9	19.121	58.815	4.874	58.244	99.5	4.874	4.312	2.998	20.7	54.0	2–00
16	10	18.134	58.753	4.932	58.175	99.4	4.932	3.328	1.867	12.9	71.3	2–01
32	11	17.112	58.727	4.960	58.146	99.3	4.960	2.307	.702	4.8	89.2	2–02
64	12	16.951	58.050	5.531	57.402	97.8	5.531	2.195	.360	2.4	94.4	2–03
128	13	15.693	57.111	4.658	56.565	96.3	4.658	1.328	−.287	−1.9	104.4	2–04
256	14	15.555	56.275	4.886	55.703	94.6	4.886	1.342	−.360	−2.4	105.5	2–05

Figure 20-5
Part 3 of the program. The data for the standard curve are read from the punched paper tape and recorded.

nanograms of CEA by means of a *K* value, which is manually stored in register 4 before starting the program. The calculator computes the percent binding of CEA for each tube, compares it to the percent bound in tube 5, computes the percent inhibition, and stores the inhibition in a register as indicated in Fig. 20-5 for later recall when calculating unknown data.

In part 4 of the program, a plot of the standard curve is made on the Wang 701 Output Writer (Fig. 20-6). This plot is made by using the spacing mechanism of the typewriter.

The data for the unknown samples are calculated in part 5 of the program (Fig. 20-7). The nanograms of CEA in a given unknown are calculated by interpolation of the two points on the standard curve closest to the percent inhibition given by that sample.

A repeat of the standard curve is usually included at the beginning

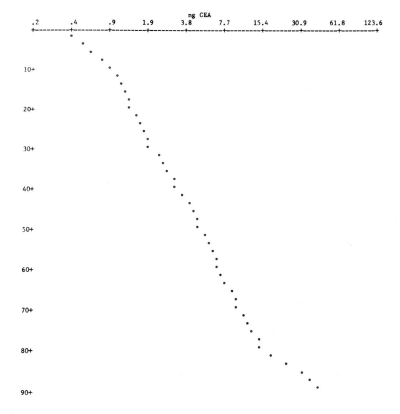

Figure 20-6
Part 4 of the program. The standard curve is printed out by means of the spacing mechanism of the Wang 701 Output Writer.

Sample No	Ch 1	Ch 2	Ch 3	131I	% 131I	22Na	125I	125I Pptd	% Pptd	% Inhib	ng CEA
15	4.472	6.660	1.767	6.506	101.3	1.767	2.664	1.703	8.9	74.6	35.8
16	4.888	6.600	2.278	6.401	99.5	2.278	3.020	1.787	9.4	73.4	34.3
17	4.869	6.556	2.074	6.375	99.1	2.074	3.041	1.928	10.1	71.3	32.1
18	5.324	6.512	2.782	6.269	97.3	2.782	3.404	1.909	10.0	71.6	32.4
19	6.180	6.777	2.646	6.546	102.1	2.646	4.217	2.876	15.1	57.2	13.5
20	6.187	6.707	2.625	6.478	100.8	2.625	4.244	2.917	15.3	56.6	13.2
21	6.032	6.446	2.054	6.267	97.3	2.054	4.232	3.213	16.9	52.2	11.2
22	6.139	6.487	2.224	6.293	97.7	2.224	4.305	3.201	16.8	52.4	11.2
23	6.838	6.736	2.515	6.517	101.5	2.515	4.904	3.694	19.4	45.1	8.5
24	6.460	6.594	2.496	6.376	99.1	2.496	4.562	3.333	17.5	50.4	10.4
25	7.399	6.779	2.779	6.537	101.8	2.779	5.417	4.117	21.6	38.8	6.4
26	6.680	6.550	2.713	6.313	98.0	2.713	4.761	3.433	18.0	48.9	9.9
27	6.892	6.531	2.000	6.357	98.8	2.000	5.080	4.147	21.8	38.3	6.2
28	7.161	6.619	2.378	6.412	99.7	2.378	5.274	4.165	21.9	38.1	6.2

Figure 20-7
Part 5 of the program. The results of each assay tube are calculated and reported as nanograms CEA.

or end of the assay to check for the reproducibility of results. Controls also included are an ascitic fluid which contains a known amount of CEA, 2 tubes with normal goat serum rather than antibody to check for nonspecific precipitation of CEA, and 2 tubes with a sufficient amount of antibody to bind almost all of the CEA · ^{125}I. Nonspecific binding of CEA in the assay is usually 0–2%. Freshly iodinated CEA is 90% bound by anti-CEA. Two weeks after iodination the value is down to 64–70%.

Typical Protocol for Triple Isotope Double Antibody Assay of CEA

REAGENTS
A. Phospate-buffered saline solution (PBS)—pH 7.2; sodium phosphate 0.075 M; sodium chloride 0.075 M
B. PBSE (PBS + 73.4 mM disodium (ethylenedinitrilo)tetraacetate)
C. PBSG (PBS + gelatin (Knox)—1 mg/ml)
D. CEA Cocktail: 0.5 ng/10 λ CEA · ^{125}I
       ~ 1 μg/10 λ goat IgG · ^{131}I
       ~ 40,000 cpm/10 λ ^{22}Na
E. Inhibitor: serial doubling dilutions of CEA in PBSG. Concentration range ~ 0.5 ng/10 λ to ~ 120 ng/10 λ

MATERIALS
A. Series of Eppendorf tubes
B. Automatic pipettor (Micromedic)
C. Microcentrifuge tubes—50
D. Microfuge
E. Incubator at 37° C; at −4° C

TITRATION OF ANTI-CEA
1. Dilute normal goat serum 1:20 in PBSE (this dilution will vary, depending on the normal goat serum and the horse anti-goat IgG). 500 λ normal goat serum + 9.5 ml PBSE.
2. Dilute anti-CEA 1:20 in PBSE; 100 λ anti-CEA + 1.9 ml PBSE.
3. Place 0.5 ml 1:20 normal goat serum in a series of Eppendorf tubes. Add 0.5 ml 1:20 anti-CEA to first tube and mix well (1:40 dilution); transfer 0.5 ml to next tube and mix well (1:80 dilution); continue to make serial dilutions until serum is diluted 1:40,960 (more or less, depending on titer of serum).
4. Pipette 10 λ CEA cocktail with the Micromedic pipettor into each of 50 microcentrifuge tubes. Give tubes 41–50 a quick spin in Microfuge (these are set aside to check reproducibility of the Micromedic pipettor for each assay).
5. Add 200 λ PBSG to microcentrifuge tubes 1–40.
6. Add 50 λ of the serial dilutions of anti-CEA to the first 36 tubes. Test each serial dilution in triplicate:

Tube No.	Material
1–3	50 λ 1:20 anti-CEA
4–6	1:40
	1:80
	.
	.
	.
34–36	1:40,960

7. Add 50 λ 1:40 normal goat serum to tubes 37–40.
8. Mix tubes well by closing caps tightly and shaking tubes upside down and right again 5 times. Incubate 2 hours or overnight at 37° C. (The assay may be completed in 5 hours but sometimes it is more convenient to set up the assay in late afternoon and add the second antibody the following morning.)
9. Add 100 λ horse anti-goat IgG to each tube.
10. Incubate 1 hour at 37° C; 15 min at −4° C.
11. Centrifuge tubes and aspirate most of the supernate, leaving approximately 20 λ.
12. Count precipitate and unaspirated supernate.

STANDARD CURVE FOR CEA DETERMINATIONS
1. Choose dilution of anti-CEA which binds 30–40% of CEA.
   a. Make 1:20 anti-CEA into PBSE
      100 λ anti-CEA + 1.9 ml PBSE
   b. Make 1:20 dilution normal goat serum
      500 λ normal goat serum + 9.5 ml PBSE
   c. Make 1:1600 anti-CEA into 1:20 normal goat serum
      50 λ 1:20 anti-CEA + 3.95 ml 1:20 normal goat serum
2. Pipette 10 λ CEA cocktail into 40 tubes. Give tubes 1–4 and 33–40 a quick spin in Microfuge.
3. Add 10 λ of serial dilutions of inhibitor (cold CEA) to the following tubes:

Tube No.		
6, 15	10 λ CEA	.48 ng/10 λ
7, 16		.96
8, 17		1.93
9, 18		3.86
10, 19		7.72
11, 20		15.41
12, 21		30.82
13, 22		61.6
14, 23		123.3

4. Add 200 λ El ascitic fluid (diluted 1:100) to tubes 27 and 28. This is a control ascitic fluid which should measure 12–15 $\mu g/ml$.
5. Add 200 λ PBSG to tubes 5–32 (except tubes 27 and 28).
6. Add 50 λ 1:1600 anti-CEA to tubes 5–28.
7. Add 50 λ 1:20 anti-CEA to tubes 29–30.
8. Add 50 λ 1:20 normal goat serum to tubes 31–32.
9. Follow steps 8 through 12 as for the titration of anti-CEA.
10. To assay serum samples, substitute 200 λ serum for the PBSG in step 5.

When a large number of assays are performed, a significant amount of time is saved by using the ^{22}Na volume marker. However, if a triple channel counter is not available, the assay may be performed without the ^{22}Na volume marker. If the ^{22}Na is omitted, the precipitate should be washed once with 200 λ PBSG and then counted.

Conclusion

The description of CEA by Gold and Freedman represents a major advance in the field of tumor immunology. Clinical testing has defined the questions which remain to be answered concerning the use of a CEA assay to detect cancer. Hopefully, the elucidation of the structure of CEA will aid in the production of more specific reagents which will enable the assay to discriminate among different types of malignant diseases as well as between malignant and nonmalignant disease states.

References

1. Abeyonnis, C. J., and Milgrom, F.   Studies on carcinoembryonic antigen. *Fed. Proc.* (abstract) 31:786, 1972.
2. Banjo, C., Gold, P., Freedman, S. O., and Krupey, J.   Immunologically active heterosaccharides of carcinoembryonic antigen of human digestive system. *Nature [New Biol.]* 238:183, 1972.
3. Berson, S. A., Yallow, R. S., Bauman, A., Rothschild, M. A., and Newerly, K.   Insulin • I^{131} metabolism in human subjects: Demonstration of insulin binding globulin in the circulation of insulin treated subjects. *J. Clin. Invest.* 35:170, 1956.
4. Burtin, P., von Kleist, S., and Sabine, M. C.   Loss of a normal colonic membrane antigen in human cancers of the colon. *Cancer Res.* 31:1083, 1971.
5. Burtin, P., Martin, E., Sabine, M. C., and von Kleist, S.   Immunological study of polyps of the colon. *J. Natl. Cancer Inst.* 48:25, 1972.
6. Burtin, P., Sabine, M. C., and Chavanel, G.   Presence of carcinoembryonic antigen in children's colonic mucosa. *Int. J. Cancer* 10:72, 1972.
7. Chu, T. M., Reynoso, G., and Hansen, H. J.   Demonstration of carcinoembryonic antigen in normal human plasma. *Nature [New Biol.]* 238:152, 1972.

8. Chu, T. M., and Reynoso, G.   Evaluation of a new radioimmunoassay method for carcinoembryonic antigen in plasma, with use of zirconyl phosphate gel. *Clin. Chem.* 18:918, 1972.

9. Coligan, J. E., Lautenschleger, J. T., Egan, M. L., and Todd, C. W. Isolation and characterization of carcinoembryonic antigen. *Immunochemistry* 9:377, 1972.

10. Coligan, J. E., Egan, M. L., and Todd, C. W.   Detection of carcinoembryonic antigen by radioimmune assay. *Natl. Cancer Inst. Monogr.* 35.427, 1972.

11. Coligan, J. E., Henkart, P. A., Todd, C. W., and Terry, W. D.   Heterogeneity of the carcinoembryonic antigen. *Immunochemistry* 10:591, 1973.

12. Denk, H., Tappeiner, G., Eckerstorfer, R., and Holzner, J. H.   Carcinoembryonic antigen (CEA) in gastrointestinal and extragastrointestinal tumors and its relationship to tumor-cell differentiation. *Int. J. Cancer* 10:262, 1972.

13. Egan, M. L., Lautenschleger, J. T., Coligan, J. E., and Todd, C. W. Radioimmune assay of carcinoembryonic antigen. *Immunochemistry* 9:289, 1972.

14. Egan, M. L., Coligan, J. E., Lautenschleger, J. T., and Todd, C. W. The triple isotope double antibody assay: Application to the carcinoembryonic antigen. In M. G. Anderson and J. H. Coggin (eds.), *Proceedings of the 1st Conference and Workshop on Embryonic and Fetal Antigens in Cancer*. Springfield, Va.: Oak Ridge National Laboratory, National Technical Information Service, 1971.

15. Egan, M. L., and Todd, C. W.   Instrumentation for the triple isotope double antibody assay. (Postgraduate course at Harvard Medical School) Radioimmune Assay: Principles and Practical Applications. (November), 1973.

16. Egan, M. L., Coligan, J. E., and Todd, C. W.   Radioimmune Assay for the Diagnosis of Human Cancer. *Cancer* (in press, 1974).

17. Freed, D. L. J., and Taylor, G.   Carcinoembryonic antigen in faeces. *Br. Med. J.* 1:85, 1972.

18. Gold, P., and Freedman, S. O.   Demonstration of tumor-specific antigens in human colonic carcinomata by immunological tolerance and absorption techniques. *J. Exp. Med.* 121:439, 1965.

19. Gold, P., and Freedman, S. O.   Specific carcinoembryonic antigens of the human digestive system. *J. Exp. Med.* 122:467, 1965.

20. Gold, P.   Embryonic origin of human tumor-specific antigens. *Prog. Exp. Tumor Res.* 14:43, 1971.

21. Goldenberg, D. M., Tchilinguirian, N. G. O., Hansen, H. J., and Vandevoorde, J. P.   Carcinoembryonic antigen present in meconium: The basis of a possible new diagnostic test of fetal distress. *Am. J. Obstet. Gynecol.* 113:66, 1972.

22. Gotschlich, E. C.   A simplification of the radioactive antigen binding test by a double label technique. *J. Immunol.* 107:910, 1971.

23. Hall, R. R., Laurence, D. J. R., Darcy, D., Stevens, U., James, R., Roberts, S., and Neville, A. M.   Carcinoembryonic antigen in the urine of patients with urothelial carcinoma. *Br. Med. J.* 9:609, 1972.

24. Krupey, J., Gold, P., and Freedman, S. O.   Purification and character-

ization of carcinoembryonic antigens of the human digestive system. *Nature* 215:67, 1967.

25. Krupey, J., Gold, P., and Freedman, S. O. Physicochemical studies of the carcinoembryonic antigens of the human digestive system. *J. Exp. Med.* 128:387, 1968.

26. Kupchik, H. Z., and Zamcheck, N. Carcinoembryonic antigen(s) in liver disease: II. Isolation from human cirrhotic liver and serum and from normal liver. *Gastroenterology* 63:95, 1972.

27. Laurence, D. J. R., Stevens, U., Bettelheim, R., Darcy, D., Leese, C., Turberville, C., Alexander, P., Johns, E. W., and Neville, A. M. Role of plasma carcinoembryonic antigen in diagnosis of gastrointestinal, mammary, and bronchial carcinoma. *Br. Med. J.* 9:605, 1972.

28. LeBel, J. S., Deodhar, S. D., and Brown, C. H. Evaluation of a radio-immunoassay for carcinoembryonic antigen of the human digestive system. *Cleve. Clin. Q.* 39:25, 1972.

29. Lo Gerfo, P., Krupey, J., and Hansen, H. J. Demonstration of an antigen common to several varieties of neoplasia. *N. Engl. J. Med.* 285:138, 1971.

30. Lo Gerfo, P., Lo Gerfo, E., Herter, F., Barker, H. G., and Hansen, H. J. Tumor-associated antigen in patients with carcinoma of the colon. *Am. J. Surg.* 123:127, 1972.

31. Lo Gerfo, P., and Herter, F. P. Demonstration of tumor associated antigen in normal colon and lung. *J. Surg. Oncol.* 4:1, 1972.

32. Luzzi, M., and Depieds, R. Methodes d'obtention d'immunserums anti-antigene carcinoembryonnaire a partir de tumeur colique. *Ann. Inst. Pasteur* 122:341, 1972.

33. Martin, F., and Martin, M. S. Demonstration of antigens related to colonic cancer in the human digestive system. *Int. J. Cancer* 6:352, 1970.

34. Martin, F., and Martin, M. S. Radioimmunoassay of carcinoembryonic antigen in extracts of human colon and stomach. *Int. J. Cancer* 9:641, 1972.

35. Martin, F., Martin, M. S., Bordes, M., and Bourgeaux, C. The specificity of carcino-foetal antigens of the human digestive tract tumours. *Eur. J. Cancer* 8:315, 1972.

36. Moore, T. L., Kupchik, H. Z., Marcon, N., and Zamcheck, N. Carcino-embryonic antigen assay in cancer of the colon and pancreas and other digestive tract disorders. *Am. J. Dig. Dis.* 16:1, 1971.

37. Moore, T. L., Kantrowitz, P. A., and Zamcheck, N. Carcinoembryonic antigen (CEA) in inflammatory bowel disease. *J.A.M.A.* 22:944, 1972.

38. Moore, T., Dhar, P., Zamcheck, N., Keeley, A., Gottlieb, L., and Kupchik, H. Z. Carcinoembryonic antigen(s) in liver disease: I. Clinical and morphological studies. *Gastroenterology* 63:88, 1972.

39. Morgan, C. R., and Lazarow, A. Immunoassay of insulin using a two-antibody system. *Proc. Soc. Exp. Biol. Med.* 110:29, 1962.

40. National Cancer Institute of Canada and American Cancer Society Investigation. A collaborative study of a test for carcinoembryonic antigen (CEA) in the sera of patients with carcinoma of the colon and rectum. *J. of Canadian Med. Assoc.* 107:25, 1972.

41. Page, L., Dessaulles, E., Lagg, S., and Haber, E. Interference with immunoassays of angiotensin I and II by proteins in human plasma. *Clin. Chim. Acta* 34:55, 1971.

42. Reynoso, G., Chu, T. M., Holyoke, D., Cohen, E., Nemoto, T., Wang, J. J., Chuang, J., Guinan, P., and Murphy, G. P.   Carcinoembryonic antigen in patients with different cancers. *J.A.M.A.* 220:361, 1972.
43. Reynoso, G., Chu, T. M., Guinan, P., and Murphy, G. P.   Carcino-embryonic antigen in patients with tumors of the urogenital tract. *Cancer* 30:1, 1972.
44. Rodbard, D.   Statistical aspects of radioimmunoassays. In W. D. Odell and W. H. Daughaday (eds.), *Principles of Competitive Protein Binding Assays.* Philadelphia: Lippincott, 1971, p. 204.
45. Rosai, J., Tillack, T. W., and Marchesi, V. T.   Membrane antigens of human colonic carcinoma and non-tumoral colonic mucosa: Results obtained with a new isolation method. *Int. J. Cancer* 10:357, 1972.
46. Sorokin, J. J., Kupchik, H. Z., Zamcheck, N., and Dhar, P.   A clinical comparison of two radioimmunoassays for carcinoembryonic antigen (CEA). *Immunol. Communications* 1:11, 1972.
47. Terry, W. D., Henkart, P. A., Coligan, J. E., and Todd, C. W.   Structural studies of the major glycoprotein in preparations with carcino-embryonic antigen activity. *J. Exp. Med.* 136:200, 1972.
48. Thomson, D. M. P., Krupey, J., Freedman, S. O., and Gold, P.   The radioimmunoassay of circulating carcinombryonic antigen of the human digestive system. *Proc. Natl. Acad. Sci. U.S.A.* 64:161, 1969.
49. Todd, C. W., Egan, M. L., Lautenschleger, J. T., and Coligan, J. E.   Dosage, isolement et characterisation de l'antigene carcinoembryonnaire. *Ann. Inst. Pasteur* 122:841, 1972.
50. Turner, M. D., Olivares, T. A., Harwell, L., and Kleinman, M. S.   Further purification of perchlorate-soluble antigens from human colonic carcinomata. *J. Immunol.* 108:1328, 1972.
51. Von Kleist, S., and Burtin, P.   Isolation of a fetal antigen from human colonic tumors. *Cancer Res.* 29:1961, 1969.
52. Zamcheck, N., Moore, T. L., Dhar, P., and Kupchik, H.   Immunologic diagnosis and prognosis of human digestive-tract cancer: Carcinoembryonic antigens. *Med. Intelligence* 286:83, 1972.

IV

Supplemental Information and Methods

21

Other Useful Immunologic Methods

Carol A. Bell

Numerous other procedures not covered in the preceding chapters have found use in the diagnosis of immunologic disease. Many of these are modifications of agar gel precipitin reactions and are in common laboratory use, e.g., immunoelectrophoresis (IEP) and radial immunodiffusion (RID), while others are simple enough to perform so that they can be used with little additional time or equipment, e.g., electroimmunodiffusion or disc electrophoresis.

Basics of Gel Precipitin Reactions

Since many of the new techniques in immunology are based on some phase of agar gel precipitin reactions, it is worthwhile to review the pertinent features of such systems. Precipitin reactions depend upon combining of antigen and its specific antibody in an insoluble, complex lattice of large molecular size. Gel diffusion techniques use a high solvent content (98% buffer) so that migration of the reactants is primarily by diffusion; addition of electrical current only increases that diffusion [1, 11].

Gel pore size acts as a sieve, allowing free diffusion of substances of less than MW 200,000; large MW serum proteins, α_2 macroglobulin, α_2 liproprotein, fibrinogen, and IgM diffuse poorly. Similarly, the antigen-antibody complexes over MW 200,000 diffuse in gel poorly. Most precipitins are IgG antibodies which are diffusible, whereas polymerized IgA and IgM antibodies are less so, and IgG antibodies comprise approximately 80% of all antibodies [11].

In the antigen-antibody reaction, if the antibody starts as excess (zone of antibody excess), increasing amounts of antigen increase the amount of precipitate until the point of equivalence. In the zone of equivalence, which can be rather narrow, increasing antigen no longer increases the precipitate; and when antigen becomes the excess reagent, the reaction not only halts (zone of inhibition), but the precipitate may dissolve

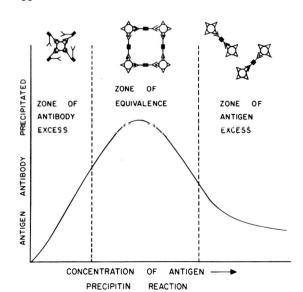

Figure 21-1
Changing antigen concentration resulting in precipitins with a fixed concentration of antibody.

(Fig. 21-1). Once formed, the precipitate acts as a barrier to further diffusion of its reactants. In most systems, however, excess antigen acts as a solvent to the precipitin barrier. As long as antigen remains in excess, it alternately dissolves and reforms the precipitin barrier as it diffuses toward antibody, until equilibrium is reached, and a final well-defined precipitin line is formed (Fig. 21-2). Antibodies made in rabbit, goat, or guinea pig are not solvents when they are in excess; thus, the

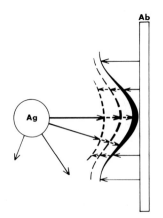

Figure 21-2
Precipitin formation in gel diffusion. Antigen diffuses radially from the well toward antibody. Precipitin arcs dissolve in antigen excess migrating outward until equivalence. Dense precipitin barrier prevents further diffusion of specific antigen and antibody.

antibody edge of the precipitin barrier tends to be less well defined and more diffuse. This is not the case for horse antisera, in which antibody excess does act as a solvent [11]. As a consequence, if horse antisera are selected for use, although the precipitin arcs are sharply defined, the equivalency of antibody to antigen is critical, and some experimentation may be necessary for this equivalency to be achieved. The importance of antigen excess is that it results in soluble prozones which may wash away in the later stages of preparation.

Some techniques use variations of simple gel diffusion with or without the addition of electrophoresis or radioisotopes. When current is employed, the ions in the supporting medium (ionic strength or μ) contribute to migration of protein reactants.

Immunoelectrophoresis (IEP)

General Background
Initially divided into albumin and globulin on the basis of solubility, serum proteins were further subdivided by zone electrophoresis [49], first at pH 7.0 and then at pH 8.6. At such pH, proteins are negatively charged and migrate to the anode (+). At the more alkaline pH, α_1 globulin separates from albumin (Fig. 21-3). Serum proteins can be evaluated and quantitated by electrophoresis by supporting them in a

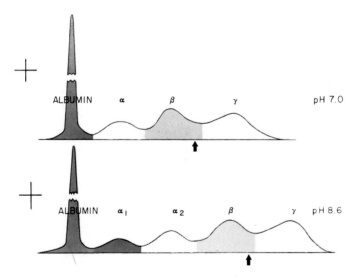

Figure 21-3
Serum protein electrophoresis. At pH 8.6 proteins assume greater negative charge than at pH 7.0. They migrate from inoculation point (↑) to anode (+). At pH 8.6 α_1 globulin separates from albumin.

Table 21-1. Immunoglobulin Nomenclature.

	WHO[a] Terminology	Older Terminology
	IgG, or γG	γ, γ_{ss}, 7Sγ
	IgA, or γA	γ, A, β_2A
	IgM, or γM	γ, M, β_2M, 19Sγ
	kappa light chain or κ	I, 1, B
	lambda light chain or λ	II, 2, A

[a] *Bull. WHO* 30:447 (1964).

variety of solid media including paper, starch, cellulose acetate, and acrylamide gel.

Bacteriologists have been long familiar with the technique of immune precipitation, and in 1953 Grabar and Williams [21, 52] combined this technique with electrophoresis as immunoelectrophoresis, allowing a further division of globulins into more than 40 precipitin arcs in approximately 12 zones. Of these arcs, 3 were found to be associated with serum antibody activity and were thereafter termed immunoglobulins.

Nomenclature of Immunoglobulins

The immunoglobulins were originally named by their location relative to standard protein electrophoresis (Table 21-1), but since this functional group of globulins underlaps several globulins from α_2 to γ (Fig. 21-4), such classification proved unsatisfactory. Using human and mouse myeloma proteins, information on the structure of the immunoglobulins was obtained which has led to changes in the nomenclature attached to

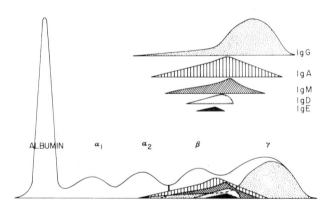

Figure 21-4
Distribution of immunoglobulins after electrophoresis.

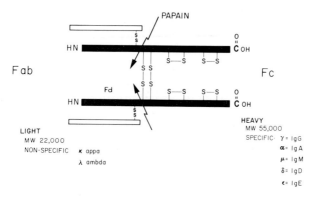

Figure 21-5
The immune globulin molecule. Papain disrupts disulfide bonds, producing
fragments Fab and Fc. Further denaturation of Fab produces Fd, a heavy
chain fragment.

them. The immunoglobulins are units composed of four polypeptide
chains, two heavy chains (MW approximately 55,000), and two light
chains (MW approximately 22,000) joined by disulfide bridges (Fig.
21-5). The heavy chain is specific for the particular immunoglobulin
labeled γ, α, μ, δ, or ε. Thus, for any immunoglobulin (Ig) a shorthand
notation of IgG, IgA, IgM, etc. may be applied. As of 1971, only 2
globulins had been completely sequenced for amino acid constituents,
although many have been partially sequenced [13, 39]. Immunologic
differences apparently correlate with differences in the sequence of approximately 450 amino acids in each heavy chain and have determined
4 subtypes for IgG (G_1, G_2, G_3, and G_4) and 2 for IgA (A_1, A_2).

The two types of light chains, called kappa (κ) and lambda (λ), are
bound to the heavy chains by disulfide bonds. They are not specific in
that they may attach to any heavy chain, the only requirement being that
on any one molecule they must be the same. Hence, two γ heavy chains
may combine with 2 κ light chains as $\gamma_2 k_2$ to constitute an IgG molecule.
Similarly, 2 μ heavy chains may combine with 2 λ chains as $\mu_2\lambda_2$ to
constitute one unit in an IgM molecule.

The immunoglobulin molecule may be broken into specific fragments
by proteolytic enzymes, papain, trypsin, or pepsin. Papain fragments
the molecule into three parts, two Fab and one Fc. The Fab is composed of one heavy chain fragment and one light chain fragment. Degradation of the light chain leaves a heavy chain fragment alone, termed
Fd, which has advantages in immunologic work of acquiring narrower
specificity. The Fc fragment determines the physicochemical properties
of the molecule, including its complement-binding capabilities. Hence
the Fc of the μ pentamer is many times more efficient in binding the $C'1q$
portion of complement than are the monomers of IgG_2 or IgG_4. IgA,

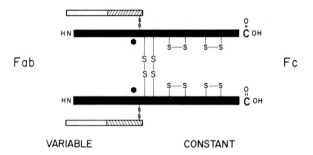

Figure 21-6
The antibody combining site is in the hypervariable zone near the hinge portion of the molecule, marked by a diamond. It may involve both heavy and light chains or the heavy chain only. Both heavy and light chains have constant and variable parts, seen on light chain as striped and clear area respectively.

IgD, and IgE do not have Fc receptors for complement [2]. Determinants on the Fc fragment also correspond to cell membrane receptor sites of macrophages, the mechanism of reticuloendothelial system destruction of antibody-coated cells, including blood cells, bacteria, or viruses [12].

Partial amino acid sequences of many proteins have shown that the carboxyl portion of the molecule (C-terminus) is relatively constant in its constituents, whereas the opposite (N-terminus) end is more variable (Fig. 21-6). Near the hinged area of the molecule, the amino acid differences are hypervariable [13, 39], possibly in the zone of antibody binding. This latter area may be composed of dominant and subdominant zones of 3 to 8 amino acids on both heavy and light chains [30] or on the heavy chain only [8].

The immunoglobulins function as units specific for the particular

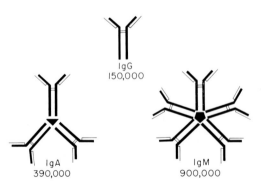

Figure 21-7
Structure of immune globulins. Immunoglobulins appear as monomers (IgG), dimers or trimers (IgA), or pentamers (IgM). They appear as a T, becoming Y-shaped on combination with antigen.

immunoglobulin, thereby determining their molecular weight. IgG, IgD, and IgE function as monomers, IgA as a dimer (but also as monomer or trimer), and IgM as a pentamer (Fig. 21-7). The configuration of the molecule is apparently a T which becomes a Y on combination of antibody with antigen, molecular binding occurring at the hinge area.

The IgA molecule has certain features that distinguish it from the other immunoglobulins. Primary among these is the addition of a secretory piece (SP) acquired in the ductal epithelium as the globulin is transferred to its functional areas of secretion and surface areas. The SP lies between the α heavy chains of the IgA dimer and is apparently responsible for molecular binding to viruses at cell surfaces. Without the SP, IgA is not functional, despite the fact it can be quantitated [4]. More recently, other molecular pieces (J piece, i.e., joining) have been found for both IgA and IgM, but their significance is unknown [29] (Fig. 21-8).

All serum proteins are manufactured in the liver except the immunoglobulins, which are manufactured in plasma cells of the bone marrow and in the lymphoid tissue of the reticuloendothelial system and gut. The level of immunoglobulins depends upon antigenic stimulation and is, therefore, age dependent.

Although much of the discussion is directed to the immunoglobulins, many of the following techniques can be used with other proteins. Commercial antisera are available for investigation of an extensive array of globulins, and in many cases agar gel plates for quantitation are also available (Table 21-2).

Principles of the Technique

By combining electrophoresis with immunodiffusion, the quality and a rough estimation of the quantity can be made of the immunoglobulins. No matter what analytic system is ultimately used, the basic principles remain the same. The protein for analysis (antigen), be it whole human serum, spinal fluid, or concentrated eluate from a red cell, is placed in a well in or on some support medium, and separated into its component

Figure 21-8
Secretory piece manufactured in epithelial lining cells of gland is added to IgA molecule as it passes into secretion.

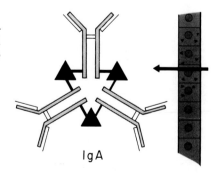

IgA

Table 21-2. Commercial Antisera and Immune Diffusion Materials Available for Investigation of Clinically Significant Serum Proteins.

Serum Protein	Protein Electrophoretic Migration	IEP Antiserum	Radial Immunodiffusion	Disease Correlation
α_1-antitrypsin	$\alpha 1$	X	X	Decreased in familial pulmonary emphysema
Ceruloplasmin	$\alpha 2$	X	X	Decreased in Wilson's disease, increased in infection or inflammation
Haptoglobin	$\alpha 2$	X	X	Decreased in hemolysis or liver disease—increased in infection
α_2 macroglobulin	$\alpha 2$	X	X	Increased in nephrotic syndrome
Cholinesterase	$\alpha 2$	X	O	Decreased in abnormal sensitivity to succinyl choline derivatives
Hemopexin	$\beta 1$	X	X	Decreased in hemolysis
Transferrin	$\beta 1$	X	X	Decreased in hereditary atransferrinemia
$\beta_1 C$ globulin (C_3)	$\beta 1$	X	X	Decreased in active lupus nephritis or active glomerulonephritis
$\beta_1 E$ globulin (C_4)	$\beta 1$	X	X	
C1 esterase inhibitor	$\beta 1$	X	X	Decreased in hereditary angioneurotic edema

Immunoglobulin G	$\gamma_2\text{--}\alpha_2$	X	X	Decreased or absent in acquired or congenital dysgamma globulinemia
Immunoglobin A	$\gamma_1\text{--}\alpha_2$	X	X	Increased polyclonal in collagen disease or infection
Immunoglobulin M	$\gamma_2\text{--}\beta_2$	X	X	Increased monoclonal in myeloma or macroglobulinemia
Immunoglobulin D	$\gamma_1\text{--}\beta_2$	X	X	Increased in rare myelomas
Immunoglobulin E	$\gamma_1\text{--}\beta_2$	X	O	Increased in allergy, or rare myelomas; decreased in chronic sinopulmonary infection?
Light chains (κ, λ)	$\gamma\text{--}\alpha_2$	X	O	Monoclonal in urine—Bence Jones protein; monoclonal in serum—light chain myeloma

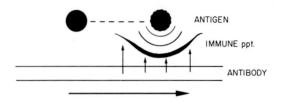

Figure 21-9
Serum proteins (antigen), placed in a well, are migrated in an electrical field, distributing themselves on the basis of net charge and size. Antibody is placed in a trough parallel to the migration path. Antigen and antibody diffuse radially depending on concentration, molecular size, temperature, etc. At points of equivalence immune precipitates are formed. Minimal variations in charge and molecular size permit discrimination among quite similar proteins.

parts by allowing it to migrate in a buffered electrical field at pH 8.6 for 45 min (Fig. 21-9).

Electrophoretic migration is dependent on protein charge at pH 8.6, the molecular size of the antigen relative to the pore size of the support medium, the ion concentration (usually 0.05), and the voltage. At pH 8.6, all proteins are negatively charged and are carried toward the anode (+); however, those of slow mobility have relatively little charge and are carried passively in the opposite direction, by electroendosmosis [11].

Support media include dilute solutions of agar, agarose, or ion agar, and have lately included cellulose acetate or acrylamide gel. A recent innovation is an agarose film (Marine Colloids) that requires only rehydration in the Veronal buffer before it is ready to use. The choice of medium varies, but agar or agarose are the easiest to use. Agar is a mixture of agarose and agaropectin, linear sulfated polysaccharides containing Na^+, K^+, Ca^{++}, and Mg^{++} ions. Sulfate bridges interlink to produce the gelling effect. During electrophoresis these ions move with the solvent to the cathode $(-)$, creating an effect known as electroendosmosis. Very weakly charged proteins are carried passively to the cathode as well. Agarose is neutral, lacking significant ions, so that electroendosmosis is minimized; however, the material is more expensive. Agar of high quality (i.e., Noble agar) has some increase in ions but the effect can be managed, and it usually proves quite satisfactory. Since the ion content of different batch lots varies, be prepared for shifts in the degree of endosmosis with lot changes [11, 31].

Cellulose acetate as a support medium is satisfactory, but it requires some experience to apply antiserum evenly between the electrophoretic pathways [11].

Starch and acrylamide gel have a marked sieving effect, retarding larger molecules more than either paper or agar. Polyacrylamide gel is inert, so electroendosmosis provides no problem. Although only 20 min are required for electrophoresis, the diffusion phase is greatly increased. It is useful for very acid or alkaline reactants and certain enzymatic systems [11].

The ionic strength of the buffer and the ion concentration of the agar or agarose determine the degree of electroendosmosis, the latter being most important [31]. Heat is generated in providing sufficient current to allow adequate protein migration, and this is increased when the ion concentration is high, > 0.5. Once a method has been selected, however, these factors can be standardized. Following electrophoretic migration, a trough is excavated parallel to the path of electrical migration, and antiserum is placed in it. The type of antiserum used is dependent on the protein, or proteins, under investigation; thus one may use antiserum to whole human serum, to the 3 immunoglobulins, to one immunoglobulin or other protein, or to part of a globulin (e.g., heavy chain, light chain, Fab, etc.). Antiserum diffuses toward antigen, creating precipitin arcs where antiserum recognizes homologous antigen in optimum concentration, a process requiring 24–72 hours.

The rate of diffusion is dependent on temperature, molecular size of antigen and antibody, and concentration. Due to the heterogeneity of even a single class of proteins, the precipitin arcs tend to be symmetrically curvilinear. Yet if pH, temperature, voltage, and gel concentration are kept constant, their appearance and location are remarkably stable. Proteins that are abnormal due to a monoclonal population (paraproteins) have irregular contours or "shoulders" for the arcs, and/or appear in locations differing from the control [11, 35].

Following diffusion, the slides are washed free of unreacted proteins and buffer salts. Since prozones are soluble, it is advisable to evaluate the slides, or photograph them, before the washing phase. This latter phase requires 12–16 hours to prevent excessive nonspecific binding of dye in the background. Following the washing phase, the 2% agar is allowed to air dry, depositing the arcs in a thin film on the solid support of glass or Mylar film. The arcs can be fixed and stained for ease in reading and to retain a permanent record for later comparison. Stains commonly used are Amido black, Azo carmine, or Thiazine red R. The Amido black is the best stain when black and white photographs for publication are desired.

ANTISERA.   Antisera are available as polyvalent reagents active toward all serum proteins, to all three immunoglobulins, or they may be monovalent. Of the monospecific antisera, some are made heavy chain specific by absorbing out the light chain activity with specific Bence Jones proteins from myelomatous urines. However, antigenic determinants between the pathologic Bence Jones and normal light chains may not be the same, and absorption will be incomplete. This leads to false identifications due to cross-reactions of the light chain portions of IgA and IgG or IgM [7, 35, 37].

Quality control of antisera requires some ingenuity and a high index of suspicion. It is fairly obvious that good antisera (a) react specifically with the stimulating antigen, or its appropriate polypeptide chain, in normal as well as abnormal proteins, (b) do not cross-react with antigenic determinants shared by other immunoglobulins, (c) do not react with nonimmune components, and (d) do not show excessive tendency to prozone. It has been shown that many antisera are contaminated with antibodies other than the stated monospecificity, or fail to react with one or more immune globulins [7, 35].

The number of precipitin arcs produced by any antiserum to whole human proteins is dependent on the animal in which the antiserum is made. The horse recognizes many more antigenic differences in human proteins than the goat or rabbit, so more arcs are expected. However, antigen-antibody concentration is much more critical for horse-derived antisera than for goat or rabbit, and prozones are more common [1, 11].

Micromethod of Scheidegger [44] (See Procedures)
Although the macromethod of Grabar and Williams [21, 52] is very sensitive, it requires great quantities of antisera which can greatly increase the expense. Therefore, a microtechnique is commonly used, using 1–2% agar or agarose supported on glass microscopic slides or Mylar film. Since there is greater overlapping in the α_2 and β zones, investigation of globulins in these areas requires monospecific antisera [35].

A control serum should be run with every test serum, preferably on the same slide, but certainly in the same run. The source of the control serum can be any relatively normal outpatient or prenatal patient where 5–6 ml of serum are available. The single source control provides fewer variables than a serum pool. Protein electrophoresis is obtained and immunoglobulin quantitation performed to verify relative normalcy, particularly for IgA and IgM. The serum is preserved with 0.1% sodium azide or 1:10,000 merthiolate powder (Lilly) and refrigerated. Using the same control for 2–3 months allows some stability in interpretation. Unfortunately IgM withstands storage at 4° C poorly, and this arc will gradually fade. Either additional IgM (parasitized from immunodiffusion kits) is added or a new control is obtained.

Some general comments can be made which make the technique easier to use. (a) Never attempt immunoelectrophoresis, particularly interpretation, without a standard serum protein electrophoretic pattern. This prevents the embarrassment of stating that there is no globulin when in reality 10 gm per 100 ml of it have created a soluble prozone. (b) Not all antisera from the same manufacturer are of equal quality and effectiveness. Therefore, use more than one manufacturer's materials and use adequate controls. This is less of a problem for standard IEP antiserum for whole human protein than for specific fractions, particularly light chains. Furthermore, in a period of one to two years the precipitin quality of an antiserum from a manufacturer may change as the individual animals in which it is made change, so be wary of discrepant results, and confirm them by another antiserum or a different technique. (c) Do not be afraid to combine the techniques of standard protein electrophoresis, IEP, and immunodiffusion to arrive at the correct interpretation. This is more a testament to one's thoroughness than to lack of ability. Table 21-3 lists some of the manufacturers of antisera and immunodiffusion equipment.

Gel cutting die patterns commonly employed are

although other combinations including interrupted troughs, are used [7, 34]. For most standard patterns, the antibody-containing trough contains 30–50 times the volume of the antigen well, which helps in avoiding prozones due to antigen excess. When spinal fluid or urine is tested the excess reagent may be antibody so that concentration of the specimen will be necessary before immunoelectrophoresis.

Protocol for IEP Analysis

A flow sheet for the analysis of protein abnormalities in the adult is shown in Fig. 21–10. Infants and children do not have paraproteins so that quantitation is usually all that is necessary. In the adult, the type of protein abnormality (hyperglobulinemia, monoclonal gammopathy, hypoglobulinemia) is decided by protein electrophoresis on cellulose acetate.

Polyclonal (i.e., broad) elevations show a smooth electrophoretic arc and are compatible with chronic inflammation, collagen disease (especially rheumatoid arthritis) or neoplasm. Abnormal shapes raise the possibility of biclonal gammopathies.

Monoclonal spikes suggest IgG or IgA myeloma, rarely IgM macroglobulinemia (Waldenström's) and very rarely IgE myeloma. IgD myelomas are more often associated with hypogammaglobulinemia. The location of M (i.e., monoclonal) spikes is rarely helpful in guessing what the specificity of the M protein will be. It is helpful in deciding how much the serum must be diluted before immunoelectrophoresis; the protein should be approximately 2 gm/100 ml after dilution with normal saline. In general, sharply spiked M proteins on cellulose acetate are more likely to be IgG, while broader spikes in the beta-gamma zone may be IgA, rarely IgM.

A monoclonal protein is shown to be a single population by virtue of its dominance over other immunoglobulins, and a single light chain type. The absence of the other immunoglobulins is seen on immunoelectrophoresis and can be confirmed by quantitation on immunoplates. Use of the two trough and one well pattern, with light chain antiserum in one

Table 21-3. Commercial Sources for Immunodiffusion and Immunoelectrophoresis Equipment.

Company	Address	Antisera[a]	Radial Immunodiffusion[a]	Ouchterlony Double Diffusion	Disc Electrophoresis
Antibodies, Inc.	Route 1, Box 1482 Davis, Calif. 95616	6, 7	0	0	0
Behring Diagnostics	400 Crossways Park Dr. Woodbury, N.Y. 11797	1, 3, 5, 6, 7	1, 2, 5, 6	0	0
Bioware, Inc.	P.O. Box 8152 Wichita, Kan. 67208	1, 2, 3, 4, 6 ($G_1G_2G_3G_4$)	1	X	0
Burroughs Wellcome Co.	Research Triangle Park, N.C. 27709	1, 3, 6	1	X	0
Canalco, Inc.	5635 Fisher Lane Rockville, Md. 20850	0	0	0	X
Cordis Laboratories	P.O. Box 684 Miami, Fla. 33137	1, 2, 3, 4, 5 heavy chain specific ($G_1G_2G_3G_4$)	0	X	0
Dade	Delaware Parkway Miami, Fla. 33125 3300 Hyland Ave. Costa Mesa, Calif. 92626	1, 2, 3, 4, 6	1, 2, 3	0	0
Hyland Laboratories	Costa Mesa, Calif. 92626	1, 2, 3, 4, 5	1, 2 high/low level, 6	X	0
IBL	451 S. Stonestreet Ave. Rockville, Md. 20850	1, 4, 6	0	0	0
ICL	18249 Euclid St. Fountain Valley, Calif. 92708	1, 2–5, 6	1, 6	0	0

Company	Address				
Kallestad Laboratories, Inc.	4005 Vernon Avenue Minneapolis, Minn. 55416	1, 2, 4, 5, 6, 7	1, 2, 6	X	0
Mann Research Laboratories	136 Liberty Street New York, N.Y. 10006	1, 4, 6, 7 IgM-fast/slow	0	0	0
Marine Colloids, Inc.	Rockland, Me. 04841			X	0
Meloy Laboratories	6714 Electronic Dr. Springfield, Va. 22151	1, 2, 4	1, 2	0	0
Melpar Biological Products Laboratory	7700 Arlington Blvd. Falls Church, Va. 22046	1, 2, 4, 6	1, 2	0	0
Miles Laboratories, Inc.	Res. Products Div. Elkhart, Ind. 46514	1, 2, 4, 5, 6 heavy chain specific	6	X	0
Pentex, Inc. (also see Laboratories, Inc.)	P.O. Box 272 Kankakee, Ill. 60901	7	0	X	0
Pfizer Diagnostics Div.	235 E. 42nd Street New York, N.Y. 10017	1, 2, 3, 4	1, 2	0	0
Spectrum Medical Industries, Inc.	60916 Terminal Annex Los Angeles, Calif. 90054	5, 6	0	0	0

[a] Antisera available for the following groups: 1—IgG, IgA, IgM; 2—IgD; 3—IgE; 4—BJ-κ, λ; 5—β1C, β1E and other complement fractions; 6—miscellaneous other human proteins; 7—animal antisera.

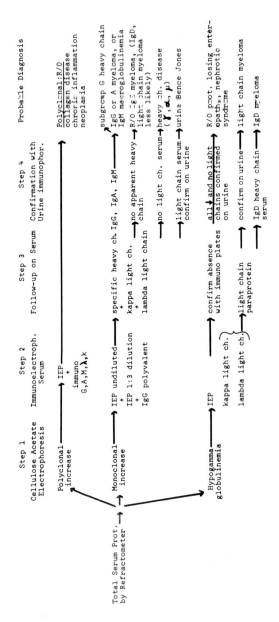

Figure 21-10

Flow sheet for evaluation of abnormal protein electrophoretic patterns in the adult. Step 1: General assessment of abnormality and its zone by cellulose acetate electrophoresis. Step 2: Immunoelectrophoresis using the indicated antisera. Helpful when both normal and abnormal patient sera are tested in a single run. Step 3: Confirmatory immunodiffusion or immunophoresis using monospecific antisera may be combined with step 2. Step 4: Immunoelectrophoresis of urinary proteins using polyvalent anti-IEP and monospecific antisera as determined by prior findings in serum. Probable diagnoses should be supported by bone marrow aspiration, x-ray surveys, serum viscosity, and serum calcium as required.

trough and specific heavy chain antiserum in the second trough, may give a line of identity (fusion), classifying the κ or λ light chain character of the myeloma. Residual normal light chains will not give lines of fusion. IgG myeloma may be further subclassified using anti-IgG$_1$, G$_2$, G$_3$, or G$_4$ antisera. The specificity of the pathologic light chain is confirmed by finding the same solitary light chain type in urine, i.e., Bence Jones protein. Where nephrotic syndromes have become superimposed due to renal damage, albumin, other globulins, and the pathologic heavy chain are also seen in the urine. This fact can also be noted on standard protein electrophoresis of the urine. The presence of albumin in the urine usually negates heat solubility tests for Bence Jones proteinuria. In patients with serum M proteins only about 20% will have urinary Bence Jones protein [50], and about half of all patients with marrow documented myelomatosis will show urinary Bence Jones protein.

Where monoclonal gammopathies are present, plasma cell dyscrasias are the most common associated finding. These usually involve bone in multiple areas, but can be solitary or involve extramedullary sites. In cases where the M spike is small, the associated disease may be lymphoma or metastatic carcinoma, breast, prostate, colon being most common.

Failure to identify either light chain type in serum or urine raises the possibility of heavy chain disease. Retest with heavy chain specific antiserum and another source of κ and λ light chain antiserum. The mobility of the M protein in serum and urine will be the same. IgG (Fc) heavy chain disease (Franklin's disease) is a lymphoma-like disease; μ chain disease has been associated with lymphocytic leukemia; and α heavy chain disease is a steatorrhea syndrome in young adults with dense lymphoid infiltrates of the intestine, common in the Middle East [45].

Hypogammaglobulinemia in the adult may be complete loss of IgG, IgA, and IgM (protein losing enteropathy, nephrotic syndromes), isolated loss of immune globulins (congenital absence of IgA, steatorrhea, or sprue syndromes), or a reflection of plasma cell dyscrasias (light chain myelomas or IgD myeloma). The latter are confirmed by finding a single light chain with the characteristic abnormal "shoulder" in serum and usually in urine as well. Renal failure due to amyloidosis usually occurs early in light chain disease, and the bone marrow and clinical findings may be atypical. IgD myeloma is much less common, does not usually produce an M spike and should be excluded before serum is dismissed as having no identifiable paraprotein or as being light chain variant [45].

Rarely, tissue proven myelomas will have no paraprotein in serum or urine [50]. Paraproteins in serum may be idiopathic in 3–6% of older individuals, but if a similar single light chain type appears in urine, their presence should then be viewed with caution [50]. In all cases where paraproteins are found, studies should include bone marrow aspiration, x-ray studies of bone and, where indicated, gastrointestinal tract, and serum calcium if these have not already been done. Bone lesions include severe osteoporosis as well as discrete punched-out defects.

Some paraproteins have distinctive physicochemical characteristics, e.g., gel formation of serum at 4°C (cryoglobulin), gel formation of plasma at 4°C (cryofibrinogen), precipitation of 56°C (pyroglobulin) [45]. These abnormalities influence treatment as does serum viscosity, and therefore, should be evaluated. Some paraproteins have antibody activity, e.g., within blood groups, to Salmonella species, as rheumatoid factor [50], or antinuclear factor leading to false diagnoses. Any laboratory test using these sera against latex particles coated with globulin will generally give false positive results. Such tests include some mononucleosis spot tests, tests for rheumatoid factor (RF), tests for fibrinogen or fibrin degradation products, for chorionic gonadotropin as in many pregnancy tests. Tests for heterophile or RF using sheep cells, i.e., Davidsohn absorption and Rose test respectively, can avoid this problem.

Interpretation of Results

Some clinically significant arcs are seen in Fig. 21-11. Gross abnormality is the complete absence of one or more precipitin arcs or an increase in concentration, as indicated by widening or increased density of the arc or distortion of its location or shape [11, 35, 37]. IEP permits only rough estimation of a particular serum protein, as high, medium, or low, by arc proximity to the antiserum trough. Where very high concentrations are present, as in myeloma, the arc may be lost in the trough, or actually rim it, so that no abnormal curve can be seen. This problem can be avoided by diluting the serum in saline on the basis of the standard protein electrophoresis pattern. When a monoclonal protein is present or when γ-globulin is greater than 1.7–2 gm %, the IEP should be run both undiluted and with a 1:3 or 1:10 dilution of serum in saline so that the complete arc may be seen (Fig. 21-12).

Some of the more frequently seen variations in morphology of the

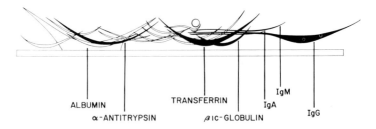

Figure 21-11
Albumin on the left (anode) and immunoglobulins to the right (cathode). Darkened protein arcs left to right, albumin; α_1 anti-trypsin, transferrin, β_1C. Above it, the last three arcs are IgA, IgM, and IgG.

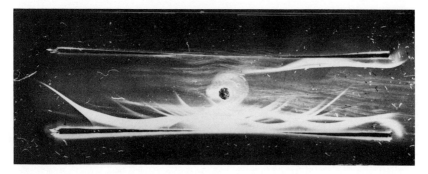

Figure 21-12
IgG paraprotein, κ chain. Lower trough contains antiserum to whole human serum. The antigen was diluted 1:3 in order to demonstrate the skewing of the paraprotein. The monospecific antiserum for IgG is in the upper trough. Residual normal IgG is seen as a line across the paraprotein arc.

precipitin arcs are listed in Table 21-4. These abnormalities may be classified as deviations in position, fusion of arcs, or spur formation [11]. As for gel reactions, in general fusion implies identity of antigen; and spur formation, partial identity. These abnormalities are due to unexpected components in either antigen or antiserum [35]. Many monospecific antisera are absorbed with antigen pools which may contain antigens which will remain unreacted. In agar patterns of two troughs and one well, the unreacted antigens contaminating the antiserum of one trough may react with antibody of the second trough, producing linear streaks in the path of migration [37]. These often fuse with a particular antibody arc allowing identification of the contaminant, usually albumin, transferrin, or IgG [1, 35].

Streaks connecting the IgG arc of patient and control at the end of the trough result when antigenic determinants of patient and normal IgG are similar. Since these are produced by increased endosmosis, they are seen more often when agar is used. Precipitates surrounding the antigen well may be lipoprotein, insoluble euglobulin if rounded, or immune complexes if tapered, and are found on the cathodal (−) side of the well, in the direction of IgG.

Spur formation is commonly due to contamination of supposedly monospecific antisera [35], but it can also be due to residual normal immunoglobulin in the presence of paraprotein. Since both molecules have a common base, a reaction of partial identity leads to spur formation. Anti-IgG antisera with antibody to both light chains will also give a split [7] arc. Where there is antigen excess, the antigen-antibody complex may react with antibody, creating a spur [11]. Bacterial contamination of test sera may result in proteolytic denaturation of proteins, which then have different electrophoretic migration of the fragments, yet which

Table 21-4. IEP Interpretation Problems.

Problem	Cause	Solution
1. Absent arc in final preparation	1. Prozone solubility due to Ag excess	1. Rerun using dilution of serum ($= Ag$)
	2. Acquired or congenital absence	2. Quantitate absent globulin to confirm its absence
		3. Do cellulose acetate protein electrophoresis
2. Flat arc near trough	1. Excess Ag	1. Dilute serum to achieve less than 2 gm per 100 ml for the specific protein
3. Arcs stacked, failure to migrate	1. Wick in electrophoresis chamber fails to contact agar	1. Use bromphenol blue albumin marker to follow electrophoretic migration before the diffusion step
	2. Current not 6 ma/cm	
	3. Old buffer	
4. Arcs duplicated	1. Antiserum reacting with Ag:Ab complex	1. Ag excess; dilute
	2. Variable temperature due to heat excess in electrophoresis	2. Check buffer ionic strength
	3. Recharging of wells	3. Concentrate antigen, do not recharge wells
5. Discoloration of agar at ends of slide	1. Excessive heating of agar during electrophoresis	1. Change buffer, ionic strength too high
	2. Excessive current	2. Check power source stability

Observation	Interpretation	Action
6. Linear ppt parallel to trough (one well, 2 troughs)	1. Antigens common to well and antisera. Antisera absorbed with excess antigen 2. Complexes between albumin and IgA or IgM paraproteins	1. Line may fuse with specific arc as line of identity
7. Spur, IgG arc (split)	1. Storage artifact 2. Minimonoclonal protein 3. Antibody to both light chains	1. Obtain fresh specimen 2. Inspect cellulose pattern
8. IgG connection around end of trough	1. Exaggerated endosmosis	1. Shorten electrophoresis time 2. Change buffer; ionic strength too high
9. White precipitate near antigen well	1. Cathodal aspect: consider immune complex of euglobulin 2. Anodal aspect: lipoproteins	1. 2-ME denaturation of serum should remove 2. Confirm with protein electrophoresis pattern, and Sia test
10. White precipitate in migration path	1. Euglobulin	1. See electrophoresis pattern
11. Arcs subtending paraprotein arc	1. Not monospecific antiserum 2. Residual normal protein with paraprotein	1. Use different antiserum on repeat and check vs. control Ig 2. Compare with protein electrophoresis, and light chain antisera

are still precipitated by the same antiserum [11], producing wavy precipitin arcs of spur formation.

Immunodiffusion

Background
Several variants of gel diffusion [34] are in common use. Simple diffusion (one dimension) is a technique commonly employed for C-reactive protein studies when antigen and antibody diffuse toward each other in a tube. Single radial diffusion, when antibody is incorporated into the agar and antigen diffuses radially into it from an inoculation well, is used to quantitate proteins. The double diffusion technique of Ouchterlony involves antigen and antibody diffusing from individual wells into untreated gel, and is useful in qualitative protein analysis.

Qualitative Evaluation of Proteins by Ouchterlony Double Diffusion
The relative advantage of double diffusion over single radial diffusion is that it requires less in reagents (particularly antiserum), since none has to be incorporated into the agar. Also, when the purity of antibody or antigen is in doubt, double diffusion can indicate to what extent contamination has taken place. It is somewhat more sensitive than radial diffusion [11, 34], and it is less susceptible to temperature change artifact.

As the reactants diffuse toward each other, precipitation patterns of antibody and antigen in the Ouchterlony technique can assume 3 basic patterns (Fig. 21-13): (a) Complete identity of two antigens produces a total fusion of precipitate with a single antibody. (b) Nonidentity causes both lines to cross. (c) Partial identity, where one determinant of several is held in common, creates spurs which elongate with time as the antigen continues to diffuse. A reaction of inhibition results when complex antigens and a related more simple antigen diffuse toward antibody for the more complex variant. The precipitate also shows antibody spur formation, but more dense than for simple partial identity [11, 34].

Quantitative Evaluation of Proteins by Radial Immunodiffusion
Current methods of quantitating immunoglobulins are based on the technique of Mancini et al. [28]. The patient serum or test antigen is inoculated into a well cut in agar containing monospecific antibody. Antigen diffuses radially, and at the point of equivalent concentration with antibody it forms a precipitin ring. The rate of diffusion is a function of antigen size and solubility; the time, temperature, and humidity; and the relative concentrations of antigen and antibody. The diameter of the ring is proportional to antigen concentration. Using control standards of "known" concentration, a semilogarithmic plot of concen-

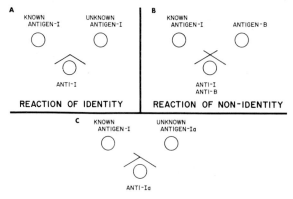

Figure 21-13
Agar gel double diffusion reaction patterns. (A) With an antigenic factor in common, there is complete fusion of lines in a reaction of identity. (B) When no determinant is held in common, there is no deviation of lines, which then cross in a reaction of non-identity. (C) Where serologically related antigens are present, there is some deviation of precipitin lines with partial fusion, leaving a fine spur in a reaction of partial identity. A variant of C is the reaction of inhibition, in which the particle has multiple non-related antigens leading to dense spur formation.

tration vs. ring diameter may be constructed. Alternatively, a linear relationship between concentration and squared diameter may be plotted (Fig. 21-14). The ring diameters for patient sera are then used to derive concentration of immunoglobulin or other specific antigen.

Diffusion is a dynamic process, and until antigen is exhausted the precipitate is dissolved and reprecipitated in ever widening rings. When final equivalency is reached, the ring diameter remains relatively fixed; this may take hours to years [34], and may require more agar than is present in the plate. Therefore it is customary to determine ring diameters at set times, depending on the antigen involved, before equivalency is reached (e.g., 4 hours for IgG; 16 hours for IgA and IgM), as is done with Hyland immunoplates [15]. If diffusion is allowed to proceed for longer periods, ring diameter is no longer proportional to concentration, and the diffuse edge to the ring is difficult to read. In some systems antigen is diluted before charging the well, and diffusion is allowed to proceed to end point (approximately 72 hours for Partigen Plates) (Behringwerke), where it should remain fixed [28]. Thus, standards need not be reapplied every time as additional test serum is added to the plate. However, it is wise to run at least the middle standard with every patient to check for differences created by changes in temperature and humidity.

Precision of quantitation depends on absolute monospecificity of the

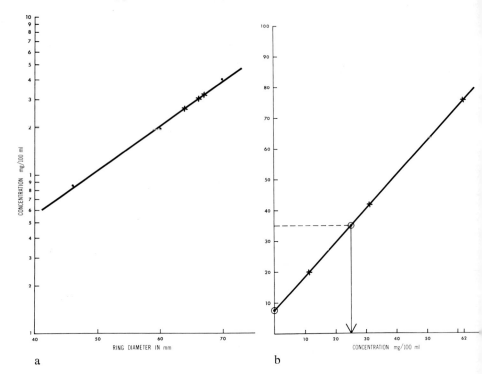

a   b

Figure 21-14
Calculation of immunoglobulin concentration in radial immunodiffusion.
(a) Kinetic determination at specified time. Ring diameter is plotted semi-
logarithmically against concentration. Linearity is not absolute, particularly
at either ends of the curve. (X indicates patients; dots indicate standards.)
(b) End point determination. A linear plot of concentration vs. squared
diameters of precipitin rings. This method of calculation can be used before
end point to derive the best straight line. (⊙ indicates patients; X indicates
standards.)

antiserum placed in the agar, and the characteristics of the antiserum
as a precipitating antibody. The need for accurate delivery of test or
control specimen to the well depends upon the method used in measurement of the precipitin ring. Visual filling of the antigen well is practical
only when ring diameters are measured before end point and at a
constant time. When the method of end point determination is used, the
delivery of patient specimen should generally be done with a micro-
pipette, since there is variation in well capacity among supplying com-
panies, and among batch lots for the same company. Immunoglobulin
determinations that fall above and below the high and low standards are
no longer in the linear parts of the curve. They should be diluted and

the determination repeated. Radial immunodiffusion is more acceptable for IgG and antigens of similar molecular size than for IgA and IgM, which have multiple polymer forms, so that diffusion is not uniformly proportional to concentration [15].

Quality Control for Radial Immunodiffusion

At present there is no precise standard for the absolute mass of any immunoglobulin by radial immunodiffusion. Instead, reference standards provided by the manufacturer must be used. The assay of these reference materials has been accomplished by various methods under different conditions such that there has been no uniformity of standards, and the values expressed in milligrams per milliliter differ widely from laboratory to laboratory. The World Health Organization [41, 42, 43, 51] has recently developed an international reference standard for IgG, IgA, and IgM with which manufacturers may compare their working standards, either directly or with secondary standards. The concentration of these standards is expressed in terms of international units (IU) per milliliter. National standards for IgD and IgE are now available as well.

INTERNATIONAL STANDARDS. As an example, the international standards for IgG, IgA, and IgM and recent standards for IgD and IgE suggest the following equivalences [24, 41, 42, 43]

IgG 1 unit = 0.8147 mg lyophilized specimen 67/86
IgA 1 unit = 0.8147 mg lyophilized specimen 67/86
IgM 1 unit = 0.8147 mg lyophilized specimen 67/86
IgD 1 unit = 0.8188 mg lyophilized specimen 67/37
IgE 1 unit = work not completed yet   68/341

Some difficulties have been encountered in the assay of IgE, which requires the more sensitive technique of radioimmunoassay [24].

It is hoped that these standards, acting as a benchmark for manufacturers of immunoglobulin plates, will produce more uniform results from laboratory to laboratory. Attempts to evaluate the standards of one company on the plates of another are usually unsuccessful, due to variations in agar and antibody. The coefficient of variation for 2 standard deviations is 6–10% for IgG, IgA, IgM, and IgD as measured in mg/100 ml [7, 31].

Interpretation of Results

NORMAL IMMUNOGLOBULIN CONCENTRATIONS (Age Variation). Normal immunoglobulin concentrations show distinct age variation as shown by Stiehm and Fudenberg [48] and others [5]. The normal newborn begins life with only passively acquired maternal IgG, which is catabolized by age 2½ to 3 months. His own globulin production begins soon after birth, and since it is due to primary immune stimuli, it is usually IgM (80% of adult level by age 2). By 3 months, production of IgG is evident, but IgA lags behind (80% of adult only at 10 or 11 years). Deficiencies in one or more globulins are discussed in Chapter 2. In addition, it has been shown [6] that adults do not have fixed levels of immunoglobulins, but show a peak in the second and third decade with some decrease thereafter.

Since neither standard protein electrophoresis nor immunoelectrophoresis are sensitive enough to detect the normally low levels of individual immunoglobulins in children, they should be evaluated by radial immunodiffusion on children 3 years or younger. In infants less than 3 months of age low level plates are useful, especially for IgA and IgM. All reports should include the normal levels for age (see Fig. 3-4 in Chapter 3).

Immunoglobulin concentrations in adults have been categorized for a wide range of diseases [27] but are pathognomonic for none.

DIFFUSION PATTERNS.   Again prozones are the pit for the unwary. Antigen excess causes a hazy background in the agar, which may not be appreciated and thus interpreted as negative in the presence of 8–10 gm/100 ml of abnormal protein. Standard protein electrophoresis should be done simultaneously. In some cases where serum proteins have genetic polymorphisms (e.g., transferrin, haptoglobin), the polyvalent antiserum may not have specificity for a rare genotype which results in no precipitation [17]. Double diffusion rings are seen where there have been wide variations in temperature or humidity, and in serum containing two proteins with common antigenic determinants. Rarely, double rings result from antiserum that is not monospecific. In these cases, measure the outer ring diameter.

MONOCLONAL GAMMOPATHIES.   It is hazardous to attempt identification of an M protein by quantitation of immunoglobulins. In part, this is because excessive amounts of protein (antigen excess) may fail to precipitate. Further, since paraproteins do not diffuse readily due to their large molecular size or molecular aggregation, true concentration cannot be calculated. The antisera in the agar may not be specific for the antigenic determinants of the abnormal protein and thus may not precipitate.

Electroimmunodiffusion

This technique is applicable where very small amounts of antigen are available. If immunoelectrophoresis is performed with the antibody already present in the agar, both antigen and antibody migrate in the electrical field, which creates a flame-shaped line of precipitation. This technique of Laurell [26] is termed *electroimmunodiffusion*. The only

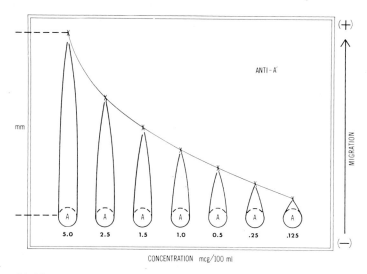

Figure 21-15
Electroimmunodiffusion. Antigen is inoculated into wells cut in antibody containing agar. The length of the flame at point of closure (mm) is proportional to antigen concentration and can be plotted as a semilogarithmic function. An arithmetic plot results in a curve as shown schematically on the agar.

requirements are that antigen be in excess, have greater mobility then its antibody, and have a different isoelectric point [3]. As the flame forms, it is redissolved by antigen excess diffusing through it and is sequentially reprecipitated, the tip of the flame moving in the direction of antigen migration until equivalence is reached. The length of the flame is related to the amount of antigen, and serial antigen dilutions can result in a rough quantitation of the amount of antigen (Fig. 21-15). The method can quantitate micrograms of protein. The standard error of the method is said to be ± 2–3% if wells are filled carefully [18, 46]. This method has recently been applied to quantitation of albumin-globulin ratios in CSF. It can be modified to use cellulose acetate as a support [18] (see Procedures).

Radioimmunoelectrophoresis

Radioimmunoelectrophoresis is a variant of antigen-antibody complexing. Radiolabeled antigen (Ag*) is allowed to react with specific antibody (Ab) and the Ag*-Ab complex is electrophoresed in an agar medium. Free Ag* migrates more efficiently than the larger Ag*-Ab complex. The relative radioactivity of the two zones is measured by autoradiography or cutting out the appropriate agar zones, eluting the reactants and counting them to give a ratio of bound:free antigen. Of importance are the specificity of the antiserum, and the specific activity of the radioactive label to be applied to the antigen [10].

Radioimmunoassay (RIA)

A variation of radioimmunoelectrophoresis, this technique without the supporting agar medium has found wide application. The utilization of RIA and its variants is not truly within the field of tissue immunology, for it finds its greatest use in hormone analysis, and the interested reader is referred to several recent works for applications and methods [3, 16, 19, 22, 25, 32, 36, 38]. One application in immunology rests in the assay for serum IgE, which is normally at too low a level to be detected by radial immunodiffusion.

Disc Electrophoresis

Disc electrophoresis, first devised by Orenstein [33] and Davis [14], combines electrophoresis in a glass column with the molecular sieving effect of polyacrylamide gel. The technique has the capacity to separate serum proteins (or other biologic fluids) from a 1 μl specimen into at least 20 components in 20 min [33]. At pH 8.6 if a mixture of ions, all similarly charged, is applied near the boundary of two ions also of like charge, and current applied with a polarity such that the fastest ion is ahead in the order of migration, the mixture will separate, as in all electrophoretic systems, with the greatest charge moving ahead of all others. The ion mixture is placed in a large-pore (sample) gel to reduce convection. The proteins will layer in disks of like charge, with concentration not dependent on their initial concentration but on their concentration relative to that of the fastest ion. If now the conditions of the experiment are altered—pH, gel pore size, etc.—the layers will redistribute. This is usually accomplished by an abrupt change in gel pore size. Ions now redistribute by virtue of size more than charge, and some of weaker charge pass through those of greater charge distributing in approximately 20 bands [14] (Fig. 21-16).

The original buffer system is tris-glycine-HCl [14]. Acrylamide gel, 5% in aqueous solution, is polymerized with N,N′-methylenebisacrylamide, a cross-linking agent [9, 31]. The anode is at the bottom of the column, and albumin appears lowest. The gel columns are stained with Amido black, and the excess dye either washed or electrophoresed away. Due to diffusion, the colored bands may alter with time. There are several bands constant for most sera, but many are peculiar to only some sera [9, 14]. Furthermore, comparisons of migration distance in one column may not be comparable to a second, which may make interpretation difficult [31].

The technique has been advocated for investigating serum protein polymorphisms, including β-lipoproteins, and general study of minute

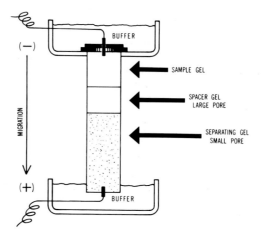

Figure 21-16
Disc electrophoresis. The antigen sample gel is placed on the polymerized gel column. The spacer gel permits stacking of antigens dependent on charge. Further separation depends on molecular seiving in gel of smaller pore size.

(0.1 mg) specimens. The classic technique is described by Davis [9], but more simplified procedures are available [31], and Canalco provides an easy system which is adaptable to several different types of analysis.

Conclusion

Other useful techniques not involving gel diffusion or its electrophoretic variations include passive hemagglutination [20, 47] and hemagglutination inhibition. Haptens may be conjugated [20] to red cells tanned by several methods [23, 46]. These techniques have already been discussed in preceding chapters.

Procedures

Immunoelectrophoresis

REAGENTS
A. Agar, special (Difco), 2% solution
    1. Dissolve 4 gm in 100 ml cold water in 250 ml beaker.
    2. Bring to a boil in water bath. When clear
    3. Add 100 ml Veronal buffer (pH 8.6, μ 0.05).
    4. Add 40 mgm Thimerosol powder (Lilly).
    5. Can be stored at 4° C for 3 months.
    Optional: Lyophilized agar plates (Marine Colloids) can be rehydrated in Veronal buffer diluted 1:2 with distilled water.
B. Veronal buffer, pH 8.6 μ 0.1
    1. 6.30 gm diethylbarbituric acid
    2. 38.5 gm sodium barbiturate
    3. 2000 ml distilled water

Store in refrigerator. Before use, dilute 1:2 with distilled water to give ionic strength 0.05, and allow to come to room temperature.

C. Agar-coated slides
1. Alcohol wipe and dry glass slides.
2. Etch patient number on end of slide.
3. Melt 2% agar until clear.
4. Apply 3 ml smoothly to each slide. Do not allow agar to run off the edge as it siphons the remaining agar away.
5. Allow to gel 15 min at room temperature. Can be stored for 48 hours in humidor at room temperature.

D. Antisera: Polyvalent anti-human—in goat, polyvalent anti-IgG (heavy chain and light chain specific); anti-IgG (heavy chain specific); anti-IgA (heavy chain specific); anti-IgM (heavy chain specific)
anti-κ, anti-λ
anti-B_1C, anti-IgD, anti-IgE, anti-Fc, are also useful for categorizing paraproteins.

E. 30% bovine albumin, filter paper wicks (Beckman No. 319329, Model R).

F. Amido black dye—0.5% w/v in 9:1 methanol:glacial acetic acid.

G. Bromphenol blue dye marker for albumin migration.

EQUIPMENT
A. Electrophoretic chamber (National, Helena, etc.)
B. Stable power source
C. Hot plate or 100° C water bath
D. Clean, etched glass slides—8
E. Dies to cut agar
F. Filter wicks
G. Filter paper strips
H. Pasteur pipettes
I. Humidifying chamber

PROCEDURE
1. Either rehydrate lyophilized agar membranes or melt 2% agar in 100° C water bath. Layer 8 clean, etched glass slides with 3 ml agar and allow to gel at room temperature.
2. Dilute 600 ml Veronal buffer with 600 ml distilled water and fill electrophoresis chambers to equal levels.
3. Moisten slide holder and allow agar-coated slides to adhere, agar side up, by capillary action.
4. Cut agar with dies for desired well and trough patterns.
5. Apply patient serum (test antigen) to one well and control serum to other well, slides 1–7.
6. Slide 8, add 30% bovine albumin and a few crystals of Bromphenol blue dye.

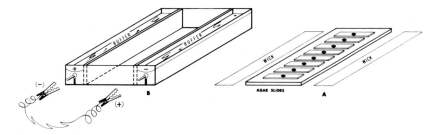

Figure 21-17
Immunoelectrophoresis chamber and slide carrier. Wicks draw buffer onto agar slides from the buffer wells of the electrophoresis chamber.

7. After 5–10 min, add a small button of melted agar to seal each well.
8. Place slide carrier in electrophoresis chamber. Use filter wicks lengthwise from buffer compartment to ends of all 8 slides. Apply small filter paper strips between slides to allow better flow (Fig. 21-17).
9. Electrophorese at 100 mA, or approximately 150 V, for 60 min, or until albumin marker moves ⅔ the distance to the anode.
10. Shut off current. Carefully remove prescored trough agar without damaging the agar.
11. Fill trough with antiserum using Pasteur pipette.
12. Place slides in humidifying chamber for 24–48 hours. Any longer time allows precipitin lines to blur.
13. Examine and/or photograph before washing, to avoid loss of prozones.
14. Rinse with tap water 10–12 hours, then allow to air dry.
15. Stain for 20 min in Amido black, and destain in running tap water for 20–30 min or until background dye is removed.

NOTES
A. Difficulties in electrophoretic migration arise if buffer is not fresh and pH exactly 8.6. Change buffer every two or three uses.
B. Levels in electrophoretic chambers must be equal to prevent siphoning effect.
C. Avoid distortion of antiserum trough or distortions of precipitin arcs will result.
D. Rinse water should be cold to prevent lifting of agar off the slides.
E. Too rapid drying permits cracking of agar.

Electroimmunodiffusion [40]

EQUIPMENT
A. Electrophoresis as used for IEP
B. Power supply: stabilized current type

C. Plastic agar gel holders (Hyland immuno kit) alcohol cleansed
D. Hamilton Microliter Syringe, 1 µl with guide and with Teflon tube tip
E. Magnetic stirrer
F. Blotters
G. Forceps
H. Glass rods

REAGENTS
A. Veronal buffer pH 8.6, ionic strength 0.05 for preparation of agar, ionic strength 0.1 for electrode chambers.

	For Agar ($\mu = 0.05$)	For Cell ($\mu = 0.1$)
Diethylbarbituric acid	0.55 gm	2.76 gm
Sodium barbital	3.50 gm	17.52 gm
Thimerosol	0.10 gm	0.20 gm
Distilled water to	1 liter	2 liter

B. Noble agar (Difco) made as 1% solution in Veronal buffer (μ 0.05) by heating to 100° C in a water bath until clear.
C. Antisera (monospecific, goat or rabbit)
D. Reference samples (normal pooled serum)

PROCEDURE
1. Heat agar 1% in barbital buffer (μ 0.05) in water bath until clear.
2. Add monospecific 1.5 ml antiserum, to 15 ml cooling (50° C) agar.
3. In alcohol-cleansed plastic template carefully layer 11 ml agar-antiserum mixture and allow to gel. (Plates can be stored at 4° C for 2 weeks if desired.)
4. Immediately before use, cut antigen wells 2 mm in diameter along short edge of plate. Wells are 3 mm apart and 10 mm from each end, 30 mm from edge.

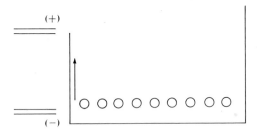

5. With syringe carefully add 2 µl of antigen. Use 3 wells for standard serum; radial immunodiffusion standards are satisfactory.

6. After 2–3 min, seal the wells with agar buffer solution; let gel.
7. Electrophoresis: Fill electrode chambers with phosphate buffer (μ 0.1). Place agar gel in chamber, agar surface up. Wet filter paper wicks and drape them from buffer onto agar, held in place by glass rods. Place clear plastic cover on electrophoresis chamber. Use 50 mA current for 1–3 hours. When tips of the "flame" close over, end point has been reached.
8. Evaluation: Look at precipitates as is, or stain as in IEP. Measure lengths of "rockets." Construct a standard curve on semilog paper, concentration vs. mm length.

Electrodiffusion Method Using Cellulose Acetate [18, 40]

EQUIPMENT AND REAGENTS
A. Plastic electrophoresis chamber with sponges (Hyland Immuno kit) (e.g., LDH isoenzymes or haptoglobin).
B. Plastic application template: In empty plastic agar holder of Immuno kit (Hyland), drill 16 holes (0.9 mm diameter) 3.5 mm apart, no closer than 1.6 cm to the long edge and 2.4 cm from the ends.
C. Barbital buffer (μ 0.075) pH 8.6:

Diethylbarbituric acid	2.76 gm
Sodium diethylbarbiturate	15.4 gm
Distilled water	1000 ml

for all antisera except transferrin, IgG, IgA, and IgM. Use diluted 1:4 in distilled water.
D. Phosphate buffer (μ 0.15) pH 7.4:

Na_2HPO_4	12.8 gm
$NaH_2PO_4–H_2O$	2.62 gm
Distilled water	1000 ml

Dilute 1:8 in distilled water. Use to dilute IgG, IgA, IgM, or transferrin antisera.
E. Ponceau S 3 mg/liter of 5% acetic acid.
F. Cellulose acetate membrane—3 × 3″ on Mylar backing (Helena).

METHOD
1. Soak cellulose acetate membrane in antiserum for transferrin, IgG, IgA, or IgM, diluted 1:20 with 1:8 dilution of phosphate buffer (μ 0.15) for 10 min as for any microzone technique. Avoid bubbles and wet evenly. Blot firmly on filter paper.
2. Place cellulose acetate surface up on moist wet paper towels and cover with plastic template. Center and allow to stand for 3 min to equilibrate. Keep moist at all times.

3. Apply antigens: Using 1 μl Hamilton syringe fitted with Teflon tube tip, apply 0.25 μl through holes in template onto membrane. Apply sample slowly. After all samples are applied remove template. Test sera and standard sera are diluted to the following concentrations [18]:

	Concentrations of Standard, mg/100 ml				Dilutions of Test Serum for Protein Determination		
IgG	10.00	5.00	2.50	1.25	1:128	256	512
IgA	15.00	7.50	3.75	1.88	16	32	64
IgM	27.00	13.50	6.75	3.38	8	16	32

4. Electrophoresis: Fill electrode chambers with 35 ml undiluted buffer and place sponges in compartments.
5. Place membrane cellulose side down on chamber bridging the two sponges. Equilibrate 1 min. Electrophorese at 50 mA for 25 min for all proteins; except IgA and transferrins, 45 min; IgG and IgM, 60 min.
6. Remove membrane from cell, wash in 3 liter beaker containing phosphate buffer (μ 0.15) diluted 1:4 in distilled H_2O. Rinse for 10–15 min.
7. Stain with Ponceau S 4 min. No destaining is necessary. Air dry at room temperature.
8. Measure "rockets" to nearest 0.1 mm with a measuring magnifier, and construct standard curve as semilog of protein concentration vs. length of rocket in mm.

NOTE: Care must be used in application of sample not to nick cellulose or agar, or peaks will be badly distorted.

References

1. Arquembourg, P. C., Salvaggio, J. E., and Bickers, J. N. *Primer of Immunoelectrophoresis.* Ann Arbor and London: Ann Arbor-Humphrey, 1970.
2. Augener, W., Grey, H. M., Cooper, N. R., and Müller-Eberhard, H. J. The reaction of monomeric and aggregated immunoglobulins with C1. *Immunochemistry* 8:1011, 1971.
3. Berson, S. A., and Yalow, R. S. Quantitative aspects of the reaction between insulin and insulin binding antibody. *J. Clin. Invest.* 38:1996, 1959.
4. Brandtzaeg, P., Fjellanger, I., and Gjeruldsen, S. T. Human secretory

immunoglobulins: I. Salivary secretions from individuals with normal or low levels of serum immunoglobulins. *Scand. J. Haematol. Suppl.* 12, 1970.

5. Buckley, R. H., Dees, S. C., and O'Fallon, W. M.   Serum immunoglobulins: I. Levels in normal children and in uncomplicated childhood allergy. *Pediatrics* 41:600, 1968.

6. Buckley, C. E., and Dorsey, F. C.   Serum immunoglobulin levels throughout the life span of healthy man. *Ann. Intern. Med.* 75:673, 1971.

7. Cawley, L. P.   Serum protein electrophoresis. In ASCP Commission on Continuing Education, *Clinical Immunology and Immunochemistry.* Chicago, 1972.

8. Cebra, J. J., Ray, A., Benjamin, D., and Birshtein, B.   Localization of affinity label within the primary structure of γ_2 chain from guinea pig IgG (2). In B. Amos (ed.), *Progress in Immunology.* 1st International Congress in Immunology. New York and London: Academic Press, 1971, p. 269.

9. Clarke, J. T.   Simplified "disc" (polyacrylamide gel) electrophoresis. In H. E. Whipple (ed.), *Gel Electrophoresis. Ann. N.Y. Acad. Sci.* 121:428, 1964.

10. Clausen, J., and Munkner, T.   Immunoelectrophoresis and autoradiography. In H. Peeters (ed.), *Protides of the Biologic Fluids,* Elsevier Publishing Company, Amsterdam 1960, pp. 147–151.

11. Clausen, J.   Immunochemical techniques for the identification and estimation of macromolecules. In T. S. Work and E. Work (eds.), *Laboratory Techniques in Biochemistry and Molecular Biology.* Amsterdam and London: North-Holland, 1969, vol. 1.

12. Cooper, N. R.   Complement in cell survival and destruction. In P. J. Schmidt (ed.), *Progress in Transfusion and Transplantation.* Proceedings of the 25th Annual Meeting of the American Association of Blood Banks and 13th Congress of the International Society of Blood Transfusion. Washington, D.C.: American Association of Blood Banks, 1972, p. 191.

13. Cunningham, B. A., Gottlieb, P. D., Pflumm, M. N., and Edelman, G. M.   Immunoglobulin structure: Diversity, gene duplications and domains. In B. Amos (ed.), *Progress in Immunology.* 1st International Congress in Immunology. New York and London: Academic Press, 1971, p. 3.

14. Davis, B. J.   Disc electrophoresis: II. Method and application to human serum proteins. In H. E. Whipple (ed.), *Gel Electrophoresis. Ann. N.Y. Acad. Sci.* 121:404, 1964.

15. Fahey, J. L., and McKelvey, E. M.   Quantitation determination of serum immunoglobulins in antibody-agar plates. *J. Immunol.* 94:84, 1965.

16. Federlin, K., Hales, C. N., and Kracht, J. (eds.)   *Immunologic Methods in Endocrinology.* New York and London: Academic Press, 1971.

17. Giblett, E. R.   *Genetic Markers in Human Blood.* Philadelphia: Davis, 1969.

18. Gill, C. N., Fischer, C. L., and Holleman, C. L.   Rapid method for protein quantitation by electroimmunodiffusion. *Clin. Chem.* 17:501, 1971.

19. Gleich, C. J., Averbeck, A. K., and Swedland, H. A.   Measurement of IgE in normal and allergic serum by radioimmunoassay. *J. Lab. Clin. Med.* 77:690, 1971.

20. Gold, E. R., and Fudenberg, H. H.   Chromic chloride: A coupling reagent for passive hemagglutination reactions. *J. Immunol.* 99:859, 1967.

21. Grabar, P., and Williams, C. A., Jr.   Méthode permettant l'étude conjugée des propriétés électrophorétiques et immunochimiques d'une mélange de protéines. Application au serum sanguin. *Biophys. Acta* 10:193, 1953.

22. Hunter, W. M.   The preparation of radioiodinated proteins of high activity, their reaction with antibody in vitro: The radioimmunoassay. In D. M. Weir (ed.), *Handbook of Experimental Immunology.* Oxford: Blackwell, 1967, p. 608.

23. Ingraham, J. S.   The preparation and use of formalized erythrocytes with attached antigens of haptens to titrate antibodies. *Proc. Soc. Exp. Biol. Med.* 99:452, 1958.

24. Johansson, S. G. O., Bennich, H. H., and Berg, T.   The clinical significance of IgE. *Prog. Clin. Immunol.* 1:157, 1972.

25. Kirkham, K. E., and Hunter, W. M. (eds.)   *Radioimmunoassay Methods.* London: Churchill Livingston, 1971.

26. Laurell, C. B.   Quantitative estimation of proteins by electrophoresis in agarose gel containing antibodies. *Anal. Biochem.* 15:45, 1966.

27. Leonardy, J. G., and Peacock, L. B.   Evaluation of quantitative serum immunoglobulin determinations in clinical practice. *Ann. Allergy* 30:378, 1972.

28. Mancini, G., Carbonara, A. O., and Heremans, J. F.   Immunochemical quantitation of antigens by single radial immunodiffusion. *Immunochemistry* 2:235, 1965.

29. Mestecky, J., Zikan, J., and Butler, W. T.   Immunoglobulin M and secretory immunoglobulin A: Presence of a common polypeptide chain different from light chains. *Science* 171:1163, 1971.

30. Metzger, H., Chesebro, B., Hadler, N. M., Lee, J., and Otchin, N.   Modification of immunoglobulin combining sites. In B. Amos (ed.), *Progress in Immunology.* 1st International Congress of Immunology. New York and London: Academic Press, 1971, p. 253.

31. Nerenberg, S. T.   *Electrophoresis: A Practical Laboratory Manual.* Philadelphia: Davis, 1966.

32. Odell, W. D., and Doughaday, W. H. (eds.)   *Principles of Competitive Protein Binding Assays.* Philadelphia: Lippincott, 1971.

33. Orenstein, L.   Disc electrophoresis: I. Background and theory. In H. E. Whipple (ed.), *Gel Electrophoresis. Ann. N.Y. Acad. Sci.* 121:321, 1964.

34. Ouchterlony, O.   *Handbook of Immunodiffusion and Immunoelectrophoresis.* Ann Arbor: Ann Arbor Science, 1968.

35. Palmer, D. F., and Woods, R.   *Qualitation and Quantitation of Immunoglobulins.* Department of Health, Education, and Welfare, Procedural Guide No. 3, Publication No. (HSM) 72–8102. Atlanta: Center for Disease Control, 1972.

36. Parker, C. W.   Radioimmunoassays. In M. Stefanini (ed.), *Progress in Clinical Pathology.* New York: Grune & Stratton, 1972, vol. 4, p. 103.

37. Penn, G. M., and Davis, T.   Clinical immunoelectrophoresis. In

L. Cawley, G. Penn, R. Nakamura, E. Tucker, S. Deodhar, V. Agnello (eds.), *Clinical Immunology and Immunochemistry*. Chicago: American Society of Clinical Pathologists, Commission on Continuing Education, 1972, p. 57.

38. Peron, F. G., and Caldwell, B. V. (eds.) *Immunologic Methods in Steroid Determination*. New York: Appleton, 1970.
39. Putnam, F. W., Shimizu, A., Paul, C., and Shinoda, T.   Tentative structure of human IgM immunoglobulin. In B. Amos (ed.), *Progress in Immunology*. 1st International Congress of Immunology. New York and London: Academic Press, 1971, p. 292.
40. Ritzmann, S. E., Fischer, C. L., Cobb, K. E., Gill, C. W., and Daniels, J. C.   Electroimmunodiffusion. In American Society of Clinical Pathologists, *Workshop in Clinical Chemistry*. (Director, John B. Fuller, M. D.) 1972.
41. Rowe, D. S., Anderson, S. G., and Grab, B.   A research standard for human serum immunoglobulins IgG, IgA, and IgM. *Bull. WHO.* 42:535, 1970.
42. Rowe, D. S., Anderson, S. G., and Tackett, L.   Research standard for human serum immunoglobulin D. *Bull. WHO.* 43:607, 1970.
43. Rowe, D. S., Tackett, L., Bennich, H., Ishizaka, K., Johansson, S. G. O., and Anderson, S. G.   A research standard for human serum immunoglobulin E. *Bull. WHO.* 43:609, 1970.
44. Scheidegger, J. J.   Une micro-méthode de l'immunoelectrophorese. *Int. Arch. Allergy Applied Immunol.* 7:103, 1955.
45. Snapper, I., and Kahn, A.   *Myelomatosis: Fundamentals and Clinical Features*. Baltimore: University Park Press, 1971.
46. Spiegelberg, H.   Principles of methods. In Meischer, P. A. and Müller-Eberhard, H. (eds.), *Textbook of Immunopathology*. New York and London: Grune & Stratton, Vol. II, 1968, p. 789.
47. Steffen, C.   Antibodies in tissues. *Prog. Clin. Pathol.* 3:326, 1970.
48. Stiehm, E. R., and Fudenberg, H. H.   Serum levels of immune globulins in health and disease: A survey. *Pediatrics* 37:715, 1966.
49. Tiselius, A.   Electrophoresis of serum globulin. *Biochem. J.* 3:13, 1937.
50. Waldenström, J.   *Diagnosis and Treatment of Multiple Myeloma*. New York and London: Grune & Stratton, 1970.
51. WHO Expert Committee on Biologic Standardization. Measurements of concentrations of human serum immunoglobulins. *J. Immunol.* 107: 1798, 1971.
52. Williams, C. A., Jr., and Grabar, P.   Immunoelectrophoretic studies on serum proteins: I. The antigens of human serum. *J. Immunol.* 74:158, 1955.

22

Fluorescent Antibody Methods

Fluorescent compounds are illuminated by light of short wavelengths, and after absorption of energy they emit a second light of a longer wavelength. When the emission of light following absorption is extremely short, it is generally called *fluorescent,* while *phosphorescence* requires a longer period between absorption and emission. Most fluorescent compounds have a ring structure. When the compound absorbs light, there is an excitation of electrons which oscillates in resonance. With the absorption of light of shorter wavelength, the energy can be emitted in the form of light of longer wavelength with only a short time lapse between absorption and emission of light. If the excitation light is very strong and causes irreversible displacement of electrons of the molecules, there will be a fading of the emission light. Thus, the fluorescent compound may fade under continued exposure to excitation light.

Fluorescent-labeled antibody was first used by Coons and associates [13] in 1941, for studying localization of antigens in tissues. The fluorescent dye was used as a chemically linked marker on the specific antibody and did not alter its immunologic reactivity. The two fluorochromes most widely used are fluorescein and rhodamine, or some stable derivative of each of the dyes. Fluorescein has a yellowish-green fluorescence with a maximum at about 520 nm, and rhodamine has a reddish-orange fluorescence with a maximum at about 620 nm (Figs. 22-1, 2). These compounds have been the fluorochromes of choice because of intensity or efficiency of fluorescence [15, 22, 25].

The green fluorescence of fluorescein offers two important advantages over the red fluorescence of rhodamine. (a) The human eye is more sensitive to the apple-green color than to the reddish-orange color, and (b) red autofluorescence is more common in nature than green autofluorescence (Fig. 22-3). The most popular conjugate used in the laboratory is the fluorescein isothiocyanate-conjugate antiserum. The isothiocyanate derivative is stable and is coupled to the free amino groups of the protein to form a carbamido linkage. Tetramethylrhodamine isothiocyanate can be conjugated in a similar manner as fluorescein isothiocyanate for the reddish-orange fluorescent reagent [8, 29].

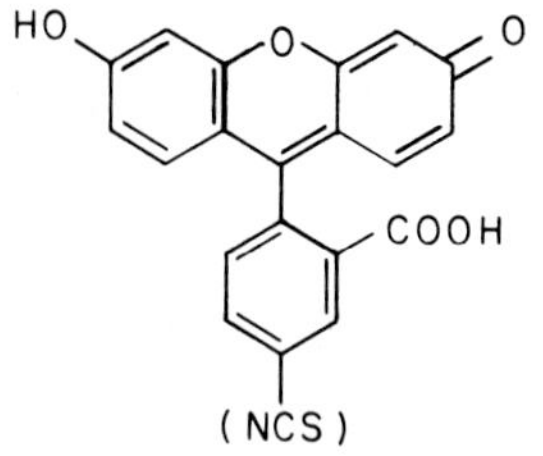

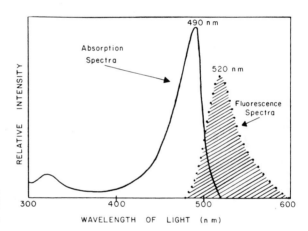

Figure 22-1
Fluorescein isothiocyanate (FITC) $C_{21}H_{11}O_6N$ $(C_{21}H_{15}O_5NS)$. Absorption peak, 490 nm; emission peak, 520 nm.

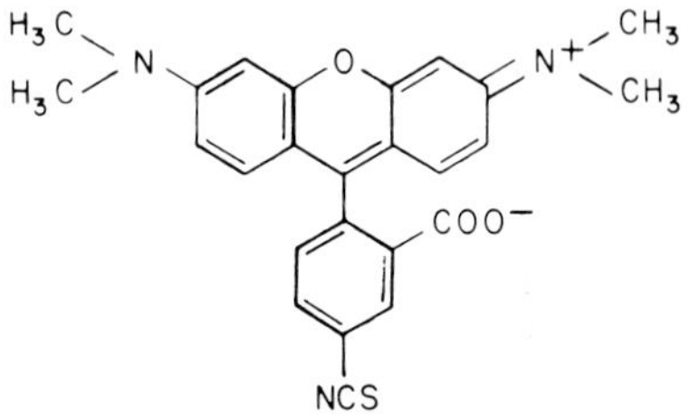

Figure 22-2
Tetramethyl rhodamine isothiocyanate $(C_{25}H_{21}O_3NaS)$. Absorption peak, 550 nm; emission peak, 620 nm.

Figure 22-3
Absorption and fluorescence spectra of fluorescein at pH 7.1.

Application of Fluorescent Antibody Methods

The technique is helpful in the localization of antigen and antibody reactions at a cellular level. Fluorescent methods have been used to study numerous immunologic problems such as [6, 11, 15, 22, 25] (a) the detection of specific antibodies in patients' sera by use of appropriate antisera and antigen substrate; (b) the localization of antigen, antibody, complement, and immune complexes in host tissues; (c) determining the site of localization and fate of injected foreign antigens; (d) the localization and site of multiplication of infectious agents for use in the rapid diagnosis of microbial infections; and (e) studies on the localization of various hormones and enzymes in tissues.

General Methods for Use of Fluorescent Antibody

In the use of fluorescent antibody there are several methods which can be used to detect the presence of unknown antigens and tissues or smears, and the presence of unknown antibodies in the patient's serum. Some of the more common methods are the direct, indirect, inhibition, and complement-staining methods.

The Direct Method

The antibody is labeled with the fluorescent compound and is used to detect the presence of antigen fixed in tissue fixed to a slide. The fluorescent-labeled antibodies are added to the antigen in its optimal dilution and allowed to react at least 30 min at room temperature or 37° C. The preparation is next washed to remove the labeled γ-globulins which do not react with the antigen. The smear tissue sections are blotted and the preparation mounted with buffered glycerol for examination with the fluorescence microscope (Fig. 22-4).

Indirect Method

This method is utilized for detection of either unknown antigen in tissue sections or unknown antibody in the patient's serum. It is based on the principle that a specific antigen-antibody reaction may be visualized by addition of labeled anti-antibody globulin directed against the antibody globulin in the specific immune reaction. The antigen plus antibody globulin plus labeled anti-antibody complex results in fluorescence of the coated antigen. The indirect method has the advantage of utilizing a single labeled anti-antibody globulin to detect many different specific antigen-antibody reactions occurring within a given species, such as the human. For example, fluoresceinated rabbit or goat anti-human globulin may be used to detect a wide variety of human antibody-antigen reactions.

In the detection of the unknown antigen or antibody the tissue sections or smear is processed with unlabeled antiserum specific for the antigen being tested and allowed to react for at least 30 min at room

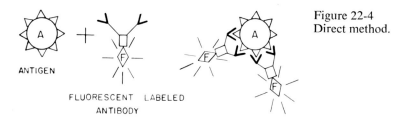

ANTIGEN

FLUORESCENT LABELED ANTIBODY

Figure 22-4
Direct method.

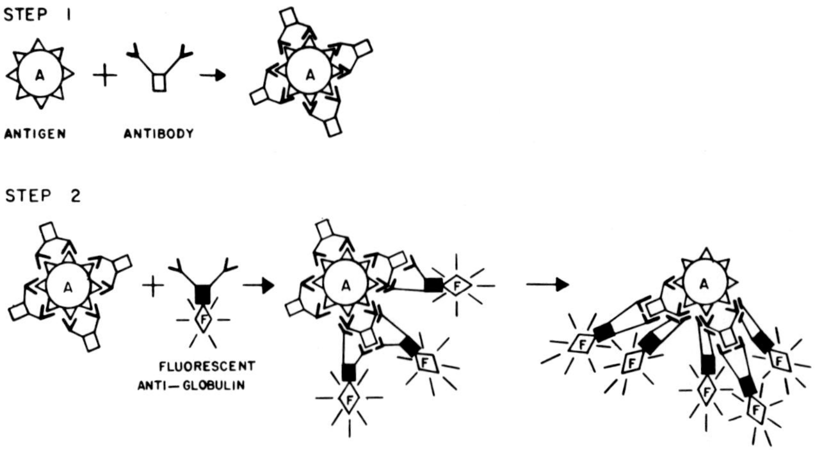

Figure 22-5
Indirect method.

temperature or 37° C. The preparation is thoroughly washed to remove unlabeled antibody unattached to the antigen. Then labeled anti-antibody globulin is employed and allowed to incubate similar to the direct technique (Fig. 22-5).

Inhibition Method

This method is often employed as a control for testing the specificity of the antibodies in the direct fluorescent procedure. It has been applied for detection of certain microorganisms such as *Toxoplasma gondii* in serum [14]. These tests are based on the principle that antigen when treated with unlabeled specific antibody becomes saturated, and subsequent exposure to specific labeled antibody results in negative fluorescence. Treatment of the antigen with unlabeled normal serum and subsequent exposure to specific labeled antibody should result in no fluorescence of the antigen. Optimal concentrations of both labeled and unlabeled antibodies should be determined (Fig. 22-6).

Mixed Antiglobulin Method

In this method, an anti-immunoglobulin is first allowed to combine with tissue antibody that has become attached to the tissue substrate similar to the indirect method. The free antibody-combining sites of the antiglobulin are then reacted with fluorescent-labeled immunoglobulin (antigen) [3].

The mixed immunofluorescent staining procedure offers certain advantages and disadvantages over the indirect method. The mixed method can be performed in the first step with impure antiserum as long as the fluorescent-labeled immunoglobulin antigen is pure and free of contami-

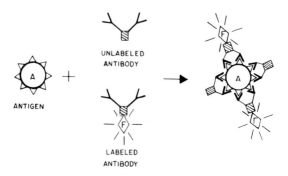

Figure 22-6
Competitive inhibition method. The procedure consists of a one-step inhibition reaction. The antigen substrate is exposed to a mixture of fluorescent-labeled and nonlabeled antibodies and shows a reduced fluorescence.

nants. The mixed antiglobulin method facilitates quantitative analysis since the antiglobulins and the labeled immunoglobulin antigen can be varied independently.

The disadvantages of the mixed antiglobulin method are [3]: (a) the methods require one extra step and a longer time than the indirect method, and (b) the concentration of the antiglobulin required to obtain constant plateau titers is greater for the mixed than for the indirect immunofluorescent-staining method (Fig. 22-7).

Complement-Staining Method
This is similar to the indirect technique except that the labeled antibody is directed against the species-binding complement used in the test. Often guinea pig complement is used. The method is useful to detect either unknown antigen or unknown antibody in patient's serum. The antibody must be able to fix complement. The test is based on the principle that the antigen sensitized with specific antibody will bind the complement to a complex. The addition of labeled anti-guinea pig complement globulin will result in fluorescence of the specific antigen-antibody complex bound with complement (Fig. 22-8).

Controls in the Fluorescent Antibody Methods
Controls in the staining with labeled antibodies, as in any standard laboratory procedure, are a necessary part of the procedure.

Some of the most useful controls include:
A. Absorption of the antibody from the labeled antiserum by the specific antigen before staining the preparation.
B. Comparison of the fluorescence of the experimentally positive slide with similar tissue material known to be unreacting, e.g., a tissue exhibiting a different pathological process.

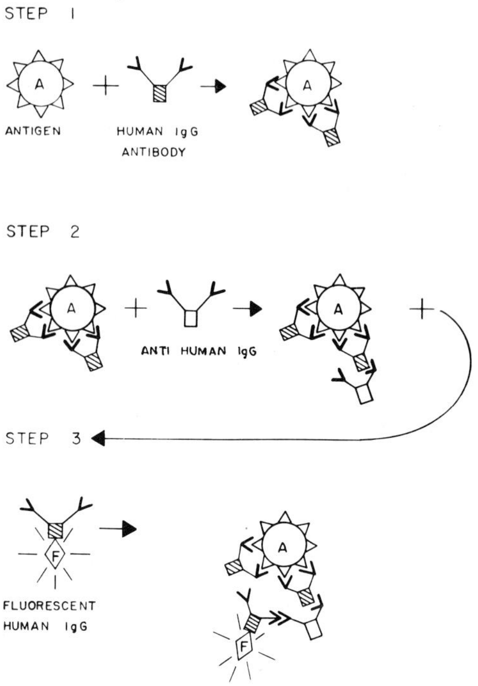

STEP   1

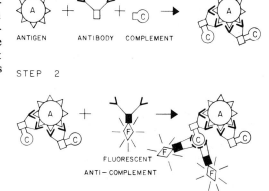

ANTIGEN   HUMAN IgG
                ANTIBODY

STEP   2

ANTI HUMAN IgG

Figure 22-7
Mixed immunofluorescence.
This procedure requires an
additional step over the indirect method. The procedure
has certain advantages in that
the fluorescein label is not
placed on an antibody, and
the antiserum employed in
the second step can contain
other extraneous antibodies
besides anti-human IgG.

STEP   3

FLUORESCENT
HUMAN IgG

Figure 22-8
Anticomplement staining.
The advantage of the anticomplement staining reaction
is that a single labeled anticomplement serum may be
used to detect many different
antigen-antibody reactions
which bind complement.

STEP   1

ANTIGEN   ANTIBODY   COMPLEMENT

STEP   2

FLUORESCENT
ANTI-COMPLEMENT

C. The use of unrelated fluorescent antisera or fluorescent normal
   globulin on the experimental tissue.
D. Inhibition of the "blocking" of fluorescence by prior application of
   unlabeled antibody. This method may yield only partial inhibition.

Antibody Preparation, Labeling, and Adsorption

Preparation of Antiserum

Methods of purification of antigen and production of antisera will not
be discussed here, for there are many different acceptable published
procedures. Purification of the antigen is extremely important before
antiserum production to avoid the production of contaminating antibodies.

Determination of Antibody Concentration

Antibody concentration may be roughly determined by the units of
precipitating antibody [3]. By a double diffusion gel method, the reciprocal of the highest dilution of the antiserum giving a precipitin line with
1 mg of the antigen is considered to be the number of units of precipitating antibody [3, 5]. Good antiserum should have greater than 4
units/ml or 1 mg antibody protein/ml [4, 19, 20]. Quantitative determination of the precipitating antibody may be determined by the classic
procedure [21].

Isolation of the γ Globulin Fraction of Antiserum by
Salt Fractionation: Ammonium Sulfate Precipitation

MATERIALS AND REAGENTS
A. 0.85% isotonic saline solution
B. Refrigeration to 0° C
C. Cold saturated $(NH_4)_2SO_4$ (pH 7.0)
D. Agitator
E. Centrifuge
F. Equipment for dialysis
G. Buffered saline solution, .01 M phosphate buffered saline, pH 7
H. Saturated $BaCl_2$—1 or 2 drops
 I. 0.1 N HCl—0.5 ml
J. Merthiolate
K. Freezer at 4° C (for storage if desired)

PROCEDURE
1. Dilute antiserum with an equal volume of 0.85% isotonic saline
   solution. Cool to 0–4° C.
2. Slowly add sufficient volume of cold saturated $(NH_4)_2SO_4$, ph 7.0,
   with constant stirring to effect 33.3–40% saturation. Continue stirring
   for 2 to 3 hours at 4° C.
3. Centrifuge mixture at 4° C at 1,400 g for 30 min.
4. Discard supernatant.
5. Dissolve precipitate in minimum amount of cold saline solution.
   Repeat steps 2, 3, 4.

6. Collect precipitate and dialyze in the cold against buffered saline solution until dialyzing solution is free of sulfate, and then dialyze 10 to 24 hours against nonbuffered saline solution. The loss of $(NH_4)_2SO_4$ is noted when no precipitate forms when one or two drops of saturated $BaCl_2$ solution are added to approximately 100 ml dialysate acidified with 0.5 ml 0.1 N HCl.

7. Add merthiolate to a final concentration of 1:10,000 and store at 4° C.

Isolation of γ-Globulin by DEAE Cellulose Chromatography

The γ-globulin fraction is a much better fraction for fluorescent labeling. A pure γ-globulin fraction will help in minimizing the nonspecific fluorescence. This may be done by dialyzing the $(NH_4)_2SO_4$ fraction against 0.01 M phosphate buffer pH 7.5, and then passing the protein solution over N,N-diethylamino-ethyl (DEAE) cellulose [28]. The slow γ-fraction is eluted in the first peak.

   Preparation of DEAE cellulose column.   The weight of DEAE cellulose used should be at least 20 times the weight of protein applied to the column.

SUPPLIES AND REAGENTS
A. 0.1 N NaOH solution
B. Sintered glass Buchner funnel attached to a vacuum suction device
C. Large beaker
D. Distilled H_2O
E. Large Buchner funnel
F. Phosphate buffer (pH 7.5; 0.2 M; 0.01 M)
G. 2.5 cm diameter column
H. Solution containing 0.4 M NaH_2PO_4 and 2 M NaCl (for reuse of DEAE cellulose if desired)

PROCEDURE
1. The DEAE cellulose is first washed with a 0.1 N NaOH solution.
2. DEAE is collected on a sintered glass Buchner funnel attached to a vacuum suction device. The resulting DEAE mat is transferred to a large beaker and resuspended in several volumes of distilled H_2O. The DEAE is repeatedly washed about 3 times with several changes of distilled H_2O. The sintered glass Buchner funnel is used to separate the DEAE sediment from the supernate. The DEAE may be resuspended and stirred with the next washing of distilled water in a large Buchner funnel.
3. The DEAE cellulose is then equilibrated with 0.2 M phosphate buffer.
4. The DEAE, which has been equilibrated with 0.2 M buffer, is then initially washed with distilled H_2O and then with a 0.01 M phosphate buffer.
5. The DEAE is added to a 2.5 cm diameter column after removal of

air bubbles by a vacuum suction. The 0.01 M phosphate buffer is allowed to run through the column, and the conductance of the eluate is measured to check equilibration with the 0.01 M buffer before application of the protein sample.

NOTE: After fractionation and isolation of the γ-globulin, the DEAE cellulose can be used again, provided that all protein is stripped from the column with a solution containing 0.4 M NaH_2PO_4 and 2 M NaCl [28].

Determination of Protein Concentration

Since the conjugation of fluorescein to antibody globulin is done on a weight-to-weight basis, the quantity of protein in the globulin solution must be determined. This may be done by one of several methods, such as a protein measurement at 280 nm with an ultraviolet spectrophotometer or by the Nesslerization [23] or Folin [24] methods.

Preparation of Fluorescein Conjugate

Several fluorescent compounds now exist that are easily conjugated to proteins, the commonest among them being fluorescein isothiocyanate (greenish-yellow fluorescence) and tetramethylrhodamine isothiocyanate (orange-red fluorescence). The isothiocyanate derivatives are stable, with a good labeling efficiency.

STANDARD METHOD FOR FLUORESCEIN CONJUGATION.   The following protocol may be used for the conjugation procedure with fluorescein isothiocyanate.

REAGENTS
   Preparation of buffer solutions.   Carbonate buffer stock solution (pH 9.5, 0.5 M)
A. Na_2CO_3 13.25 gm dissolved in 250 ml distilled H_2O
B. $NaHCO_3$ 10.50 gm dissolved in 250 ml distilled H_2O
Phosphate-buffered saline solution 0.15 M with pH 7.0 and phosphate 0.01 M.
A. NaCl—80 gm
B. NaH_2PO_4—13.8 gm
C. NaOH (40%)—7.0 ml
D. Make to 10 liters with distilled H_2O
E. The pH of the final solution should be checked.
Before conjugation, add $NaHCO_3$ solution to Na_2CO_2 to about 1:9 ratio. Check pH and add enough Na_2CO_3 solution for a final pH of 9.5 at 4° C.
   The reagents should be added in the order given below (4° C with constant agitation):
1. 0.15 M NaCl (nonbuffered) 42.5 (ml) volume of protein solution to give 500 mg of globulin (enough to dilute the protein up to the final concentration of 1%)
2. Carbonate buffer 0.5 M, pH 9.5 (15% vol./vol.)—7.5 ml

3. Protein (globulin fraction) 500 mg dry globulin or an appropriate volume of protein solution to give 500 mg globulin. Final concentration 1% wt/vol
4. 0.1 N NaOH should be added to adjust pH to 9.5 at 4° C
5. Fluorescein isothiocyanate (added slowly)
    a. Mixing is done at 0°–4° C with constant stirring. After the protein is added, sprinkle in the fluorescein slowly. The solution will quickly take on a greenish-yellow color.
    b. Stirring should continue for 18 hours in the cold. Then the conjugated protein is dialyzed against phosphate-buffered saline solution until the dialysate is free from green color.
    c. Two to three days may be needed for clearing. When dialysis is is terminated, add merthiolate (1:10,000) and divide into 4 ml portions in test tubes. These may be stored frozen and removed one at a time for use.

MATERIALS AND REAGENTS
A. Crystalline $(NH_4)_2SO_4$, analytical grade
B. Distilled H_2O
C. Burner for heating
D. Refrigeration to 4° C
E. Diluted NaOH (to adjust pH to 7.0)
F. Dialysis bag
G. Bicarbonate buffer (pH 9.5, 0.25 M)
H. Fluorescein isothiocyanate
 I. Phosphate buffered saline solution, 0.15 M with phosphate 0.01 M, pH 7.0
J. Sephadex G–25 or G–50 (Pharmacia; medium grade satisfactory)
K. Physiologic saline solution
L. Glass column approximately 2.5 cm in diameter, with sintered glass disc
M. Protein γ globulin for labeling
N. Fraction collector
O. Freezer (for storage if desired)

PREPARATION OF SATURATED AMMONIUM SULFATE SOLUTION.   Add approximately 375 gm analytical grade crystalline $(NH_4)_2SO_4$ to about 500 ml distilled water while heating over a burner. Large amounts are required for a saturated solution. The supersaturated solution is cooled and crystals will form at 4° C. The saturated $(NH_4)_2SO_4$ solution is decanted from the bottom layer of crystals and adjusted to a pH of 7.0 by addition of diluted NaOH. The pH should be checked again just prior to use.

CONJUGATION WITH FLUORESCEIN BY THE DIALYSIS TECHNIQUE [12]
1. The γ globulin is brought to a concentration of 1% (wt P/vol).
2. Place protein solution in dialysis bag and dialyze against 10 vol

bicarbonate buffer at pH 9.5, 0.25 M (1:20 of the usual 0.5 M bicarbonate buffer) for 1 hour.
3. Then add fluorescein isothiocyanate to the dialysate (0.1 mg per ml of dialysate) and allow conjugation to proceed for 24 to 48 hours.
4. Replace the dialysate with buffered saline solution and remove all unbound fluorescein from the protein solution.

PREPARATION OF A SEPHADEX COLUMN FOR SEPARATION OF LABELED PROTEIN FROM UNLABELED FLUORESCEIN.   A Sephadex column G-25 or G-50 is set up so that the ratio of the volume of column to volume of conjugate is at least 5 to 1 and the conjugate is layered carefully on the top.
1. 25 grams of G-25 is suspended in 250 ml physiologic saline solution. The suspension is mixed and allowed to settle and the suspension of fine particles is decanted. This procedure is repeated 3 times.
2. The suspension is then poured into a glass column approximately 2.5 cm in diameter with a sintered glass disc, and the column is filled to at least a height of 25 cm.
3. The column will handle 10 to 15 ml labeled protein.
4. The protein conjugate is collected on a fraction collector; elution occurs in the void volume.
5. The labeled protein is concentrated and characterized, and may be stored in aliquots in a freezer at $-20°$ C or lower.

Removal of Nonspecific Fluorescence

In the fluorescein-conjugated antibody solution there are substances which can cause nonspecific tissue staining. Such substances present in high concentrations can be adsorbed with tissue powders. Also with the use of DEAE cellulose chromatography bright and specific fluorescent antibodies may be isolated following fluorescein conjugation [29].

MATERIALS AND REAGENTS
A. Thawed fluorescent antibody—4 ml
B. Liver powder—100 mg/ml to 400 mg
C. Agitator
D. Centrifuge in cold, or funnel and filter paper

METHOD OF TISSUE POWDER ADSORPTION.   The choice of species that may be used is dependent upon the antibody to be adsorbed. For example, one should not use a powder of human liver to adsorb fluorescent anti-human IgG, since it contains some of the homologous antigen, which may react despite being denatured. For this reason, it is good to have on hand stocks of powders from several species. Bovine or rabbit liver powder may be used to adsorb conjugated antisera to human immunoglobulins.
1. Thaw a tube containing 4 ml fluorescent antibody. Add to this 100 mg powder per milliliter, or a total of 400 mg powder.
2. Agitate 40 min with a shaker at room temperature.

3. Then centrifuge at high speed in the cold (16,000 rpm for 20 min) to recover the supernatant. Carefully remove the supernate from the sedimented powder.
4. Repeat step 3 so as to remove all powder. Complete separation is visibly observable because the powder particles will have a brilliant fluorescence. Keep supernatant refrigerated.
5. Alternatively, the conjugated antibody may be separated from the tissue powder following the adsorption procedure by filtration through a funnel with filter paper. The powder is washed with a small volume of phosphate-buffered saline solution to increase recovery of the conjugated protein.

MATERIALS AND REAGENTS
A. Waring blender
B. Fresh or freshly thawed liver tissue—100–400 gm
C. Saline solution
D. Large beaker
E. Acetone
F. Buchner funnel with suction
G. Air evaporation
H. Storage at 4° C or less

PREPARATION OF BOVINE LIVER TISSUE POWDERS
1. Place in a blender 100 to 400 gm fresh or freshly thawed liver tissue with a little saline solution. Homogenize with short bursts.
2. Then add the homogenate to a large beaker and after marking the volume, add 4 vol. acetone with stirring.
3. Wash the denatured protein with saline solution by repeated centrifugation until the supernatant is free of hemoglobin.
4. The precipitate is then mixed with a minimum of saline solution and 4 vol. acetone.
5. Repeat step 4 once more and allow the precipitate to stay in the acetone 1 hour.
6. Wash several times in acetone in a Buchner funnel with suction, and finally remove the acetone by air evaporation at room temperature or 37° C.
7. Store the powder at 4° C or less.

FRACTIONATION OF SPECIFIC FITC-LABELED ANTIBODIES WITH DEAE CELLULOSE CHROMATOGRAPHY. The conjugation of fluorescein isothiocyanate (FITC) with antibody globulin changes the electrical charge of the protein molecule. If too few FITC groups are coupled, the conjugate does not emit sufficient light for visualization; whereas if excess numbers of FITC molecules are coupled to antibody protein, the staining is bright but the molecule may attach to nonspecific sites. DEAE cellulose chromatography may be used to isolate coupled and uncoupled FITC-labeled antibody (method of Wood et al. [29]).

1. After conjugation of the antibody protein with fluorescein isothiocyanate, the entire reaction mixture may be diluted ten-fold with 0.01
   M sodium phosphate buffer, and applied to a DEAE cellulose column, equilibrated with the same buffer.
2. The lightly coupled globulin does not bind to the DEAE and is
   eluted with 0.01 M sodium phosphate buffer.
3. Stepwise elution is then performed with 0.03 M sodium phosphate
   buffer.
4. Again stepwise elutions are done with 0.05 M and 0.1 M sodium
   phosphate buffer.
5. Each fraction eluted at a given salt concentration is pooled and
   checked for protein concentration.

Procedure for Tetramethylrhodamine Isothiocyanate (TRITC)
Conjugation of Antibody Globulin [8]

A. Tetramethylrhodamine isothiocyanate may be conjugated to antibody globulin similar to the procedure outlined for fluorescein isothiocyanate. The amounts of rhodamine isothiocyanate which can
   be used in the direct conjugation method may be 20–40 μg per milligram of protein. Rhodamine isothiocyanate can be used in the same
   weight ratio as fluorescein isothiocyanate to label by the dialysis
   method of Clark and Shepard [12].
B. Following the labeling procedure with TRITC, the unreacted rhodamine isothiocyanate must be separated from the coupled protein by
   passage through a column of Sephadex G–50. This is contrary to the
   fluorescein isothiocyanate procedure, in which a 10 times dilution
   of the reaction mixture of fluorescein isothiocyanate and immunoglobulin can be applied directly to a DEAE cellulose column [29].
C. Following separation of TRITC labeled globulins from free unlabeled
   TRITC with Sephadex G–50, the conjugated globulins may be fractionated on DEAE cellulose in accordance with the method outlined by Cebra and Goldstein [8]. In their method, the TRITC
   globulins were fractionated on DEAE with 0.01 M phosphate buffer
   pH 7.5, followed by stepwise elution with 0.04, 0.1, and 1.0 M
   NaCl in the phosphate buffer.
D. Fractions of conjugated globulins eluted at different salt concentrations may be pooled and concentrated to small volume.

Preparation, Storage, Sectioning, and Fixation of Substrate Tissue for Fluorescent Studies

Preparation of Frozen Tissues

MATERIALS AND REAGENTS
A. Fresh tissue to be frozen
B. Aluminum foil

C. Optimal temperature cutting compound (OCT, Lab-Tek)
D. Liquid nitrogen or dry ice and acetone (for snap freezing)
E. Precooled screw-cap bottles
F. Freezer at $-70°$ C (for storage)
G. Pressed polystyrene boxes containing solid carbon dioxide, or small bottles or test tubes containing isoprene and snap frozen
H. Forceps
 I. Test tubes and sealant
 J. Cryostat

PROCEDURE
1. Fresh tissue to be frozen is cut into small cubes approximately 3 mm^3 in dimension.
2. The cubes are placed on aluminum foil and covered with optimal cutting temperature compound (OCT, Lab-Tek) and snap frozen by immersion into liquid nitrogen or dry ice and acetone.
3. Then they are wrapped in aluminum foil and placed in a precooled screw cap bottle for storage in a $-70°$ C freezer. Stomach mucosa is carefully separated from the muscle layers and cut into small rectangles and folded into a loop with the mucosal surface upwards before freezing.
4. A composite block containing several tissues is prepared by placing small folds and pieces of tissue close together on one plate.
5. The frozen section, wrapped in aluminum foil, is best stored in a tightly sealed bottle with a screw cap at $-70°$ C.
6. The chuck and tissue sections can be carried from the freezer to the cryostat in pressed polystyrene boxes containing solid carbon dioxide.
7. The tissue should not be allowed to thaw before sectioning since the slightest degree of thawing would allow sections to become unrecognizable.
8. Alternatively, the tissue may be placed in a test tube or small bottle containing isopentane and frozen by immersion into liquid nitrogen or dry ice and acetone. A few minutes should be sufficient for freezing. The tissue should not be left in the solvent for a long period of time since it dries out and becomes very difficult to section. After the tissue is completely frozen it is removed from the test tube with forceps and placed in another test tube, sealed, and stored in a freezer, preferably at $-70°$ C. Tissue may be stored in a regular freezer at $-20°$ C or below but should not be stored in an automatic frost free freezer.

Preparation of Needle Biopsy Material
Small needle biopsies of kidney, thyroid, or other excisional biopsies of the skin can be collected directly from the operation and carried to the laboratory and mounted upon a section of tongue blade or small sponge (Onko Sponge No. 1) (Histo-Med) with the optimal cutting tempera-

ture compound (OCT) (Lab-Tek) and quickly frozen by immersion in liquid nitrogen. The OCT has not been found to interfere with the immunochemical studies.

Cryostat Sectioning of Tissues
The sections are cut from 4 to 6 μ on a standard cryostat. The optimum temperature for cutting most tissues depends on the amount of fatty tissue and may vary from $-22°$ C to lower than $-30°$ C for tissues with a large amount of lipids. Cleaned microscopic slides should be used. The sections are placed on the slide after drying and may be stored in a $-70°$ C cabinet.

Fixation of Tissue Sections
In order to prevent the loss of water soluble antigens or antibodies, the tissue or other material on the microscope slide is placed in a mild fixative. One may employ an equal mixture of absolute ethyl alcohol and ethyl ether at room temperature for 10 min, followed by 95% ethyl alcohol at room temperature for 10 min. However, other agents such as acetone and methyl alcohol have been used. In certain studies, fixatives are not used, since they may destroy the immunologic reactivity of the antigen.

Fluorescent Staining Procedures

MATERIALS AND REAGENTS
A. Glass slides and test tubes
B. Cold buffered saline solution (pH 7.0, 0.01 M)
C. Conjugated antibody (of several types)
D. Moist chamber
E. Glycine buffer mounting medium, pH 8.6, glycine buffer 0.1 M
F. Petri dish with moistened filter paper, or plastic box constructed with glass rods and moistened cheesecloth cover
G. Serum
H. Pipette
I. Guinea pig complement

MOUNTING MEDIUM [10, 26].   Fluorescence is optimal at buffer pH 0.1 M, glycine pH 8.6.
   a. Glycine   14.0 gm
   b. Sodium hydroxide   0.7 gm
   c. Sodium chloride   17.0 gm
   d. Sodium azide   1.0 gm
   e. Distilled water to 1 liter.

For mounting 1 part of buffer to 2 parts glycerol. For semipermanent mounting the stained and washed slides may be first dipped into 1%

photographic gelatin (Kodak) and dried. The slides are then mounted and the coverslip is sealed with wax or nail varnish [10, 26].

Semipermanent mounting medium (elvanol-buffered glycerine mixture) [22]

a. Elvanol (polyvinyl alcohol, 51–05 grade)   10 ml
b. Carbonate buffer, pH 9.0, 0.5 M   40 ml

The two ingredients are mixed with a magnetic stirrer for 16 hours. One volume of reagent grade glycerine is mixed with two volumes of the above mixture. The final mixture is stirred again with a magnetic stirrer for 16 hours, centrifuged for 60 min at 12,000 rpm to remove any sediment. The pH of the supernate is checked and adjusted to 8.5.

Although 0.01 M phosphate-buffered saline solution pH 7.0–7.2 has been satisfactory for various procedures, at times Coons' buffered saline solution pH 7.2 is preferred.

Direct Method
1. The tissues are rinsed for 10 to 20 min in 2 to 3 changes of cold buffered saline solution to remove extraneous protein.
2. After drying the slide around the tissue, the wet tissue is covered with the conjugated antibody.
3. The fluorescein conjugate is incubated at room temperature with the antigen substrate for 30 min in a moist chamber to prevent evaporation and drying.
4. Then the excess fluorescein conjugate is washed off with 2 to 3 8-min rinses with 0.01 M phosphate-buffered saline solution.
5. The section is then mounted with glycine buffer mounting medium.

To avoid evaporation, it is well to place over the slide a petri dish with moistened filter paper attached to its inner surface. For greater convenience, though, a plastic box may be constructed. Fixed parallel glass rods support the slides and well-moistened cheesecloth may be taped to the cover to prevent evaporation.

Indirect Method
1. Various dilutions of the serum sample being tested for antibody are applied to sections containing the antigen and incubated for 30 min in a moist chamber so that the section will not dry from evaporation.
2. The excess serum is removed with an initial rinse and followed by two 8-min washes with buffered saline solution.
3. Then the fluorescein-conjugated antibody to the serum immunoglobulin, i.e., FITC rabbit anti-human IgG is applied to the section and incubated for 30 min.
4. The excess fluorescein conjugate is removed with a rinse and followed by two 8-min washes in buffered saline solution.
5. The section is then mounted with glycine buffer mounting medium.

Inhibition Method [15]

This procedure can be performed in two steps as a control for the direct staining procedure; however, the one-step method is often used for serologic testing.

1. 0.1 ml serial dilutions of test serum are made in a set of test tubes.
2. An equal volume of diluted conjugated antiserum (0.1 ml) is pipetted into each tube containing various dilutions of test serum.
3. The tubes are mixed and a few drops of each mixture are placed on different sections or smears containing antigen substrate.
4. The sections are incubated 1 hour in a moist chamber to prevent drying and evaporation.
5. The sections are washed of the excess serum and conjugated reagent with two 8-min rinses of buffered saline solution.
6. The sections are mounted with buffered glycerol.

In the inhibition procedure, the presence of antibody in the test serum is indicated by the absence or reduction of fluorescence at the higher serum concentrations. With increasing dilutions of serum, the fluorescence of the section should reach the level of the normal serum control. Previously titrated positive and negative control serum should be included with each run.

Mixed Antiglobulin Method

1. Various dilutions of the serum sample containing antibody (i.e., human IgG) are applied to the sections containing antigen substrate and incubated for 30 min in a moist chamber.
2. The excess serum is removed with several washes of buffered saline solution.
3. Unlabeled heterologous antiserum rabbit and anti-human IgG is then applied to the section with antigen substrate previously reacted with specific human IgG antibody for 30 min.
4. The excess rabbit antiserum is removed with an initial rinse and followed by two 8-min washes with buffered saline solution.
5. Then fluorescein-conjugated human IgG is added to the section to react with free antibody-combining sites of the rabbit anti-human IgG and allowed to incubate in a moist chamber for 30 min.
6. The excess fluorescein conjugate is removed with a rinse and followed by two 8-min washes in buffered saline solution.
7. The section is then mounted with glycine buffer mounting medium.

    Optimal mixed antiglobulin immunofluorescent staining may be obtained with 4 units or more of an antiglobulin-precipitating antibody (i.e., anti-human IgG) and with 1 unit of fluorescein-labeled immunoglobulin antigen (fluorescein-labeled human IgG), if the fluorescein-to-protein ratio of labeled immunoglobulin is in the range of 1 to 3 [3].

Anticomplementary Method

The procedure is similar to the indirect method. The test is sensitive but requires carefully titrated complement and labeled anticomplement reagents.

1. Test serum is inactivated at 56° C for 30 min. 0.1 ml serial dilutions of serum are placed in test tubes.
2. A constant amount of guinea pig complement is added to each tube and mixed.
3. Drops of mixture from each tube are placed on different slides with the antigen substrates. The slides are incubated for 30 min to 1 hour in a moist chamber.
4. After an initial rinse and two 5-min changes of buffered saline solution, labeled anticomplement antiserum is placed on the section for 30 min.
5. The section is then rinsed and washed 2 times for 8 min each with buffered saline solution and mounted.
6. Positive and negative controls provide baseline fluorescence against which the serum titration is evaluated.

Equipment for Fluorescence Microscopy

If the laboratory possesses a microscope with reasonable objectives, the basic equipment needed would be an ultraviolet light source and a few filters. The low degree of illumination in fluorescence microscopy makes it necessary to keep the equipment in a special darkened room [6].

Illumination

In the past, the most widely used light source was the Osram HB 200 lamp. This is a high pressure mercury lamp which provides a steady powerful source of ultraviolet light. It should be employed with a special housing unit. More recently, a halogen quartz lamp has been made available by many manufacturers. This light source provides a high intensity emission in the 400–500 nm range. Thus, the halogen quartz lamp would be convenient for working with fluorescein isothiocyanate-labeled compounds since the peak absorption of fluorescein isothiocyanate is 490 nm (Fig. 22-9).

Primary and Secondary Filter Systems

A heat filter system is necessary with any intense source of illumination. It is usually located in the lamp housing between the lamp and the collecting lens. In addition, two basic filter systems are necessary for fluorescence microscopy.

PRIMARY FILTERS.   There are generally two types of primary filters: (a) the absorption filter, which absorbs light of a certain wavelength and allows light of another wavelength to pass, and (b) the interference

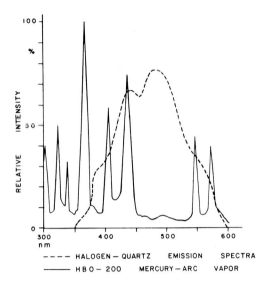

Figure 22-9
Lamp emission spectra. The halogen quartz lamp emission is maximal in the range of 400 to 500 nm and is useful for work with fluorescein-labeled compounds. The absorption peak for fluorescein is 490 nm.

filter, which selects the desired band of light by reflection and dispersion of the undesired light. The advantage of the interference filter is that the light passed has a higher intensity than the light passed by the absorption filters.

The primary absorption filters usually have a pale sky-blue appearance and are approximately 2 to 4 mm thick. Common filters used are the Schott Filter BG–12 (3 to 4 mm thickness) or No. 5840 Corning filter. The transmission maximum for these filters is frequently in the 366 nm region, near ultraviolet. Another set of primary absorption filters looks dark blue and is used for a blue light excitation. Their transmission includes the blue portion of the visible spectrum from 420 to 450 nm. Blue light excitation filters are used in conjunction with secondary filters of a yellow-orange color.

Special fluorescein isothiocyanate (FITC) primary interference filters are now available and are recommended for most of the fluorescent work using FITC.

In addition to the above primary exciter filters and heat-absorbing filter, one can use a sky-blue Schott BG 38 filter. The BG 38 suppresses the transmission in the far red spectrum given by many primary filters. The purpose of the BG 38 is to make the background in the field of view completely black (Fig. 22-10).

SECONDARY OR CONTRAST FILTERS.   In general, a dark field condenser is used and the secondary filters are inserted in the body of the tube or the eye pieces, or a variety of filters can be utilized in the rotating device in the body of the microscope. Barrier filters serve to remove remnants of exciting light so that only the fluorescent light reaches the observer's

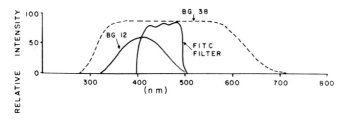

Figure 22-10
Primary filter transmission curves. FITC filter is an interference filter used specifically for work with fluorescein isothiocyanate (FITC)-labeled compounds. The FITC interference filter will allow a higher intensity of light to pass than the BG 12 primary absorption filter. A BG 38 filter is used to remove light in the red region.

eyes. They are inserted between the objective and the observer's eyes either above the nose piece or in the rotating disk in the stands. Various filters are complementary to the primary filters. For use with FITC-labeled compounds, the secondary filter which can be used is a Zeiss 53, which has a peak cut-off point near the maximal emission peak of FITC, which is 525 nm. A No. 50 filter is useful in other applications (Fig. 22-11).

Filter System for Double-Staining Studies
Tissue may be stained with either fluorescein-conjugated antibody (green) or rhodamine-conjugated antibody (red), or both. Cebra and Goldstein [8] used an Osram HB200 mercury lamp, KGl heat-absorbing filter, with a 2 mm No. 5840 Corning primary filter.
    Objective discrimination of green, red, and mixed color was made with sequential use of Kodak Wratten K2 filter, and Kodak Wratten filters No. 23A and No. 57A. The filters were mounted in a metal slide

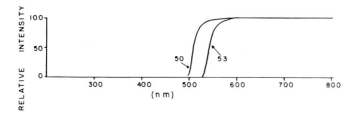

Figure 22-11
Secondary filter transmission curves. The Zeiss 53 filter helps in the elimination of the background when fluorescein-labeled compounds are examined as the emission peak is 520 nm.

insert which fits into the barrel of the fluorescence microscope and acts as a secondary filter. Filter No. 23A is a red barrier filter which blocks the yellow-green light of the fluorescein conjugate. Filter No. 57A is a green filter which excludes most of the red-orange light of the rhodamine conjugate when used in double thickness. The Wratten K2 filter allows transmission of both conjugates, and a mixture will show an intermediate shade of yellow.

Microscope Condenser System
Dark field condensers render images of very high contrast. They transmit considerably less light than do light field condensers. The dark field has an advantage that none of the exciting light enters the objective of the microscope, with the exception of whatever small light is scattered by the specimen. The dark field condensers afford the best protection for the observer's eyes.

Photomicrography
The Wratten No. 3 light yellow filter may be used for black and white photography. With Pan F film, exposure time varies from 1 to 2 min. For color photography, high speed Ektachrome with special processing may be used with the Wratten 2-E yellow filter. Exposure time will vary from 15 sec to 3 min, according to the brightness of the preparation. Anscochrome 500 is often used for color photography in a similar manner as high speed Ektachrome color film.

Evaluation and Recommendations for Use of Fluoresceinated Antibody Conjugates

Standards and procedures for evaluation of conjugated antisera are given below. The guidelines are especially important in the evaluation of commercially prepared antisera.

Recommendations for Manufacturing of Anti-Human IgG Fluorescein Conjugates
The following section comprises subcommittee recommendations at a Round Table Conference sponsored by the Permanent Section for Microbiological Standardization of the International Association of Microbiological Societies in London, October 11, 1968 [19].

MODE OF PREPARATION
A. Immunize animals with purified human IgG prepared by DEAE cellulose chromatography.
B. Fractionate the resulting antiserum and use the IgG fraction for conjugation.

C. The anti-human IgG antibody content of a satisfactory conjugate should be no less than 1 mg protein/ml and at least 10% of the total protein in the conjugate should be specific antibody.
D. For a given conjugate, the level of fluorescein labeling is specified. The method by which the F:P ratio is determined should be supplied, along with the methods of assay.
E. It is desirable that the leaflet describing the product give details of preparation and information of further processing, such as additions and absorptions. For anti-IgM, and anti-IgA, anti-B_{1c} conjugates, the same recommendations are applicable, except that the appropriate immunizing antigens are used respectively.

Recommended Specification and Labeling for Fluorescein Anti-Human IgG Conjugates [2, 4]

A. Conjugates shall be free of unbound fluorescein.
B. The conjugates and original raw antisera should yield a single IgG line by immunoelectrophoresis without absorption.
C. Conjugates should contain at least 4 units of antibody/ml which is approximately equal to 160 μg antibody nitrogen/ml or 1 mg specific antibody/ml.
D. Lyophilized conjugates should be labeled as conjugated anti-human IgG (unabsorbed, free of unbound fluorescein):

Dry weight _____ mg.
Reconstituted with distilled water _____ ml.
Properties of reconstituted conjugates:
_____ mg/ml protein _____ molar F:P ratio
_____ μg/ml fluorescein _____ units/ml
_____ molar F:P ratio _____ μg antibody N/ml.

Several detailed recommendations on the characterization and clinical use of immunologic reagents were recently made by the Medical Research Council Subcommittees on (a) fluorochrome-labeled antibodies and (b) antisera for gel diffusion studies [19].

Methods of Evaluation and Testing for Specificity of Fluorescein Isothiocyanate Anti-Human IgG Conjugates

TESTING OF CONJUGATES FOR FREE UNBOUND FLUORESCEIN
AND PROTEIN ADDITIONS
Dialysis. Conjugates may be checked by dialysis for absence of unbound fluorescein. Also, the conjugates may be separated from unbound fluorescein by gel filtration. Protein concentrations may be determined by the Biuret reaction with readings at 560 nm, instead of the usual 540

nm, to avoid interference from fluorescein absorbency as described by Goldwasser and Shepard [16]. An alternative method for determination of the protein concentration is according to the procedure of Wood et al. [29].

$$\text{Protein (mg/ml)} = \frac{\text{O.D. 280 nm} - 0.35 \ (\text{O.D. 495 nm})}{1.4}$$

Cellulose acetate electrophoresis. This procedure may be used to evaluate for the presence of unbound fluorescent material and protein added to previously conjugated protein. A routine cellulose acetate strip electrophoresis can be performed similar to the procedure utilizing Beckman Microzone equipment. After electrophoresis, the strip is examined under a Woods' light (366 nm) for fluorescence of separated proteins. The location and brightness of each band should be noted and sketched [17]. The strip is then stained with an appropriate protein stain as Ponceau S and scanned by a densitometer. The Ponceau S-stained strip is compared with the sketch of fluorescence made before protein staining. A fluorescent band beyond the albumin position indicates the presence of unreacted fluorescein. A strong fluorescence in the γ-globulin region with no fluorescence in the β area denotes a high concentration of labeled γ-globulin and indicates that the γ-globulin fraction alone was labeled with fluorescein. The absence of fluorescein in bands stained by Ponceau S as α_1, α_2, or albumin indicates that protein has been added to FITC-labeled protein.

TESTS FOR SPECIFICITY OF CONJUGATES

Immunoelectrophoresis. This procedure is performed in which the fluoresceinated antiserum reacted against normal whole human serum. A heavy line of precipitation in the IgG region should be obtained. Additional lines with antibodies to serum proteins other than immunoglobulins are often seen in commercial antisera. The extraneous antibodies may not necessarily interfere with the specificity of the immunofluorescence test; however, they contribute to increased nonspecific staining.

Also, the presence of contaminant antibodies casts doubt on the purity of the antigen used for immunization. Spurs from the IgG line produced by cross-reaction of the anti-IgG conjugate with IgM or IgA in the electrophoresed normal human serum may be expected in the presence of antibodies to the light chain of IgG. The light chain antibodies may be specifically removed by absorption with purified human IgM or IgA preparations. Cross-reactions of antibodies to the light chain in antisera to IgG with light chain antibodies of IgM and IgA do not usually occur in immunofluorescent staining, providing (a) that the immunization is carried out with purified IgG, and (b) that the conjugate is diluted to ¼ unit/ml [5]. Thus, at ¼ unit/ml anti-IgG no visible immunofluorescent staining occurs with IgA or IgM immunoglobulins in indirect immunofluorescent staining reactions. If a concentration of 1 unit/ml of labeled anti-IgG is used and there are present anti-light chain antibodies, then the IgG antiserum will detect the presence of IgA and IgM immunoglobulins.

The gel diffusion precipitin test.   This test is performed with a reference anti-serum to IgG; and the test conjugate against normal human serum should give precipitin lines of complete identity. Cross-reactions of antihuman IgG conjugate with human IgM and IgA may be detected by the precipitin test.

DETERMINATION OF IMMUNOLOGIC SENSITIVITY OF THE CONJUGATE. This is determined by measuring the level of specific precipitating antibodies which can be expressed in units per milliliter. The units of conjugate is based on the titer of antiglobulin determined in the standard gel diffusion precipitin test using 1 mg IgG/ml antigen and two-fold dilutions of the conjugate [3]. The conjugate is more specific for purified IgG than for normal human serum. However, the units of antibody may be determined with normal human serum diluted to contain 1 mg IgG (normal serum diluted 1:12). The agar gel template [4, 5] recommended for determining the units of antibodies was a horizontally placed line of wells 2.8 mm in diameter placed 7.5 mm apart in a gel with a depth of 1.5 mm. Titration is performed by serial two-fold dilutions of the conjugates, which are placed opposite the wells containing the antigen test in a concentration of 1 mg/ml. Pipettes are changed with each dilution, and plates are incubated at room temperature for 24 hours and read for the highest dilution giving a visible line of precipitation. This titer is the unit. A linear pattern agar gel template for gel diffusion should be used instead of one with a circular pattern. Acceptable conjugates should have at least 4 units per 1% protein when the unit assay is employed. This is approximately equivalent to 1 mg precipitating antibody per 10 mg protein. Conjugates with lower antibody levels are not recommended for use.

Figure 22-12
Agar gel template for unitage assay of precipitating antibodies in fluorescent-labeled conjugates. The thickness of the gel should be at least 1.5 mm.

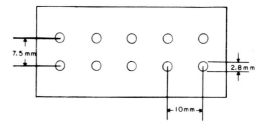

DETERMINATION OF FLUORESCEIN PROTEIN RATIO BY THE
METHOD OF W. D. BRIGHTON [7]

$$\text{Molecular F:P ratio} = \frac{2.87 \times E_{(495 \text{ nm})}}{E_{(280 \text{ nm})} - 0.35 E_{(495 \text{ nm})}}$$

The F:P ratio is not valid if it is determined after the addition of un
labeled protein for adsorption of contaminant antibodies. In an indirect
antinuclear antibody test utilizing mouse liver, a molar F:P ratio of 3 to
5 was found to be optimal for conjugates with 4 units of antibody per
milliliter [4, 5]. However, different molar F:P ratio may be optimal for
other systems.

Evaluation of Anti-IgM and Anti-IgA Conjugates [5]
   Immunoelectrophoresis.   An immunoelectrophoresis should be performed with normal adult serum and in addition tested against other
preparations of IgA or IgM or IgG. The adult serum should, of course,
yield lines in expected regions with the anti-IgA or anti-IgM conjugate,
but the IgG preparation should be negative with monospecific absorbed
conjugate.
   Gel precipitation tests.   These tests are performed to determine the
lack of cross-reactivity of anti-IgA or anti-IgM conjugates with IgG or
other heterologous immunoglobulins. Immunologic sensitivity ratios of
anti-IgM or anti-IgA conjugates can be expressed as units per 1% protein. Units are assayed by gel precipitin titrations for IgA since normal
human serum levels of IgA are about 3.5 mg/ml. A dilution of 1:3 whole
serum can be used for antigen for unit antibody assay of monospecific
anti-IgA conjugates. Unit assay of the monospecific anti-IgM conjugates
can be performed with use of normal serum (undiluted normal serum
IgM concentration is about 1 mg/ml). Titers of unit of anti-IgM conjugates should be read after a 72-hour incubation at room temperature
because of the slow diffusion rate of IgM. If the antisera do not contain
4 units of antibody per 1% protein/ml either anti-IgA or anti-IgM, it
is not considered to be an acceptable reagent. The F:P ratio may be
determined as above for anti-human IgG conjugates.
   Chantler and Haire evaluated two anti-IgM fluorescein conjugates by
gel diffusion and direct immunofluorescent techniques on characterized
bone marrow preparations taken from patients with myeloma, and by
an indirect method with virus-infected cells and selected postinfection
human sera [9]. It should be emphasized that neither gel diffusion nor
direct immunofluorescent methods appears to provide a reliable index of
specificity for fluoresceinated anti-human IgM conjugates to be used in
indirect procedures [9].
   Indirect techniques are preferable to direct tests for defining the
specificity of anti-human immunoglobulin IgG and IgM conjugates be-

cause of the sensitivity of the indirect method. The presence of unwanted anti-IgG and anti-IgM reactivity in the conjugates may be detected by appropriate selection and fractionation of the test serum in the indirect method so that the sample will contain only anti-IgM or anti-IgG antibodies. At present a convenient test system is not available for indirect assessment of anti-IgA activity.

Use of Conjugates

EVALUATION.   Fluoresceinated anti-human IgG can be evaluated in the indirect antinuclear antibody tests with rat kidney substrate tissue [27]. Chessboard titrations should be carried out with different unit dilutions of fluoresceinated antisera against different high and lower titered sera known to contain antinuclear antibodies. With good fluoresceinated antiserum, a plateau endpoint of $\frac{1}{16}$ or $\frac{1}{64}$ units may be seen when reacted against a high titered serum. A working dilution of the fluorescein conjugate should be $\frac{1}{4}$ to $\frac{1}{8}$ unit/ml. In the antinuclear antibody test, a working dilution of $\frac{1}{4}$ unit/ml is recommended provided that the F:P ratio is approximately 3 to 5:1. This provides for a satisfactory background and will ensure detection of the low titered sera containing antinuclear antibodies. Also reproducible titers can be obtained on the same serum containing antinuclear antibodies when tested with a different source of conjugated antisera. This working dilution has been previously recommended by Beutner, Barnett, and co-workers with the use of mouse liver in the indirect antinuclear factors test [4, 5].

WORKING DILUTIONS.   Usually the working dilutions of the anti-IgA and anti-IgM conjugate being used should be at least 1 unit/ml. The use of polyvalent anti-immunoglobulin conjugate should be used at the dilution of 1 unit/ml. In fluorescent kidney biopsy studies, anti-IgM and anti-IgA are recommended for use at a concentration of 1 unit/ml. In the use of conjugated anti-B_{1C}, a working dilution of $\frac{1}{2}$ unit/ml is satisfactory for use in kidney biopsies. A chessboard titration may be performed in a test system, and if a plateau endpoint of $\frac{1}{16}$ unit/ml is seen, then a working dilution of $\frac{1}{4}$ unit may be used [4]. Criteria for evaluation of anti-B_{1C} conjugates are the same as above, and the conjugates should also have 4 units antibody per 1% protein/ml.

Available Standards

Two research standards have been made available from the Director of the Division of Biological Standards, National Institute for Medical Research, Hampstead Laboratories, Holly Hill, London, NW 3 6RB, England [1, 20]. They are (a) code No. 66/233 homogeneous antinuclear serum factor, and (b) code No. 68/45 fluorochrome-labeled antibody to human serum immunoglobulins (sheep anti-human). This conjugate reacts strongly with human IgG with some weak cross-reactions [20].

A Paraffin Embedding Method for Immunofluorescence
Studies of Tissue
(Method of Heron [18])
Since many pathologists consider the routine histologic examination to be very important, it would be extremely useful to them to employ this convenient paraffin embedding technique, which would allow tissue to be processed for immunofluorescence studies. This technique is primarily useful for kidney biopsies, to which it has been successfully applied; it can be used also to process synovial tissue.

MATERIALS AND REAGENTS
A. Tissue biopsy material
B. 95%, 99%, 96%, 70% ethanol, all precooled to 4° C
C. Xylol precooled to 4° C
D. Paraffin
E. Heat to 58° C
F. Microtome
G. Water bath at less than 4° C
H. Acid wash glass slides for mounting
 I. Buffered saline solution

PROCEDURE
1. Tissue biopsy material is placed in 95% ethanol, precooled to 4° C, and left overnight at 4° C in 95% ethanol, then dehydrated with 99% ethanol at 4° C for 3 hours, and cleared in 4° C cold xylol through 2 consecutive baths for 3 hours. While still containing the tissue, the last bath is allowed to rise to room temperature.
2. The specimens are placed in paraffin and heated in the oven at 58° C overnight.
3. On the third day, the blocks are sectioned with an ordinary microtome and the sections are floated on a water bath with the temperature at less than 4° C.
4. Sections are mounted on acid wash glass slides and processed as follows:
    a. 60 sec in xylol at 4° C, 2 changes
    b. 60 sec in 99% ethanol at 4° C, 2 changes
    c. 10 sec in 96% ethanol at 4° C, 2 changes
    d. 10 sec in 70% ethanol at 4° C, 1 bath
    e. 60 sec in buffered saline solution, changed 3 times
5. After deparaffinization, as described below, the section is reacted with the immunologic reagents in the usual manner for use of antibody fluorescence conjugates.

Summary

The fixation and deparaffinization procedure:

Day 1: The biopsy is placed in 95% ethanol at 4° C overnight.

Day 2: Place in 99% ethanol, 4° C for 3 hours. Two changes of xylol at 4° C for 3 hours. The last bath is allowed to rise to room temperature and the section is placed in paraffin at 58° C overnight.

Day 3: The section is embedded in the paraffin block and sectioned, deparaffinized, and incubated with the immunological agent.

DISADVANTAGES OF THE PROCEDURE

A. There is an increased background in the connective tissue over the conventional procedure with use of frozen sections.

B. The detection of C3 complement is weak and may be due to the inactivation of some of the complement fraction by the fixatives and heat resulting from paraffin embedding.

ADVANTAGES OF THE PROCEDURE

A. Convenience

B. The tissue blocks may be stored for months and still be suitable for immunofluorescent investigation.

C. The immunohistologic examinations are possible without interference with routine histologic studies.

References

1. Anderson, S. G., Addison, I. E., and Dixon, H. G.   Antinuclear factor serum (homogeneous): An international collaborative study of the proposed research standard 66/233. *Ann. N.Y. Acad. Sci.* 177:337, 1971.

2. Barnett, E. V.   Staining activity of conjugates in relation to their antibody content. In E. J. Holborow (ed.), *Standardization of Immunofluorescences.* Oxford: Blackwell, 1970.

3. Beutner, E. H., Holborow, E. J., and Johnson, G. D.   Quantitative studies of immunofluorescent staining: I. Analysis of mixed immunofluorescence. *Immunology* 12:327, 1967.

4. Beutner, E. H., Sepulveda, M. R., and Barnett, E. V.   Quantitative studies of immunofluorescent staining: II. Relationships of characteristics of unabsorbed anti-human IgG conjugates to their specific and nonspecific staining properties in an indirect test for antinuclear factors. *Bull. WHO.* 39:587, 1968.

5. Beutner, E. H., Chorzelski, T. P., and Jordon, R. E.   *Autosensitization in Pemphigus and Bullous Pemphigoid.* Springfield, Ill.: Thomas, 1970, pp. 131–159.

6. Blundell, G. P.   Fluorescent antibody techniques. In M. Stefanini (ed.), *Progress in Clinical Pathology.* New York: Grune & Stratton, 1970, vol. 3, p. 211.

7. Brighton, W. D.   Fluorochromes and labeling: II. In E. J. Holborow (ed.), *Standardization in Immunofluorescence*. Oxford: Blackwell, 1970, p. 55.

8. Cebra, J. J., and Goldstein, G.   Chromatographic purification of tetra-methylrhodamine-immune globulin conjugates and their use in the cellular localization of rabbit γ-globulin polypeptide chain. *J. Immunol.* 95:230, 1965.

9. Chantler, S., and Haire, M.   Evaluation of the immunological specificity of fluorescein-labeled anti-human IgM conjugates. *Immunology* 23:7, 1972.

10. Chapman, J. C.   Immunofluorescent techniques. *Can. J. Med. Technol.* 32:147, 1970.

11. Cherry, W. B., and Moody, M. D.   Fluorescent-antibody techniques in diagnostic bacteriology. *Bacteriol. Rev.* 29:222, 1965.

12. Clark, H. F., and Shepard, C. C.   A dialysis technique for preparing fluorescent antibody. *Virology* 20:642, 1963.

13. Coons, A. H., Creich, H. J., Jones, R. N., and Berliner, E.   The demonstration of pneumococcal antigen in tissues by the use of fluorescent antibody. *J. Immunol.* 45:159, 1942.

14. Goldman, M.   Staining *Toxoplasma gondii* with fluorescein-labeled antibody: II. A new serological test for antibodies to toxoplasma based upon inhibition of specific staining. *J. Exp. Med.* 105:557, 1957.

15. Goldman, M.   *Fluorescent Antibody Methods*. New York: Academic Press, 1968.

16. Goldwasser, R. A., and Shephard, C. C.   Staining of complement and modification of fluorescent antibody procedures. *J. Immunol.* 80:122, 1958.

17. Hebert, G. A., Pittman, B., and Cherry, W. B.   The definition and application of evaluation techniques as a guide for the improvement of fluorescent antibody reagents. *Ann. N.Y. Acad. Sci.* 177:54, 1971.

18. Heron, I.   A paraffin embedding method in kidney immunofluorescent studies. *Acta Pathol. Microbiol. Scand.* 78:444, 1970, section B.

19. Holborow, E. J., Lachmann, P. J., and Batty, I.   Report by a subcommittee on the discussion of requirements for specification of anti-immunoglobulin conjugates that took place during the conference. In E. J. Holborow (ed.), *Standardization of Immunofluorescences*. Oxford: Blackwell, 1970, p. 275.

20. Humphrey, J. H. et al.   Characterization of antisera as reagents. Recommendations made by the MRC Working Party on the Clinical Use of Immunological Reagents. *Immunology* 20:3, 1971.

21. Kabat, E. A., and Mayer, M. M.   *Experimental Immunochemistry*. Springfield, Ill.: Thomas, 1961, chap. 2, p. 22.

22. Kawamura, A.   *Fluorescent Antibody Techniques and Their Application*. Baltimore: University Park Press, 1969.

23. Lanni, F., Dillon, M. L., and Beard, J. W.   Determination of small quantities of nitrogen in serological precipitates and other biological materials. *Proc. Soc. Exp. Biol. Med.* 74:4, 1950.

24. Lowry, O. H., Rosebrough, M. J., Farr, A. C., and Randall, R. J.   Protein measurement with the Folin reagent. *J. Biol. Chem.* 193:265, 1951.

25. Nairn, R. C.   *Fluorescent Protein Tracing*. Williams & Wilkins, 1969, 3rd ed.
26. Roitt, I. M.   Immunofluorescent tests for detection of autoantibodies. In World Health Organization, *Manual of Autoimmune Serology*. Geneva, Switzerland, 1970.
27. Tan, E. M.   Relationship of nuclear staining patterns with precipitating antibodies in systemic lupus erythematosus. *J. Clin. Lab. Med.* 70:800, 1967.
28. Whittingham, S.   Serological methods in autoimmune disease. In J. B. G. Kwapinski (ed.), *Research in Immunochemistry and Immunobiology*. Baltimore: University Park Press, 1972, vol. 1, p. 173.
29. Wood, B. T., Thompson, S. H., and Goldstein, G.   Fluorescent antibody staining: III. Preparation of fluorescein-isothiocyanate labeled antibodies. *J. Immunology* 95:225, 1965.

23

Immunoenzyme Histochemical Methods

Coons and co-workers [10] introduced an extremely powerful tool to study immunologic problems with fluorescent-labeled antibodies. Singer and Schick [28] have shown that ferritin-conjugated antibodies can be used for electron microscopic studies. More recently, enzymes have been used as markers by the covalent coupling of various enzymes such as peroxidase and alkaline phosphatase to antigens and antibodies. Nakane and Pierce [18] and Avrameas and Uriel [1] were the first workers to propose the use of enzyme-coupled antibodies for the detection of tissue antigen-antibody reactions. The enzyme may be used as an antigen or can be coupled to antibodies similar to fluorescent-labeled antibodies. The enzyme marker can be identified by histochemical techniques because of its catalytic effect on specific substrates.

The peroxidase-conjugated antibody is commonly used in the clinical laboratory for demonstration of tissue autoantibody such as anti-basement membrane and immune complexes in the kidney [12], antinuclear antibodies [8, 11], and antibodies in pemphigus and bullous pemphigoid [14]. The method has been used for detection of antibodies to *Treponema pallidum* [24] and other autoimmune antibodies such as antibodies to parietal cells [16, 24] and neurons [32].

Immunoenzyme Methods

Although enzyme markers may be used similar to the fluorescent marker for antigen-antibody reactions, the protein and antigenic nature of the enzyme allows for a wide variation in available methods to study specific antibody-antigen reactions in tissues. For example, the enzyme is immunogenic and may be used as an antigen for experimental studies. The antigenic nature of the enzyme marker has made possible the production of specific antienzyme antibodies with the synthesis of unique hybrid antibody, and specificity to specific antigen as well as to the enzyme. Immunoenzyme methods may be broadly classified into (a) direct methods and (b) indirect methods.

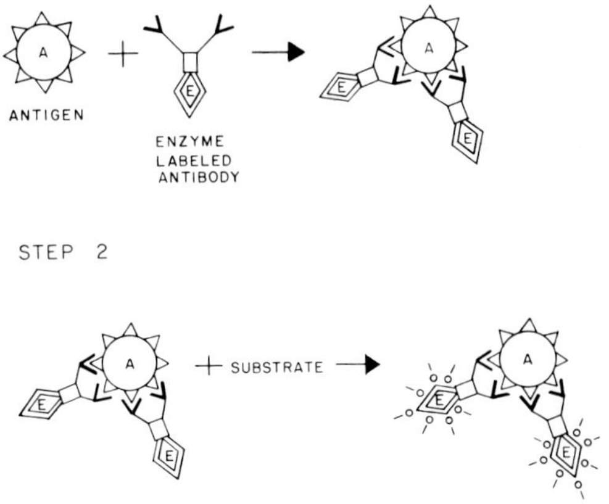

Figure 23-1
Direct immunoenzyme method. Detection of an antigen by enzyme-labeled antibody and reaction of enzyme with specific substrate produce a chromogenic or electron dense product which can be visualized.

Direct Methods

In the usual direct immunoenzyme method, one detects an antigen or another antibody by the use of an enzyme-labeled antibody (Fig. 23-1). The localization of the enzyme-labeled antibody is detected by the action of the enzyme on a specific substrate which produces chromogenic or electron dense substrates. If the enzyme-labeled antibody is an anti-immunoglobulin, then the enzyme-labeled antibody may be employed similar to a fluorescent-labeled anti-immunoglobulin and may be used to detect specific autoantibodies in serum such as antinuclear antibodies [8, 11]. When the method involves detection of spec fic antibodies in a serum sample with use of specific substrate and fluorescent-labeled anti-immunoglobulin, it is often referred to as an indirect fluorescent method similar to an indirect Coombs' test. To avoid confusion, the direct immunoenzyme method refers only to the specific immunohistochemical reaction.

A variation of the direct immunoenzyme method is the detection of antienzyme antibody by use of the homologous enzyme antigen (Fig. 23-2). The methods are quite similar whether an enzyme-labeled antigen is used to detect an antigen, or whether the enzyme serves an antigen for immunization and one wishes to detect production of antienzyme antibody. Both techniques can be used for localization of antigen or antibody at the light or electron microscopic level.

Indirect Methods

Of the indirect methods, Avrameas [6] has described three types: (a) the hybrid antibody method, (b) the mixed antibody method, and (c) the amplification antibody method.

THE HYBRID ANTIBODY METHOD. In the indirect hybrid antibody method, a hybrid antienzyme antiprotein antigen-antibody is used to

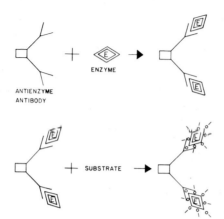

Figure 23-2
Detection of antienzyme by use of its homologous enzyme antigen.

detect protein antigen in tissues (Fig. 23-3). Hybrid antibodies of double specificity [13, 22, 23] are prepared from purified preparations of antienzyme and antiprotein antibodies. The antibodies are first reduced and subsequently recombined, and the specific hybrid antibodies are isolated by use of specific immunoadsorbent columns.

THE MIXED ANTIBODY METHOD.   The indirect mixed immunoenzyme technique is used to detect the presence of an immunoglobulin by the use of an anti-immunoglobulin and antienzyme antibody [6]. The anti-immunoglobulin reacts with specific species A immunoglobulin on the cell (Fig. 23-4). The anti-immunoglobulin reacts on the cell surface with only one of its active sites and leaves the other available. The available site can then react subsequently with added antienzyme antibodies

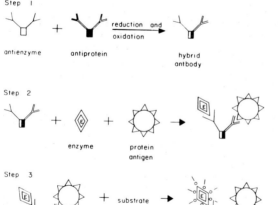

Figure 23-3
Hybrid antibody-indirect immunoenzyme method. A hybrid antienzyme antiprotein antibody is used to detect the protein antigen. The antienzyme portion of the hybrid antibody reacts with the enzyme, which is used as the localization marker.

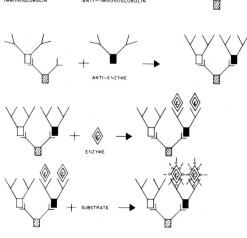

Figure 23-4
Indirect immunoenzyme-mixed antibody method. The anti-immunoglobulin antibody reacts with immunoglobulin of species A which may be present in the cell. The anti-immunoglobulin can then react with an antienzyme immunoglobulin made in species A. The addition of enzyme will then allow localization of the immunoglobulin of species A.

of species A antienzyme immunoglobulin. The final addition of the enzyme allows localization of the immunologic reaction.

THE AMPLIFICATION ANTIBODY METHOD.   The third indirect immunoenzyme technique is the amplification antibody method. This is essentially an enhanced direct technique in which the sensitivity of the enzyme-labeled antibody is enhanced by the use of an antienzyme antibody with subsequent layering of uncoupled enzyme (Fig. 23-5). In this way, the specific immunologic reaction is amplified with the presence of a greater amount of enzyme for the histochemical reaction.

Enzymes Commonly Used for Labels

For the regular microscopic slide histochemistry, any enzyme which does not modify the structure of the cell can be used as a marker. The enzyme must not interfere with the immunologic specificity of the antibody reaction. For electron microscopic studies, the enzyme when reacted with substrates must produce electron dense reaction products. The enzyme which has been most often used as a marker is horseradish peroxidase. Other enzymes which have been used and may later show wider application are alkaline phosphatase, acid phosphatase, glucose oxidase, and lactic dehydrogenase [6].

Some of the desirable features of an ideal enzyme are [6, 7, 21] (a) availability of preparation with high specific activity; (b) low molecular weight so that the coupled antibodies allow easy penetration into tissues; (c) noninterference with specific immunologic reaction; (d)

STEP 1

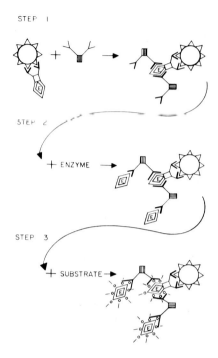

STEP 2

STEP 3

Figure 23-5
Indirect immunoenzyme-amplifica-
tion antibody method. The sensitivity of the reaction of an enzyme-
labeled antibody is markedly increased by the use of antienzyme
antibody. The number of enzyme
molecules localized is increased.

allowance of formation of electron dense reaction product with formation of different colors when reacted with different substrates; and (e)
low or absent concentrations of interfering enzymes in tissues studied.

Advantages and Disadvantages of Immunoenzyme Methods Over Fluorescent Antibody Methods

Immunoreactivity of tissues by enzyme immunohistochemical technique
has certain advantages over fluorescent antibody methods [3, 24]. With
use of peroxidase-labeled antibody, some of the advantages are as
follows:

A. The slide may be examined by ordinary light microscopy.
B. The preparations are permanent, and the localization of the enzyme
   marker can be compared against the remaining histologic background more accurately than by the fluorescent technique.
C. The preparations can be studied in more detail by staining with a
   radiolabeled antibody or with another antibody labeled with a different enzyme.
D. Ultrastructural studies may be performed with the peroxidase-

labeled antibody as a marker, since the reaction product of the enzyme and substrate is electron dense.

E. The peroxidase-labeled antibody is able to penetrate to intracellular antigens more effectively than ferritin-labeled antibodies because of its smaller size.

Avrameas [4, 6] has found that isolated pure antibody is important in the preparation of an effective enzyme-labeled antibody. Thus, the enzyme procedure may seem more time consuming; however, the examination of cellular preparations under the microscope is easier with the immunoenzyme method.

The enzyme-labeled antibody method still requires much investigation to standardize the reagents and procedures such that comparable reproducible results can be obtained by different clinical laboratories. In the area of standardization of reagents and quantitation of procedures, the fluorescent antibody methods are far more advanced than are the enzyme-labeled antibody methods.

Methods for Isolation of Antibodies and Antibody Fragments for Use in the Immunoenzyme Methods

It is necessary to obtain antisera of high titers to the specific antigen. Nakane and Pierce [19] first described use of a γ-globulin which was isolated by ammonium sulfate precipitation from immune serum. However, in many cases, reproducible satisfactory results were obtained only when purified antibody was isolated from immunoadsorbent columns and then coupled to the enzyme marker [4].

Purification and isolation of specific antibodies such as antibodies to human IgG may be performed in the following way:

1. A water insoluble immunoadsorbent is prepared by the aggregation of a mixture of human IgG and carrier protein such as bovine serum albumin with ethyl chloroformate [2] or glutaraldehyde [5]. More recently, proteins have been coupled to polyacrylamide beads with glutaraldehyde [29, 30]. Preliminary results indicate that an immunoadsorbent made of polyacrylamide coupled to protein with glutaraldehyde is a convenient technique.
2. The anti-human IgG antibodies are then reacted with the immunoadsorbent.
3. The immunoadsorbent is washed to remove uncoupled serum proteins.
4. The adsorbed antibody (anti-human IgG) is then eluted from the immunoadsorbent with a low pH buffer or with a high salt solution.
5. The antibody eluate is neutralized and dialyzed with isotonic buffer, and concentrated and stored.

Preparation of Insoluble Immunoadsorbent for Isolation of
Anti-Human IgG Antibodies
(Method of Avrameas and Ternynck [2])

MATERIALS AND REAGENTS
A. Human IgG—50 mg
B. Bovine serum albumin—450 mg
C. 10 ml beaker
D. Acetate buffer (pH 5.1, 0.2 M)
E. Chemically pure ethyl chloroformate (Merck)—0.3 ml
F. 1 N NaOH
G. Homogenizer (Sorvall)
H. Phosphate-buffered saline solution (pH 7.0–7.2, 0.01 M)
 I. Sintered glass funnel
J. 0.1% Na_2CO_3—200 ml
K. Glycine-HCl buffer (pH 2.2, 0.2 M, or tris buffer, pH 8.2, 0.05 M)
L. Potassium iodide (5.5 M)

PROCEDURE
1. 50 mg human IgG and 450 mg bovine serum albumin (BSA) are dissolved in 5 ml acetate buffer in a 10 ml beaker.
2. 0.3 ml chemically pure ethyl chloroformate is added with gentle stirring to the mixture of human IgG and BSA. The pH is maintained between 4.5 and 5 with 1 N NaOH. After 10–15 min, there is formation of a gel and the mixture is allowed to stand for 30 more min at room temperature without stirring.
3. The polymerized protein is homogenized at 15,000 rpm for 30–45 sec and dispersed in 200 ml phosphate-buffered saline solution.
4. The suspension is filtered on a sintered glass funnel and washed successively with 2 liters phosphate-buffered saline solution, 200 ml 0.1% Na_2CO_3, 300 ml phosphate-buffered saline solution, and glycine-HCl buffer until the optical density of the eluate is 0 at 280 nm. Potassium iodide in tris buffer may be used for elution of antibodies in place of the glycine HCl buffer.
5. The immunoadsorbent is then washed with 1 liter phosphate-buffered saline solution until eluates show a neutral pH.

Isolation of Specific Anti-Human IgG Antibodies
with Use of Insoluble Immunoadsorbent [2, 7]

MATERIALS AND REAGENTS
A. Whole immune serum containing anti-human IgG
B. Insoluble immunoadsorbent polymer
C. Centrifuge
D. Agitator
E. Phosphate-buffered saline solution, pH 7.0–7.2, 0.01 M
F. Glycine-HCl buffer, pH 2.2, 0.2 M, or potassium iodide 5.5 M in tris buffer pH 8.2, 0.05 M
G. NaOH 0.1 M

H. Equipment for dialysis
I. Storage at 4° C

PROCEDURE
1. Appropriate volumes of whole immune serum containing anti-human IgG are mixed in a large centrifuge tube with the insoluble immunoadsorbent polymer prepared above. The immunoadsorbent has a capacity of approximately 100 mg antibodies.
2. The mixture is stirred gently for 2 hours and then centrifuged at 5,000 g for 20 min. The supernatant is kept to test for nonadsorbed antibodies.
3. The precipitate is washed 6 times or more with 150 ml phosphate-buffered saline solution and centrifuged at 5,000 g for 20 min. The supernatant of the final washing should show an optical density (O.D.) of zero at 280 nm.
4. The antibody is eluted by either glycine-HCl buffer or potassium iodide in tris buffer. The immunoadsorbent is washed repeatedly with 10 ml fractions and centrifuged. The elution is continued until the O.D. of the eluate is less than 0.05 at 280 nm.
5. The eluates are neutralized with NaOH immediately and dialyzed against several changes of phosphate-buffered saline solution, concentrated to at least 1–2 mg protein per milliliter and stored at 4° C. The protein preparation may be lyophilized.

Preparation of Fab Antibody Fragments
MATERIALS AND REAGENTS
A. Whole antiserum
B. Bovine serum albumin
C. Human IgG
D. NaOH 1 N (to adjust pH)
E. Sephadex G-200, G-100 columns (Pharmacia)
F. Papain 2%
G. DEAE cellulose column
H. Phosphate buffer (pH 6.9, 0.0175 M)

PROCEDURE
1. Anti-human IgG can be isolated by passage of whole antiserum over immunoadsorbent prepared by copolymerization at pH 5 with four parts bovine serum albumin and one part of IgG by the method of Avrameas and Ternynck [2].
2. The antibody preparation subsequently is passed through a Sephadex G–200 column and the IgG-containing fractions are pooled.
3. The Fab fragments are prepared by the method of Porter [25]. Papain is added to the Fab fragments at a concentration of 2% and digested for 2 hours at 37° C.
4. Fab and Fc fragments are separated from nondigested antibodies by gel filtration of the reaction mixtures through a Sephadex G-100 column, which is 90 × 1.5 cm.

5. The Fab fragment is separated from the Fc component with a DEAE cellulose column equilibrated with phosphate buffer. Under these conditions, the Fab fragment is eluted in the void volume.

Use of Polyacrylamide Protein Immunoadsorbent Prepared with
Glutaraldehyde for Isolation of Anti-Human IgG Antibodies
(Method of Weston, Ternynck, and Avrameas [29, 30])
Glutaraldehyde contains 2 active aldehyde groups. When polyacrylamide gels are treated with an excess of glutaraldehyde, one of the 2 aldehyde groups of the glutaraldehyde will react with the free amino groups in the polyacrylamide gel. The remaining free active aldehyde is able to combine with the amino groups of any protein added in the second step.

MATERIALS AND REAGENTS
A. Bio-Gel column P–300, 400 mesh (BioRad)
B. Distilled water
C. 6% solution of gluteraldehyde—500 ml/100 ml hydrated gel
D. Phosphate buffer (pH 7.0, 0.1 M; pH 7.4, 0.1 M; pH 7.0, 0.01 M; containing 0.01% sodium azide) (for storage at 4° C)
E. Incubator
F. Storage at 4° C
G. Acrylamide gel particles—10 ml
H. Centrifuge at 4° C
 I. Human IgG—15–30 mg
J. Lysine (pH 7.4, 0.1 M)
K. Glycine-HCl buffer (pH 2.8, 0.2 M) (chilled and unchilled); (pH 2.2, 0.2 M)
L. K_2HPO_4 (0.2 M)—20 ml
M. Immunoadsorbent gel—10 ml
N. Whole immune serum or sheep anti-human IgG—5–20 ml
O. 0.45 μ millipore filter
P. Equipment for dialysis; vacuum dialysis
Q. Sodium azide (0.01 M)

PREPARATION OF GLUTARALDEHYDE-ACTIVATED POLYACRYLAMIDE BEADS
1. Bio-Gel, P-300, P-400 mesh is allowed to hydrate for 24 hours in distilled water and is washed several times with distilled water.
2. To 100 ml hydrated gel, 500 ml 6% solution of glutaraldehyde in phosphate buffer pH 7, 0.1 M is added. The suspension is then incubated overnight.
3. The gel is then washed 10–20 times with distilled H_2O with use of 500 ml H_2O per wash.
4. The activated gel may be stored at 4° C for at least 1 week without loss of activity.

PREPARATION OF IMMUNOADSORBENT CONTAINING HUMAN IgG
1. 10 ml activated acrylamide gel particles (centrifuged 3,000 g for 10 min at 4° C) are mixed with 10 ml phosphate buffer pH 7.4, 0.1 M containing 15–30 mg human IgG.
2. The suspension is allowed to rotate slowly at room temperature overnight or for 48 hours at 4° C.
3. The suspension is centrifuged 3,000 g for 10 min at 4° C and the supernatant removed. The sediment is washed by repeated centrifugations with phosphate-buffered physiologic saline solution, pH 7.0, 0.01 M until the optical density (O.D.) of the supernatant is less than 0.05 at 280 nm.
4. The first supernatant and that of the two following washes are pooled and the protein content is determined. The amount of protein conjugated can be determined by the difference between the protein added and the amount found in the pooled supernates.
5. Free active aldehyde groups on the gels are blocked by suspending the gel in an equal volume of lysine pH 7.4, 0.1 M and left at room temperature for 18 hours.
6. The gel particles are washed 3 to 4 times with 0.01 M phosphate-buffered physiologic saline solution, pH 7.0, 0.01 M. This is followed by two washes with 50 ml chilled glycine-HCl buffer, pH 2.8, 0.2 M and one with 20 ml K_2HPO_4, 0.2 M.
7. Washing with phosphate-buffered physiologic saline solution, pH 7.0, 0.01 M is then repeated until the O.D. of the washings is 0 at 280 nm.
8. The immunoadsorbent is stored at 4° C in buffered saline solution containing 0.01% sodium azide.

PREPARATION OF PURIFIED ANTIBODIES TO HUMAN IgG
1. 10 ml immunoadsorbent gel is mixed with 5–20 ml whole immune serum or sheep anti-human IgG. The suspension is gently stirred at room temperature for 1 hour and centrifuged 3,000 g for 10 min at 4° C. The supernatant is reserved to estimate the amount of non-adsorbed antibodies.
2. The gel particles are suspended in buffered physiologic saline solution (pH 7.0, 0.1 M) and washed by successive centrifugations until the supernatant has an O.D. of less than 0.02 at 280 nm.
3. Adsorbed antibodies are eluted with two washings of 20–30 ml HCl-glycine buffer, pH 2.8, 0.2 M and one washing with HCl-glycine pH 2.2, 0.2 M. The eluted antibodies are immediately neutralized with K_2HPO_4, 1 M, filtered on a 0.45 μ millipore filter, and dialyzed against 2 changes of phosphate-buffered saline solution pH 7.0, 0.01 M (5 liters each).
4. The antibody solution is concentrated by vacuum dialysis, stored at 4° C with sodium azide 0.01 M.

5. The purified antibody may be checked for titer and quantity of pre-cipitating antibody and homogenicity of the preparation by immuno-electrophoresis.

Preparation of Enzyme-Labeled Antibody

Several techniques for the coupling of enzyme to antibody have been reported. The reagent, p,p'-difluoro-m,m' dinitrodiphenyl sulfone (FNPS) was first used to couple ferritin to antibody [26] and subsequently em-ployed to conjugate peroxidase or acid phosphatase to antibody [19]. Nakane and Pierce [21] employed l-ethyl-3-(3-dimethyl aminopropyl) carbodiimide (CDI) to conjugate peroxidase and acid phosphatase to antibody. Glutaraldehyde has been used successfully in conjugating a wide variety of enzymes to antibodies. The glutaraldehyde initiates cross-linking of the enzyme to antibody with formation of a heterogeneous population of conjugates. Avrameas [4] feels that glutaraldehyde as a coupling agent gave the most satisfactory and reproducible results. The glutaraldehyde technique has been used to couple peroxidase, phospha-tase, tyrosinase, glucose oxidase, and lactic dehydrogenase to antibodies of various species. The glutaraldehyde-coupled enzyme-labeled antibody preparation stored at 4° C was found to be active at least 3 months with-out appreciable loss in catalytic and immunological specificity.

Peroxidase Conjugation Method with p,p'-difluoro-m,m'-dinitrodiphenyl Sulfone (FNPS)
(Method of Nakane and Pierce [19])

MATERIALS AND REAGENTS
  A. 0.5% FNPS (General Biochemicals)—0.25 ml
  B. Acetone
  C. Carbonate buffer (pH 10, 0.5 M)
  D. Horseradish peroxidase (Type II or VI, Sigma)—50 mg
  E. IgG fraction prepared from rabbit anti-human IgG—50 mg
  F. Agitator at 4° C
  G. Equipment for dialysis
  H. Phosphate-buffered saline solution (pH 7.0–7.2; 0.01 M, 0.15 M)
   I. Centrifuge at 4° C
  J. Saturated ammonium sulfate—50%
  K. Distilled water
  L. 0.1 N NaOH
  M. Refrigeration, storage at 4° C
  N. Saturated barium chloride solution

PROCEDURE
1. 0.25 ml 0.5% p,p'-difluoro-m,m'-dinitrodiphenyl sulfone (FNPS) is dissolved in acetone and added to 2 ml carbonate buffer containing

50 mg horseradish peroxidase and 50 mg IgG fraction prepared from rabbit anti-human IgG.

2. The mixture is gently agitated at 4° C for 6 hours and dialyzed against phosphate-buffered saline solution, pH 7.0–7.2, 0.01 M overnight.

3. The small amount of precipitate formed upon dialysis is removed by centrifugation at 1,000 g for 20 min.

4. An equal amount of saturated ammonium sulfate in distilled water which has been neutralized with 0.1 N NaOH is added, and the solution is mixed gently by inversion. After standing for 30 min at 4° C the mixture is centrifuged for 20 min at 2,000 g at 4° C. The supernatant containing free horseradish peroxidase is discarded.

5. The precipitate is washed with 50% saturated ammonium sulfate and is suspended in phosphate-buffered saline solution, 0.15, pH 7.0–7.2 and dialyzed against phosphate-buffered saline solution to remove the ammonium sulfate. The dialysate is tested until free of sulfate with a few drops of saturated barium chloride solution.

6. The preparation is concentrated and stored at 4° C after determination of the protein concentration.

Coupling of Peroxidase to Antibody with
Glutaraldehyde Technique
(Method of Avrameas [4])

MATERIALS AND REAGENTS
A. Horseradish peroxidase (Sigma type VI)—12 mg
B. IgG fraction of serum antibody—5 mg
C. Phosphate buffer (pH 6.8, 0.1 M)
D. 1% glutaraldehyde (Polyscience)—0.05 ml
E. Agitator
F. Equipment for dialysis
G. Refrigeration, storage at 4° C
H. Centrifuge (Spinco preparative with 40 rotor) at 4° C
 I. Sephadex G–200 column (Pharmacia)

PROCEDURE
1. 12 mg horseradish peroxidase is added to 5 mg IgG fraction in 1 ml phosphate buffer pH 6.8, 0.1 M.

2. 0.05 ml 1% glutaraldehyde is then added while stirring, and the mixture is left at room temperature for 2 hours.

3. After dialysis overnight against 2 changes of 5 liters of phosphate-buffered saline solution at 4° C, the conjugate is centrifuged at 20,000 rpm for one-half hour, at 4° C with a 40 rotor in a Spinco preparative ultracentrifuge.

4. The conjugates are stored undiluted at 4° C up to 3 months.

5. Alternatively the antibody may be separated from uncoupled peroxidase with a Sephadex G–200 column. The protein concentration can be monitored at 280 nm, and the peroxidase unit can be roughly

monitored at 403 nm (absorption due to hemin group) [17]. Evaluation and determination of the peroxidase activity is discussed below.

Two Step Conjugation of Peroxidase to IgG or Fab Fragment
(Method of Avrameas and Ternynck [7])

MATERIALS AND REAGENTS
A. Peroxidase (Worthington)—10 mg (15 mg for high ratio)
B. Phosphate buffer, pH 6.8, 0.1 M
C. 1.25% glutaraldehyde
D. Incubation at room temperature at 4° C
E. Sephadex G–25 column (Pharmacia)
F. Sodium chloride (0.15 M)
G. Diaflow PM 10 membrane
H. Anti-IgG antibody—5 mg or Fab fragments—2.5 mg
I. Carbonate-bicarbonate buffer (pH 9.5, 1.0 M)—0.1 ml
J. Solution of lysine, 0.2 M
K. Equipment for dialysis at 4° C
L. $(NH_4)_2SO_4$ (saturated neutral; half-saturated)
M. Distilled water
N. Centrifuge
O. Storage at 4° C

PROCEDURE
1. 10 mg peroxidase is dissolved in 0.2 ml phosphate buffer pH 6.8, 0.1 M containing 1.25% glutaraldehyde.
2. The solution is allowed to stand for 18 hours at room temperature and then passed through a Sephadex G–25 column equilibrated with sodium chloride, 0.15 M.
3. The brown-colored fractions containing the activated peroxidase are pooled and concentrated to 1 ml with a Diaflow PM 10 membrane.
4. To the peroxidase solution, 1 ml NaCl containing either 5 mg of IgG antibody or 2.5 mg Fab fragments is added and followed by the addition of 0.1 ml carbonate-bicarbonate buffer, pH 9.5, 1.0 M. The mixture is allowed to stand for 24 hours at 4° C.
5. After 24 hours at 4° C, 0.1 ml solution of lysine 0.2 M is added and the mixture is then allowed to stand for an additional 2 hours at 4° C.
6. The preparation is then dialyzed at 4° C against several changes of buffered saline solution.
7. The labeled antibody preparation is precipitated at 4° C with an equal volume of saturated neutral solution of $(NH_4)_2SO_4$.
8. The precipitate is washed twice with half saturated $(NH_4)_2SO_4$ and dissolved in a minimal volume of distilled water and dialyzed against large volumes of buffered saline solution.
9. Both antibody and Fab peroxidase label preparation are centrifuged at 20,000 g for 20 min and stored at 4° C. The preparation has been

reported to last at least 3 months without any loss of immunologic and enzyme activity [7].

When a high ratio of peroxidase to antibody is desired, as in the case of electron microscopic studies, 15 mg peroxidase instead of 10 mg may be used to couple with 5 mg IgG or 2.5 mg Fab fragments. Although the peroxidase-labeled antibody or labeled Fab can be separated from uncoupled antibody or Fab by filtration of the preparation on a Sephadex G–200 column, this procedure has not been found to be necessary.

Assay of Peroxidase Enzyme Activity

The purity of the horseradish peroxidase (Sigma or Worthington) is often expressed in terms of RZ (Reinheitszahl) values. This is determined by the ratio of the optical density at 403 nm (due to the hemin group) to the protein at 275 nm. The RZ value for pure crystalline horseradish peroxidase MW 40,000 was found to be 3.04 [9, 17]. The enzyme activity is dependent on the pH, type of buffer, and properties of the isoenzyme of horseradish peroxidase [27].

The concentration of pure horseradish peroxidase may be determined in aqueous solution at pH 6–7 by multiplying the absorbency at 403 nm by 0.4 [31]. The RZ value does not give any guarantee of enzyme activity since it indicates primarily the hemin content. The reference assay used in the past is the formation of purpurogallin from pyrogallol by the enzyme action of peroxidase [9, 17]. The assay is cumbersome and difficult since the purpurogallin is extracted with organic solvents after the chemical reactions. The concentration of purpurogallin is determined spectrophotometrically at 430 nm, and the activity of peroxidase has been expressed by units equivalent to amount of purpurogallin formed under specified conditions [9].

Recommended Assay of Peroxidase Activity of Enzyme
Before and After Conjugation to Antibody Protein
(Method described in Worthington Manual [31])

The peroxidase enzyme acts upon H_2O_2, the o-dianisidine acts as the hydrogen donor, and the resulting color formation is measured at 460 nm. One unit of peroxidase enzyme activity is defined as the amount capable of decomposing 1 μM of peroxide per minutes at 25° C.

ENZYME STANDARD STOCK SOLUTION
1 mg/ml in water and dilute stock just before use, 0.1 ml to 250 ml

SUBSTRATE.   Stock—1 ml 30% H_2O_2 (Merck) diluted to 100 ml with H_2O. Just before use dilute 1 ml of stock H_2O_2 to 100 ml with phosphate buffer, pH 6.0, 0.01 M.

DYE.   1% o-dianisidine in methyl alcohol (fresh in dark bottle).

MATERIALS AND REAGENTS
A. Test cuvette
B. Control cuvette
C. Pipette
D. Parafilm
E. Equipment for O.D. measurement
F. 5 N HCl
G. Water

PROCEDURE
1. Add 0.05 ml dye to 6 ml substrate.
2. Transfer 2.9 ml to test cuvette and place remainder in control cuvette.
3. At zero time add 0.1 ml dilute enzyme into cuvette with pipette tip below surface of substrate.
4. Cover cuvette with parafilm and mix solution gently.
5. Measure optical density at 460 nm at 15-sec intervals for 1 to 2 min.

$$\text{Units/mg} = \frac{\text{A460/min}}{11.3 \times \text{mg enzyme/ml reaction mixture}}$$

6. Rinse cuvette with 5 N HCl and water between tests. The test is very sensitive, and less than 0.005 μg of enzyme should be used in preparations with a RZ value of 2.

After coupling of peroxidase to antibody, the preparation should be standardized as to units of precipitating antibody activity per milliliter as well as to the peroxidase enzyme activity. The units of antibody activity are defined as the reciprocal of the highest dilution of the conjugate demonstrating a precipitin reaction with the antigen at a concentration of 1 mg per milliliter by the double gel diffusion test.

Preparation and Fixation of Tissue Specimens

Tissue preparations are handled differently depending upon the type of study.

Light Microscopy
Good fixation of various cell suspensions and sections of frozen tissue is obtained with a 10 min fixation at 4° C in acetone, absolute methanol, 95% alcohol, or alcohol:ether (60:40) and 10% neutralized formalin and saline solution. A fixative should not be used if the tissue antigen studied is altered or made immunologically unreactive upon fixation [4].
When cell preparations are treated with enzyme-labeled antibody, good results are obtained with an antibody concentration of 0.1 to 0.5 mg per milliliter with incubation times of the enzyme and substrate of 30 min to 3 hours [4, 19]. The molar ratio of enzyme to the antibody in active complexes should be at least 1:1 [7].

Electron Microscopy
Because of difficulties of penetration of the cells with enzyme-labeled antibodies, good results are obtained when mild fixatives are used. Enzymes which were coupled to Fab antibody fragments were found easily to penetrate into the interior of fixed cells [7]. Usually 0.5 mm blocks of tissue were fixed at 4° C for 15 min to 1 hour in 1.25% paraformaldehyde [6] or by 1 to 3 hours in 10% phosphate-buffered formalin [19].

Cytochemical Reaction of Various Enzymes and Substrates

Light Microscopy
Two different substrates may be used for peroxidase enzyme activity. The first substrate is 3,3′-diaminobenzidine and hydrogen peroxide according to the method described by Graham and Karnovsky [15]. The section may be processed with postincubation of stained preparations with osmium tetroxide [24]. The peroxidase activity can also be detected with 4-chloro-1-naphthol, which results in a grayish-blue stain [20]. The 3,3′-diaminobenzidine will yield dark brown precipitate, and the 4-chloro-1-naphthol will yield brilliant blue reaction products. The diaminobenzidine reaction products are insoluble in both aqueous and organic solution, whereas the 4-chloro-1-naphthol reaction product is insoluble in aqueous but soluble in organic media.

Alkaline phosphatase activity can be detected by different substrates such as naphthol-AS-MX phosphate and fast red PL-diazonium salt [4]. Acid phosphatase can be stained with Gomori's medium followed by ammonium sulfide [19].

Glucose oxidase activity can be localized by incubating the cells in a mixture of D-glucose, tetrazolium salt, and phenazine methosulfate [4]. The various sections and cell preparations on slides after staining and washing can be dehydrated, cleared, and mounted in suitable media.

Electron Microscopy
Mainly peroxidase and alkaline and acid phosphatases are used as enzyme markers for electron microscopic studies. Peroxidase is best revealed by the diaminobenzidine and hydrogen peroxide method. Phosphatase can be detected by Gomori's medium as modified for electron microscopic localization [19].

The Histochemical Localization of Horseradish Peroxidase
(Method of Graham and Karnovsky [15])
1. Preparation of substrate solution.
   a. 3,3′-diaminobenzidine tetrahydrochloride (Sigma) 25 mg.
   b. Tris-HCl buffer pH 7.6, 0.05 M, 50 ml.
   c. 3% hydrogen peroxide, 0.15 ml (layer of propylene glycol will

help preserve stock solution of H_2O_2). Stock solution 30% H_2O_2 (Superoxol, Merck).

2. The substrate is freshly prepared for each batch of sections, fixed, and the hydrogen peroxide is added immediately before use.
3. The sections are incubated 10–30 min at room temperature in the substrate solution for the histochemical reaction.
4. The sections are washed briefly in buffered saline solution followed by distilled water, dehydrated in absolute alcohol, and clarified in xylol.
5. The sections are mounted with permount and covered with a glass coverslip.

Localization of Different Constituents

By different techniques it is possible to localize two or more tissue antigens or antibodies on the same cell or tissue section. This can be done in the following ways:

A. Using different enzymes.
B. Using the same enzyme with different substrates, such as peroxidase with 3,3′-diaminobenzidine and 4-chloro-1-naphthol.
C. Use of fluoresceinated marker as a fluorochrome and an enzyme.
D. Use of ferritin and enzyme for markers on different antibodies.

Sensitivity and Specificity of Enzyme-Labeled Antibody Methods

It appears that the sensitivity for detecting antigens of the enzyme-labeled antibody technique is equivalent to the fluorescein-labeled antibody [8, 11, 24]. Several studies have been performed in comparing the detection of antinuclear antibodies and other autoimmune antibodies [8, 11, 24].

Nonspecific Staining

For control, the tissue preparations under investigation should be incubated in the following solutions:

1. Enzyme-labeled antibody previously reacted and adsorbed with specific homologous antigen.
2. Unrelated antibody coupled with the enzyme.
3. The enzyme alone.

The above controls should be negative except for endogenous enzyme activity expected in some cells. Leukocytes, erythrocytes, and macrophage granules can show a positive peroxidase stain due to endogenous enzyme activity. The polymorphonuclear leukocytes and macrophages may show positive staining for alkaline phosphatase. Glucose oxidase is not present in the above cells. Nonspecific staining is increased with a preparation containing specific low antibody activity and/or containing impure enzyme preparations [24].

The enzyme conjugates may be adsorbed with acetone-dried liver powder similar to fluorescein-conjugated antibodies just prior to use.

Examples of Practical Application of Immunoenzyme Methods

Test for Antinuclear Antibodies with Peroxidase-Labeled Anti-Human IgG

PREPARATION OF SUBSTRATE SOLUTION
a. 50 mg 3,3′-diaminobenzidine free base (Sigma)
b. Tris buffer pH 7.6, 0.05 M in sucrose, 0.25 M—50 ml
c. 0.01% H_2O_2—add 0.15 ml 3% H_2O_2 (layer of propylene glycol will help preserve stock solution of 30% H_2O_2) (Superoxol) (Merck).

The substrate solution is made fresh and filtered through Whatman No. 40 filter paper just before use.

MATERIALS AND REAGENTS
A. Rat kidney sections
B. Slides and coverslips
C. 1.25% paraformaldehyde (optional)
D. Phosphate buffer (pH 7.2, 0.1 M)
E. Acetone (optional)
F. Coons' buffered saline solution (alternative to phosphate buffer)
G. Blotter (to remove excess moisture from around slides)
H. Test serum—various dilutions
 I. Moist chamber
J. Peroxidase-labeled anti-human IgG—1 drop per slide
K. 2% osmium tetroxide (optional)
L. 0.5% methyl green (optional)
M. Alcohol (95%; 100%)
N. Xylene
O. Permount

PROCEDURE
1. Rat kidney sections may or may not be fixed in 1.25% paraformaldehyde in phosphate buffer pH 7.2, 0.1 M for 5 min, prior to peroxidase reaction [24]. Acetone fixation for 1 to 2 min [12] may also be employed as a fixative.
2. The sections are rinsed and washed 2 times for 8 min each, with Coons' buffered saline solution or phosphate-buffered saline solution.
3. Drain slides and blot excess fluid from around the tissue. Incubate 30 min with various dilutions of test serum in a moist chamber.

4. Rinse and wash the slide 2 times for 8 min each, with buffered saline solution.
5. Drain the slides and remove the excess fluid from around the tissue. One drop of peroxidase-labeled anti-human IgG is added to cover each entire section. Incubation is carried out in a moist chamber at room temperature.
6. Rinse and wash slides 2 times for 8 min each with buffered saline solution.
7. Incubation of the slide with the substrate may be from 10–30 min for the staining reaction. Specific staining relative to the background stain should be checked.
8. Wash slide for 1 min with buffered saline solution.
9. The staining reaction can be enhanced by postfixation in 2% osmium tetroxide for 5 min. This is recommended for only pale staining sections.
10. The slides may be counterstained with 0.5% methyl green.
11. Slides are successively processed through 1–2 min changes of 95% alcohol, 100% alcohol, and 2 changes of xylene.
12. Sections are mounted in permount with a coverslip.

Summary

The enzyme-labeled antibody methods not only can be used to demonstrate a wide variety of tissue autoantibodies but also have potential application to most of the techniques which currently employ fluorescent-labeled antibodies. A complete test kit including reagents, substrate, and buffer to perform the test for antinuclear antibodies by the peroxidase enzyme method is available from BioWare. The reagents work well and the kit is very convenient for the busy clinical laboratory. Various peroxidase-conjugated antibodies are also available from Cappel.

References

1. Avrameas, S., and Uriel, J.   Methode de marquage d'antigènes et d'anti-corps avec des enzymes et son application en immunodiffusion. *Comp. Rend. Acad. Sci.* 262:2543, 1966.
2. Avrameas, S., and Ternynck, T.   Biologically active water insoluble protein polymers: I. Their use for isolation of antigens and antibodies. *J. Biol. Chem.* 242:1651, 1967.
3. Avrameas, S., and Bouteille, M.   Ultrastructural localization of antibody by antigen label with peroxidase. *Exp. Cell Res.* 53:166, 1968.
4. Avrameas, S.   Coupling of enzymes to proteins with glutaraldehyde. Use of the conjugates for the detection of antigens and antibodies. *Immunochemistry* 6:43, 1969.
5. Avrameas, S., and Ternynck, T.   The cross-linking of proteins with glutaraldehyde and its use for the preparation of immunoadsorbents. *Immunochemistry* 6:53, 1969.

6. Avrameas, S. Immunoenzyme techniques: Enzymes as markers for the localization of antigens and antibodies. *Int. Rev. Cytol.* 27:349, 1970.
7. Avrameas, S., and Ternynck, T. Peroxidase labeled antibody and Fab conjugates with enhanced intracellular penetration. *Immunochemistry* 8:1175, 1971.
8. Benson, M. D., and Cohen, A. S. Antinuclear antibodies in systemic lupus erythematosus. *Ann. Int. Med.* 73:943, 1970.
9. Chance, B., and Maehly, A. C. Assay of catalases and peroxidase. In S. P. Colewick and N. O. Kaplan (eds.), *Methods in Enzymology.* New York: Academic Press, 1965, vol. 2, p. 764.
10. Coons, A. H., Creeh, H. J., Jones, R. N., and Berliner, E. The demonstration of pneumococcal antigen in tissues by the use of fluorescent antibody. *J. Immunol.* 45:159, 1942.
11. Darling, J., Johnson, G. D., Webb, J. A., and Smith, M. E. Use of peroxidase conjugated antiglobulin as an alternative to immunofluorescence for the detection of antinuclear factor in serum. *J. Clin. Pathol.* 24:501, 1971.
12. Davey, F. R., and Busch, G. J. Immunohistochemistry of glomerulonephritis using horseradish peroxidase and fluorescein-labeled antibody: A comparison of two technics. *Am. J. Clin. Pathol.* 53:531, 1970.
13. Fudenberg, H. H., Drews, G., and Nisonoff, A. Serologic demonstration of dual specificity of rabbit bivalent hybrid antibody. *J. Exp. Med.* 119:151, 1964.
14. Fukuyama, K., Douglas, S. D., Tuffanelli, D. L., and Epstein, W. L. Immunohistochemical method for localization of antibodies in cutaneous disease. *Am. J. Clin. Pathol.* 54:410, 1970.
15. Graham, R. C., and Karnovsky, M. J. The early stages of absorption of injected horseradish peroxidase into the proximal tubules of mouse kidney. *J. Histochem. Cytochem.* 14:291, 1966.
16. Hoedemacker, P. J., and Ito, S. Ultrastructural localization of gastric parietal cell antigen with peroxidase-coupled antibody. *Lab. Invest.* 22:184, 1970.
17. Maehly, A. C., and Chance, B. The assay of catalases and peroxidase. In D. Glick (ed.), *Methods of Biochemical Analysis.* New York: Interscience, 1954, p. 357.
18. Nakane, P. K., and Pierce, G. B. Enzyme-labeled antibodies: Preparation and application for the localization of antigens. *J. Histochem. Cytochem.* 14:929, 1966.
19. Nakane, P. K., and Pierce, G. B. Enzyme-labeled antibodies for the light and electron microscopic localization of tissue antigens. *J. Cell Biol.* 33:307, 1967.
20. Nakane, P. K. Simultaneous localization of multiple tissue antigens utilizing peroxidase-labeled antibody method: A study on pituitary glands of the rat. *J. Histochem. Cytochem.* 16:557, 1968.
21. Nakane, P. K. Peroxidase-labeled antibody method. In W. Montagna and R. E. Billingham (eds.), *Advances in Biology of the Skin.* Vol. II, *Immunology of the Skin.* New York: Appleton, 1971, p. 283.
22. Nisonoff, A., and Rivers, M. M. Recombination of mixture of univalent antibody fragments of different specificity. *Arch. Biochem. Biophys.* 93:460, 1961.

23. Nisonoff, A., and Palmer, J. L.　Hybridization of half molecules of rabbit gamma globulin. *Science* 143:376, 1964.
24. Petts, V., and Roitt, I. M.　Peroxidase conjugates for demonstration of tissue antibodies: Evaluation of technique. *Clin. Exp. Immunol.* 9:407, 1971.
25. Porter, R. R.　The hydrolysis of rabbit gamma globulin and antibodies with crystalline papain. *Biochem. J.* 73:119, 1959.
26. Ram, J. S., Taude, S. S., Pierce, G. B., and Midgley, A. R.　Preparation of antibody ferritin conjugates for immunoelectron microscopy. *J. Cell Biol.* 17:673, 1963.
27. Shannon, L. M., Kay, E., and Lew, J. Y.　Peroxidase isoenzymes from horseradish roots: I. Isolation and physical properties. *J. Biol. Chem.* 241:2166, 1966.
28. Singer, S. J., and Schick, A. F.　The properties of specific stains for electron microscopy prepared by the conjugation of antibody molecules with ferritin. *J. Biophys. Biochem. Cytol.* 9:519, 1961.
29. Ternynck, T., and Avrameas, S.　Polyacrylamide-protein immunoadsorbents prepared with glutaraldehyde. *F.E.B.S. Letters* 23:24, 1972.
30. Weston, P. D., and Avrameas, S.　Proteins coupled to polyacrylamide beads using glutaraldehyde. *Biochem. Biophys. Res. Comm.* 45:1574, 1971.
31. Worthington Biochemical Corp., *Enzyme Manual.* Freehold, N.J., 1972.
32. Zeromski, J.　Immunological findings in sensory carcinomatous neuropathy. Application of peroxidase labeled antibody. *Clin. Exp. Immunol.* 6:633, 1970.

24

Ferritin-Labeled Antibody
Techniques

In obtaining an ideal electron-scattering label for antibodies, the label
should possess the following characteristics:

A. The label should be attached to the antibody by a stable covalent
   linkage without alteration of biologic activity of the antibody.
B. The label should possess sufficient density with electron-dispersing
   property and still not interfere with mobility of the antibody in tissue.
C. The label should remain stable throughout the procedure involved
   in the fixation and preparation of the tissue specimen.

Various labels have been utilized including ferritin, which was first
proposed by Singer [24]; other heavy metals including mercury [19] and
uranium [25] have also been used. Mercury was first used by Pepe [19],
who successfully employed antimyosin antibodies labeled with mercury
for localizing myosin in tissues. The difficulties involve a variable coupling of an organic mercurial compound such as tetra-acetoxymercuriar-
sanilic acid. The amount of mercury which can be introduced is often
insufficient to provide significant contrast during electron microscopic examination. Another drawback is that mercury can sublimate and form
dense globules which can migrate in the section when subjected to an
intense electron beam.

Sternberger et al. [25] suggested uranium-labeled antibodies containing up to 30% weight of uranium may produce a great degree of electron capacity. In addition, the uranium-labeled antibodies are smaller
than ferritin-labeled antibodies, and the problems of cellular penetration
are less serious; however, direct treatment of antibodies with uranyl
acetate results in case of antibody activity. Therefore, the antibody
should be protected in the presence of antigen during the labeling procedure followed by elution of the labeled antibody. It may be used for a
system in which an insoluble antigen is used, and the antibody after
labeling may be disassociated from the antigen with ease. The method is
cumbersome and is not the one most widely used.

Singer and Schick [24] were the first to suggest the use of a bifunctional agent for the conjugation of antibodies to ferritin. Ferritin is a protein which has a molecular weight in excess of 650,000 and which contains an average of 23% iron in the form of ferritin hydroxide micelles [8, 11]. It can be identified under the electron microscope by its characteristic fine structure, and it can be seen in an electromicrograph. One of the disadvantages of ferritin antibody conjugates is that they diffuse sluggishly in formalin fixed tissue and cellular membranes.

Preparation of Ferritin-Conjugated Antibody

There are numerous published procedures for the preparation of ferritin-conjugated antibody [2, 21, 22]. The ferritin must be first purified by recrystallization and reprecipitation. If the antibody is purified with the use of an immunoadsorbent before ferritin coupling, then it is possible to obtain a more active and specific reagent. The ferritin may be conjugated to the antibody in a two-step reaction with toluene, 2,4-diisocyanate [24] or by a one-step procedure with p,p′-difluoro-m,m′-dinitrodiphenyl sulphone (FNPS) [22]. Numerous other coupling agents have also been used [2, 21]. Ferritin-conjugated antibody may be obtained from a commercial source (Cappel).

Characterization and Testing of Ferritin Conjugate Before Use

Each lot of ferritin-labeled conjugate should be tested for specificity and purity, and characterized before use by the following procedures [2, 7, 13, 17]:

Immunoelectrophoretic Analysis
This test is performed to ascertain whether a ferritin conjugate is present and whether the conjugated antibody can react with the specific antigen. Ferritin-labeled globulin is faster than γ-globulin and slower than the ferritin covalently linked to the coupling agent (treated ferritin) alone upon electrophoretic analyses. The conjugated and treated ferritin are colored.

Studies with Immunofluorescent Labeling of
Ferritin Conjugate [17]
The ferritin conjugate globulin antibody can be labeled with fluorescein, and the technique of double labeling of the antibody permits the relatively simple method of immunofluorescence to be used as a screen for selecting optimal conjugates of ferritin and antibody for subsequent use in electron microscopic studies.

A second alternate procedure is labeling the immunoglobulin antibody with fluorescein before it is sequentially coupled to ferritin. The potency and the specificity of the antiserum can be readily determined with the immunofluorescence technique; therefore, a thorough study of the immunofluorescence technique should precede most experiments in which electron microscopy is used.

Use of Radioiodine-Labeled Antibody Globulin
for Calculation of Molecular Ratio of Ferritin
and γ-Globulin in Isolated Conjugates

The antibody is first labeled with radioiodine [17] for conjugation with ferritin. The ferritin conjugate is isolated from uncoupled ferritin and globulin by ultracentrifugation and electrophoresis [17]. The amount of γ-globulin can be determined by comparison of radioactivity with the known protein concentration of I-labeled γ-globulin prior to labeling. The percentage of coupled ferritin is determined densimetrically after electrophoresis and staining of the strip with the Prussian blue reaction. The number of molecules of labeled ferritin can then be calculated from the known molecular weight and nitrogen content.

By the determination of the ferritin-to-globulin molecular ratio of the conjugates, the reaction can be quantitated with counting of the ferritin molecules if [24] the ferritin used for conjugation is free of apo-ferritin, and if [19] the isolated conjugate is free of uncoupled antibody.

Preparation of Specimens and Use of Ferritin-Labeled Antibody

The methods used for tissue preparation should preserve the cellular architecture and antigenic determinants and still allow penetration of the heavy ferritin-labeled antibody.

Prefixation

A. Fixatives such as osmium tetroxide which have been satisfactory for conventional electromicroscopy may destroy the specificity of many antigens [2]. Exposure to 6.5% gluteraldehyde for 20 min reduced the capacity of the antigens in renal tissue to react with antibody and prevent penetration of conjugates [18].

B. Dilute formalin has proved to be the fixative which has most adequately fulfilled the requirements for immunoferritin technique. Five % formalin in phosphate-buffer, pH 7.2 when used to prefix cultured cells of small pieces of tissue at 0° C will maintain the fine structure without inactivating the antigen [23]. After treatment with ferritin-conjugated antibody, further fixation with osmium tetroxide and/or gluteraldehyde is essential to preserve the fine structure.

Localization of the surface antigens may be accomplished by immersion in these specific ferritin conjugates for 5 to 20 min at room temperature. A prior fixation in 10% buffered formalin, pH 7.2 is helpful in preserving the internal structures and preventing pinocytosis of the conjugate [2, 23].

Localization of Intercellular Antigens and Free Cells

Ferritin-labeled antibodies do not penetrate untreated cells because of their large size. Pretreatment of infected cells with digitonin solution in phosphate-buffered saline solution, pH 7 has been reported to be effective in permitting penetration of conjugated antiviral antibody [9, 16]. For localization studies of intracellular or intercellular antigens in tissue, the tissue may be quickly frozen in a dry ice alcohol bath and sectioned on the cryostat in 10 μ sections. The sections are then immersed in ferritin-conjugated antibody, washed, fixed in gluteraldehyde and osmium tetroxide, and embedded in plastic [2, 21].

Methods and Controls

The direct method of ferritin-labeled antibody, in which the labeled antibody reacts directly with the substrate, is performed because of its ease in establishing controls.

The indirect method has certain advantages in that only one ferritin conjugate is required for the study of many specific antibodies providing they are prepared in the same species [6]. There are many variations in the use of ferritin-labeled antibody as in the use of hybrid antibody with specific antihost antigen and antiferritin activity. For example, hybrid antibody with anti-IgG and antiferritin specificity in locating cell surface antigens was used for electron microscopy study. Ferritin-conjugated antibody fragments have been used in electron microscopic study of viruses [4, 5, 12, 14].

Controls to determine the specificity of the immunoferritin method should be established as follows:

A. Duplicate tissue is treated first with unconjugated specific antibody and then is washed and treated with ferritin-conjugated antibody. The unconjugated antibody should block the binding of the conjugated antibody almost completely.

B. The ferritin-labeled antigen is first absorbed with specific antigen before use, and the absorbed conjugate should not result in binding in tissue in contrast to the section treated with specific unabsorbed conjugate.

C. Treatment of the tissue section with ferritin-labeled antibody is not specific for antigens in the test tissue.

D. Similar tissues with different antigens can be used with the specific ferritin conjugate. For example, in the localization of viral antigens the same tissue infected with other viruses which do not cross-react with viruses being studied, may be used for a control study.

Applications. The immunoferritin technique has been used for the localization of surface and intercellular tissue antigens as well as for the

identification of viral and other microbial antigens. The technique may
be used for the study of a wide variety of problems, including experimental and human glomerulonephritis [1, 3, 26], blood cells [10, 15],
basement membrane antigens [20], and coagulation proteins [27].

References

1. Andres, G. A., Accini, L., Hsu, K. C., Zabriskie, J. B., and Seegal, B. C.
Electron microscopic studies of human glomerulonephritis with ferritin-
conjugated antibody. *J. Exp. Med.* 123:399, 1966.
2. Andres, G. A., Hsu, K. C., and Seegal, B. C.   Immunoferritin technique
for the identification of antigens by electron microscopy. In D. M. Weir
(ed.), *Handbook of Experimental Immunology*. Oxford: Blackwell,
1967, chap. 15, p. 527.
3. Andres, G. A., Seegal, B. C., Hsu, K. C., Rothenberg, M. S., and
Chapeau, M. L.   Electron microscopic studies of experimental nephritis with ferritin conjugated antibody. Localization of antigen-anti-
complexes in rabbit glomeruli following repeated injections of bovine
serum albumin. *J. Exp. Med.* 117:691, 1963.
4. Aoki, T., Hammerling, U., deHarven, E., Boyse, E. A., and Old, L. J.
Antigenic structure of cell surfaces: An immunoferritin study of the
occurrence and topography of H–2, 0, and TL alloantigens on mouse
cells. *J. Exp. Med.* 130:979, 1969.
5. Aoki, T., and Takahashi, T.   Viral and cellular surface antigens of
murine leukemiae and myelomas. Serological analysis by immunoelectron microscopy. *J. Exp. Med.* 135:443, 1972.
6. Baxandall, J., Perlmann, P., and Afzelius, B. A.   A two layer technique
for detecting surface antigens in the sea urchin egg with ferritin-conjugated antibody. *J. Cell Biol.* 14:144, 1962.
7. Borek, F., and Sliverstein, A. M.   Characterization and purification of
ferritin antibody globulin conjugates. *J. Immunol.* 87:555, 1961.
8. Crichton, R. R.   Ferritin: Structure, synthesis and function. *N. Engl.
J. Med.* 284:1413, 1971.
9. Dales, S., Gomatos, P. J., and Hsu, K. C.   The uptake and development
of reovirus in strain L cells followed with labeled viral ribonucleic acid
and ferritin-antibody conjugates. *Virology* 25:193, 1965.
10. Easton, J. M., Goldberg, B., and Green, H.   Immune cytolysis: Electron
microscopic localization of cellular antigens with ferritin-antibody conjugates. *J. Exp. Med.* 115:275, 1962.
11. Farrant, J. L.   An electron microscopic study of ferritin. *Biochim.
Biophys. Acta* 13:569, 1954.
12. Hammerling, U., Aoki, T., deHarven, E., Boyse, E. A., and Old, L. J.
Use of hybrid antibody with anti γG and anti-ferritin specificities in
locating cell surface antigens by electron microscopy. *J. Exp. Med.* 128:
1461, 1968.
13. Hsu, K. C., Rifkind, R. A., and Zabriskie, J. B.   Immunochemical
studies with fluorescein and ferritin doubly-labeled antibodies. *J. Histochem. Cytochem.* 12:7, 1964.
14. Isliker, H., LeMaire, B., and Morgan, C.   The use of ferritin-conjugated

antibody fragments in electron microscopic studies of viruses. *Pathol. Microbiol.* 27:521, 1964.

15. Lee, R. E., and Feldman, J. C.   Visualization of antigenic sites of human erythrocytes with ferritin antibody conjugates. *J. Cell Biol.* 23:396, 1964.

16. Levinthal, J. D., Cerrottini, J. C., Ahmad-Zadek, C., and Wicker, R. The detection of intracellular adenovirus type 12 antigens by indirect immunoferritin technique. *Int. J. Cancer* 2:85, 1967.

17. Marinis, S., Vogt, S., and Brandner, G.   Isolation and characterization of immunoferritin conjugates. *Immunology* 17:77, 1967.

18. Morgan, C., Rifkind, R. A., Hsu, K. C., Holden, M., Seegal, B. C., and Rose, H. M.   Electron microscopic localization of intracellular viral antigen by the use of ferritin-conjugated antibody. *Virology* 14:292, 1961.

19. Pepe, F. A.   The use of specific antibody in electron microscopy: I. Preparation of mercury labeled antibody. *J. Biophys. Biochem. Cytol.* 11:515, 1961.

20. Pierce, G. B., Beals, T. F., Ram, J., S., and Midgley, A. R., Jr.   Basement membranes: IV. Epithelial origin and immunological cross reactions. *Am. J. Pathol.* 45:929, 1964.

21. Pierce, G. B., Jr., Ram, J., and Midgley, A. R., Jr.   The use of labeled antibodies in ultrastructural studies. *Int. Rev. Exp. Pathol.* 3:1, 1964.

22. Ram, J., S., Tawde, S. S., Pierce, G. B., Jr., and Midgley, A. R., Jr. Preparation of antibody-ferritin conjugates for immune electron microscopy. *J. Cell Biol.* 17:673, 1963.

23. Rifkind, R. A., Hsu, K. C., and Morgan, C.   Immunochemical staining for electron microscopy. *J. Histochem. Cytochem.* 12:131, 1964.

24. Singer, S. J., and Schick, A. F.   The properties of specific stains for electron microscopy prepared by the conjugation of antibody molecules with ferritin. *J. Biophys. Biochem. Cytol.* 9:519, 1961.

25. Sternberger, L. A., Donati, E. J., and Wilson, C. E.   Electron microscopic study on specific protection of isolated *Bordetella bronchiseptica* antibody during exhaustive labeling with uranium. *J. Histochem. Cytochem.* 11:48, 1963.

26. Vogt, A., Bockhorn, H., Kozima, K., and Sasaki, M.   Electron microscopic localization of the nephrotoxic antibody in the glomeruli of the rat after intravenous application of purified nephritogenic antibody ferritin conjugates. *J. Exp. Med.* 127:867, 1968.

27. White, J. E., Krivit, W., and Vesnier, R. C.   The platelet-fibrin relationship in human blood clots: An ultrastructural study utilizing ferritin-conjugated anti-human fibrinogen antibody. *Blood* 25:241, 1965.

25

Radioiodine Labeling of Proteins, Radioimmunodiffusion, and Radioimmunoelectrophoresis

Radioactive Labeling of Proteins: Trace Labeling with Radioiodine

The proteins for use in the clinical laboratory and research are commonly labeled with ^{125}I or ^{131}I. The advantages of radioiodine as a trace label are:

A. The labeling can be performed in vitro with labeled proteins of very high specific activity.

B. The label is firmly covalently linked to the protein molecule and there is no exchange with other protein molecules. If the iodination is under careful control conditions, many proteins can be labeled such that the native protein is indistinguishable from the labeled protein. However, in certain cases such as insulin, the iodination process may result in the loss of immunologic and biologic activity unless there is selective labeling of a certain portion of the insulin molecule [1].

^{131}I is a β and γ-ray emitter with a half-life of 8 days that can be obtained carrier free [9]. ^{125}I has a half-life of 57 days [2] with low energy γ-emission and is useful for (a) paired label experiments with ^{131}I, (b) work with radioautography, radioimmunodiffusion, and radioimmuno-electrophoresis, and (c) labeling valuable proteins available only in small quantities since the half-life is much longer than ^{131}I.

Methods of Iodination

The radioiodine is stored as a radioactive iodide ion. The iodide ion is converted to free iodine with an oxidant. The free iodine then reacts with the tyrosine ring on the protein or may enter in the histadine molecule. The reaction is stopped with the addition of a reducing agent. All direct protein iodination procedures require the formation of free iodine but conditions may vary [7].

The common techniques which are available include the following.

IODINE-MONOCHLORIDE TECHNIQUE. This technique has some difficulties when less than 2–5 mg of protein is available for labeling.

ELECTROLYTIC METHOD [16]. This method requires small amounts of protein; however, when very high specific activities are required the time taken for electrolytic labeling may result in denaturation.

CHLORAMINE-T METHOD [5, 8, 10, 17]. This system has certain advantages over the other labeling methods as follows [5, 8, 10]:

a. The manipulations do not require a large amount of skill.
b. Little or no iodine is volatilized and the procedure is rapid.
c. Efficiency of labeling for most proteins varies between 40 and 90%.
d. No carrier iodine is needed, and it allows labeling of proteins with labels of high specific activity.
e. The amount of protein labeled can be as small as 5 μg.

This procedure has been widely used for labeling small quantities of proteins for radioimmunoassays.

LACTOPEROXIDASE IODINATION [4, 13, 14, 18]. This method provides a means of using an automatic titrator to follow the incorporation of iodine into the protein. Very low concentrations of oxidant and iodide 1×10^{-6} M may be used in enzymatic iodination, and the extent of iodination can be calculated at any time during the course of the reactions [14]. This procedure is very promising and can be used to label proteins with radioiodine in a very short time while maintaining very low levels of hydrogen peroxide oxidant. The concentration of the lactoperoxidase enzyme used in the reaction is less than 1% of the total protein, to avoid iodination of the enzyme.

The lactoperoxidase procedure has been very successfully used to label and isolate the highly immunologically and biologically active monoiodinated insulin [6] and other polypeptide hormones [18]. A clever technique which can be used involves the radioiodination of proteins with bovine lactoperoxidase coupled to cyanogen bromide-activated Sepharose 4B [4]. The enzyme is readily removed by centrifugation after iodination.

A well-radiolabeled protein preparation should have the following properties: (a) no free iodine activity; (b) radioactivity covalently linked to protein; (c) the labeled protein should not be denatured, but should have identical immunochemical as well as biologic properties in vitro and in vivo.

Methods

Trace Iodination of Proteins by a Chloramine-T Method
(Method of McConahey and Dixon [10])

MATERIALS AND REAGENTS

A. Phosphate buffer (pH 7.0, 0.05 M)
B. Chloramine-T—highest purity grade (Distillation Products)
C. Sodium metabisulfite, sodium chloride, potassium phosphate, and sodium hydroxide. All reagents are of certified or analytical grade quality.
D. Distilled water
E. Carrier free Na ^{125}I in 0.1 M NaOH, free from preservatives or reducing substances (Schwartz).
F. 30 ml beakers containing 2.5 cm polyethylene-coated magnetic stirring rods—1 for each protein solution
G. Crystallizing dishes containing cracked ice—1 for each beaker
H. Magnetic stirrers—1 for each dish
I. 1 ml glass syringes with 22 gauge needles
J. Dialysis tubing (20/100 or 22/100) (Union Carbide). Soak and wash in distilled H$_2$O and buffer before use to remove any possible interfering substances.
K. Sephadex G–25 column and Dextran blue–2000 (Pharmacia)
L. Plastic tubes which fit into counting and fraction-collecting equipment
M. Carrier protein (used in control as serum)
N. 20% trichloracetic acid (TCA) (used in control)
O. Centrifuge
P. Fraction collector with UV monitor
Q. Gamma well scintillation counter

PROCEDURE

1. Proteins are dissolved in or dialyzed against phosphate buffer prior to iodination.
2. Fresh chloramine-T and sodium metabisulfite are prepared for each iodination in distilled H$_2$O at a concentration of 200 microgram per milliliter.
3. Protein solutions containing 1 to 5 mg protein per 4 ml phosphate buffer are placed in 30 ml beakers each containing a 2.5 cm polyethylene-coated magnetic stirring rod.
4. Each beaker is placed in a crystallizing dish containing cracked ice to keep the reactant cooled, and the crystallizing dish with beaker is then placed on a magnetic stirrer.
5. The appropriate quantity of radioactive iodine is added and the mixture is stirred. For example, to 1 mg human IgG protein is added 500 μCi of Na ^{125}I.

6. While the mixture is stirring, 100 μg chloramine-T (0.5 ml) is injected via a 22 gauge hypodermic needle to ensure prompt mixing.
7. Five minutes after the addition of chloramine-T, an equal amount of sodium metabisulfite is added (100 μg [0.05 ml]) with a 22 gauge needle to neutralize the oxidizing agent and stop the reaction.
8. The nonprotein iodine is removed by dialysis in the cold against phosphate buffer by either continuous flow or several changes over a 12–18 hour period.
9. Removal of nonprotein-bound radioiodine may be done by passage of the solution through a G–25 Sephadex column presaturated with buffer and precalibrated with 1% Dextran blue–2000 which is used as a marker for the determination of void volume.
10. Labeled proteins collected after passage through the Sephadex G–25 are often dialyzed against 3 changes of buffer in a 2–3 liter volume that is changed every 4 hours.
11. Suitable duplicate dilutions of the labeled proteins are made. To one sample is added a small amount of carrier protein as serum, and 20% trichloracetic acid (TCA) is added to a final concentration of 10%. To a second tube no serum or TCA is added. The tube with the TCA should form a white precipitate. It is centrifuged and the supernatant is removed.
12. The tubes are then counted in gamma well scintillation counters to determine the amount of TCA precipitable counts. The preparation should have at least 98% TCA precipitable counts.
13. For prolonged storage, the dilute labeled protein should be protected with either some unlabeled protein or a different protein to prevent radiolysis.

When smaller amounts of proteins are labeled, appropriate reduction in buffer volume, chloramine-T, and metabisulfite are employed. Five to 50 μg of proteins are dissolved in 1 ml phosphate buffer; 10–25 μg of chloramine-T and metabisulfite are employed.

Radioiodination of Proteins with Lactoperoxidase (Insulin)
(Method of J. Hamlin and E. R. Arquilla, Department of Pathology, University of California, Irvine)
The enzyme lactoperoxidase is being used increasingly for the iodination of polypeptide hormones [18], largely due to the efficiency of iodination, and to the apparent lack of deleterious side effects during the course of the reaction. The iodination of insulin by lactoperoxidase has been examined with a view towards obtaining preparations with high specific radioactivity (greater than 100 millicuries/mg) and complete retention of biological activity.

MATERIALS AND REAGENTS
A. Crystalline insulin (Elanco or Novo)—25 μg
B. HCl, 0.01 N; 1.0 N

C. EDTA 5×10^{-3} M
D. Sodium citrate (pH 5.2; 0.1 M, 0.05 M)
E. Na ^{125}I—5 μCi
F. H_2O_2, 2.3×10^{-9} M
G. Lactoperoxidase (Sigma)
H. Distilled water
 I. Small vial
 J. Centrifuge

PROCEDURE

1. 25 μg micrograms crystalline insulin are dissolved in 10 μl 0.01 N HCl containing 5×10^{-3} M EDTA, and the insulin is precipitated iso-electrically by the addition of 10 μl sodium citrate, pH 5.2, 0.1 M.
2. The suspension is kept intact and no precipitate is removed. 5 μCi carrier-free Na ^{125}I (2.3×10^{-9} M) is prepared in a final volume of 15 μl containing 2.3×10^{-9} M H_2O_2. Na ^{125}I is ordinarily supplied in a 0.1 N NaOH solution, and should be adjusted to pH 7.0 by the addition of an appropriate volume of 1 N HCl.
3. The enzyme lactoperoxidase is dissolved in water to an absorbancy of 0.084 at 412 nm, and is diluted 1/10 before use (final concentration is 7.4×10^{-8} M).
4. At 0, 15, and 30 min, 5 μl each of the enzyme and H_2O_2–Na ^{125}I solutions are added to the insulin suspension in a small vial, and the contents mixed by swirling.
5. 15 min after the third addition, the reaction mixture is centrifuged at 2,000 g for 15 min, the supernatant fluid is removed, and the precipitated insulin is washed 3 times with 20 μl sodium citrate, pH 5.2, 0.05 M.
6. The precipitate is finally suspended in 50 μl sodium citrate, pH 5.2, 0.05 M, and stored at 4° C. In this condition, the iodinated insulin should be stable for several weeks.
7. The combined supernatant and washed precipitate should be counted for radioactivity and the approximate percentage uptake determined. Incorporation of radioactivity by insulin should be from 80–90% of the total input.

It is recommended that a pilot experiment be performed exactly as above, employing a solution which contains 2.3×10^{-9} mole H_2O_2 and 2.3×10^{-9} moles cold potassium iodide containing a trace of Na ^{125}I, in order to verify that the enzyme and peroxide activities are correct. If satisfactory incorporation is obtained, the experiment is repeated with the carrier free Na ^{125}I, employing the same stock enzyme and peroxide solutions.

This procedure for labeling insulin has been demonstrated to produce monoiodinated insulin to the virtual exclusion of higher order iodinated derivatives. The final iodinated mixture should consist of an approximately equal mixture of unlabeled and labeled insulin. Monoiodinated insulin retains essentially full biological activity in both the mouse convulsion and mouse blood sugar depression assays, and is completely cross-reactive with anti-insulin antibodies. This preparation can therefore be used in radioimmunoassays for insulin, and as a biological tracer.

Indirect Radioimmunoelectrophoresis [12, 19]

MATERIALS AND REAGENTS
A. Slides for electrophoresis for both test and control sera
B. Test and control sera
C. Moist chamber
D. Phosphate-buffered saline solution (0.01 M)
E. ^{125}I-labeled antigen
F. Distilled water
G. Fan (for air drying)
H. Sticky tape long and wide enough to leave margin of ½ inch around slides placed on it
I. Darkroom and photographic developing and fixing supplies
J. x-ray film (Kodak Industrial type KK)
K. Sealed light-tight container with Drierite

PROCEDURE
1. Immunoelectrophoresis is performed on regular slides as described in the preceding chapter or by other acceptable methods [3, 15]. Serum containing the specific antibody to be evaluated is placed in the upper well, and the control serum sample is placed in the lower well. For example, human serum containing antibodies to insulin is placed in an upper well.
2. After immunoelectrophoresis, the specific anti-immunoglobulin is placed in the trough (i.e., rabbit anti-human immunoglobulin).
3. The antiserum is allowed to diffuse for 24 hours at room temperature in a moist chamber.
4. The slide is washed in phosphate-buffered saline solution for 24 hours.
5. At least 1 μCi of ^{125}I-labeled antigen is then added to the trough and allowed to react for 24 hours in a moist chamber at room temperature.
6. The slides are washed repeatedly in changes of phosphate-buffered saline solution for 6 to 48 hours, the last wash consisting of distilled H_2O.
7. The slides are air dried and placed on a piece of sticky tape with gel side up. The sticky tape should be sufficiently long and wide enough to leave a ½ inch margin around the edges.
8. In the darkroom, the slide with adhering tape is placed gel side down on a piece of x-ray film. The slide is secured to the film with the free margin of the tape.

9. The film with attached slide is placed in a sealed container which has some Drierite. The box should be light tight and stored at room temperature, so that the film remains in a flat position.
10. After exposure for 24 to 36 hours, carefully pull the tape from the film in a darkroom.
11. Develop and fix, following instructions on the film package.
12. Control slides to establish specificity of antibody with normal serum, unlabeled antigen, and other antigens.

Indirect Radioimmunodiffusion
(Method of Minden et al. [12])

MATERIALS AND REAGENTS
A. Slides coated with agar 1 mm thick, with 2% Ionager (Consolidated Laboratories)
B. Template to punch wells in agar-coated slides
C. Sera and antigens
D. Moisturized closed plastic chamber
E. Phosphate-buffered saline solution (0.01 M)
F. ^{131}I or ^{125}I
G. Moist chamber
H. Distilled water
 I. 2% acetic acid solution
 J. 10 B Amido black (Roboz)—0.5 gm/100 ml dye
K. Absolute methanol—90 ml
L. Glacial acetic acid—10 ml
M. Fan (for air drying)
N. Sticky tape, x-ray film (Kodak Industrial type KK), and photographic developing and fixing supplies as in preceding procedure

PROCEDURE
1. 1 mm layer agar coated slide with 2% Ionagar. Appropriate wells are punched with a template.
2. The sera and appropriate antigens are applied and slides are incubated at room temperature for 24 hours in a moisturized closed plastic chamber.
3. The slides are washed with phosphate-buffered saline with several changes for 24 hours after which about 1.5 $\mu Ci/\mu g$ N of I* antigen (^{131}I or ^{125}I) is added to the appropriate well and allowed to react in a moist chamber at room temperature for 24 hours.
4. Slides are then washed in phosphate-buffered saline several times ranging from 6 to 48 hours, then washed in distilled water.
5. Slides are first placed in 2% acetic acid solution for 5 min to decrease the solubility of the specific immune precipitates and then stained.
6. Convenient all purpose stain is used, a 10 B Amido black stain made

by dissolving 0.5 gm of dye in 100 ml of a solution of 90 ml absolute methanol and 10 ml glacial acetic acid [14]. The slides are then placed in the dye for 20 min and then destained with 3 to 5 washings of 5 to 10 min each with the 90:10 methanol-acetic solution without dye.
7. The slides are then dried at room temperature.
8. Slides are air dried, placed on sticky tape, and layered onto x-ray film (Kodak Industrial type KK) for 24 to 36 hours in a dark room or placed in a closed dark container and developed by conventional methods as described above for the procedure on indirect radio-immunoelectrophoresis.

Direct Radioimmunodiffusion and Direct Radioimmunoelectrophoresis [12]
These procedures are performed using the same methods described above except the I* antigen is added directly to the antiserum to be placed in the trough. The radioactivity should be adjusted so that 1 mg of antisera contains 1 μg radiolabeled antigen.

References

1. Arquilla, E. R., Miles, P. V., and Morris, J. W.   Immunochemistry of insulin. In D. F. Steiner and N. Freinkel (eds.), *Handbook of Physiology–Endocrinology*. Washington, D.C.: American Physiological Society, 1972, vol. 1, p. 159.
2. Campbell, D. H., Garvey, J. S., Cremer, M. E., and Sussdorf, D. H. *Methods in Immunology*. New York: Benjamin, 1970, 2nd ed., p. 142.
3. Cawley, L. P. *Electrophoresis and Immunoelectrophoresis*. Boston: Little, Brown, 1969.
4. David, G. S.   Solid state lactoperoxidase: A highly stable enzyme for simple, gentle iodination of proteins. *Biochem. Biophys. Res. Comm.* 48:464, 1972.
5. Greenwood, F. C., Hunter, W. M., and Glover, J. S.   The preparation of ^{131}I labeled human growth hormone of high specific radioactivity. *Biochem. J.* 89:114, 1963.
6. Hamlin, J. L., and Arquilla, E. R.   Monoiodo insulin. Preparation, purification, and characterization of a biologically active derivative substituted predominantly on tyrosine A14. *J. Biol. Chem.* 249:21, 1974.
7. Hughes, W. L.   The chemistry of iodination. In S. P. Masouredis (ed.), *The Role of [131]I Labeled Proteins in Biology and Medicine. Ann. N.Y. Acad. Sci.* 70:1, 1957.
8. Hunter, W. M., and Greenwood, F. C.   Preparation of iodine ^{131}I labelled growth hormone of high specific activity. *Nature* 194:495, 1962.
9. Masouredis, S. P. (ed.)   *The Role of [131]I Labeled Proteins in Biology and Medicine. Ann. N.Y. Acad. Sci.* 70:1, 1957.
10. McConahey, P., and Dixon, F. J.   A method of trace labeling of proteins for immunologic studies. *Int. Arch. Allergy Appl. Immunol.* 29:185, 1966.
11. McFarlane, A. S.   Efficient trace labelling of proteins with iodine. *Nature* 182:53, 1958.

12. Minden, P., Grey, H. M., and Farr, R. S.   False positive radioimmuno-autograph lines associated with immunoglobulins from normal sera. *J. Immunol.* 99:304, 1967.
13. Morrison, M., and Sisco Bayse, G.   Catalysis of iodination by lacto-peroxidase. *Biochemistry* 9:2995, 1970.
14. Morrison, M., Sisco Bayse, G., and Webster, R. G.   Use of lacto-peroxidase catalyzed iodination in immunochemical studies. *Immuno-chemistry* 8:289, 1971.
15. Ritzmann, S. E., Lawrence, M. C., and Daniels, J. C.   Serum protein analysis and immunoelectrophoresis. In J. B. Fuller (ed.), *Selected Topics in Clinical Chemistry*. Chicago: American Society of Clinical Pathologists, Workshop Manual, 1972.
16. Rosa, V., Scassellati, G. A., Pennsis, F., Riccioni, M., Giagnoni, P., and Giordani, R.   Labelling of human fibrinogen with ^{131}I by electrolytic iodination. *Biochim. Biophys. Acta* 86:519, 1964.
17. Sonoda, S., and Schlamowitz, M.   Studies of ^{125}I trace labelling of immunoglobulin G by chloramine-T. *Immunochemistry* 7:885, 1970.
18. Thorell, J. I., and Johansson, B. G.   Enzymatic iodination of polypep-tides and ^{125}I to high specific activity. *Biochim. Biophys. Acta* 251:362, 1972.
19. Yagi, Y., Maier, P., Pressman, D., Arbesman, C. W., Reisman, R. E., and Lenzner, A. R.   Multiplicity of insulin binding in human sera. *J. Immunol.* 90:760, 1963.

26

Quality Control, Standards, and Reference Centers for Immunologic Tests

Problems of Standardization

Standardization and quality control in immunologic methods have not reached the state of precision and accuracy achieved in certain clinical chemical and hematologic assays. One of the major reasons for the difficulties in standardizations is that each antiserum to a specific antigen may vary even within the same laboratory [5]. The antisera may vary as to their (a) animal source, (b) specificity, and (c) sensitivity. A given antiserum contains antibodies to a given antigen which contains many different antigenic determinants.

Often the characteristics of the antigen have not been well established. One example is the carcinoembryonic antigen found in gastrointestinal and other tumors. Various investigators have used different assay methods which cannot be fully understood until the characteristics of the antigen are well defined (see Chapter 20).

Immunofluorescence tests are widely used in the study of immunologic problems. The immunofluorescence tests are only as good as the specificity of the antibody used. Often the specificity is tested by antibody-precipitating methods such as agar gel diffusion or immunoelectrophoresis. The immunofluorescence test is probably more than 100 times as sensitive as the precipitin test, and specific fluorescent reagents established by precipitin reactions will give cross-reactions in the fluorescent antibody tests [5]. In the evaluation of fluorescein-labeled anti-human IgM conjugates, Chantler and Haire [4] have shown that neither gel diffusion nor direct immunofluorescent methods provided a reliable index of specificity for conjugates used in indirect tests.

Unless the antiserum used in the tests is carefully standardized, titration values in various tests have very little correlation from one laboratory to another. Further, it is almost impossible to standardize the instrumentation, filters, substrates, and other variables in a test, such as indirect fluorescent antinuclear antibody test.

Various immunologic test values of a particular laboratory may be considered relative rather than absolute. As a result, each test often requires interpretation relative to normal and positive controls and in relationship to other laboratory tests. As expressed in Chapter 1, the immunologic tests should be clustered in a disease oriented basis and interpreted in light of clinical findings. One should pursue meaningful answers in relation to the problem whether the test is used in the evaluation of the diagnosis, prognosis, or therapy.

Quality Control of Reagents and Procedures

Unless specific international standards are available, the results of a particular laboratory may be considered relative rather than absolute. However, each laboratory should strive for precision, reproducibility, and accuracy in a particular test.

There are two major areas in the establishment of a quality control program for laboratory tests in immunopathology: (a) standardization of specificity and sensitivity of immunologic reagents, and (b) establishment of control procedures which yield maximal precision and accuracy.

Standardization of Specificity and Sensitivity of
Immunologic Reagents
Each laboratory should carefully standardize and evaluate the reactivity and potency of the immunologic reagents whether they are purchased from a commercial source or individually made. For each reagent or test the following check points should be considered:

A. Certification of the specificity and antibody content of a given antiserum. It should be checked against a reference preparation.
B. The reagents should be stored with proper preservatives. Antiserum following absorption is not as stable as unabsorbed antiserum. The antiserum is preferably stored in a lyophilized state or at $-70°$ C. After prolonged storage, the potency and specificity should be rechecked. The reagents should not be stored in a diluted state for prolonged periods since dilute solutions of proteins are unstable.
C. Antigen preparations in various tests should be carefully checked for purity and quality with reference antigen and antiserum. Care should be exercised in the storage of antigen preparations similar to the storage of antiserum.
D. Each lot number of commercial reagents and each batch of individually manufactured reagents should be checked against a known panel of reference serum samples in which the values are known. In this manner, each laboratory may be able to standardize a particular test. The evaluation of each lot of reagents with reference

samplès can be easily done with tests such as the quantitative immunoglobulin test and the latex test for rheumatoid factor.

Control Procedures Which Yield Maximal Precision and Accuracy

A. One should employ only technical personnel who are thoroughly familiar and experienced with the performance of the procedures.
B. If possible, test procedures which are selected should be well standardized.
C. In the testing of unknown samples, positive and negative controls should be included with each run.
D. Each laboratory should establish criteria for a normal range for a particular test.
E. In addition to negative and positive controls, replicate split specimens and unknown controls should be included in the determinations for the day.
F. The reliability of the assays should be periodically checked by unknown check samples and referred to a reference laboratory.
G. The customary quality control program must be established to monitor equipment such as the incubator and temperature monitoring apparatus.

Immunologic Standards Established by the World Health Organization

The various international immunology societies and the World Health Organization are attempting to provide standards [2, 3, 5, 11] for various immunologic tests. This has been a difficult task, but a certain amount of progress has been made. With the use of international reference standards, it may be possible to compare and contrast results from different laboratories. The desired end result is the standardization of certain tests with similar reproducible results from different laboratories with the same biologic sample. Only then can the computer analysis of immunologic tests be meaningful [5].

Recommendations of the WHO Expert Committee on Biological Standardization for the Use of Reference Standards and Expression of Immunoglobulin Concentrations in Terms of International Units [3]:

A. Concentrations of IgG, IgA, and IgM working standards should be expressed in international units per milliliter. The working standards should be directly compared and calibrated with the International Reference Preparation or other suitably calibrated preparation.
B. Concentrations of IgG, IgA, and IgM in human sera should be expressed in IU per ml following comparison of human sera with the calibrated working standards.
C. To ensure continuity with established practices for a transitional period, the estimated immunoglobulin content of their standards should be expressed by weight as well as international units. The

relationship between estimated weight and international units for a given immunoglobulin may be different among different standard lot numbers. Therefore, each lot of standards must be calibrated directly with a primary or secondary international reference standard.

Immunoglobulins

PRIMARY STANDARD.   World Health Organization 67/86 standard for the measurement of IgG, IgA, and IgM immunoglobulins by methods of immunodiffusion [8]: Concentrations of immunoglobulins are expressed as IU per unit volume rather than on a weight per volume basis.

The WHO Expert Committee on Biological Standardization defined the IU for human immunoglobulins IgG, IgA, and IgM and the activity of each of these contained in 0.8147 mg of their freeze dried International Reference Preparation [8]: Each ampule of the International Reference Preparation contains an average of 100 IU of IgG, 100 IU of IgA, and 100 IU of IgM, which is 81.47 mg per ampule.

The primary standard is available in limited amounts and reserved for the calibration of national standards. For such purposes, the primary international standard can be obtained from: Director, WHO International Laboratory for Biological Standards, Statens Seruminstitut, Amager-Boulevard 80, Copenhagen S, Denmark.

SECONDARY STANDARD.   In the United States, a secondary standard (67/95) is available from the Director, NCI Immunoglobulin Reference Center, 6715 Electronics Drive, Springfield, Virginia 22151 [3]. In the United Kingdom, preparation 67/99 is available from the Director, Division of Biological Standards, National Institute for Medical Research, Mill Hill, London, N.W. 7 1AA, England. Reference preparation 67/97 is available from the Director, WHO International Reference Centre for Immunoglobulins, 21 rue du Bergnon,.1011 Lausanne, Switzerland.

RESEARCH STANDARDS.   Research standards for IgD (67/37) and IgE (68/341) may be obtained from the Immunoglobulin Reference Centers in the United States, England, and Lausanne, Switzerland [9, 10]. The research standards do not have the official status of the standard reference preparations of the WHO. The research standards are prepared and calibrated with the same precautions as the international standards. It is anticipated that research standards may eventually be accepted and established as official international standards after careful study by the Expert Committee on Biological Standardization of WHO.

The IgD research standard 67/37 has been defined so that 1 unit of activity of IgD is the activity present in 0.8188 mg of the freeze dried powder. Each ampule contains 81.88 mg and 100 units of activity of IgD [9].

The IgE research standard (68/341) is defined so that one unit of activity of IgE is the activity present in 0.009284 mg of the freeze dried powder. Each ampule contains 92.84 mg of the freeze dried preparation or 10,000 units of activity of IgE [10].

STANDARDS FOR FLUORESCENT REAGENTS.   The recommendations for the manufacture of fluorescent reagents by various standards committees and the methods of evaluation of fluorescent reagents are discussed in Chapter 22.

Currently the following research standards are available from: Division of Biological Standards, National Institute for Medical Research, Hampstead Laboratories, Holly Hill, London N.W. 3 6 RB, England.
A. Research standard A for antinuclear factor serum (homogeneous) 66/233 [2]
B. Research standard A for fluorochrome-labeled antibody to human immunoglobulins (sheep anti-human) 68/45

INTERNATIONAL REFERENCE PREPARATION OF RHEUMATOID ARTHRITIS SERUM.   The IU of rheumatoid arthritis serum has been defined as the activity contained in 0.171 mg of the international reference preparation [1]: For practical purposes, each ampule of the international reference preparation contains 100 international units.

Information may be obtained from: Director, Division of Biological Standards, National Institute for Medical Research, Mill Hill, London N.W. 7 1AA, England.

World Health Organization Reference Centers for Immunology [13]

Immunoglobulins
International Reference Center for Immunoglobulins, Institute of Biochemistry, University of Lausanne, Switzerland.
Regional Reference Center for Immunoglobulins, National Cancer Institute, 6715 Electronics Drive, Springfield, Virginia 22151.

Genetic Factors of Human Immunoglobulins
International Reference Center for Genetic Factors of Human Immunoglobulins, Centre départemental de Transfusion sanguine et de Génétique humaine, Bois-Guillaume, Seine-Maritime, France.
Regional Reference Center for Genetic Factors of Human Immunoglobulins, Department of Medical Microbiology, University of Lund, Sweden.
Regional Reference Center for Genetic Factors of Human Immunoglobulins, Department of Biology, Western Reserve University, Cleveland, Ohio 44106.

Serology of Autoimmune Disorders
International Reference Center for the Serology of Autoimmune Disorders, Department of Immunology, Middlesex Hospital Medical School, London, England.
Regional Reference Center for the Serology of Autoimmune Disorders, The Center for Immunology, State University of New York at Buffalo, New York 14214.
Regional Reference Center for the Serology of Autoimmune Disorders, The Walter and Eliza Hall Institute of Medical Research, Melbourne University, Australia.

Tumour-Specific Antigens
International Reference Center for Tumour-Specific Antigens, Division of Immunology and Oncology, Gamaleja Institute of Epidemiology and Microbiology, Moscow, U.S.S.R.

Testing of Natural Resistance Factors
International Reference Center for Testing of Natural Resistance Factors, Department of Immunology, Institute of Microbiology, Prague, Czechoslovakia.

Use of Immunoglobulin Anti-D in the
Prevention of Rh Sensitization
International Reference Center for the Use of Immunoglobulin Anti-D in the Prevention of Rh Sensitization, Medical Research Council Experimental Haematology Research Unit, St. Mary's Hospital Medical School, London, England.

References

1. Anderson, S. G., Bentzon, M. W., Houba, V., and Krag, P. International reference preparation of arthritis serum. *Bull. WHO.* 42:311, 1970.
2. Anderson, S. G., and Dixon, H. G. Antinuclear factor serum (homogeneous): An international collaborative study of the proposed research standard 66/233. *Ann. N.Y. Acad. Sci.* 177:337, 1971.
3. Anderson, S. G., et al. (World Health Organization Expert Committee on Biological Standardization). Measurement of concentrations of human serum immunoglobulins. *J. Immunol.* 107:1798, 1971.
4. Chantler, S., and Haire, M. Evaluation of the immunological specificity of fluorescein-labelled anti-human IgM conjugates. *Immunology* 23:7, 1972.
5. Fudenberg, H. H. Problems in standardization of immunological laboratory results. In E. R. Gabrieli (ed.), *Clinically Oriented Documentation of Laboratory Data.* New York: Academic Press, 1972, p. 359.
6. Humphrey, J. H., et al. Characterization of antisera as reagents: Recommendations made by the MRC working party on the clinical use of immunological reagents. *Immunology* 20:3, 1971.

7. Reimer, C. B., Phillips, D. J., Maddison, S. E., and Shore, S. L.   Comparative evaluation of commercial precipitating antisera against human IgM and IgG. *J. Clin. Lab. Med.* 76:949, 1970.

8. Rowe, D. S., Anderson, S. G., and Grab, B.   A research standard for human serum immunoglobulins IgG, IgA, and IgM. *Bull. WHO.* 42:535, 1970.

9. Rowe, D. S., Anderson, S. G., and Tackett, L.   A research standard for human serum immunoglobulin D. *Bull. WHO.* 43:607, 1970.

10. Rowe, D. S., Tackett, L., Bennich, H., Ishizaka, K., Johansson, S. G. O., and Anderson, S. G.   A research standard for human serum immunoglobulin E. *Bull. WHO.* 43:609, 1970.

11. Standards for immunoglobulins.   *Lancet* 2:82, 1971.

12. WHO Expert Committee on Biological Standardization, WHO Technical Report, Series No. 463. Geneva: World Health Organization, 1971.

13. WHO Scientific Group on Clinical Immunology: Clinical Immunology. WHO Technical Report Series No. 496. Geneva: World Health Organization, 1972.

Appendix

Major Manufacturers
Mentioned in the Text

Antibodies, Inc.
Davis, Calif. 95616

Aoki Co.
Long Beach, Calif. 90813

J. T. Baker Chemical Co.
Phillipsburg, N.J. 08865

Beckman Instruments, Inc.
Fullerton, Calif. 92634

Behring Diagnostics
Somerville, N.J. 08876

Bellco Glass, Inc.
Vineland, N.J. 08360

Bio-Rad Labs.
Richmond, Calif. 98404

Bioware, Inc.
Witchita, Kans. 67218

Burroughs Wellcome Co.
Research Triangle Park, N.C. 27709

Calbiochem
San Diego, Calif. 92112

Canalco, Inc.
Rockville, Md. 20852

Cappel Labs Inc.
Downington, Pa. 19335

Clay Adams Corp., Div. of
Becton, Dickinson & Co.
Parsippany, N.J. 07054

Coleman Instruments, Div. of
Perkin-Elmer Corp.
Maywood, Ill. 60153

Consolidated Laboratories, Inc.
Chicago Heights, Ill. 60411

Cooke Engineering Co.
Laboratory Products Div.
Alexandria, Va. 22314

Cooper Labs., Inc.
Wayne, N.J. 07470

Cordis Laboratories
Miami, Fla. 33137

Curtin-Matheson Scientific
Houston, Tex. 77001

Dade Reagents, Inc.
Miami, Fla. 33125

Difco Laboratories
Detroit, Mich. 48232

Distillation Products Industries,
Div. of Eastman Kodak Co.
Rochester, N.Y. 14650

Dolan Scientific Instruments
Houston, Tex. 77042

Eastman Chemical, Div. of
Guardian Chemical Corp.
Hauppage, N.Y. 11787

Eastman Kodak Co.
Rochester, N.Y. 14650

Elanco Products Co.
Indianapolis, Ind. 42606

Felon Laboratories
Rockville, Md. 20852

Fenwal Labs, Div. of Travenol
Labs.
Morton Grove, Ill. 60053

Fernwood Laboratories
Pittsburgh, Pa. 15232

Fisher Scientific Co.
Pittsburgh, Pa. 16219

Gallard-Schlesinger Chemical
Corp.
Carle Place, N.Y. 11514

Gamma Biologicals
Houston, Tex. 77018

General Biochemical
Chagrin Falls, Ohio 44022

Gibco (Grand Island Biological
Co.)
Grand Island, N.Y. 14072
Berkeley, Calif. 90608

Hamilton Company
Whittier, Calif. 90608

Harleco, Div. of American
Hospital Supply Corp.
Philadelphia, Pa. 19143

Harvard Apparatus Co.
Millis, Mass. 02054

Helena Laboratories
Beaumont, Tex. 77704

Otto Hiller
Madison, Wisc. 53701

Hollister-Steir Laboratories
Spokane, Wash. 99220

Hyland Laboratories
Costa Mesa, Calif. 92626

IBL
Rockville, Md. 20850

ICL Scientific
Fountain Valley, Calif. 92708

International Products Corp.
Trenton, N.J. 08601

Jefferson Drug Co.
Beaumont, Tex. 77701

K & K Laboratories
Plainview, N.Y. 11803

Kallestad Laboratories, Inc.
Minneapolis, Minn. 55416

Laboratoire Roger Bellon
Neuilly, Seine, France

Lab-Tek Products
Naperville, Ill. 60540

Life Instrumentation
Glenville, Ill. 60025

Eli Lilly
Indianapolis, Ind. 46206

Linbro of the Pacific
Van Nuys, Calif. 91406

Mann Research Laboratories
New York, N.Y. 10006

Marine Colloids
Rockland, Maine 04841

McNeil Laboratories, Inc.
Fort Washington, Pa. 19034

Medical Chemical Corp.
Santa Monica, Calif. 90404

Meloy Laboratories, Inc.
Biological Products Div.
Springfield, Va. 22151

Melpar Biological Products
Laboratory
Falls Church, Va. 22046

Merck Sharp & Dohme
West Point, Pa. 19486

Micromedic Systems, Inc.
Philadelphia, Pa. 19905

Miles Laboratories, Inc.
Elkhart, Ind. 46514

National Instrument Laboratories, Inc.
Rockville, Md. 20852

New England Nuclear
Boston, Mass. 02118

Novo Industries
Copenhagen, Denmark

Nuclear Chicago
Plaines, Ill. 60018

Nutritional Biochemical
Cleveland, Ohio 44218

Nyegaard and Co.
Oslo 4, Norway

Osram G.m.b.H.
Berlin, West Germany

Packard Instruments
Downersgrove, Ill. 60515

Parke-Davis & Co.
Detroit, Mich. 48232

Pentax, Inc.
Kankakee, Ill. 60901

Pfizer Diagnostics Div.
New York, N.Y. 10017

Pharmacia Fine Chemicals, Inc.
Piscataway, N.J. 08854

Polyscience, Inc.
Warrington, Pa. 18976

Riker Laboratories
North Ridge, Calif. 91324

Roboz Surgical Instruments Co.
Washington, D.C. 20006

Schering Corp.
Bloomfield, N.J. 07003

Schott Optical Glass, Inc.
Duryea, Pa. 18642

F. W. Schumacher Co.
Sandwich, Mass. 02563

Schwartz Bioresearch
Orangeburg, N.Y. 19062

Schwartz-Mann, Div. of Becton,
Dickinson & Co.
Orangeburg, N.Y. 19062

Scientific Products
Houston, Tex. 77055

G. D. Searle & Co.
Chicago, Ill. 60680

Sigma Chemical Co.
St. Louis, Mo. 63178

Ivan Sorvall
Newtown, Conn. 06470

Spectrum Medical Industries, Inc.
Los Angeles, Calif. 90054

E. R. Squibb & Sons
Princeton, N.J. 08540

Travenol Laboratories, Inc.
Morton Grove, Ill. 60053

Union Carbide Corp.
New York, N.Y. 10017

Wang Laboratories
Tewksbury, Mass. 01876

Waring Products Div. of Dynamics Corp. of America
New Hartford, Conn. 06057

Wellcome Reagents Division, Burroughs Wellcome Co.
Research Triangle Park, N.C. 27709

Winthrop Laboratories
New York, N.Y. 10016

Worthington Biochemical Co.
Freehold, N.J. 07728

Carl Zeiss, Inc.
New York, N.Y. 10018

Index

Index

701

uric acid levels in, 436
vasculitis in, 425–426
viral factors in, 216
x-ray studies in, 432
tumors with, 219
Arthus reaction, 119
complement role in, 116–117
immune complexes in, 170
skin reactions in, 148
Aspermatogenesis, autoimmune mechanisms in, 210
Asthma, 144–145
anti-smooth muscle antibody in, 301–
302, 303
Ataxia-telangiectasia, 30–31
malignancies with, 33
mixed lymphocyte culture reaction
in, 483
Atopic or reaginic disorders, 138–164
acute reactions in, 104–105
biochemical factors in, 105
anaphylaxis, 139, 147–148
in autoimmune disorders, 212
biochemical mediators in, 104, 143,
158–161
clinical patterns of, 143–144
complement-mediated reactions, 140–
141
cutaneous, 145–147
diagnosis of, 161–162
familial occurrence of, 143, 161
gastrointestinal, 147
granulomatous hypersensitivity, 214
laboratory tests in, 148–164
leukocyte histamine release tests in,
150–154
pathophysiology of, 138–143
release of biochemical mediators in,
143
detection of, 158–161
in respiratory tract, 144–145
shock organs in, 143
skin tests in, 148–150
Australia antigen. See also Hepatitis-
associated antigen
and anti-smooth muscle antibody,
301, 302
in chronic hepatitis, 290, 302, 305
in immune complexes, 213
in vasculitis, 216
Autoimmunity, 201
abnormal immune mechanisms in,
205–206
age factors in, 219–220, 234
altered body constituents in, 206–
207

anaphylactic or atopic mechanisms
in, 212
antiadrenal antibodies in, 235–236
antibody formation in, 201, 235–237
antigastric antibodies in, 235
antimitochondrial antibodies in, 236
antimuscle antibodies in, 236
antinuclear antibodies in, 236–237
antireticulin antibodies in, 236, 356
anti-salivary gland antibody in, 236
antithyroid antibodies in, 235
and bioassay for LATS, 233
and cancer, 217–219
cellular mechanisms in, 201
characteristics of disorders in, 209,
225–226
in collagen diseases, 209
complement fixation test in, 232
Coombs' test in, 232
cross-reacting antigen in, 206
cytotoxic or cytolytic mechanisms in,
212
delayed cellular or sensitivity mechanisms in, 213
and detection of antibody to intrinsic
factor, 233
diagnosis of disorders in, 225–240
drug-induced disorders, 398–415
in endocrine diseases, 210
enzyme-labeled antibody tests in,
227–231
in gastrointestinal diseases, 210
genetic factors in, 216
granulomatous sensitivity in, 214
hemagglutination test in, 232
in hematologic diseases, 209
hemolytic anemias, 367–394
humoral mechanisms in, 201
and immune deficiency diseases, 33–
34, 214–215
immunofluorescence tests in, 227–232
immunopathologic mechanisms in,
210
interpretation of tests in, 234–235
in kidney diseases, 210
laboratory tests for, 225
latex agglutination test in, 233
level of autoantibodies in, 234
liver disorders, 289–305
lupus group of disorders, 226–227
and malignancies, 527–528
in neuromuscular diseases, 209
and neutralization of biologically
active molecules, 210
non-organ specific disorders, 208, 226
organ specific disorders, 207, 226

immunoglobulin levels in, 296
positive LE cell tests in, 290, 292, 294
lupoid, 290, 292
  antibody detection in, 228
  antiglomerular antibody in, 295, 296
  antinuclear antibodies in, 237
  anti-smooth muscle antibodies in, 236, 237, 301
  autoimmune mechanisms in, 208, 210
Hepatitis-associated antigen. *See also* Australia Antigen
  detection of, 4
  in liver disorders, 301, 304
  in lupus erythematosus, 270
Heterocytotropic antibodies, 142
Histamine release
  in anaphylaxis, 139
  in atopic or reaginic reactions, 104, 143
  complement affecting, 114
  from leukocytes, tests for, 150–154
  from platelets, 173
  tests for, 150–154
Histocompatibility antigens, 461–479
  ABO blood group, 462, 463–467
  HL–A system, 462–463, 469–475
  Rh blood group, 467–469
  and tissue typing techniques, 508–525
History-taking, in diagnosis, 43–44
HL–A system, 462–463, 469–475
  antigens in, 469
    cross-reactivity of, 469
    nature of, 469
    population distribution of, 471
  and contamination of blood transfusions, 516–517
  diseases associated with, 478–479
  and tissue typing procedures, 512–525
  in transfusions, 474
  in transplantations, 473–474, 476–477
Hodgkin's disease, 31
  mixed lymphocyte culture reaction in, 483
  tumor-associated antigen in, 535
  viral factors in, 528, 530
Homocytotropic antibodies, 142
Humoral immunity, 17–21
  deficiency in, diagnosis of, 63

to glomerular basement membrane, 340–341
mechanisms, in autoimmunity, 201
tests for evaluation of, 50–60
in thyroiditis, 309
Hydantoins, and antinuclear antibody formation, 266
Hypersensitivity, delayed, 14
  in autoimmunity, 201, 213
  skin tests in, 60–61, 66–69, 149
  in tumors, 534
Hyperthyroidism. *See* Thyrotoxicosis
Hyperviscosity syndrome, 187–188
Hypocomplementemic nephritis, and complement system, 120, 126, 337
Hypogammaglobulinemia, acquired, 31

Immune adherence, 25
Immune complexes, 168
  in Arthus reaction, 170
  Australia antigen in, 213
  in biopsy material, 184, 230
  column chromatography of, 182
  detection of, 169, 180–184, 192–195
  DNA-antiDNA complexes, 248
    detection of, 269
    in lupus erythematosus, 296
  in drug-induced hematologic disorders, 403–405
  in glomerulonephritis, 184, 334–337
  immunoelectrophoretic patterns of, 181–182
  in joint lesions, 178, 184, 435–436
  laboratory tests for, 169
  localization of, factors in, 119–120, 172, 213
  in lupus erythematosus, 174–178, 296
  platelet aggregation test for, 184
  reaction to, 171–172
  reaction with C1q component of complement, 183
  reaction with rheumatoid factor, 183–184
  in renal tubular disorders, 340
  in rheumatoid arthritis, 178–180, 184, 418–422
    reactivity of, 421–422
  in serum sickness, 170–174
  toxic, 213
  ultracentrifugation studies of, 182–183
  in vasculitis, 119